D1687741

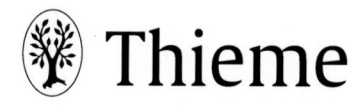

Spinal Trauma—
An Imaging Approach

Victor N. Cassar-Pullicino, M.D.
Consultant Radiologist and Clinical Director
Department of Radiology
The Robert Jones & Agnes Hunt Orthopaedic Hospital
Oswestry, Shropshire
U.K.

Herwig Imhof, M.D.
Professor of Radiology and Nuclear Medicine
Head of the Department of Radiodiagnostics
University and General Hospital Vienna
Austria

With contributions by
R. Bodley, V.N. Cassar-Pullicino, A. Chevrot, R. Daffner, S.D. Daffner, J.L. Drapé, S. Ehara, G.Y. El-Khoury, W.S. El Masry, A. Feydy, S. Grampp, J.H. Harris, A.M. Herneth, H. Imhof, F. Kainberger, G. Kernbach-Wighton, P.H. Lander, F.C. Oner, A.E. Osman, P. Peloschek, J.J. Rankine, K.S. Saternus, D.J. Short, B. Tins, J.M. Trivedi, P.N.M. Tyrrell, C. Vallée, M.L. White

439 illustrations

Thieme
Stuttgart · New York

Library of Congress Cataloging-in-Publication Data

Cassar-Pullicino, V. N. (Victor N.), 1954-
Spinal trauma : an imaging approach/Victor N. Cassar-Pullicino, Herwig Imhof ; with contributions by R. Bodley… [et al.].
  p. ; cm.
Includes bibliographical references.
ISBN 3-13-137471-3 (alk. paper) – ISBN 1-58890-348-6 (alk. paper)
1. Spine–Wounds and injuries. 2. Spine–Wounds and injuries–Imaging. 3. Spine–Diseases–Diagnosis.
[DNLM: 1. Spinal Injuries. 2. Spinal Cord Injuries. 3. Spinal Injuries–diagnosis. WE 725 C343s 2006] I. Imhof, H. (Herwig) II. Title.
RD533.C33 2006
617.5'6044–dc22
                    2006000850

Chapter 2 translated by John Grossman, Berlin, Germany

Illustrator: Salvador Beltran, M.D., E-mail: sa221237@terra.es

Important note: Medicine is an ever-changing science undergoing continual development. Research and clinical experience are continually expanding our knowledge, in particular our knowledge of proper treatment and drug therapy. Insofar as this book mentions any dosage or application, readers may rest assured that the authors, editors, and publishers have made every effort to ensure that such references are in accordance with **the state of knowledge at the time of production of the book.**

Nevertheless, this does not involve, imply, or express any guarantee or responsibility on the part of the publishers in respect to any dosage instructions and forms of applications stated in the book. **Every user is requested to examine carefully** the manufacturers' leaflets accompanying each drug and to check, if necessary in consultation with a physician or specialist, whether the dosage schedules mentioned therein or the contraindications stated by the manufacturers differ from the statements made in the present book. Such examination is particularly important with drugs that are either rarely used or have been newly released on the market. Every dosage schedule or every form of application used is entirely at the user's own risk and responsibility. The authors and publishers request every user to report to the publishers any discrepancies or inaccuracies noticed. If errors in this work are found after publication, errata will be posted at www.thieme.com on the product description page.

© 2006 Georg Thieme Verlag,
Rüdigerstrasse 14, 70469 Stuttgart, Germany
http://www.thieme.de
Thieme New York, 333 Seventh Avenue,
New York, NY 10001, USA
http://www.thieme.com

Typesetting by primustype Hurler GmbH, Notzingen
Printed in Germany by Grammlich, Pliezhausen
10-ISBN 3-13-137471-3 (GTV)
13-ISBN 978-3-13-137471-4 (GTV)
10-ISBN 1-58890-348-6 (TNY)
13-ISBN 978-1-58890-348-8 (TNY)   1 2 3 4 5

Some of the product names, patents, and registered designs referred to in this book are in fact registered trademarks or proprietary names even though specific reference to this fact is not always made in the text. Therefore, the appearance of a name without designation as proprietary is not to be construed as a representation by the publisher that it is in the public domain.

This book, including all parts thereof, is legally protected by copyright. Any use, exploitation, or commercialization outside the narrow limits set by copyright legislation, without the publisher's consent, is illegal and liable to prosecution. This applies in particular to photostat reproduction, copying, mimeographing, preparation of microfilms, and electronic data processing and storage.

Dedication

To:

Wendy, my wife, my secretary, and best friend
Amy and James, my children
Guze and Celine, my parents

       Victor Cassar-Pullicino

Ilse, my wife
Andrea, Klaus and Nini, my children
Grete, my mother

       Herwig Imhof

and
to all the patients whose injuries have taught us,
so we can teach others.

Foreword

Diagnostic imaging of spinal trauma has been revolutionized: findings obscured in the shadows of radiography have been brought to light by computed tomography (CT) and magnetic resonance imaging (MRI). CT and MRI illuminate much that was previously unseen and still more that was unsuspected. The pace of change has been swift and the cumulative impact of imaging on the initial diagnosis and subsequent treatment of patients with spinal cord injury has been enormous.

While these contributions have been chronicled in numerous reports in the radiologic, orthopedic, and neurosurgical scientific literature, there is great need for a compilation and integration of these advances in a single text. Drs. Cassar-Pullicino and Imhof have admirably fulfilled this need by putting together a major, cutting-edge, integrated resource on imaging the injured spine.

The editors assembled a cast of internationally recognized authorities in diagnostic radiology, orthopedic surgery, and neurosurgery to contribute to this text. Anatomic, pathophysiologic, clinical considerations and surgical treatment of spinal injuries are presented to provide an essential background for the proper performance and accurate interpretation of CT and MRI, as well as radiographic examinations, in those suspected of spinal injury.

The indications and contraindications for the use of various imaging modalities in the assessment of spinal injury are thoroughly explained. In keeping with their importance, the roles of CT and MRI in the detection and evaluation of spinal injury are emphasized. The text and illustrations admirably provide the how, where, and what to look for when imaging those who either have or may have sustained a spinal injury.

The text is profusely illustrated with outstanding illustrations of the pertinent imaging findings. Most chapters cite from 40 to 100 references that include essentially all the classic articles as well as the important recent scientific publications devoted to spinal trauma.

The entire range of spinal cord injury is covered; from low-impact to high-impact trauma and in all ages from childhood to the elderly. The underlying pathology and imaging assessment of patients with spinal cord injury without radiographic abnormalities (SCIWORA) is fully explored.

Controversial topics are presented in a non-dogmatic fashion: classifications of injury are described and their advantages and disadvantages discussed; the problems of interobserver variability and other potential difficulties encountered with the use of classification systems are acknowledged. The concept of stability is explored and both the potential and limitations of imaging in the determination of spinal stability are explained.

Chapters are devoted to injuries that may occur in the ankylosed, rigid spine and in the elderly with degenerative changes and osteoporosis. The text also contains interesting and informative chapters on spondylolysis and stress injuries as well as Scheuermann's disease. The vexing problems of Charcot's spine and benign versus malignant vertebral collapse are the subject of separate chapters.

There is also a chapter devoted to imaging the long-term multisystem effects of spinal cord injury. This includes the pulmonary, genitourinary, and gastrointestinal as well as spinal, neurologic, musculoskeletal complications. The role of CT and MRI in such patients is outlined and the cause and appearance of the lesions encountered are described.

Spinal trauma is a significant health problem in modern society. Spinal cord injury carries with it substantial morbidity and mortality, and the resources and expenditures required for the treatment and care of the spinal injured are considerable. Motor vehicle accidents (MVAs) are the plague of high-speed auto travel and the most frequent cause of spinal cord injury in developed countries the world over. Aging of the global population carries with it an increased risk of because those with degenerative changes in the spine are susceptible to spinal injury from even low-impact trauma, usually no more than simple falls. As a result, radiologists and their clinical colleagues worldwide are now commonly called upon to assess and treat spinal cord injuries.

The primary objectives of the assessment and treatment of patients with potential spinal injury are to either accurately exclude or correctly identify injuries, to preserve neurologic function when injuries are present, and to restore spinal stability in those so afflicted. Imaging plays an essential role in these endeavors. The editors have produced a work that will aid radiologists and all other physicians in achieving these objectives. To that end, this book should be on the shelves, if not in the hands, of all physicians involved in the care of patients with spinal injuries.

Drs. Cassar-Pullicino and Imhof and their collaborators are to be congratulated on this superb and timely text.

Lee F. Rogers, M.D.

Contributors

R. Bodley, M.D.
Consultant Radiologist
Department of Radiology
Stoke Mandeville Hospital
Aylesbury, Bucks
U.K.

Victor N. Cassar-Pullicino, M.D.
Consultant Radiologist and Clinical Director
Department of Radiology
The Robert Jones & Agnes Hunt Orthopaedic Hospital
Oswestry, Shropshire
U.K.

Alain Chevrot, M.D.
Professor and Head
Department of Radiology B
Cochin Hospital
Paris
France

Richard H. Daffner, M.D.
Professor of Radiologic Sciences
Department of Diagnostic Radiology
Drexel University College of Medicine
Allegheny General Hospital
Pittsburgh, Pennsylvania
U.S.A.

Scott D. Daffner, M.D.
Department of Orthopedic Surgery
Thomas Jefferson University School of Medicine
Philadelphia, Pennsylvania
U.S.A.

J.L. Drapé, M.D.
Department of Radiology B
Cochin Hospital
Paris
France

Shigeru Ehara, M.D.
Professor and Chair
Department of Radiology
Morioka
Japan

Georges Y. El-Khoury, M.D.
Professor of Radiology and Orthopedics
Director of the Musculoskeletal Radiology Section
University of Iowa Hospitals and Clinics
Department of Radiology
Iowa City, Iowa
U.S.A.

W.S. El Masry M.B., B.Ch., F.R.C.S. (Ed.)
Director of Midland Centre for Spinal Injuries
The Robert Jones & Agnes Hunt Orthopaedic Hospital
Oswestry, Shropshire
U.K.

A. Feydy, M.D.
Department of Radiology B
Cochin Hospital
Paris
France

S. Grampp, M.D.
a.o. Professor
Section of Osteology
Department of Radiodiagnostics
University and General Hospital
Vienna
Austria

J.H. Harris, Jr., M.D., D.Sc.
Professor Emeritus
Radiology and Emergency Medicine
Sedona, Arizona
U.S.A.

A. Herneth, M.D.
a.o. Professor
Section of Osteology
Department of Radiodiagnostics
University and General Hospital
Vienna
Austria

Herwig Imhof, M.D.
Professor of Radiology and Nuclear Medicine
Head of the Department of Radiodiagnostics
University and General Hospital
Vienna
Austria

F. Kainberger, M.D.
a.o. Professor
Section of Osteology
Department of Radiodiagnostics
University Hospital
Vienna
Austria

Gerhard Kernbach-Wighton, M.D., D.R.M., S.F.M., Ph.D.
Professor
Head of the Institute of Forensic Medicine
University of Edinburgh Medical School
Teviot Place – Wilkie Building
Edinburgh
U.K.

Philip H. Lander, M.D.
Associate Professor
Department of Radiology
University of Alabama Health Services
The Kirklin Clinic
Birmingham, Alabama
U.S.A.

F.C. Oner, M.D.
Orthopedic Surgeon
University Medical Center Utrecht
Utrecht
The Netherlands

A.E. Osman, M.B., Ch.B., M. Med. Sci., F.R.C.S.
Centre for Spinal Injuries
The Robert Jones & Agnes Hunt Orthopaedic Hospital
Oswestry, Shropshire
U.K.

Philipp Peloschek, M.D.
Department of Radiodiagnostics
University and General Hospital
Vienna
Austria

James Julian Rankine, M.D., M.R.C.P., M.Rad., F.R.C.R.
Consultant Musculoskeletal Radiologist
Chancellor Wing X-ray Department
St. James' University Hospital
Leeds
U.K.

Klaus-Steffen Saternus, M.D.
Professor and Head
Institute of Forensic Medicine
Georg-August-University of Göttingen
Göttingen
Germany

D.J. Short, F.R.C.P.
Centre for Spinal Injuries
The Robert Jones & Agnes Hunt Orthopaedic Hospital
Oswestry, Shropshire
U.K.

Bernhard Tins, M.D.
Consultant Radiologist
Department of Radiology
The Robert Jones & Agnes Hunt Orthopaedic Hospital
Oswestry, Shropshire
U.K.

J.M. Trivedi M.Ch. (Orth.), F.R.C.S. (Tr. & Orth.)
Director Centre of Spinal Disorders
Consultant Orthopaedic Surgeon
The Robert Jones & Agnes Hunt Orthopaedic Hospital
Oswestry, Shropshire
U.K.

P.N.M. Tyrrell, M.D.
Consultant Radiologist
Department of Radiology
The Robert Jones & Agnes Hunt Orthopaedic Hospital
Oswestry, Shropshire
U.K.

C. Vallée, M.D.
Department of Radiology
Raymond Pointcarré Hospital
Garches
France

Matthew L. White, M.D.
Associate Professor
Department of Radiology
University of Nebraska
Nebraska
U.S.A.

Preface

"Spinal trauma" often generates a sense of unease in both trainee and experienced diagnostic clinicians owing to the potentially catastrophic implications of missing significant acute trauma. Diagnostic dilemmas and uncertainty are further encountered when dealing with other aspects of vertebral column injury. With the reader in mind, this book covers a broad spectrum of spinal trauma topics. General as well as special focus categories are comprehensively covered, each incorporating all aspects of diagnostic imaging in a practical and cohesive manner.

An Imaging Approach is fundamental to providing the crucial information that firstly aids an accurate understanding of the underlying pathology, and secondly forms the basis of therapeutic decisions. To ensure best medical practice, attending radiologists and clinicians need to understand and incorporate the clinical applications of imaging.

The international cast of expert authors are all recognized teachers. Their vast wealth of experience, logical approach, and diagnostic principles are distilled in their excellent contributions. Each chapter is designed to reflect the manner in which the authors currently regard the role of imaging in their area of expertise within the field of spinal trauma. Well-chosen illustrations complement the text throughout and enhance the understanding of the reader; this is further aided by the superb drawings of Salvador Beltran, the renowned medical illustrator.

We hope that the finished product accurately reflects the state of the art, furthers and improves the knowledge of the readers, enhancing their confidence and diagnostic skills so that they can "get it right" for the benefit of the patient.

V.N. Cassar-Pullicino and H. Imhof

Contents

1 Clinical Perspectives on Spinal Injuries 1

W. S. El Masry and A. E. Osman

Introduction 1	**Standards for Neurological Examination**
Effects of Spinal Cord Injury 1	**and Documentation** 7
Clinical and Radiological Assessment	Frankel's Classification 8
in the Acute Stage 2	The ASIA/IMSOP Classification 8
Missed Spinal injuries 2	**Management of the Spinal Injury** 9
Clinical Diagnosis of SCI in the Conscious	The Secondary Injury 9
Patient 2	Biomechanical Instability of Injuries
Clinical Diagnosis in the Semiconscious	to the Spinal Column 9
or Unconscious Patient 3	Unstable Injuries Without Neurological
Associated Injuries 3	Damage 9
Radiological Assessment 4	Physiological Instability of the Spinal Cord 10
The Subacute Stage and Long Term 5	Stable and Unstable Injuries with
Assessment of the Cardiovascular System 5	Neurological Damage 10
Assessment of the Respiratory System 5	Canal Encroachment 10
Assessment of the Abdomen 6	Cord Compression 10
Bladder and Urinary System 6	Natural History of Complete Spinal Cord Injuries . 11
Assessment of Level of Consciousness 7	Natural History of Incomplete Cord Injuries 11
Psycho-Social Assessment of Cognitive	**The Role of Surgery** 11
Functions 7	**Conclusion** 12
Electrophysiological Assessment 7	References 12

2 Understanding Cervical Spinal Trauma: Biomechanics and Pathophysiology 15

K.-S. Saternus and G. Kernbach-Wighton

Introduction 15	**Injuries to the Intervertebral Disk and**
Atlanto-Occipital and Atlanto-Axial Joints 15	**Major Longitudinal Ligaments** 24
Condylar Fracture 15	Traumatology 24
Alar Ligaments 16	Biomechanics 24
Cruciform Ligament, Apical Ligament,	**Vertebral Injury** 28
Anterior Atlanto-Occipital Membrane, and	Compression Fracture 28
Anterior Longitudinal Ligament 17	Avulsion Fracture of the Margin
Atlas Fracture 18	of the Vertebra 30
Anterior Arch 18	Injuries to the Facet Joints and Intervertebral
Jefferson Fracture 19	Foramina 30
Lateral Mass 20	Spinous Process Fractures 32
Posterior Arch 21	**Conclusion** 32
Axis Fracture 22	References 34
Odontoid Fracture 22	
Hangman's Fracture 23	

3 Optimizing the Imaging Options — 36

B. Tins and V. N. Cassar-Pullicino

Introduction	36	Specific Scenarios and Technical Considerations	47
Imaging Modalities	38	An Approach to Imaging of Spinal Injuries	50
Pros and Cons	40	Conclusion	51
Imaging Approaches and Dilemmas	45	References	51

4 Classification: Rationale and Relevance — 55

F. C. Oner

Why Classify?	55	Influence of Imaging Modality	60
Classification of Thoracolumbar Spine Fractures	55	Problems of Reproducibility	61
The Three-Column CT Era	56	The Concept of Stability	62
The Load-Sharing Classification	57	Do We Need Any Classification at All?	63
The AO (Comprehensive) Classification	58	References	64

5 Malalignment: Signs and Significance — 66

J. H. Harris, Jr

Introduction	66	Case 7	73
Normal Alignment	67	Case 8	74
Cervicocranium (Occiput–C2–C3 Interspace)	67	Case 9	74
Lower Cervical Spine (C3–C7)	68	Case 10	75
		Case 11	75
Malalignment	69	Case 12	76
Case 1	69	Case 13	76
Case 2	70	Case 14	77
Case 3	70	Case 15	78
Case 4	71	Case 16	79
Case 5	72	Case 17	79
Case 6	72	References	80

6 Vertebral Injuries: Detection and Implications — 81

R. H. Daffner and S. D. Daffner

Introduction	81	"Footprints" of Vertebral Injury—the ABCS	93
Indicators of High Risk for Injury	82	Vertebral Stability Following Trauma	98
Mechanisms of Injury and Their Imaging "Fingerprints"	83	Implications	98
		References	98

7 Neurovascular Injury — 100

M. L. White and G. Y. El-Khoury

Introduction	100	Vascular Injury	104
MR Imaging/Histopathological Correlation of Acute Spinal Cord Injury	100	Vertebral Artery Injury	104
MRI Features of Spinal Cord Hemorrhage	101	Conclusion	111
Prognostic Role of MR Imaging in Neurological Outcome	103	References	111

8 Trauma to the Pediatric Spine — 113

P. N. M. Tyrrell and V. N. Cassar-Pullicino

Introduction	113	Atlanto-Axial Dislocation	121
Development of the Vertebral Column	113	Atlanto-Axial Rotatory Fixation	121
Normal Variants	114	Thoracolumbar Spine Injury	123
Birth Injury	117	Physeal Injury	126
Nonaccidental Injury (NAI)	118	SCIWORA	131
Cervical Spine Injuries	118	Slipped Vertebral Apophysis	133
Atlanto-Occipital Dissociation (AOD)	118	Spondylolysis	133
Fractures of C1	118	Prognosis	133
Injury of C2	119	References	133
Os Odontoideum	119		

9.1 Sports Injuries: Spondylolysis — 137

F. Kainberger

Introduction	137	Image Interpretation	143
Indications for Imaging	138	Imaging Anatomy	143
Investigation Techniques	139	Signs	144
Radiography	139	Differential Diagnosis	146
Computed Tomography	139	Conclusion	148
Magnetic Resonance Imaging	139	References	148
Nuclear Medicine Studies	139		
Ultrasound	139		

9.2 Sports Injuries: Diskovertebral Overuse Injuries — 149

J.J. Rankine

Introduction	149	Disk Degeneration	152
Anatomy	149	References	153
Scheuermann's Disease	150		

10 The Rigid Spine — 155
P. H. Lander

Introduction 155	Mechanisms and Imaging Techniques 155
Ankylosing Spondylitis 155	Cervical Spine Injuries 157
Disseminated Idiopathic Skeletal Hyperostosis (DISH) 155	Thoracolumbar Spine Injuries 160
	References 165

11 Spinal Trauma in the Elderly — 166
S. Ehara

Background 166	Thoracolumbar Spine 170
Cervical Spine 166	Biomechanical Characteristics 170
Biomechanical Characteristics 166	Clinical Features 170
Clinical Features 166	Imaging Techniques 171
Imaging Techniques 167	Imaging Features 172
Radiological Features 167	Conclusion 174
	References 174

12 Therapy—Options and Outcomes — 175
J. M. Trivedi

Introduction 175	Management 178
Epidemiology of Spinal Trauma 175	Initial Management 178
Pathophysiology of Spinal Cord Injury 175	Pharmacological Intervention 180
Anatomical Classification of Spinal Fractures 175	Nonsurgical Management of Spinal Fractures ... 180
Patterns of Injury 176	Surgical Treatment of Spinal Fractures 181
Flexion Injury 176	Burst Fractures 183
Burst Fractures 176	Osteoporotic Vertebral Fractures 184
Flexion Distraction Injury 176	Conclusion 185
Flexion Rotation 178	References 186

13 Imaging in Chronic Spinal Cord Injury: Indications and Benefits — 188
R. Bodley

Abbreviations 188	Cord Changes Post-SCI 189
Introduction 188	Reported Series 191
Neurological System 188	Treatment 192
	Imaging 192

Urological Investigations	196	Pressure Sores	197
Surveillance	196	Ectopic Ossification	199
		Pain	199
Imaging in Specific Conditions	197	Muscular Spasms	199
Deteriorating Neurology	197	Airway Problems	199
Spinal Instability	197	Elective Management of the Renal Tract	199
The Acutely Unwell Patient	197		
Deteriorating Renal Function and Renal Tract		**Conclusion**	199
Complications	197	References	201

14 Vertebral Fractures and Osteoporosis   203

P. Peloschek and S. Grampp

Introduction	203	Dual X-ray Absorptiometry	206
		Quantitative Computed Tomography	207
Definition	203	Quantitative Ultrasonography of Bone	207
Osteoporosis	203	Radiographic Absorptiometry	207
T-Score and Z-Score	203	Single-Photon Absorptiometry	207
Vertebral Fragility Fracture	204		
		The Radiologist's Role in Therapy—Percutaneous	
Epidemiology and Outcome of Osteoporotic		**Vertebroplasty**	208
Spinal Fractures	204		
		Conclusion	208
The Radiologist's Role in Diagnosis	204		
Screening during Routine Chest Radiography	204	**Ten Things to Remember**	208
Diagnosis of Osteoporosis on Lateral			
Radiographs of the Spine	205	**Case Study**	209
Bone Densitometry	205	References	211

15 Vertebral Collapse—Benign or Malignant   213

A. M. Herneth

Introduction	213	Imaging Findings	214
		New Imaging Methods	218
Clinical Evaluation	213	Biopsy	220
Age	213		
History of Trauma	213	**Conclusion**	220
		References	221

16 Neuropathic Osteo-Arthropathy of the Spine   223

A. Chevrot, A. Feydy, C. Vallée, J. L. Drapé

Introduction	223	Differential Diagnosis	228
Mechanism	223	Treatment	230
Clinical Findings	225	References	230
Imaging Findings	225		

17 The Future: Trends and Developments in Spinal Cord Regeneration — 231

A. E. Osman, D. J. Short, V. N. Cassar-Pullicino, H. Imhof, W. S. El Masry

Introduction 231	**Future Trends—Role of Imaging** 233
Spinal Cord Research 231	**Conclusion** 233
Neuroprotection 232	References 233
Regeneration 232	
Transplantation 232	
Rehabilitation 232	

Index — 235

1 Clinical Perspectives on Spinal Injuries

W. S. El Masry and A. E. Osman

Introduction

Traumatic spinal column injuries are potentially catastrophic events in an individual's life. When associated with neurological damage they result in devastating medical, psychological, social, emotional, financial, vocational, environmental, and economic consequences.

The impact of the effects of the neurological damage on the individual and those related to him/her can, however, be minimized. With good management of all aspects of paralysis from the time of the injury, many initially paralyzed patients can make significant neurological recovery and walk again. With ongoing expert monitoring, care, and support, those who do not recover are able to lead fulfilling and fruitful lives, as well as contribute to society.

A thorough assessment of the patient, including full neurological examination, appropriate radiological investigations, and accurate documentation of the findings, is of paramount importance in initiating good management and in monitoring progress.

As spinal cord injury (SCI) affects the physiology of almost all systems of the body, any assessment should encompass more than spinal column or spinal cord functions.

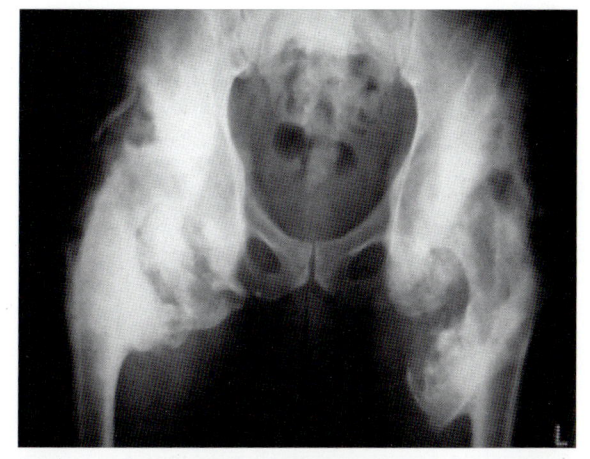

Fig. 1.**1 Heterotrophic ossifications in a tetraplegic patient**. They can be detected early with an ultrasound scan. Early treatment with biphosphonates and anti-inflammatory medication minimizes the severity of the outcome.

Effects of Spinal Cord Injury

A spinal cord injury results in a generalized physiological impairment that involves most systems of the body either directly or indirectly.

The physiological impairment and the consequent multi-system malfunction caused by SCI are dynamic in nature throughout the patient's life. The rate of change in the functioning of the various systems of the body is more rapid, though predictable, in the early stages (first 4–6 months) following injury.

Unpredictable changes in functions will inevitably occur throughout the patient's life, when the condition is likely to be perceived by most clinicians as being stable. The importance of frequent reassessments and repeated documentation at all stages following injury cannot be overemphasized. The only difference in the requirement for monitoring between the acute stage and the lifelong follow-up is the frequency of the monitoring.

In the absence of complete neurological sparing or full neurological recovery, the majority of patients with spinal cord injuries have sensory impairment or sensory loss below the level of their injury. Associated injuries and/or pathological complications can, therefore, develop in the absence of the conventional symptoms and signs, resulting in delay of diagnosis often with unpleasant consequences (Fig. 1.**1**).

When a complication develops, the interruption of the higher coordinating and moderating functions of the brain at the site of the spinal cord injury usually results in multiple and/or cascading intersystem effects, which are rarely seen in other conditions and which are seldom easy to manage. For example, an anal fissure, while painless, may nevertheless cause excess spasticity, which in turn may cause a fall and fracture of a long bone. Alternatively, excess spasticity involving the pelvic floor muscles may result in urinary retention, autonomic dysreflexia, and possibly a cerebrovascular accident.

The multi-system malfunction caused by the spinal cord injury is not only a source of multiple disabilities, but also a potential source of a wide variety and range of complications. What is perhaps not widely appreciated is that almost all complications following spinal cord injury are preventable.

Fortunately, the incidence of spinal cord injuries is the lowest of all major traumas. However, a combination of low incidence and high complexity necessitates an even more thorough and time-consuming systematic assessment than usual. The management of such patients, once they are stable for transfer, is therefore easier and safer to conduct in spinal injuries centers. These centers are usually equipped with the infrastructure of both the required expertise of adequately trained multidisciplinary teams and the necessary equipment. They are geared to provide comprehensive management, while giving equal attention to details that are necessary to ensure safety, comfort, and a good outcome for the patient, as well as medico-legal protection for the clinician and the institution.

Clinical and Radiological Assessment in the Acute Stage

Missed Spinal Injuries

Missed spinal injuries are regularly reported in the literature.[1-4] It is probable that in a significant number of patients the diagnosis of a spinal cord injury is delayed without being reported. Delaying diagnosis can result in increased neurological impairment.[4,5] This is likely to result in more paresis or paralysis, increased disability, more disturbance of function of the various systems of the body and more complications. It is indeed a disaster to miss a spinal fracture or delay its diagnosis. It can easily be alleged that the neurological impairment has been caused or at best aggravated by failure to diagnose the fracture promptly. A delay in diagnosis is not unusually perceived by some patients and lawyers as having led to delays in ensuring appropriate precautions and adequate treatment. It is therefore paramount that no effort is spared in making as accurate a diagnosis in the accident and emergency department as possible. A high level of suspicion is a major prerequisite to early diagnosis in patients presenting following major trauma. The knowledge that a small group of patients with certain bone conditions, for example ankylosing spondylitis, osteoporosis, osteogenesis imperfecta, is more vulnerable to spinal injuries following minor trauma is at least equally important.

A thorough assessment of the patient including a full neurological examination together with appropriate radiological investigations, and accurate documentation of the findings are of paramount importance for initiating good management and monitoring progress.

Clinical Diagnosis of SCI in the Conscious Patient

A conscious alert patient, who is able to communicate and has symptoms of neck or back pain, rigidity, or tenderness in the spine following trauma is likely to have sustained a spinal column injury.[6] There are, however, some rare exceptions. Pain may not be a feature in elderly patients with pure cervical ligamentous injuries without major vertebral damage in spondylotic spines. The author has personally witnessed this in a small number of patients, some of whom successfully pursued litigation. Extreme pain from other associated injuries may also mask pain from a spinal fracture with consequences to the timely diagnosis of a spinal injury.[7] Neck pain, loss of consciousness following injury (regardless of duration), and/or neurological deficit are clinical predictors of unstable cervical spinal injuries requiring immediate radiological investigation of the cervical spine.[8,9] The clinical diagnosis of a spinal cord injury in the conscious patient, who has no associated major injuries can be made without difficulty. Loss or impairment of motor power, sensation, and reflexes are indicative (individually or in combination) of damage to the spinal cord or the cauda equina depending on the level of impairment. Extra care should be taken in patients with L2 injuries and below. A traumatic injury below the level of S1 without injury to the cauda equina is rare. If present, it can, however, present with normal tendon reflexes and unimpaired motor power.

It is essential to determine at the earliest stage possible both the level and the density of the neural tissue damage.

The level of the injury is defined by the last normal dermatome and myotome. It is now internationally accepted by all experts in the field that the dermatomal and myotomal distributions may be abnormal for three segments below that level. In other words both sensation and motor power could be present but impaired in three segmental distributions below the last normal segment. For example if the last normal sensation is at the dermatomal distribution of C5 but there is hypoesthesia or analgesia in the dermatomal distribution of C6, C7, and C8 the level of the injury should be defined as C5. The impairment of sensation in the dermatomal distribution of C6, C7, and C8 can be explained by the logical assumption that the spinal cord segments C6, C7, and C8 are not completely damaged. Damage of these segments is incomplete; hence these segments represent the "zone of partial preservation."

The density of the deficit from the damaged area in the spinal cord is defined by the presence or absence of sparing of sensation with or without sparing of motor power below the zone of partial preservation.

Absence of motor power including voluntary contraction of the anal sphincter and loss of sensation including loss of anal sensation below the zone of partial preservation are usually indicative of a clinically complete cord injury at the time of the examination. It is important, however, to appreciate that not all clinically complete injuries in the early hours or days following SCI remain clinically complete.[10,11] Spinal shock can also mimic an initially complete injury following which significant recovery can occur.

The presence of sensation, however patchy or impaired, below the level of the zone of partial preservation is indicative of some anatomical sparing of sensory tracts and possibly also of corticospinal tracts which may be dormant in function at the time of the examination. Sensory sparing limited to the anal canal without motor sparing below the zone of partial preservation is also indicative of an incomplete SCI. A number of such patients can subsequently recover significantly. A rectal examination to elicit sensation in the S5 dermatome and voluntary/involuntary contraction of the anal sphincter is therefore an essential component of the neurological examination of patients diagnosed or suspected to have sustained an SCI.

An accurate and thorough neurological examination at an early stage following the injury is paramount for monitoring purposes and for prognosis.

A repeated accurate neurological assessment, with thorough documentation initially at frequent intervals (3–4 hours), is not only essential for the adequate clinical management of any neurological deterioration, it would also help resolve some of the controversies around the indications and effectiveness of the various methods of management of the SCI (conservative versus surgical decompression and/or stabilization).

It is not advisable to rely entirely on the neurological and general examination carried out in the accident and emergency department to make a definitive diagnosis of the density of the spinal cord injury. The patient's attention can, at this early stage, be distracted by anxiety, confusion, and pain. These may also limit performance of motor functions and responses to sensory testing. It is therefore possible that the neurological examination in the first few hours may not be very accurate with a tendency to underscore the motor power and underscore or overscore the sensory sparing. The documentation of the state of consciousness and cooperation of the patient during the neurological examination is understandably essential.

Clinical Diagnosis in the Semiconscious or Unconscious Patient

Unconscious or semiconscious patients with head injuries and the intoxicated patient present particular problems to the clinician which can result in delays of the diagnosis of a spinal injury.[12] It is therefore, in my opinion, imperative that such patients, following major trauma, are nursed as having sustained a spinal injury until otherwise proven clinically and radiologically when the patient becomes alert.

In such patients a clear entry should be made in the medical records that the patient's neurological assessment could not be made because of the poor level of consciousness. This fact should also be communicated verbally to the nursing staff looking after the patient.

I would strongly advise that a written instruction "NOT TO SIT THE PATIENT UP IN BED OR OUT OF BED PRIOR TO THE EXCLUSION OF A SPINAL INJURY CLINICALLY AND RADIOLOGICALLY AND UNTIL THE PATIENT REGAINS CONSCIOUSNESS" **is clearly documented in the medical records and communicated verbally to the nursing staff**.

This simple, logical, and easy documentation can result in the prevention of paralysis or further neurological deterioration as well as the prevention of litigation against the clinician and/or the institution.

The general examination of the unconscious patient can also yield a number of clinical signs that, in combination, can increase the clinician's level of suspicion regarding the presence of a neurological impairment of spinal cord origin.

During a systematic examination of the patient the following signs can be strongly suggestive of a cervical spinal cord injury:

- Facial or scalp lacerations;
- Miosis of one or both pupil(s);
- Bruising or swelling of the neck;
- Absence of chest expansion during inspiration associated with increasing abdominal girth and retraction of intercostal muscles (diaphragmatic breathing);
- Differences in the pattern of spontaneous movement of the limbs;
- Difference in tone between the proximal and distal muscles in the upper limbs and between the muscles of the upper and the lower limbs;
- Response to painful stimuli by pressure over bony prominences along the segmental dermatomal distribution of the cord throughout the body;
- The combination of hypotension and bradycardia;
- The presence of priapism.

Bruising over the chest or thoracolumbar spine in association with the presence of normal breathing, the absence of responses to painful stimuli applied to the bony prominences of the lower limbs, and the absence of reflexes in the lower limbs, could be indicative of a lower thoracic cord or cauda equina injury.

Unlike a patient with head injury who is likely to be incontinent of urine on presentation at the accident and emergency department, a patient with combined head and spinal cord injury is likely to be dry for some time before developing overflow incontinence. In the author's experience, a palpable bladder in a semiconscious or unconscious patient following trauma is a highly suspicious sign of a spinal injury with neurological damage.

Associated Injuries

Double injury and occasionally multiple noncontiguous injuries of the spinal axis are not uncommon following major trauma. Following the diagnosis of a primary injury in the spinal axis, the diagnosis of a secondary injury is often delayed. The incidence of multi-level spinal injuries is reported to be as high as 16.7%.[13]

Early recognition is important for the assessment and planning of the treatment in order to avoid further neurological damage when the nondamaging second spinal fracture is proximal to the primary injury. In our series, 55% of patients with multi-level injuries had incomplete neurological lesions on admission.[14] Although no definite pattern of injury could be identified in terms of the relationship between the primary and the secondary level, the lower cervical and cervicothoracic lesions were the most frequently involved followed by the upper cervical region. Once a spinal injury has been identified we strongly recommend that the whole spine be examined clinically and radiologically.

The incidence of extra-spinal fractures associated with spinal cord injuries is reported to be about 28%.[15,16] When all levels of spinal cord injuries were pooled the most common areas of fracture reported were chest followed by lower extremity, upper extremity, head, and pelvis.[15]

Loss or impairment of sensation below the level of the spinal cord injury presents one of the greatest challenges to the clinician in the diagnosis of the associated injuries. A thorough clinical examination is paramount to the diagnosis.

The importance of bruises, lacerations, or swellings in these patients cannot be overestimated. Facial bruises with or without bruises on the neck in an unconscious patient should heighten the suspicion of a cervical spinal injury with associated facial, dental, or mandibular injuries. Although there could be any combination of associated injuries with the injury of the spinal axis, there are nonetheless certain patterns of association.

Head injuries, facial injuries, dental, and mandibular injuries can be associated with cervical injuries, and vice versa.[17] Thoracic injuries can be associated with fractures of the sternum,[18] fracture ribs, hemothorax, fracture clavicle, or fracture scapula.[19] A case of upper thoracic spine fracture was reported to be associated with tracheo-esophageal perforation.[20]

Abdominal injuries are not uncommonly associated with thoracolumbar fractures and lumbar fractures.[21,22] Children involved in motor vehicle collisions are particularly at high risk. In one series, almost 10% of adults with blunt trauma of the thoracolumbar spine had associated abdominal injuries.[22] Solid organs and viscus injuries (spleen, kidneys, adrenals, liver, small intestine, and mesentery) have been reported. Patients who sustained multi-level vertebral fractures were more severely injured and had a higher number of solid organ injuries.[22] Blunt, abdominal, aortic trauma in association with thoracolumbar spine fractures have been reported mainly when the fracture was caused by a distractive mechanism with or without translation.[23]

Injuries of the upper limbs including shoulders, wrists, and hands are worthy of specific mention. In the paraplegic and tetraplegic patients the upper limbs will also substitute the functions of the lower limbs during transfer and some activities of daily living, personal care, and hygiene.

Radiological Assessment

In the accident and emergency department, AP and lateral radiographs of the spine are still the commonest procedures and probably the most practical for the diagnosis or the exclusion of an injury of the spinal axis. It is important that the transfer and positioning of the patient is supervised by an experienced clinician and is documented to have been supervised. The absence of a fracture radiologically does not exclude a serious ligamentous injury of the spine nor indeed serious cord damage. An enlarged prevertebral soft tissue shadow can be the only radiological manifestation of a serious spinal injury. The cervicodorsal junction and upper thoracic vertebrae are usually difficult to visualize despite pulling on the arms of the patient while taking a lateral radiograph. The quality of the exposure is likely to improve if an attendant gently pushes the shoulders downward while two other attendants hold a gentle pull on the arms from both the elbow and the wrist. Swimmer's views are helpful in patients with short thick necks.

Spinal cord injuries without radiologic abnormality (SCIWORA) have been reported in the literature for many decades and may have contributed to a delay in diagnosis in some patients. Although SCIWORA is generally expected in some children, it can also occur in elderly patients with central cord syndrome due to hyperextension injuries of the cervical spine. In the author's opinion the term SCIWORA needs to be reviewed in the light of the advanced radiological investigations (CT and MRI).

Once a traumatic injury to the spinal axis has been suspected and/or confirmed, in my opinion it is imperative that the whole of the spinal column is radiologically investigated. There is a significant incidence of double injury of the spinal column that ranges between 9.5% and 17%.[13,14]

Although the CT scan is the investigation of choice for assessing spinal fractures, an MRI scan is usually essential to assess ligamentous injuries, stability, and cord damage. MRI scans are also very valuable in detecting single or multiple vertebral contusions adjacent or noncontiguous to the fracture. The prognostic value of the MRI scan (in terms of neurological recovery) in the acute stage is discussed elsewhere. A baseline MRI scan is, however, essential to compare with subsequent MRI scans in case of neurological deterioration. This deterioration does not only occur in the acute stage, it can also occur anytime throughout the patient's life. The incidence of MRI-evident posttraumatic syringomyelia is up to 30% in these patients.[24] Fortunately, the clinically manifested effects occur in a much smaller percentage. El Masry and Biyani discussed the pathophysiology and documented the incidence of posttraumatic syringomyelia at various levels and for various densities of lesions.[25,26]

A baseline chest radiograph is highly advisable especially in tetraplegic/paretic patients and patients with thoracic injuries. Most patients with cervical cord injuries will have impaired respiratory functions. Those patients with thoracic spinal injuries are likely to have associated rib fractures, and/or sternal fractures both of which may add to the biomechanical instability of the thoracic spinal fracture. A lateral radiograph of the sternum is therefore also advisable in all patients with thoracic spinal injuries.

The interpretation of the film taken in the supine position requires radiological expertise. A hemothorax may not result in blunting of the costophrenic angle, but the collection is likely to be seen over the apex of the lungs.

Most patients with thoracic fractures will develop an increase in the paravertebral shadow and an appearance of widening of the mediastinum. Further radiological investigations may be required to exclude mediastinal damage.

Caution needs to be exercised during any procedure undertaken on patients with suspected cord damage, especially those with higher thoracic or cervical cord injury. Because during the stage of spinal shock the sympathetic nervous system is areflexic, patients are usually poikilothermic. In a cold environment they can readily become hypothermic. Hypothermia in patients with cord injury above the level of T5 can result in bradycardia and cardiac arrest. Radiology departments in trauma centers are advised to keep some atropine ready to administer if the pulse of the patient drops below 45/min. In a hot environment the patient can easily become pyrexial.

The Subacute Stage and Long Term

A repeat radiograph of the chest should be considered on the second, third, or fourth post-injury day in patients with thoracic spinal injuries. In the author's experience about 40–50% of these patients are likely to have an increase in the size of the hemothorax 24–48 hours following the injury.

Patients with spinal cord injuries, at all levels, are at risk of developing a delayed ileus and care should be taken not to commence hydration and oral feeding before normal bowel sounds are heard at least 24 hours following injury.

Patients with thoracolumbar and lumbar injuries are likely to develop a retroperitoneal hematoma and a paralytic ileus for a period of time even when the spinal cord has not been damaged. An associated intra-abdominal injury is not easy to exclude clinically. Often the radiologist has to come to the rescue. An abdominal ultrasound scan and/or a CT scan are likely to be required if the bowel sounds do not return by the fourth or fifth day post injury. A perforation in the lesser sac can remain undiagnosed for a number of days and requires a high degree of suspicion for exclusion.

In the absence of normal sensation, the combination of vomiting and a distended abdomen with or without pyrexia offer a great diagnostic challenge to the clinician treating spinal cord injury patients. This can happen on a number of occasions during the patient's life. Although constipation is likely to be the commonest cause, this diagnosis can only be made by exclusion.

Assessment of the Cardiovascular System

The combination of: bradycardia (pulse of 45–60/min), hypotension (systolic blood pressure of 80–90), warm peripheries, visible veins, and good peripheral pulse volume in a patient presenting to hospital following trauma is indicative of a spinal cord injury until otherwise proven. Unlike patients with hemorrhagic shock who exhibit tachycardia in association with hypotension, cold peripheries, and poor volume pulse, and who require bigger intravascular volume replacements, great care should be taken with intravenous fluid administration to patients with bradycardia and hypotension due to SCI. The impaired sympathetic system of the patient, which is responsible for the hypotension and partly responsible for the bradycardia, is usually unable to cope with any excess amount of fluid. The patient can easily develop pulmonary edema and respiratory failure.

Bradycardia can be aggravated by hypoxia, hypothermia, and tracheal suction all of which can cause cardiac standstill. The highest risk is during the stage of spinal areflexia "spinal shock" when the vagus nerve activity is unopposed by the sympathetic nervous system activity. The patient without a previous history of cardiac disease responds readily to cardiac massage and atropine 0.3 mg intravenously provided the cause of the cardiac standstill is effectively treated.

Following the stage of spinal shock (return of reflex activity) patients with tetraplegia and paraplegia above T5 are at risk of developing autonomic dysreflexia. This is one of the major emergencies in spinal injuries. Patients develop a pounding headache associated with high blood pressure in the magnitude of 220/110 or over, and can also develop cerebrovascular accidents. Viscus distension as in urinary retention or bowel obstruction; or painful stimuli below the level of the injury as in appendicitis, diskitis, severe urinary infection, or fracture of a long bone are likely to send volleys of afferent stimuli which travel unsuppressed up and down the spinal cord and initiate this sympathetic mega-discharge.

Assessment of the Respiratory System

The presence of diaphragmatic breathing (absence of chest expansion during inspiration associated with increasing girth with or without retraction of intercostal muscles) in a trauma patient is strongly suggestive of a cervical or upper thoracic cord injury. Frequent clinical examinations of the chest to ensure good air entry throughout the lung and exclude associated chest injuries, hemothorax or pneumothorax, are of paramount importance. These should be combined with monitoring of the vital capacity and oxygen saturation. An initial chest radiograph is advisable in all patients suspected of having sustained an SCI. Patients with dorsal column injuries are at higher risk of developing hemothorax than patients with cervical or thoracolumbar injuries. Frequently, the hemothorax does not become apparent until the third or fourth day following the injury, hence the need for the repeat chest radiograph.

A vital capacity below one liter in a tetraplegic patient requires intensive monitoring and chest physiotherapy. If, despite these measures, the vital capacity drops further (below 600 mL) and the oxygen saturation cannot be maintained ventilation may have to be considered.

With these simple measures the great majority of patients with C5 lesions or below do not require ventilation unless they have associated major chest trauma, an ascending lesion involving the phrenic nerve motor neurons or indeed a respiratory problem prior to their injury. Ventilation should, whenever possible, be avoided since during tracheal suction stimulation of the vagus nerve can result in further bradycardia and cardiac standstill. It is also difficult to wean tetraplegic patients off ventilators. Intensive physiotherapy, frequent assessment of the neurology and breathing, as well as timely intervention can prevent death from hypoxia due to retention of secretions and respiratory failure. Hypoxia can cause death by aggravating the bradycardia to a cardiac standstill. Hypoxia can also destabilize the physiologically impaired, traumatized spinal cord further, resulting in further neurological deterioration.[27] In a patient with a C5 lesion, ascent of the neurological lesion by one or two segments due to edema of the spinal cord (involving the motor neurons of the phrenic nerves) will likely necessitate ventilation for 2–3 weeks and a recovery is likely.

The respiratory system of the tetraplegic and paraplegic patient due to a spinal cord injury above T6 remain impaired throughout the patient's life.

The absence of motor power in the intercostal muscles results in a marked reduction in vital capacity. Paralysis of the abdominal muscles results in a reduced ability to cough and expectorate. Patients with high cord injuries are always at risk of chest infections, lung collapse, and consolidation. They are also at risk of drowning in their own secretions. This improves a little following the stage of spinal shock in patients with upper motor neuron lesions, when spasticity of the abdominal wall becomes established.

Assessment of the Abdomen

A conscious, alert, and cooperative patient who is unable to cough or who is only able to effect a weak cough in the absence of rigidity or with loss of tone in the abdominal musculature is highly likely to have sustained an SCI above the level of D6. A weak cough associated with a positive Beaver's sign (movement of the umbilicus proximally in the process of coughing) indicates paralysis of the lower abdominal muscles with some function of the upper abdominal muscles. In Brown–Sequard syndrome patients, the umbilicus can be seen shifting laterally from the mid-line opposite the side of the hemicord lesion when the patient is asked to cough. Auscultation of the bowels may give good bowel sounds in the first few hours following injury, only to disappear later. It is therefore important to avoid oral fluids and food intake for 24–48 hours following injury. During this period monitoring of the abdomen and documentation of a girth chart and regular auscultation for bowel sounds should be ensured. Occasionally the bowel sounds remain silent for longer and parenteral feeding should be considered. Early oral intake of food and or fluid in the presence of paralytic ileus is likely to cause abdominal distension, which invariably leads to further embarrassment of respiration. Death from respiratory failure or from cardiac arrest caused by hypoxia can easily occur in tetraplegic and high paraplegic patients with paralytic ileus.

Bladder and Urinary System

A palpable distended bladder in an unconscious patient who lies in a dry bed is very suggestive of a spinal cord injury in shock or a cauda equina lesion. A distended bladder which does not cause discomfort to a conscious patient on palpation especially when the patient is unable to void urine is similarly a useful diagnostic sign of an injury. Unconscious patients with head injury and an intact spinal cord or cauda equina are likely to be incontinent in the accident and emergency department.

An indwelling catheter is inserted for 48 hours in the bladder in order to facilitate hourly or two hourly measurement of the urinary output. The presence of hematuria should be investigated with an intravenous urogram or an ultrasound scan of the urinary system in order to exclude renal damage or damage elsewhere in the urinary tract.

Oliguria is commonly observed following SCI and is expected to last for a few days. Vigorous intravenous fluid infusion should be avoided.

It is not advisable to leave an indwelling catheter in the bladder for longer than 48 hours as it is likely to be a source of urethral and bladder complications.

Following removal of the indwelling catheter four-hourly intermittent catheterization by the nursing staff should be carried out and the residual volume should be recorded on each occasion. This is to ensure that the residual urine does not exceed 500 mL in order to avoid bladder over distension. A week or two following the injury a number of patients will develop polyuria for variable periods of time. Various strategies are usually adopted including reduction of fluid intake, increase of the frequency of intermittent catheterization or the insertion of an indwelling catheter for a short period of time until the urinary output is readjusted.

Patients with upper motor neuron lesions may start to develop reflex micturition 3–4 weeks following the injury. Effective reflex micturition may not, however, be established before 3–5 months following the injury. During this period the patient on intermittent catheterization should be advised to keep an accurate record of the voided and of the residual urine.

A baseline urodynamic study (cysto-urethro-metrography) and a baseline IVU/renogram are generally recommended for all patients with spinal cord injury during their first admission. This is in order to evaluate upper and lower urinary tract functions and to use for comparison in the future.

Repeat ultrasound scans/IVU or a renogram together with plain X-rays of the urinary tract on an annual or alternate year basis are paramount in patients with spinal cord injuries as they are at risk of developing silent hydronephrosis, renal scaring, lithiasis of the upper and lower urinary tract, and lower urinary tract problems (Fig. 1.2)

There is no general consensus about the frequency of urodynamic studies in the asymptomatic patient with a normal ultrasound scan/IVU/renogram of the upper urinary tract. The author has to date reserved repeat urodynamics for patients with symptomatic infections, mild or severe symptoms of autonomic dysreflexia, or changes in the upper urinary tract.

Assessment of Level of Consciousness

It is paramount to make a clinical assessment of the level of consciousness in the accident and emergency department and with each subsequent neurological examination until the patient recovers consciousness completely. The level of consciousness influences the interpretation of the neurological findings and examination. The Glasgow coma scale is the most commonly used and useful scoring system.[28]

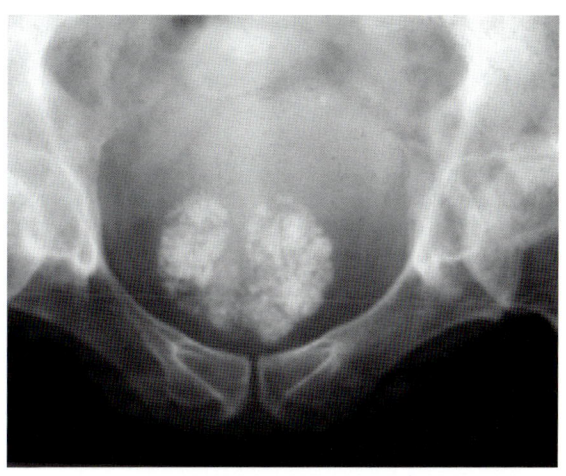

Fig. 1.2 Asymptomatic prostatic calcifications due to detrusor-sphincter dyssynergia resulting in reflux of urine into the ejaculatory ducts, the seminal vesicles, and the prostate.

Psycho-Social Assessment of Cognitive Functions

It is good practice to assess cognitive functions during the early stages of mobilization and before intensive rehabilitation commences. Cognitive functions can significantly influence the method and goals of rehabilitation, the content of the rehabilitation process as well as the outcome. The psychological state of the patient prior to and after the injury, the social, financial, and vocational background, and the adequacy of accommodation are all equally important aspects that also influence the rehabilitation process and its outcome.

Electrophysiological Assessment

Numerous electrophysiological tests are available, however, they are not widely nor routinely used except in a few clinical settings. The commonest are nerve conduction studies (NCS), somatosensory-evoked potentials (SSEP), and motor-evoked potentials (MEP).

Nerve conduction studies are commonly used and can help differentiate between upper motor neuron (UMN) and lower motor neuron (LMN) lesions in both upper and lower limbs. In a root lesion, plexus lesion, or with peripheral nerve damage both motor and/or sensory conduction are impaired. In the upper limbs study of the median and ulnar nerves can predict recovery of hand function.[29,30] In the lower limbs study of the peroneal and tibial nerves can help differentiate between conus or cauda equina and epiconal lesions.[31]

Somatosensory evoked potentials evaluate primarily the function of the dorsal columns but can also reflect function in other spinal tracts and in peripheral nerves. They may help differentiate between complete and incomplete lesions in the acute stage following injury as they are not affected by the state of consciousness of the patient or by spinal shock. In the acute SCI patient, recording of tibial and pudendal SSEP has been found to be predictive of ambulation and of the function of the somatic component of the external urethral sphincter.[32,33] They cannot, however, predict recovery of detrusor muscle functions.[34]

Motor evoked potentials can be elicited by magnetic or electrical cortical stimulation. MEP assess the function of the corticospinal tract by recording from different peripheral muscles during cortical stimulation thus enabling the assessment of both the level and extent of the lesion.[35,36] Magnetic cortical stimulation can be applied to conscious patients as it is less painful and more powerful than electrical stimulation. Unfortunately, it is not advisable to use magnetic stimulation in the presence of metal implants.

In general patients with early MEP recovery have the best chance of recovery of motor and ambulatory functions.[37,38]

Standards for Neurological Examination and Documentation

Michaelis in the late 1960s conducted an international enquiry on paraplegia and tetraplegia in order to establish an agreement on terminology and timing of examination for accurate prognosis. Unfortunately, no agreement between the specialists from 15 countries could be reached.[39] In the same year Frankel published the Frankel's classification in which the density of the neurological lesion could be described as complete or incomplete depending on the absence or presence of sensation and motor power below the level of the lesion. Patients with incomplete injuries could be further subdivided into three groups depending on the degree of sensory and motor sparing. On the basis of this classification, Frankel published the outcome of postural reduction and conservative management of a large series of patients with spinal injuries at all levels. Using Frankel's grid, Frankel et al demonstrated in 1969 for the first time that the neurological progress of groups of patients could be easily described by the assessor and easily understood by the reader.[10] Since 1980 a number of classifications have subsequently been proposed. In 1982, based on the Frankel classification, the American Spinal Injuries Association (ASIA) developed the Standards for Neurological Classification of spinal injured patients. Since 1992 the ASIA standards have become internationally accepted.[40]

The ASIA classification was revised and updated on four occasions (the last being in the year 2000).[41]

Frankel's Classification

This method of classification was developed as a system to evaluate and document the neurological progress of an individual patient, large numbers of patients, or subgroups of patients with spinal injuries following a full neurological examination. The Frankel classification is still the most commonly used classification by clinicians from all disciplines.[10]

Patients are grouped into five categories, based on their clinical neurological presentation. These categories range from patients with complete sensory and motor loss below the level of the injury (Frankel A), to patients with no somatosensory loss and no sphincter disturbance; however, abnormal reflexes may be present (Frankel E). The three categories in between describe various degrees of sparing below the level of the lesion. Frankel B describes sensory sparing only including sacral sparing, however, with complete absence of motor power. Frankel C describes sensory and motor sparing below the level of the lesion, however, the motor power is poor and of no practical use to the patient. Frankel D describes sparing of sensation and motor power below the level of the lesion which many patients could use to walk, with or without aids. Frankel E patients have normal motor power, sensation, and sphincter functions.

The advantage of the Frankel classification is that with one letter of the alphabet (from A to E) one is able to describe and/or understand in general terms both the density of neurological damage at a particular level, the presence or absence of sparing, the modality(ies) spared, and the usefulness of the motor functions spared, if any, below the level of the injury. Furthermore, any significant influence of treatment and/or time resulting in a significant change of density and function can easily be documented by repeating the assessment for the individual patient or the group of patients and documenting the findings in the Frankel grid.

The sphincter functions are not described in Frankel group A, B, C, or D. They are presumed to be undisturbed in Frankel E. Similarly, the quality of ambulation and the requirements of lower limb orthosis and/or arm support are not specified in Frankel D. Although the Frankel classification is good at measuring significant changes in neurology and function, it is not, however, sensitive enough to elicit small changes in neurology when the patient has not improved or deteriorated sufficiently to move from one Frankel grade to another. As a tool of measurement it is good at measuring most of what matters to the patient and the clinician but not necessarily what is required for the rigors of research and accurate comparison between methods of treatment. The Frankel classification, however, remains the most practical method for describing the progress of a patient or a group of patients in the clinical situation.

For research purposes the Frankel classification or its modified version by ASIA requires combination with a method to quantify loss and gain of both sensation and motor power numerically, quantitatively, and in percentage terms.[42,43] The method of percentage of loss from normal and percentage of recovery or loss following treatment were described and recommended by El Masry et al as an alternative to simple numerical calculations in order to avoid the problems of parametric measurements.[42,43]

Ambulation and sphincter functions will also require additional specific documentation.

The ASIA/IMSOP Classification

Some advantages of the ASIA classification include the limitation of motor power testing to five groups of muscles in each limb representing the myotomal distribution in each limb. It also includes a scoring system for motor power, as well as pin prick and touch sensation. This gives a total numerical score for each modality separately for both sides of the body. Progress can be monitored through repeated examination.

El Masry et al in 1996 tested the validity of testing the chosen muscles by the ASIA and the National Acute Spinal Cord Injury Study (NASCIS) group in representing the standard motor examination.[42] The assessment of the individual patient was carried out by the same examiner. Using a quantitative formula of motor deficit percentage (loss) and motor recovery percentage (gain) they concluded that the chosen muscles recommended by both ASIA and NASCIS were representative of the conventional motor scoring in the population of patients examined. It is important, however, not to miss movements in muscles other than those recommended by ASIA, such as the hip adductors that may be spared in an ASIA C patient or which may be the first to reappear.

The current guidelines, definitions, precautions, and methods of classification based on the last revision (2000) are summarized by Jonsson et al.[41]

Clinical Syndromes

The various known patterns of identifiable sparing (syndromes) in incomplete traumatic spinal injuries have been incorporated into the documentation of the ASIA classification.[44]

Management of the Spinal Injury

It is logical to suggest that since all the problems, medical and nonmedical, are caused by the cord injury; anything that can be done to reverse or minimize the pathology would in turn reduce the neurological impairment and magnitude of the effects of the spinal injury. It is also attractive to extrapolate from the results of the experimental laboratory animal and believe that certain pharmacological agents and/or surgical procedures can alter the course of the secondary injury and improve the outcome of the spinal cord injury in humans.

The Secondary Injury

Opinion is divided as to the contribution of the initial impact on the final neurological outcome following a spinal cord injury. Frankel et al and many others believe that the fate of the neurological injury is largely determined at the time of the accident.[45] Freeman and Wright in 1953 did, however, suggest that the definitive cord damage could result from the changes that occur in the spinal cord following injury rather from the initial impact.[46]

Scientists and clinicians have for a number of decades tried to direct treatment to the changes (vascular, cellular, electrophysiological, enzymatic, electrolytic, and metabolic) that occur in and around the spinal cord lesion in the hope of improving the neurological outcome. Unfortunately, the interpretation of the clinical significance of some of these changes in the spinal cord are not agreed upon.[47] In the laboratory animal, attempts at manipulating the secondary changes following sub-threshold impact within a window of opportunity can possibly be beneficial. Beyond a certain threshold of impact, however, these secondary changes cannot be manipulated successfully and neurological improvement cannot be demonstrated.[48,49] In other words, there is a threshold of magnitude of impact above which attempts at manipulating the secondary changes by surgery or other means fail and no improvement can be achieved nor demonstrated in the experimental animal.

In humans the force of the impact cannot be measured, the secondary changes cannot be directly observed nor measured; the window of opportunity could be at least theoretically different from the laboratory animal and practically difficult to take advantage of (because of associated life threatening injuries). The results from surgery and pharmacological agents such as high-dose methyl prednisolone are, therefore, more difficult to evaluate and have yet to be convincingly demonstrated in humans to parallel the experimental findings in the laboratory situation.[50]

Biomechanical Instability of Injuries to the Spinal Column

Biomechanical instability (BI) causes concern because of the potential displacement of the fractured elements at the site of the injury which can damage or further damage neural tissue. The diagnosis of BI is usually based on radiological investigations at the time of the presentation of the patient. Unfortunately, the function of the soft tissues (muscles and ligaments) and the natural history of the repair process that follows are not always taken into account. It is perhaps worthwhile noting that most vertebral fractures heal within 6–12 weeks from injury. Ligamentous injuries, however, can take much longer to heal.

In the majority of patients the biomechanical stability (BS) of the spine is usually restored once the healing of bone and/or ligament occurs. In other words, **biomechanical instability is time related**. There is no evidence to suggest that surgical stabilization enhances the speed of bony healing or achieves earlier BS. Surgical stabilization should therefore be regarded as no more than a temporary method of **containment of the BI** until natural healing occurs. The same can usually be achieved with adequate conservative treatment.

Unstable Injuries Without Neurological Damage

The biomechanical instability in patients with intact neurology can be contained by either surgical or conservative means until natural healing occurs. The risks to the intact spinal cord from surgery are minimal provided no per-operative or post-operative complications occur. In these patients, conservative treatment of 4–6 weeks of bed rest (followed by 6–8 weeks of bracing) is relatively more time consuming and probably more costly than surgical stabilization. Patients with major ligamentous injuries with no bony injuries may require even longer periods of bracing before healing occurs. It is therefore reasonable to encourage the patient who is neurologically intact to undergo surgical stabilization provided he/she understands there is a small risk of paralysis (1–3%) from surgery. Loss of surgical fixation prior to healing and prior to attainment of natural biomechanical stability due to inadequate or poor instrumentation, osteoporosis or infection is likely to add an extra risk to neural tissue.

In our practice we give all patients with and without neurological damage a choice between surgical and conservative management following adequate explanation of potential risks and benefits of each of the two methods of management.

Physiological Instability of the Spinal Cord

The injured spinal cord is **physiologically unstable**. This is due to the loss of its autoregulatory mechanisms, disruption of its brain barrier, and of the cell membrane disturbances that occur following injury.[27] This physiological instability makes the spinal cord vulnerable and unable to defend itself from nonmechanical insults such as hypoxia, sepsis, hypotension, metabolic changes, and anemia, all of which the patient is at risk of developing because of the multisystem dysfunction associated with the paralysis.

Stable and Unstable Injuries with Neurological Damage

Surgical decompression and surgical stabilization do not offer protection to the injured spinal cord against nonmechanical insults. On the contrary, hypoxia and/or hypotension, ligation of an important blood vessel, further mechanical damage during surgery, and/or post-operative complications such as chest infection, surgical wound infection, pressure sores, and septicemia can potentially cause further damage to the injured spinal cord.

One of the potentially erroneous indications for surgical stabilization is to enhance early rehabilitation and discharge from hospital. El Masry in 1993 demonstrated that early mobilization (verticalization) may not be safe nor beneficial to the neurologically impaired patient.[27] Further neurological deterioration in association with postural hypotension during mobilization has been documented in patients with BS spines and incomplete neurological injury. An immediate return of these patients to recumbency was associated with improvement of both the blood pressure and the neurology. Repeating the procedure with ephedrine challenge within 24 hours of the episode did not result in a drop of blood pressure nor neurological deterioration in these same patients.[27] It is therefore more than probable that the **physiological instability** (PI) of the injured spinal **cord** is at **least as threatening as the BI** of the spinal **column** to already impaired spinal cord functions. Early mobilization of patients with complete upper thoracic or cervical cord injuries is also associated with reduction of vital capacity and a potential drop of oxygen saturation which can impair cord functions.[51,52] Furthermore, the combination of postural hypotension and reduced vital capacity, which can occur during early mobilization, are unlikely to enhance the active process of physical rehabilitation which requires energy, motivation, and a sense of well being. Unfortunately, clinicians who manage the acute stage of injury and who are not involved with the rehabilitation process often erroneously interchange the term early mobilization and early rehabilitation. The spinal column is a segmental structure designed for maximum flexibility. Surgical stabilization with long fusions can restrict the flexibility of the spine, and interfere with the rehabilitation process and the quality of independence of the patient. Fortunately, in the last decade, instrumentation has improved to the point of involving a minimum number of units of motion (vertebra). The surgery is, however, more exacting and the complications potentially more serious.

Canal Encroachment

The first case reports to suggest that canal encroachment as demonstrated by computed tomography does not correlate with the degree of neurological impairment, does not prevent neurological recovery in patients with incomplete cord injuries, and does not result in neurological deterioration in patients without impairment of cord function were published by El Masry et al in 1992.[47,53] Since then he and his colleagues reached the same conclusions by reviewing the outcome of conservative treatment of 50 consecutive patients with canal encroachment between 10 and 90% in Frankel C, D, and E groups.[54] Other groups have since published similar findings.[55–58] It could be argued of course that the consistency of the fragments in the spinal canal cannot be determined by the radiological appearance in such cases. Only an MRI of the spinal cord could determine if the cord has been indented. Surgical decompression in patients with incomplete injuries is not necessary for neurological recovery to occur. Moreover, surgical decompression is unlikely to be beneficial if the severity of the initial impact force is beyond a certain magnitude as recovery will not occur. Furthermore, there is no evidence to suggest that surgical decompression achieves better or earlier neurological recovery than adequate conservative treatment in patients with incomplete cord injuries.

Cord Compression

Cord compression does not appear to prevent neurological recovery in patients with significant neurological impairment following spinal cord injuries.

Since the installation of the MRI scanner in our institution we have been monitoring (both prospectively and retrospectively) the neurological progress of patients with cord compression treated conservatively. The preliminary results indicate that no patient with or without neurological sparing has so far deteriorated. It appears that the same clinical prognostic indicators of recovery apply whether there is cord compression or not (Fig. 1.**3a–d**).

We would be prepared to use our data as a control for comparison of both the rate of recovery and the end point of recovery with patients who are surgically decompressed and/or stabilized.

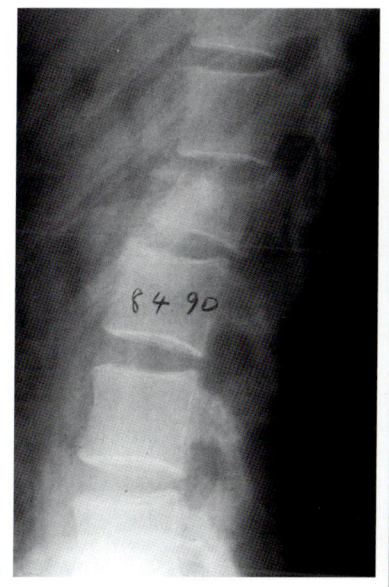

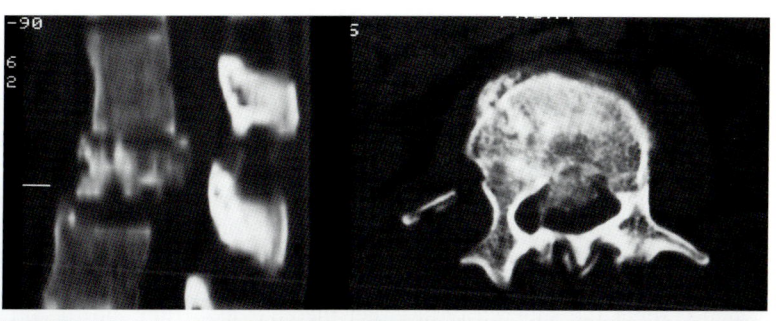

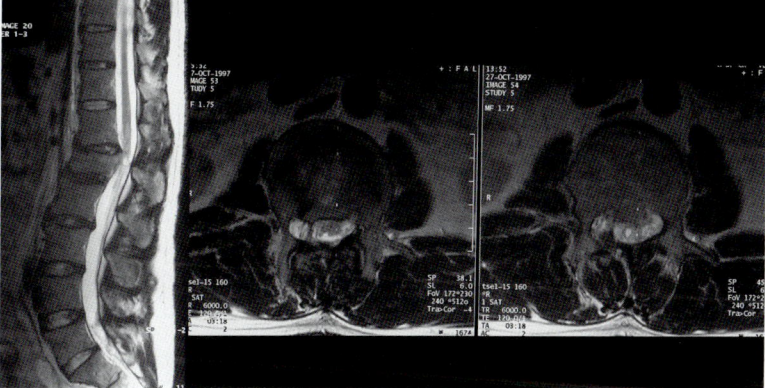

Fig. 1.3 **Paragliding accident, 1990.**
a Unstable burst fracture of L1 vertebra. Initial motor power markedly impaired in all muscle groups in the lower limbs. **b** CT scan revealing about 80% canal encroachment. The patient was treated conservatively with 7 weeks of bed rest, followed by 6 weeks of bracing. He was able to ambulate on two elbow crutches on discharge 18 weeks following the accident. **c** MRI scans in 1997 showing residual cord compression and a cord signal extending for short distances both proximally and distally. **d** Improvement continued despite residual cord compression. Patient walking without crutches 13 years post injury.

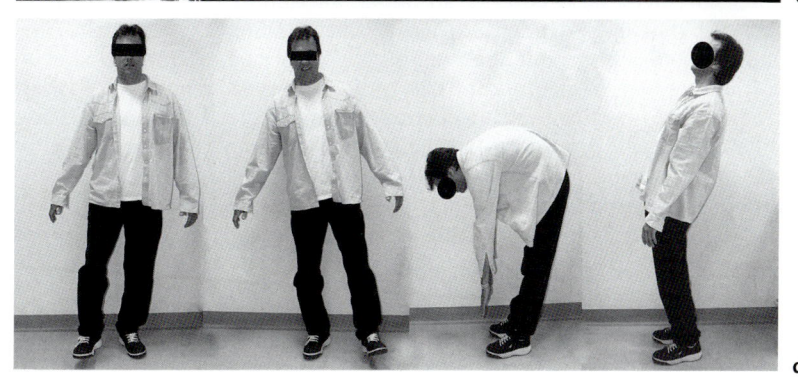

Natural History of Complete Spinal Cord Injuries

About 5–10% of patients with initially clinically complete spinal cord injuries make a significant recovery.[10] Many of these patients, however, recover cord functions for one or two myotomal distributions below the level of the injury.

Although Anderson and Bohlman in 1992 suggested that anterior surgical decompression and arthrodesis of the cervical spine result in motor zonal improvement,[59] Katoh and El Masry in 1994 demonstrated that similar results can be achieved without surgical decompression or arthrodesis.[60] In a series of 53 patients with complete traumatic tetraplegia admitted to our center within 2 days of injury, there were two good prognostic indicators for zonal motor recovery: dermatomal preservation of pin prick sensation and an initial neurological level higher than the vertebral fracture. Both were good prognostic signs for zonal motor recovery regardless of the mechanism of injury or residual canal stenosis.[60]

Natural History of Incomplete Cord Injuries

Patients with incomplete cord injuries make significant neurological recovery regardless of the degree of canal stenosis or canal encroachment provided both the BI of the spinal column and the PI of the spinal cord are well contained.[53–58,61,62]

The Role of Surgery

The role of surgery in trauma remains controversial. This is due to a number of factors which include: the relatively small incidence of traumatic cord injuries to offer adequate experience to clinicians and an adequate number of patients for randomized control trials; the differences in the background of training, experience, and expertise of clinicians involved in the management of the various effects of the paralysis; the differences between the methods of treatment of the nonspinal aspects of spinal injuries with implications on global outcome, types, and incidence of complications; the erroneous belief that surgery is beneficial to the quality of outcome and cost of treatment; the differences between the methods of funding and methods of health care provisions; the temptation to apply the principles of management of the neurologically intact to the neurologically impaired patient; the high complexity of management and multi-factorial influences on neurological recovery; and the lack of evidence about the superiority of either methods of management (surgical or conservative) in terms of outcome.

The rationale of surgery, however, is based on the belief that the BI of the fracture is difficult to contain without surgery and that the presence of canal encroachment by bony or soft tissue is detrimental to neural tissues. Those who promote conservative management of the neurologically impaired patients add more weighting to the physiological instability of the spinal cord and are able to contain the BI of the spinal column without difficulty. Most of them have on occasions witnessed neurological deterioration due to mishaps during or after surgery such as an episode of hypotension, hypoxia, ligation of an important feeding vessel, or post-operative sepsis. There are many claims and counterclaims about the superiority of various methods of management most based on retrospective studies. Retrospective evaluation of the effects of the different surgical procedures and comparison of neurological outcome with conservative management within centers and between centers did not reveal any better neurological outcome with either methods of management.[47,63] Laminectomy has a notoriously bad reputation in further destabilizing some injuries biomechanically and in causing reduction of spinal cord blood flow. The latter was shown experimentally by Anderson and Means in 1985.[64] Neurological deterioration following laminectomy is not unusual and has been documented.[65,66] There is also controversy about the rate of complications and the effect of the method of management on total hospitalization time.[63,67,68] There is evidence, however, to suggest that the incidence of complications is higher and that hospitalization is longer when the patient's transfer to a spinal injuries center (SIC) is delayed and when surgery to the injured spine is performed prior to referral to the SIC.[63,68,69]

The only prospective comparative study comparing surgical and conservative management in 208 patients with acute spinal cord injury revealed no difference in neurological outcome or length of hospitalization.[70] The only parameter found to be significant to the length of stay was the severity of the cord injury. Vocaro et al have published the only class 1 prospective randomized study comparing early surgical decompression before 72 hours vs. late surgery and found no difference in outcome.[71]

Conclusion

Patients with spinal cord injuries are small in number and their management is highly complex. The prognostic indicators of recovery have been well documented with conservative management.[61,62,72] The same clinical prognostic indicators seem to be valid in the presence of canal encroachment and cord compression. With expert care of all aspects of this condition and the prevention of secondary complications, the great majority of patients with motor sparing presenting within 24–48 hours from injury should be able to walk again. Over 60% of patients with motor paralysis but spinothalamic sensory sparing should also regain ambulation. About 10–20% of patients who have no motor power or sensory sparing at presentation will show some recovery within 24–48 hours and occasionally later. There is no evidence to suggest that surgical stabilization and/or decompression provide a better neurological outcome, or, that the same results can be achieved over a shorter period of time when compared to conservative management. The effects of the anesthetic agents (positive, negative, or neutral) on the injured spinal cord have yet to be explored.[73]

With the appropriate care and support, those patients who do not recover can continue to lead successful and fruitful lives and contribute to their community and society.

References

1. Rinaldi I, Mullins WJ, Kretz WK, Stiles TM, Stanton AC. Missed spinal fractures. A serious problem in the patient with multiple injuries. *Va Med Mon.* 1975;102:305–312.
2. Bohlman HH, Bahniuk E, Raskulinecz G, Field G. Mechanical factors affecting recovery from incomplete cervical spinal cord injury. A preliminary report. *Johns Hopkins Med J.* 1979;145:115–125.
3. Ravichandran G, Silver JR. Missed injuries of the spinal cord. *Br Med J.* 1982;284:953–956.
4. Reid DC, Henderson R, Saboe L, Miller JDR. Etiology and clinical course of missed spinal fractures. *J Trauma.* 1987;27: 980–986.
5. Rogers WA. Fractures and dislocations of the cervical spine: an end result study. *J Bone Joint Surg Am.* 1957;39A:341–376.
6. Fischer RP. Cervical radiographic evaluation of alert patients following blunt trauma. *Ann Emerg Med.* 1984;13:905–907.
7. Nichols CG, Young DH, Schiller WR. Evaluation of cervicothoracic junction injury. *Ann Emerg Med.* 1987;16:640–642.
8. Ross SE, O'Malley KF, DeLong WG, Born CT, Schwab CW. Clinical predictors of unstable cervical spinal injury in multiply injured patients. *Injury.* 1992;23:317–319.
9. Edwards MJ, Frankema SP, Kruit MC, Bode PJ, Breslau PJ, Van Vugt AB. Routine cervical spine radiography for trauma victims: does everybody need it? *J Trauma.* 2001;50:529–534.
10. Frankel HL, Hancock DO, Hyslop G, Melzack J, Michaelis LS, Ungar GH et al. The value of postural reduction in initia management of closed injuries of the spine with paraplegia and tetraplegia. *Paraplegia.* 1969–70;7:179–192.
11. Frankel H, Michaelis L, Paeslack V. Closed injuries of the cervical spine and spinal cord: results of conservative treatment of extensive rotation injuries of the cervical spine with tetraplegia. *Proceedings of the Veterans Administration Spinal Cord Injury Conference.* 1973;19:52–55.
12. Bachulis BL, Long WB, Hynes GD, Johnson MC. Clinical indications for cervical spine radiographs in the traumatized patient. *Am J Surg.* 1987;153:473–478.

13. Tearse DS, Keene JS, Drummond DS. Management of non-contiguous vertebral fractures. *Paraplegia.* 1987;25:100–105.
14. Gupta A, El Masry WS. Multilevel spinal injuries: incidence, distribution and neurological patterns. *J Bone Joint Surg Br.* 1989;71B:692–695.
15. Wang CM, Chen Y, DeVivo MJ, Huang CT. Epidemiology extraspinal fractures associated with acute spinal cord injury. *Spinal Cord.* 2001;39:589–594.
16. Norton I, Synnott K, Kenny P, McCormack D. The incidence and treatment of trauma associated with spinal injuries in Ireland. *Injury.* 2000;31:279–299.
17. Green DA, Green NE, Spengler DM, Devito DP. Flexion distraction injuries to the lumbar spine associated with abdominal injuries. *J Spinal Disord.* 1991;4:312–318.
18. Hackl W, Fink C, Hausberger K, Ulmer H, Gassner R. The incidence of combined facial and cervical spine injuries. *J Trauma.* 2001;50:41–45.
19. Gopalakrishnan KC, El Masry W. Prevertebral soft tissue shadow widening: an important sign of cervical spinal injury. *Injury.* 1986;17:125–128.
20. Folman Y, El Masry W, Gepstein R, Messias R. Fractures of the scapula associated with traumatic paraplegia: a pathomechanical indicator. *Injury.* 1993;24:306–308
21. Chen SH, Huang TJ, Chen YJ, Liu HP, Hsu RW. Flexion-distraction injury of the upper thoracic spine associated with tracheoesophageal perforation: a case report. *J Bone Joint Surg Am.* 2002;84A:1028–1031.
22. Rabinovici R, Ovadia P, Mathiak G, Abdullah F. Abdominal injuries associated with lumbar spine fractures in blunt trauma. *Injury.* 1999;30:471–474.
23. Inaba K, Kirkpatrick AW, Finkelstein J, Murphy J, Brenneman FD, Boulanger BR et al. Blunt abdominal aortic trauma in association with thoracolumbar spine fractures. *Injury.* 2001;32:201–207.
24. Wang D, Bodley R, Sett P, Gardner B, Frankel H. A clinical magnetic resonance imaging study of the traumatised spinal cord more than 20 years following injury. *Paraplegia.* 1996;34:65–81.
25. Biyani A, El Masry WS. Post Traumatic Syringomyelia: a review of the literature. *Paraplegia.*1994;32:723–731.
26. El Masry WS, Biyani A. Incidence, Management, and Outcome of Post Traumatic Syringomyelia. In memory of Mr Bernard Williams. *J Neurol Neurosurg Psychiatry.* 1996;60:141–146.
27. El Masry WS. Editorial. Physiological Instability of the Injured Spinal Cord. *Paraplegia, International Journal of the Spinal Cord.* 1993;31:273–275.
28. Teasdale G, Jennett B. Assessment of coma and impaired consciousness: a practical scale. *Lancet.* 1974;2:81–84.
29. Curt A, Dietz V. Nerve conduction study in cervical spinal cord injury: significance for hand function. *Neuro Rehabil.* 1996;7:165–173.
30. Curt A, Dietz V. Traumatic cervical spinal cord injury: Relation between somatosensory evoked potential, neurologic deficit and hand function. *Arch Phys Med Rehabil.* 1996;77:48–53.
31. Rutz S, Dietz V, Curt A. Diagnostic and prognostic value of compound motor action potentials of lower limbs in acute paraplegic patients. *Spinal Cord.* 2000;38:203–210.
32. Curt A, Dietz V. Ambulatory capacity in spinal cord injury: Significance of somatosensory evoked potentials and ASIA Protocol in predicting outcome. *Arch Phys Med Rehabil.* 1997;78:39–43.
33. Jacobs SR, Yeaney NK, Herbison GJ, et al. Future ambulation prognosis as predicted by somatosensory evoked potentials in motor complete and incomplete quadriplegia. *Arch Phys Med Rehabil.* 1995;76:635–641.
34. Curt A, Rodic B, Schurch B, et al. Recovery of bladder function in patients with acute spinal cord injury: Significance of ASIA scores and somatosensory evoked potentials. *Spinal Cord.* 1997;35:368–373.
35. McKay WB, Stokic DS, Dimitrjevic MR. Assessment of corticospinal function in spinal cord injury. Using transcranial motor cortex stimulation: A review. *J Neurotrauma.* 1997;14:539–548.
36. Curt A, Dietz V. Scientific review. Electrophysiological recordings in patients with spinal cord injury: significance for predicting outcome. *Spinal Cord.* 1999;37:157–165.
37. Curt A, Keck ME, Dietz V. Functional outcome following spinal cord injury: significance of motor evoked potentials and ASIA scores. *Arch Phys Med Rehabil.* 1998;79: 81–86.
38. Hirayama T, Tsubokawa T, Maejima S. Clinical assessment of the prognosis and severity of spinal cord injury using corticospinal motor evoked potentials. In: Shimoji K, Kurokawa T, Tamaki T, eds. *Spinal cord monitoring and electrodiagnosis.* Heidelberg, Springer, 1991:503–510.
39. Michaelis LS. International inquiry on neurological terminology and prognosis in paraplegia and tetraplegia. *Paraplegia.* 1969;7:1–5.
40. American Spinal Injury Association/International Medical Society of Paraplegia. *International Standards for Neurological and Functional Classification of Spinal Cord Injury.* 3rd ed. Chicago: ASIA; 1992.
41. Jonsson M, Tollbäck A, Gonzales H, Borg J. Inter-rater reliability of the 1992 international standards for neurological and functional classification of incomplete spinal cord injury. *Spinal Cord.* 2000;38:675–679.
42. El Masry WS, Tsubo M, Katoh S, Miligui YHS. Validation of the American Spinal Injury Association (ASIA) motor score and the National Acute Spinal Cord Injury Study (NASCIS) motor score. *Spine.* 1996;21:614–619.
43. El Masry WS, Short DJ. Current Concepts: Spinal Injuries and Rehabilitation. *Curr Opin Neurol.* 1997;10:484–492.
44. El Masry WS. Pathology of spinal cord injuries. In: Alpar EM, Gosling P, eds. *Trauma: Scientific Basis for Care.* London: Arnold Publishers; 1999:211–216.
45. Frankel H, Michaelis L, Paeslar V, Ungar G, Walsh JJ. Closed injuries of the cervical spine and spinal cord: results of conservative treatment of vertical compression injuries of the cervical spine. *Proceedings of the Veterans Administration Spinal Cord Injury Conference.* 1973a;19:29–31.
46. Freeman LW, Wright TW. Experimental observations of concussion and contusion of the spinal cord. *Ann. Surg.* 1953; 137:433–443.
47. El Masry WS, Jaffray D. Recent Developments in the Management of Injuries of the Cervical Spine. In: Frankel HL, ed. *Handbook of Clinical Neurology. Spinal Cord Trauma.* Vol 17(61). Amsterdam: Elsevier Science Publishers BV; 1992.
48. Dolan EJ, Tator CH, Endrenyi L. The value of decompression for acute experimental spinal cord compression injury. *J Neurosurg.* 1980;53:749–755.
49. Guha A, Tator CH, Endremni L, Piper I. Decompression of the spinal cord improves recovery after acute experimental spinal cord compression injury. *Paraplegia.* 1987;25:324–339
50. Short DJ, El Masry WS, Jones PW. High dose methylprednisolone in the management of acute spinal cord injury: a systematic review from a clinical perspective. *Spinal Cord.* 2000;38:273–286.
51. Cameron GS, Scott JW, Jousse AT, Botteral EH. Diaphragmatic respiration in the quadriplegic patient and the effect of position on his vital capacity. *Ann Surg.* 1955;141:451–6.
52. Morgan MDL, Silver JR, Williams SJ. The respiratory system of the spinal cord patient. In: Bloch RF, Basbaum M, eds. Management of Spinal Cord Injury. Baltimore: Williams and Wilkins; 1986: 78–117.
53. El Masry WS, Meerkotter DV. Early Decompression of the Spinal Cord following Injury: Arguments for and against. In: Illis LS, ed. *Spinal Cord Dysfunction. Intervention, Treatment.* Vol II. Oxford: Oxford University Press; 1992:7–27.
54. El Masry WS, Katoh S, Khan A. Reflections on the neurological significance of bony canal encroachment following traumatic injury of the spine in patients with Frankel C, D and E presentation. *J Neurotrauma.* 1995;10(suppl):70.
55. Limb D, Shaw DL, Dixon RA. Neurological injury in thoraco lumbar burst fractures. *J Bone Joint Surg Br.* 1995;77B:774–777.
56. Rosenberg N, Lenger R, Weisz I, Stein H. Neurological deficit in a consecutive series of vertebral fracture patients with bony fragments within the spinal canal. *Spinal Cord.* 1996;35:92–95.
57. Boerger TO, Limb D, Dickson RA. Does 'canal clearance' affect neurological outcome after thoracolumbar burst fractures? *J Bone Joint Surg Br.* 2000;82B(5):629–635.
58. Mohanty SP, Venkatram N. Does neurological recovery in thoracolumbar and lumbar burst fractures depend on the extent of canal compromise? *Spinal Cord.* 2002;40(6):295–299.

59. Anderson PA, Bohlman HH. Anterior decompression and arthrodesis of the cervical spine: Long term motor improvement. *J Bone Joint Surg Am.* 1992;74A:683–692.
60. Katoh S, El Masry WS. Neurological recovery after conservative treatment of cervical cord injuries. *J Bone Joint Surg Br.* 1994;76B:225–228.
61. Katoh S, El Masry WS. Motor recovery of patients presenting with motor paralysis, sensory sparing following cervical spinal cord injuries. *Paraplegia.* 1995;33:506–509.
62. Katoh S, El Masry WS, Jaffray D, McCall W, Eisenstein SM, Pringle RG, et al. Neurological outcome in conservatively treated patients with incomplete closed traumatic cervical spinal cord injuries. *Spine.* 1996;2:2345–2351.
63. Wilmot CB, Hall KM. Evaluation of the acute management of tetraplegia: conservative versus surgical treatment. *Paraplegia.* 1986;24:148–153.
64. Anderson DK, Means ED. Effect of laminectomy on spinal cord blood flow, energy metabolism and ATPase activity. *Paraplegia.* 1985;23:58.
65. Morgan TH, Wharton GW, Austin GN. The result of laminectomy in patients with incomplete spinal cord injuries. *Paraplegia.* 1971;9:14–23.
66. Bohlman HH. Acute fractures and dislocations of the cervical spine. An analysis of three hundred hospitalized patients and review of the literature. *J Bone Joint Surg Am.* 1979;61A:1119–1142.
67. Murphy KP, Opitz JL et al. Cervical fractures and spinal cord injury: Outcome of surgical and non-surgical management. *Mayo Clin Proc.* 1990;65:949–959.
68. Carvell JE, Grundy DJ. Complications of spinal surgery in acute spinal cord injury. *Paraplegia.* 1994;32:389–395.
69. Aung TS, El Masry WS. Audit of a British Centre for Spinal Injury. *Spinal Cord.* 1997;35:147–150.
70. Tator CH, Duncan EG et al. Comparison of surgical and conservative management of 208 patients with acute spinal cord injury. *Can J Neurol Sci.* 1987;14(1):60–69.
71. Vaccaro AR, Daugherty RJ, Sheehan TP, Dante SJ, Cotler JM, Balderston RA, et al. Neurologic outcome of early versus late surgery for cervical spinal cord injury. *Spine.* 1997;22:239–246.
72. Folman Y, El Masry WS. Spinal cord injury: prognostic indicators. *Injury.* 1989;20(2):92–93.
73. Hickey R, Albin MS, et al. Autoregulation of spinal cord blood flow. Is the cord a microcosm of the brain? *Stroke.* 1986;17:1183–1189.

2 Understanding Cervical Spinal Trauma: Biomechanics and Pathophysiology

K.-S. Saternus and G. Kernbach-Wighton

Introduction

In this chapter, osteo-articular and soft tissue injuries of the cervical spine are systematically addressed with the benefit of postmortem and experimental pathological findings. The underlying biomechanical aspects of the resultant injuries need to be appreciated as they form the foundation of correct image interpretation. At the same time the reader realizes that the vast spectrum of spinal injury poses significant challenges to the imaging modalities currently available for the diagnosis and exclusion of injury.

Atlanto-Occipital and Atlanto-Axial Joints

Condylar Fracture

Traumatology

Fractures of the occipital condyle have long been regarded as rare injuries to the atlanto-occipital joints. Less than 20 such clinical cases are discussed in the literature, from Bell's initial description of the injury in 1817 through to the mid-1980s.[1-4] In contrast, condylar fractures in fatal trauma are a familiar topic in forensic medicine.[5-9] Alker et al and Saternus each cite an incidence of 0.6% in the setting of fatal trauma.[5,7] Recent radiological reviews give an incidence of occipital condylar fracture of up to 16% of patients with craniocervical injury.[10-13]

The attention given to the alar ligaments in whiplash injuries has also increased clinical interest in the traumatology of condylar fractures.

Biomechanics

Table 2.1 lists the mechanisms of injury for a condylar fracture.[14] This does not include the horizontal avulsion fracture[6] because such a mechanism of injury in a normal joint with negligible friction would not represent plausible explanation.[15]

The most commonly used classifications of occipital condylar fractures are based on radiological criteria.[16,17] The most useful one is that of Leone and coworkers, which includes multiple new features.[12] Using a detailed review these authors point out that the clinical symptomatology of condylar fractures is so inconsistent that the diagnosis is rarely made clinically and requires dedicated cranio-cervical CT assessment.

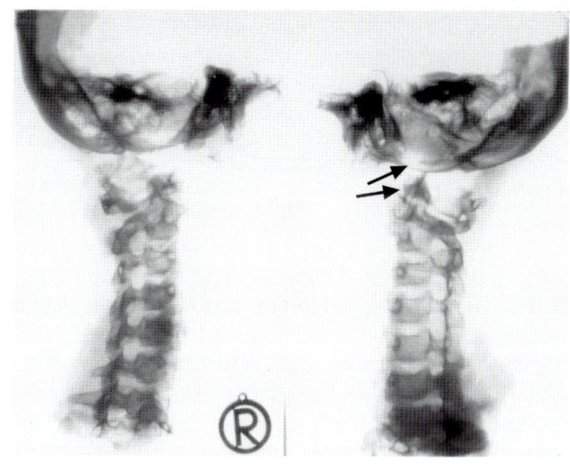

Fig. 2.1 Oblique radiographs of postmortem cervical spine showing complete atlanto-occipital dissociation (*arrows*). Transmission of the force to the base of the skull via the mandibular joints.

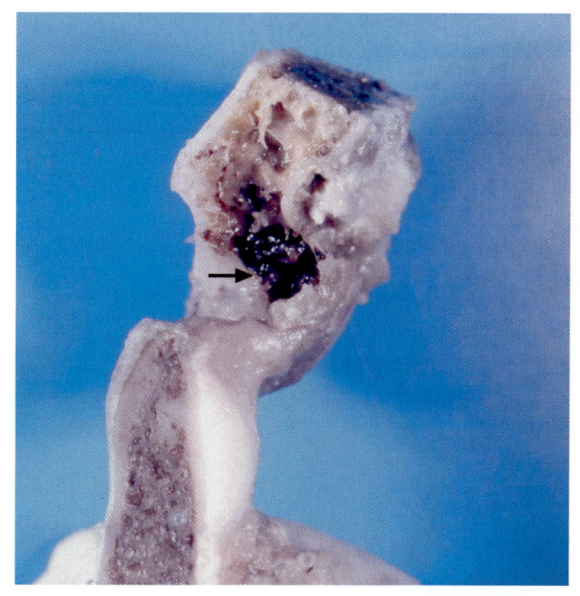

Fig. 2.2 Incomplete disruption of the occipital condyle with hemorrhage and fragment formation in the region of the insertion of the alar ligament (*arrow*).

In our own material, including over 2000 studies of fatal trauma, traction injuries in the form of condylar avulsion warrant a special mention among those constellations that lead to condylar fracture. Figure 2.1 shows an example of a complete insertion avulsion, and Figure 2.2 shows an example of an incomplete one.

Table 2.1 Classification of condylar fractures as burst fractures or injuries reflecting various degrees of force (from Saternus 1987)[14]

1. Axial compression	(Jefferson type) condylar impression
2. Axial traction	(Hangman's type) condylar retraction
3. Rotation with axial loading	Condylar retraction
4. Oblique compression	(Burst fracture of the abutment) frontal condylar fracture; contralateral
5. Oblique traction	(Horizontal shear force) a skull base fracture as in a contralateral horizontal fracture
6. Transverse shear force	(Longitudinal fracture of the base of the skull) partial condylar avulsion

Compression of the skull in the sagittal plane initially causes elastic deformation of the base of the skull. Compression exceeding the threshold value causes the bone to burst, producing transverse shear stress. The result is a sagittal fracture of the base of the skull. This transverse shear stress is resisted by a particularly stable structure at the base of the skull. This consists of the double-ring structure of the margin of the foramen magnum together with the occipital condyles and the atlas. The two rings are additionally stabilized by sturdy ligament structures (alar ligaments and the transverse ligament of the atlas) that provide stability against transverse shear stresses. A fall or blow that shatters the skull exerts traction on this exceedingly sturdy structure. This type of traction injury of the bone–ligament interface takes the form of avulsion of the insertion of the alar ligament and a fragment of variable size from the occipital condyle. Figure 2.2 demonstrates that such an insertion avulsion will not necessarily be complete.

Alar Ligaments

Topography

Many authors concur in specifying that the alar ligaments course superiorly from the odontoid process to the condyles. In contrast, Dvorac et al demonstrated significant variability in the course of the ligament in their material.[18–21] In one quarter of their cases, the alar ligaments were observed to course inferiorly from the condyle. From our group, Thrun performed dissections on forensic material (n = 31) to pursue this line of inquiry.[22] Those dissections confirmed this variability.

The ligaments normally insert into the upper two-thirds of the lateral surfaces of the odontoid process. However, individual fibers may also insert into the apex of the odontoid process. In this study too, the ligaments in one quarter of the cases coursed inferiorly from the odontoid process to the occipital condyles. Typically (in 75% of these cases), a portion of the most superior fibers passed over the apex of the odontoid process. The anterior bone spur frequently observed with the steep type of odontoid process (kyphotic odontoid process as described by Krmpotic-Nemanic and Keros) limits the anterior extent of the structure.[23]

In over one-third of the cases, the ligaments were multipartite, specifically consisting of two to five parts. In this context, we should also mention that a distinct portion between the condyle and atlas also occurs.[24]

The fan-shaped divergent angles of the alar ligaments (both to the condyle and to the odontoid process) in our own study group are significant from a functional standpoint in that they further restrict rotation in addition to the normal anatomical limitation. Such configurations occurred in 15% of the cases studied. Here, the fiber bundles were unilaterally or bilaterally twisted anteriorly toward each other.

Biomechanics

The findings presented indicate that the alar ligaments should not be regarded as compact, homogeneous ligaments and that their course may vary between individual patients. Contrary to the majority opinion expressed in the literature, it is not even true that the fibers of the structure course superiorly from the odontoid process to the condyles in most cases.

Two conclusions may be drawn from this. First, partial ruptures of the alar ligament are indeed possible; second, injury is not due solely to the unphysiological rotational stress. On the contrary, in any given injury, the patient's specific anatomical constellation is not predictable and cannot be visualized with currently available imaging modalities.

Traumatology

We have investigated in our postmortem study injuries of the alar ligaments in fatal trauma.[25] Fatal trauma can occur without any involvement of the cervical spine. Conversely, findings included every stage from lack of morphological evidence of injury to massive fracture dislocation or rupture with dislocation. Alar ligament injuries were categorized according to a semi-qualitative five-stage classification system. The individual classes do not represent a uniform distribution; there are gaps in the intermediate stages. However, the respective incidence of uninjured, moderately injured, and severely injured spines were in a comparable range.

As expected, the results demonstrate a correlation between the overall severity of the injury to the cervical spine and the extent of injury to the alar ligaments. The alar ligaments were injured in one-third of all cases of fatal trauma.

In three of 30 cases, the sole injury to the cervical spine and atlanto-occipital and atlanto-axial joints consisted of injury to the alar ligaments in the form of hemorrhage.

Most cases of massive cervical spine trauma also involved rupture of the alar ligaments. However, this was not a constant finding. With fractures of the odontoid process, findings in our own material included ligament hemorrhages but not complete ligament ruptures. Avulsion of the ligaments from the odontoid process occurred primarily in rotation. This correlation with rotation was not as clear in experimental post-mortem studies of anatomical specimens obtained from patients who had stipulated that their bodies could be used for scientific research after death.

Cruciform Ligament, Apical Ligament, Anterior Atlanto-Occipital Membrane, and Anterior Longitudinal Ligament

Anterior Atlanto-Occipital Membrane and Anterior Longitudinal Ligament

As a result of traction, the anterior longitudinal ligament is injured twice as often as the anterior atlanto-occipital membrane. This means that the anterior and posterior conditions are identical. In this regard, it should be noted that only traction, not compression, can lead to ligament injury.

Apical Ligament

Although they rarely receive clinical attention, injuries to the apical ligament are also common. A remnant of the corda dorsalis, this slender ligament courses with a small artery and veins between the clivus and the apex of the odontoid process. Although the ligament bears physiological stresses in flexion and extension,[4] it does not serve any significant functional purpose in the atlanto-occipital joint. It can rupture in combination with other soft tissue injuries. However, traumatic injury is usually only indirect (Fig. 2.3) and involves hemorrhaging from injured accompanying blood vessels.[26] Accordingly, an isolated injury to this structure is not detectable even with current imaging modalities. An important diagnostic aspect is that even bony injuries (avulsion of the insertions) practically never occur because of the small size of the ligament.

Cruciform Ligament

Rupture of the vertical portion of the cruciform ligament indicates an extensive injury. With axial traction or flexion, it often tears along with the dura, which is usually also separated from the inner surface of the adjacent skull base.

An interrelated complex of ligament rupture and ring fracture of the skull base characterizes massive traction injuries. Figure 2.4 shows an example of a marginal clivus avulsion.

Forces acting on the skull can fracture the skull base in a circular pattern emanating from the center of the injury. When this occurs (such as in a fall on the back of the head), a narrow rim is often avulsed from the clivus.[9,27–29] In cases such as a fall on the central portions of the skull or on the heels or buttocks, there is a wedge of compression pointing inward into the cranial cavity while the traction produces a fracture cone that becomes wider as one moves distally.

In forced flexion of the skull, the posterior arch of the axis acts as a lever to transfer the force of injury via the

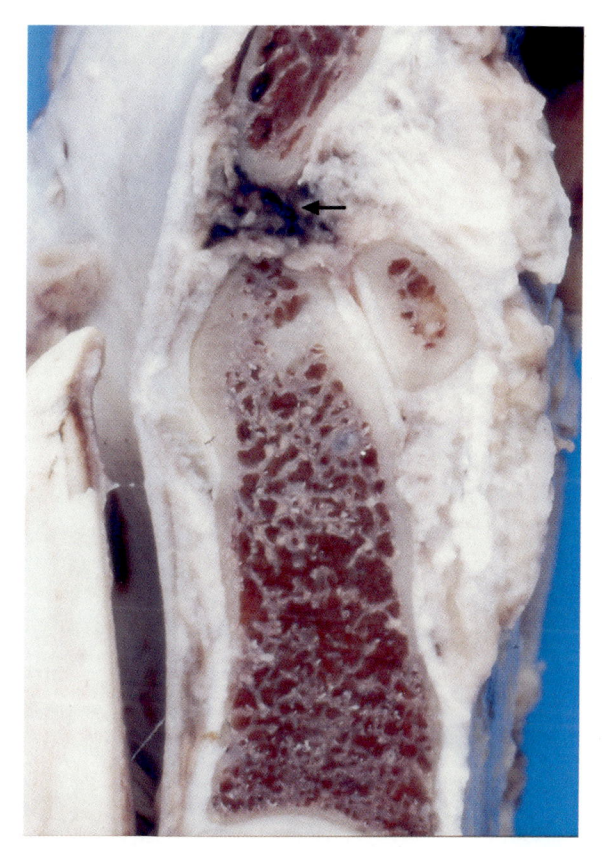

Fig. 2.3 Circumscribed hemorrhage around the apical ligament of the odontoid process due to a direct traction injury at the craniocervical junction (*arrow*).

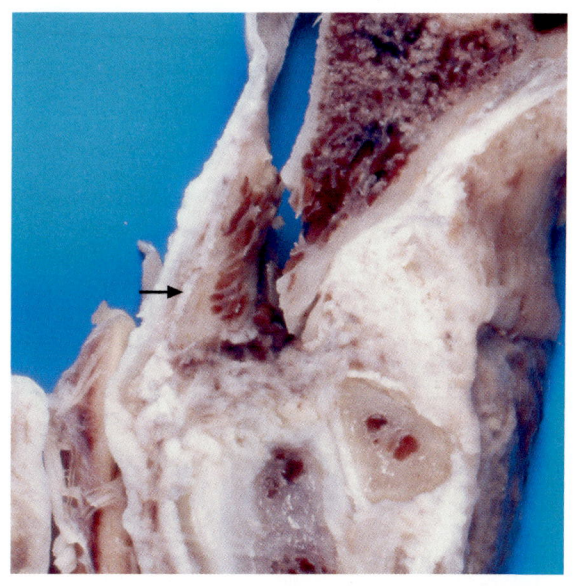

Fig. 2.4 Bone fragment (*arrow*) avulsed from the clivus by traction secondary to a ring fracture of the base of the skull.

transverse ligament of the atlas to the posterior surface of the odontoid.[30] This can produce an odontoid fracture or a rupture of the horizontal part of the transverse ligament. Several systematic studies of the strength of the ligament have been conducted and in-

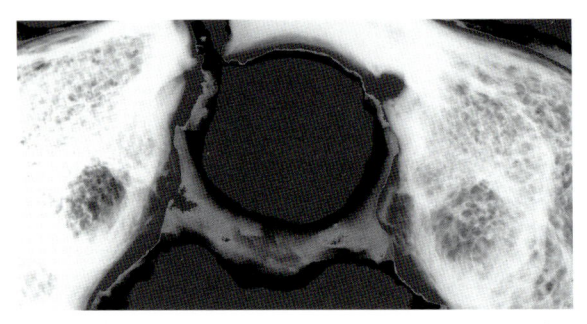

Fig. 2.5 Montage of a soft tissue radiograph superimposed on the osseous structure (C1) in a case of an experimentally induced tear of the transverse ligament of the atlas from the right lateral mass.

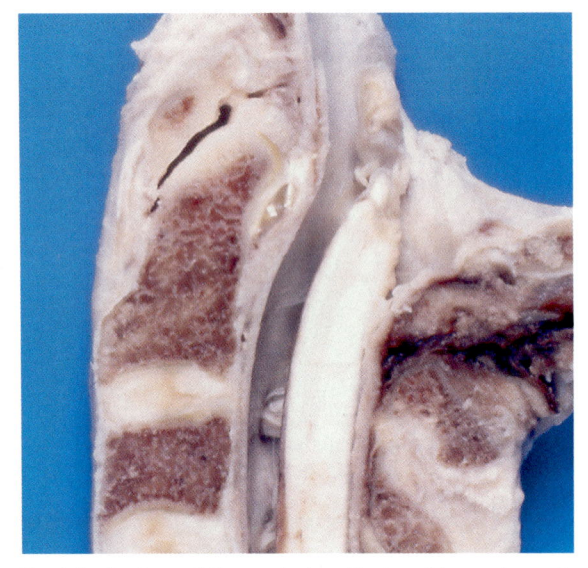

Fig. 2.6 Rupture of the posterior atlanto-axial membrane in flexion trauma.

cluded in the analysis of the injury.[31,32] This has shown that severe regressive changes in the ligament occur with increasing age. These changes are conducive to ruptures. Our own experimental studies of tearing of the transverse ligament of the atlas have demonstrated that in over half of all cases, fine avulsion of the insertions from the lateral masses had occurred (Mann, unpublished) (Fig. 2.5). There are only a few descriptions of axial avulsion of the skull with the atlas in the absence of a rupture of the transverse ligament of the atlas or odontoid fracture.[7]

Posterior Atlanto-Occipital Membrane and Tectorial Membrane, Epidural Bleeding

The most common injuries to the occipital and cervical region are ruptures and hemorrhaging deep to the posterior ligament structures. Disregarding hemorrhaging into the posterior atlanto-occipital membrane from a skull fracture (a common indirect injury), our own early studies have shown that about half as many injuries occur in the next layer, the tectorial membrane (Fig. 2.6).[33] The reason for this is the difference in strength and size of the two structures; the posterior atlanto-occipital membrane is significantly stronger than the tectorial membrane.

This means that the typical form of mechanical stress leading to rupture of the tectorial membrane occurs when the posterior arch of the atlas and the spinous process of the axis are drawn apart with the head in forward flexion. In flexion, the posterior arch of the atlas is carried along by its strong ligamentous attachment to the skull. Accordingly, a complete or partial tear of the tectorial membrane is invariably an associated injury with an odontoid fracture from flexion trauma.

This is why it appears strange that injury to the tectorial membrane occurs in the presence of stress in the opposite direction, namely with an odontoid fracture in extension trauma. Yet this too is a constant finding. This may be explained by translation, which also produces an unphysiological stress sufficient to cause a rupture. However, most actual accidents leading to injury of the tectorial membrane involve complex rotational motions.

It would be wrong to create the impression that injury to the tectorial membrane is typically associated with a bony injury. On the contrary, it is often observed as an isolated soft tissue injury to the cervical spine. Its level is determined by the size difference between the two posterior ligament systems extending between the occiput and C2. Posterior ligament injury is regularly accompanied by epidural bleeding. Epidural bleeding in the cervical spine is common in fatal trauma. The term fatal trauma could create the impression that the cervical spine is the site of the fatal injury. However, this tends to be the exception in those cases examined by coroners. On the contrary, every degree of involvement of the cervical spine may be observed, ranging from absence of injury to fatal spinal cord injury. Diffuse or circumscribed epidural bleeding may be observed with nearly every soft tissue injury to the cervical spine and with bony injuries. It most commonly occurs in the posterior epidural region.[7,34,35]

The structural differences between the posterior atlanto-occipital membrane and tectorial membrane suggest that they have different functions. At the suggestion of Dr. Nägerl (communicated personally), we are currently exploring whether these two ligament structures differ with respect to sensory elements such as lamellated corpuscles and Ruffini corpuscles. The thinking is that the posterior atlanto-occipital membrane may have more of a mechanical function whereas the tectorial membrane may also have a proprioceptive function.

Atlas Fracture

Anterior Arch

The older literature specifies the incidence of anterior arch fractures relative to posterior arch fractures as about 1:3. Several earlier postmortem studies have shown that this relation can be reversed in the case of fatal trauma,[7] namely two to one. Avulsion of the insertions of the anterior longitudinal ligament with a fragment of varying size from the anterior arch of the atlas may occur in the common extension injuries. Another mechanism, namely horizontal shear forces that cause transverse fractures of the anterior arch,[36] did not appear plausible in adults. However, in the case of an almost 2-year-old child described by Töndury and Tillmann where the odontoid and central anterior arch of the atlas were not yet ossified,[37] both the avulsion through the cartilage of the apex of the odontoid, i.e., not at the bone–cartilage interface,[38,39] and a bony avulsion of the inferior margin of the arch of the atlas may be attributed to a horizontal shear component.

In another example from our own studies, external flexion with extensive tearing of the posterior ligaments between the occiput and C2 led to a tear in the superior capsule of the median atlanto-axial joint and to bending stresses in the articular facet pressed against the anterior surface of the odontoid process. This resulted in a fracture in the margin of the median atlanto-axial joint (articular facet).

In combination with a basal odontoid fracture, such an avulsion of the inferior margin of the anterior arch of the atlas can also occur as asymmetric injuries. This has been demonstrated by an earlier study (Fig. 2.**7**).[40]

In this regard, it should be noted that in animal studies the ligaments between the occiput and C2 tend to rupture at the same kinetic energy in both extension and flexion trauma.[41,42] This means that the more common injury is not the sagittal fracture of the anterior arch of the atlas but the horizontal fracture.

Furthermore, the presence of elastic structures even permits a symmetrical avulsion of the anterior arch of the atlas (Fig. 2.**8**). The example shows step-shaped avulsion of the unossified anterior arch in a nine-year-old subjected to compression in flexion (anteriorly and inferiorly directed force vector). This type of fracture would best be described as a Jefferson fracture, which would be open to question in an adult (see the section Jefferson Fracture below).

Jefferson Fracture

Traumatology

Since Jefferson's description,[43,44] the bilateral fracture of the anterior and posterior arch of the atlas is characteristically attributed to axial loading. Lateral avulsion of the lateral masses is widely accepted as the mechanical cause of the fracture. The thinking is that compression causes the atlas to break apart like two wedges under a horizontal shear stress. The occipital condyles form the superior compressing wedge, and the two superior articular facets of the arch of the axis form the inferior wedge.

The literature repeatedly mentions that Jefferson never succeeded in reproducing this type of fracture in experiments on human anatomical specimens even when extreme force was applied.

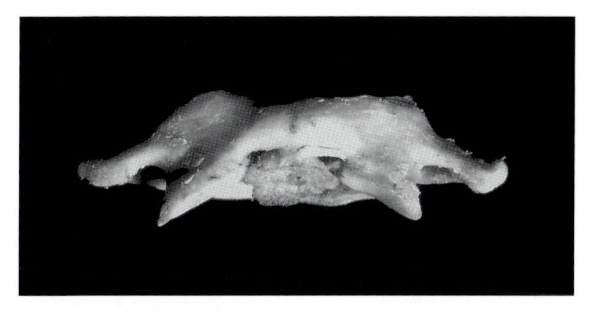

Fig. 2.**7** Anterior view of C1 with a portion of the fractured dens. This shows a C1 horizontal fracture of the lower margin of the facet for the odontoid process to the left of the mid-line extending to the left lateral mass, due to a bending strain under a ventrally flexing vector (dens fracture).

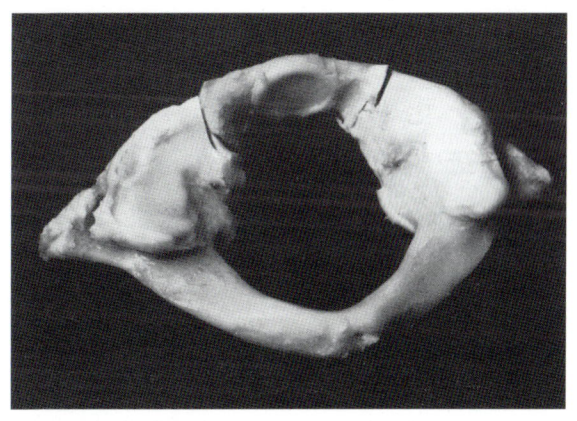

Fig. 2.**8** Avulsion of the anterior arch of C1 that is incompletely ossified with the lateral masses, from an anteriorly and inferiorly directed vector force. The transverse ligament of the atlas is intact.

The section on the Biomechanics of Condylar Fracture above describes in detail how the ring structure of the atlas and the transverse ligament that balances shear forces give the atlas a high degree of dimensional stability. Horizontal shearing of the lateral masses would require either significant elastic or plastic deformation or rupture of the ligament. Earlier experimental tests of tensile strength suggest that stretching without structural damage under actual fracture conditions is highly improbable. Tears of this ligament structure in atlas fractures are also rare. However, one would expect them according to current thinking.

In a finite element model, axial compressive pressure induces high concentration of localised stress at the anterior and posterior arch of the atlas.[45] These authors, however, did not include in their calculations the transverse ligament of the atlas which neutralizes tension.

This is sufficient cause to critically reexamine the assertion that Jefferson fractures are caused by axial compression.

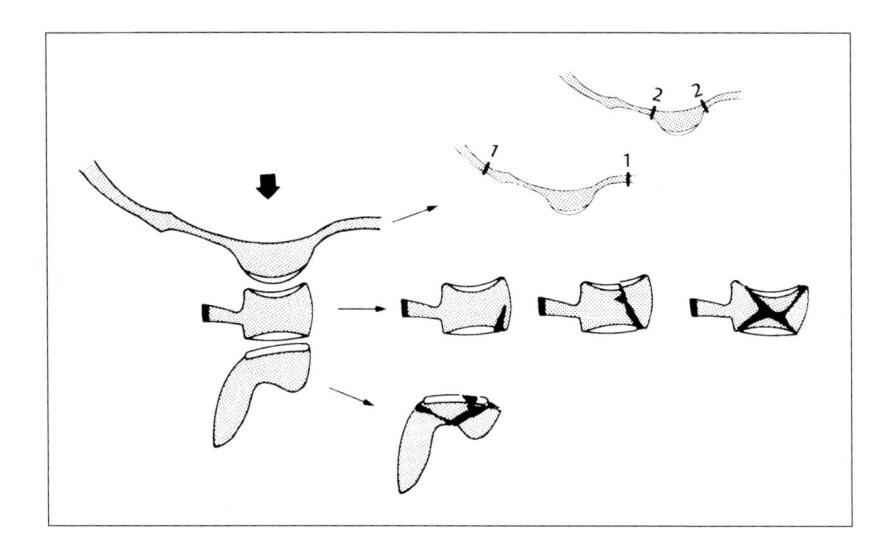

Fig. 2.**9** Traumatic sequelae from craniocervical axial compression: fractures of the occipital condyles (see Figs. 2.**1**, 2.**2**), lateral mass of C1, articular surface of C2.

Biomechanics

Our line of inquiry was to investigate whether the Jefferson fracture represents a model fracture for axial loading. Our working group performed fracture tests (n = 400) with a custom test stand of our own design.[46,47] The skull base, an indestructible structure for test purposes, was made of metal; the test specimens representing the atlas and axis were identical plaster casts.

Two real objects of different types were used as models. As regards the position of the odontoid, we used one specimen inclined 1° anteriorly and one inclined 7° posteriorly, according to Krmpotic-Nemanic and Keros and Koebke.[23,48] These authors refer to the anteriorly inclined type as kyphotic and the posteriorly inclined type as lordotic. Results of measurements of collected material and our own specimens have shown that the inclination of the odontoid's axis is indicative of the overall configuration of the region from the occiput to C2. For example, a sturdy arch of the atlas with a wide articular facet is typical for the kyphotic odontoid, whereas a slender configuration is typical for the lordotic type.[48] In terms of Jefferson's model, this would correspond to wide, flat superior and inferior wedges in the case of a kyphotic odontoid whereas the adjacent structures would correspond to narrow wedges in the case of a lordotic odontoid.

The test specimens were subjected to loading at 10 different angles until the fracture occurred; the transverse ligament of the atlas was designed not to tear. The shape and localization of these fractures (initial fractures) were recorded. Then loading was continued with a defined force until a second fracture occurred.

Using this experimental design, we produced atlas fractures in 84% of all cases with a flat wedge and in 94% of all cases with a narrow wedge. These corresponded to fracture types that actually occur. However, no Jefferson fractures occurred in 20 experiments with purely axial loading whereas seven occurred with eccentric loading. The final results of the second fractures in 200 fracture experiments included 16 fracture patterns of the Jefferson type in addition to three related forms of symmetrical atlas fractures. In two of these cases, the fracture line coursed through the center of the articular facet; in the third case, it coursed through the anterior portions of the lateral masses. In the clinical literature, this latter case is regarded as equivalent to a Jefferson fracture.

Twelve of the subsequent Jefferson fractures resulted from less extensive initial fractures. With respect to the final results after the second fracture, we found that Jefferson fractures occurred almost twice as often with axial loading than with eccentric loading. We may, therefore, conclude that these fractures occur in one of two ways. The first and more common way would be as a subsequent symmetrical fracture of the anterior and posterior arches of the atlas secondary to destabilization of the ring of the atlas at any given site under axial loading. Applied to actual clinical conditions, this frequency distribution is probably the reason for previous notions about the etiology of this type of fracture.

The second way in which a Jefferson fracture occurs is due to a bending stress on the atlas in the sagittal plane, i. e., a nonaxial stress. In this regard, the question arises as to whether such a mechanical interpretation may correctly be derived from fracture tests on plaster models.

These experimental results for the Jefferson fracture are not isolated findings. Nor is it the case that homogeneous plaster is assumed to be equivalent to bone with its functional material distribution. Nevertheless, these fracture experiments provide information about the distribution of stresses in a three-dimensional model. Our fracture experiments can build on those performed by Jefferson himself. Additionally, they provide an explanation of why the transverse ligament of the atlas usually remains intact in a Jefferson fracture.

Lateral Mass

Jefferson himself noted that axial compression at three levels can lead to bony injury.[43] Figure 2.**9** illustrates the various different types of fractures. The occipital condyles represent the upper topographic level. They are usually affected in large-scale injuries in the setting of a ring fracture of the skull base, although a narrow avulsion can occur in the form of a local impression fracture (see the section Condylar Fracture).

The middle level is the level of the lateral mass and the lower one is that of the base of the joint of the axis, the superior articular facet.[49]

The compression fracture type is primarily attributable to force acting on the central portions of the skull. However, a fracture of the lateral mass can also occur indirectly as a result of the force of the weight of the skull as can occur in a fall on the lower extremities and the buttocks.[50]

Compression fractures of the atlas include direct and indirect injuries. Even Jefferson was familiar with direct compression fractures. He refers to Ludolff in this regard.[43,51]

Indirect fractures occur where a lateral stress acts on the skull above the center of gravity with compression, for example in a car accident where a passenger is thrown against the side column of the vehicle, with a resulting compression injury. These indirect fractures are the result of high compressive forces on the contralateral side. However, ipsilateral traction and contralateral compression, i.e., bending stresses on the atlas, produce oblique fractures far more often than compression fractures. Usually these bony injuries are attributable to complex rotational motions. These eccentric stresses lead to subluxation in the atlanto-occipital joint, concentrating the load at a single point.

Incomplete avulsion of the cortex with the most anterior part of the articular surface of the lateral mass has been described.[7] This is the rare finding of a floating subtotal dislocation. Most authors describe the bony injury to the lateral mass as medial avulsion of that structure.[31,50,52–54] This type of fracture is regarded as an avulsion of the insertions of the transverse ligament of the atlas, which is difficult to imagine with an intact bony ring. Accordingly, Figure 2.**10** attempts another mechanical interpretation based on our own early case studies.[55] What had to be taken into consideration was that the transverse ligament of the atlas had remained intact while the medulla had suffered a massive shear injury. The axis and the odontoid in particular were intact.

On the basis of the fracture experiments mentioned above, we must proceed from the assumption of a Jefferson fracture with eccentric stress for our fracture analysis. This is because the findings are due to a massive extension trauma resulting from a fall from a height of 12 m on the left half of the forehead.

The oblique sagittal fracture surfaces passing through the anterior portions of the lateral masses can be explained by high compressive loads on the posterior portions of the superior articular facet with rotation around the coronal axis and collapse of the posterior arch of the atlas. This in turn represents a Jefferson fracture without the Jefferson effect. The literature includes descriptions of vertical avulsion of the anterior arch of the atlas in children without prior or concomitant fracture of the posterior arch of the atlas. Two such cases include a 2-year-old girl and a 9-year-old boy

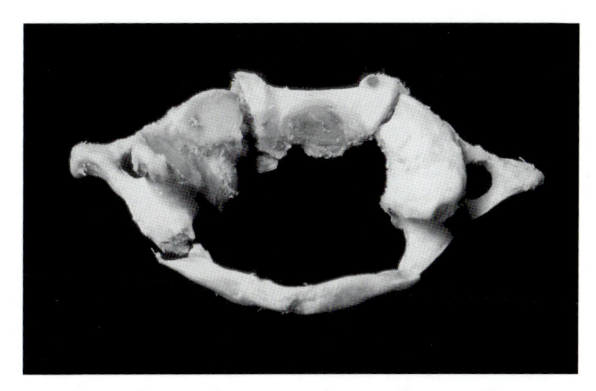

Fig. 2.**10 Jefferson fracture without Jefferson effect.** Note the course of the fracture bilaterally through the articular surfaces.

with a step-shaped avulsion in massive flexion trauma (see Fig. 2.**8**).[56,57]

Posterior Arch

Symmetrical fractures of the posterior arch of the atlas are primarily attributed to bending stresses around a coronal axis, although Sköld emphasizes the rotational component.[58]

Flexion

In flexion trauma, the traction of the strong posterior atlanto-occipital membrane flexes the posterior arch of the atlas as the skull is flexed. This opens the adjacent segment (C1–C2) posteriorly (Fig. 2.**6**), which stretches and ruptures the tectorial membrane and causes epidural bleeding and tears in the adjacent musculature of the back of the neck. The inferior margin of the anterior arch of the atlas strikes against the anterior surface of the odontoid. This can create defects in the odontoid or avulse the cortex from the inferior margin of the median atlanto-axial joint (see Fig. 2.**7**).[58] This horizontal shear force often leads to partial separation of the C2–C3 intervertebral disk. Complete separations are rare.

This section examines the typical bony injury, namely superior bending or fracture of the posterior arch of the atlas. The anterior arch can only be bent upward or twisted with the transverse ligament intact when the ring structure of the atlas has become unstable. The nature of the secondary injury depends on the direction of the force vector incident on the occiput and the distribution of material. Accordingly, this injury may take the form of a symmetrical fracture through the articular surface or bilateral arch fracture, or an asymmetrical injury with avulsion of the arch from the lateral mass or facet. These combined injuries to the arch of the atlas are common.

Extension

In the literature, it is assumed that two forms of loading are responsible for extension fractures of the poste-

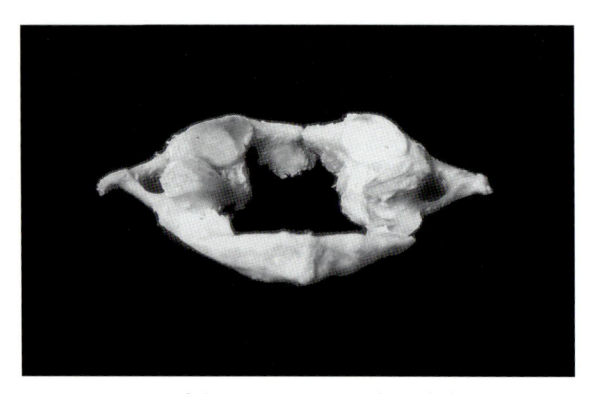

Fig. 2.11 Injury of the C1 posterior arch, with fracture of the anterior arch on the right due to a traumatic destabilization of the atlas ring with an intact transverse ligament of the atlas.

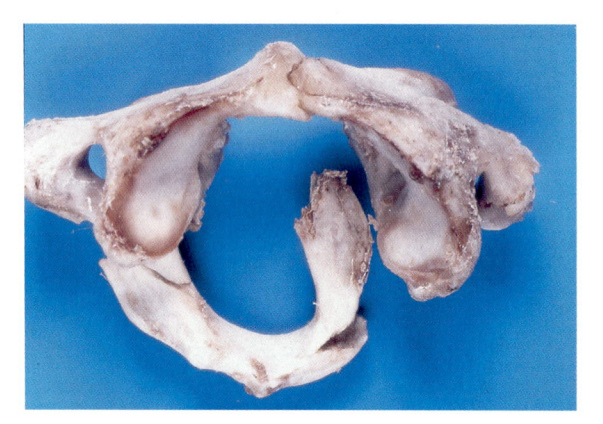

Fig. 2.12 Burst fracture of the atlas ring by compression. Fracture on the left side in the sulcus of the vertebral artery accompanied by a sagittal fracture of the anterior articulating facet for the odontoid process.

rior arch of the atlas. The first form is direct compression of the arch by the occipital bone.[43,59] The second form is thought to involve a mechanism whereby the posterior arch of the atlas is subjected to bending stress by impinging against the spinous process of the axis in an extreme superior position.[36] It remains unclear whether the occipital bone can be shaped so as to exert a concentrated stress on the posterior arch of the atlas by direct contact. In any case, this would require the posterior arch to have a point of contact on the spinous process of the axis.

The common site in the sulcus for the vertebral artery would tend to contradict this view. This applies especially where the cortex is bent superiorly as shown in Figure 2.11.

The direct compression of the arch is more evident in Figure 2.12. It determines extension fractures on the other side (sulcus of the vertebral artery and the facet of the odontoid process).

Our fracture experiments discussed in the section on the biomechanics of the Jefferson Fracture above also failed to demonstrate any contact between the occipital bone and the posterior arch of the atlas. We found no such impressions in the fractured plaster specimens. Fracture tests on actual anatomical specimens with interposed sheets for dental impressions have since confirmed contact between occipital bone and the posterior arch of the atlas but demonstrate peak compression at the lower level. Posterior arch fractures occurred only within a narrow range of extension vector angles.

Two other mechanisms probably describe the fracture mechanics better.[40] When the posterior arch of the atlas impinges against the spinous process of the axis, it is bent as long as the anterior traction persists. This bending stress is not exerted solely by anterior traction; it is also largely the result of compression of the lateral masses against the posterior portions of the superior articular facets of the lateral masses. The typical case is that of compression in extension in a car driver whose forehead strikes against the front column of the inside of the passenger compartment. The force is exerted on the atlas via the occipital condyles with the neck held in hyperextension.

The tension this creates can bend the posterior arch upward or fracture it. Clinical experience has shown that the common site for this injury is the sulcus for the vertebral artery. We confirmed that this type of mechanical loading actually occurs by examining case studies of extension trauma. This was evidenced by the medial avulsion of a narrow fragment from the posterior arch with partial superior displacement.

Axis Fracture

There is a wealth of anatomical, radiological, and traumatological literature available on axis fractures. Therefore, this overview will only briefly touch on these issues.

The special nature of the axis fracture is due to the odontoid fracture. This long lever can produce a wide bony avulsion from the body of the axis. This fracture of the body, with or without articular involvement, is still commonly but inaccurately referred to as an odontoid fracture, specifically a type III fracture according to Anderson and D'Alonzo.[60]

The issue of axial stresses in the region between the occiput and C2 with their three-level manifestation has already been discussed in detail in the section Lateral Mass.

As with any vertebral body, the anterior margin of the axis can avulse in extension. Figure 2.13 shows the different bone density axis configurations in equidensity images.[61] We may conclude from this that both the cortex and cancellous bone are relatively thin at the anterior margin.

Odontoid Fracture

Notwithstanding our objection in the previous section to the classification of odontoid fractures described by Anderson and D'Alonzo,[60] these fractures are widely discussed in the literature. For this reason, we have included them in this chapter.

In an experimental setting with isotropic material,[62,63] the kyphotic odontoid and lordotic odontoid are bent toward the horizontal in 5° increments while the loading angle is varied between 10° and 75°. This reveals similarities and differences in stress distribution. With both forms of odontoid, apical fractures (type I) predominate with small angles. Yet in the real world, this type of fracture practically never occurs. This is presumably attributable to the strong bundle of cancellous bone between the anterior and posterior joint, i.e., between the facet and the transverse ligament of the atlas. Koebke has described correlations between the shape of the odontoid and the functional configuration of this bundle.[48]

Postmortem studies of rotational trauma (see the section Traumatology of Alar Ligaments) revealed a total absence of type I fractures. Instead, bony avulsion from the apex of the odontoid occurred. Type II fractures occurred in other cases.

Our fracture experiments regularly produced hangman's fractures at the maximum loading angle (75°).

Type II fractures as described by Anderson and D'Alonzo occurred exclusively with a kyphotic odontoid.[60] The transition from a type I to type II fracture was continuous for this odontoid type, whereas the transition occurred precisely at 35° for the lordotic type in the experimental setting. This technical value must also be qualified, as it does not yet make any allowance for the distribution of material.

According to Sköld,[58] infractions of the anterior surface of the odontoid often occur with rotation. This specific correlation with rotation does not appear entirely compelling. This is because the correlation is to be expected theoretically, whereas in practice it can be shown that the anterior surface of the odontoid is subjected to a concentrated load even in flexion (see Fig. 2.**7**).

The actual odontoid fracture as such occurs where stress is applied by flexion, extension, and rotation as a result of the bending of the odontoid between the anterior arch and the transverse ligament of the atlas. This bending by the posterior arch of the atlas (a long lever) due to traction from the posterior atlanto-occipital membrane with the head in flexion, is a plausible mechanical explanation.[30]

The odontoid cannot be bent this way in extension. Anterior traction from the anterior atlanto-occipital ligament would probably be combined with compression against the posterior surfaces of the superior articular facet of the atlas. This would presumably lead to subluxation of the atlas. Once an odontoid fracture has occurred, the posterior arch of the atlas must absorb the residual kinetic energy.

According to our own studies,[64] the intense traction acting on the tectorial membrane is demonstrated by the fact that it ruptures not only under the force of flexion in an odontoid fracture, but it also invariably ruptures under extension forces of injury.

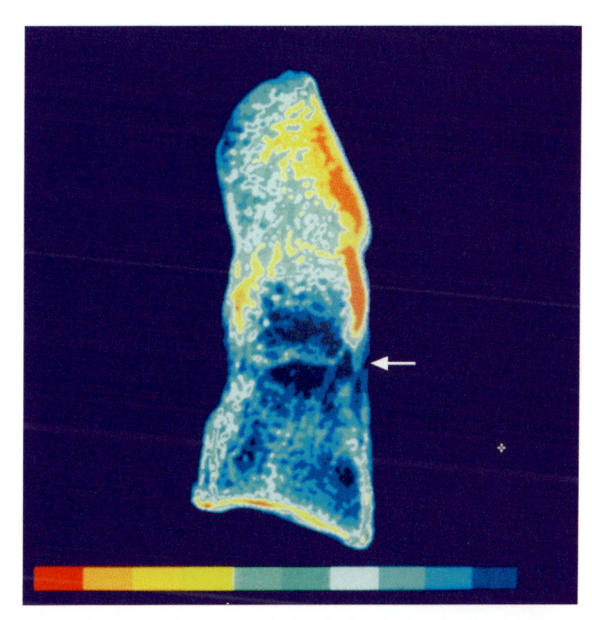

Fig. 2.**13** Bone density analysis of a lordotic odontoid process with basal dens fracture (type III) (*arrow*). Low mass distribution of the compact and spongy substance not only at the fracture site but also at the anterior lower margin of the body of the axis.

Hangman's Fracture

Wood-Jones first described the hangman's fracture in 1913,[65] and this definition still applies today. This injury has since been demonstrated even in children.[66,67] It involves a characteristic combination of bony and soft tissue injuries. It has often been noted that the soft tissue injury, namely the tear of the anterior longitudinal ligament and the avulsion of the C2–C3 intervertebral disk from the inferior and/or superior endplate, is itself a prerequisite for the bony injury. It creates space for bending stresses to act on the arch of the axis. The arch fracture usually occurs symmetrically close to the vertebral body as an extraarticular fracture in the pedicles, although it may also be intraarticular. The term pedicle fracture has been used, although it is often noted in the literature that true pedicles only exist in and distal to C3.

Studies by Schneider and Livingston have established the mode of subcranial loading described primarily for hanging as the prototype of the hangman's fracture.[68] However, it has also been shown that a blow to the upper face,[69] i.e., a different force vector, can also lead to a hangman's fracture. This compression not only causes a bilateral pedicle fracture, but also a fracture of the posterior arch of the atlas. Radiographic findings have not provided any information about the soft tissue injury.[70]

Hangman's fractures have also been described as a sequel of traction in forward flexion.[71–73] In the experimental fracture tests mentioned in previous sections, hangman's fractures in flexion regularly occurred with a large angle (75°). Accordingly, the clinical picture of a frontal fracture was observed in an injury from a fall as vertebral disk C 2/3 due to a ventral flexing force is shown in Figure 2.**14**. A deep oblique fracture in the axis body can be quoted as another example for this mechanism (Fig. 2.**15**).

Injuries to the Intervertebral Disk and Major Longitudinal Ligaments

Traumatology

In intervertebral disk injury, it is important to distinguish between functionally intact tissue and degenerative tissue on the one hand, and to identify the traumatic stresses from the various force vectors on the other. Unterharnscheidt has examined this latter aspect with exceptional clarity.[74]

To this day, clinical thinking about intervertebral disk injuries is still based largely on the stylized image of a uniform horizontal tear through the middle of the disk.

In contrast, our own systematic studies of this subject have revealed a variety of ways in which the direction of loading and degenerative changes mutually influence the pattern of disk injury.[7,75] We have defined several types.

Our experimental results have been confirmed by animal studies by Unterharnscheidt and by other groups.[22,74–77]

Thus, the basic pattern of intervertebral disk injury is not a complete horizontal tear but a more or less extensive separation of the annulus fibrosus from the inferior and/or superior endplate. Injuries to the major longitudinal ligaments are best described by classifying the type of injury according to the vector, particularly the direction of the incident force.

Biomechanics

Nondegenerative Disk Pathology

From a traumatological standpoint, the primary indicators of the presence of degenerative disk changes are not the lateral clefts in the uncovertebral joints or the posterior clefts that merge with lateral ones with advancing age.[7,8,41,78] These clefts do not in themselves significantly influence mechanical processes. The nucleus pulposus is far more important from a functional standpoint. As long as it is not yet fully compromised by cleavage, the disk itself will not tear but a partial separation will occur.

This means that the separation of part of the annulus fibrosus from the inferior and/or superior endplate requires a functional nucleus pulposus with an intact envelope. This condition can indeed be present in certain segments even in advanced age despite the fact that the composition of the extracellular matrix and the consistency of the nucleus pulposus change significantly between childhood and advanced age.[70,79,80]

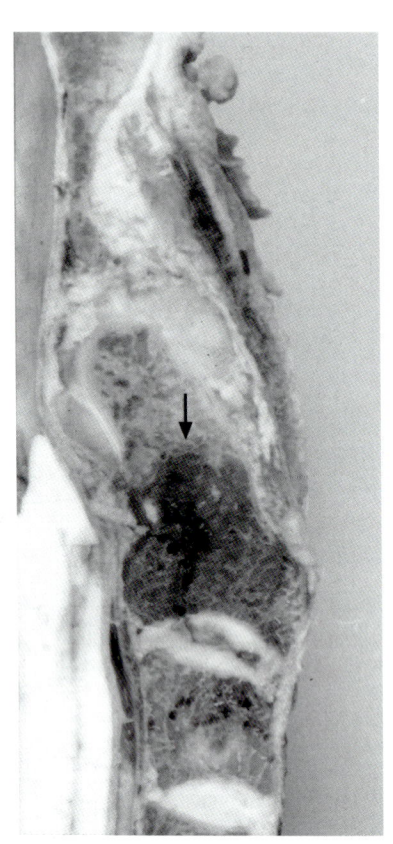

Fig. 2.**14** **Vertical fracture through the body of C2** *(arrow).* Flexion injury associated with rupture of the anterior atlanto-occipital membrane.

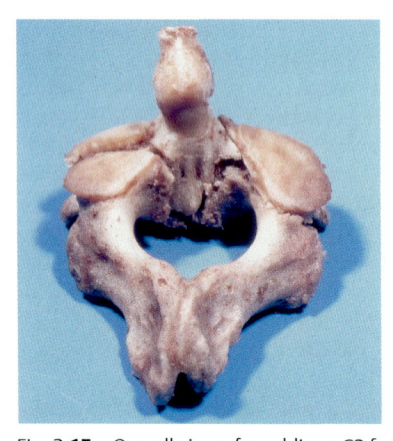

Fig. 2.**15** Overall view of an oblique C2 fracure commencing in the left superior articular facet with depression, extending to the base of the body of C2. On the right the fracture propagates inferior to the articular facet involving the pedicle and lamina.

a result of the forces involved. The fracture coursed obliquely through the superior articular facet into the vertebral body.[40] This hangman's fracture illustrated a mechanical relationship to the deep basal odontoid fracture (type III according to Anderson and D'Alonzo).[60] Such a frontal fracture through the body and thereafter through the endplate into the inter-

Axial Loading

Axial loading only differs significantly from nonaxial loading in its effect on the intervertebral disk with respect to compression. However, because the water content is higher in the nucleus pulposus than in the adjacent tissue, both compression and traction increase stress within the nucleus pulposus. Traumatic migration injection of disk material into the cancellous bone of the vertebra due to hydrostatic pressure will be discussed in greater detail in the section Degenerative Disk Pathology below.

The least common form of intervertebral disk injury occurs as a result of this increase in stress and involves a central tear.[81] However, this injury normally involves only bleeding (central bleeding) into the envelope of the nucleus pulposus. Such findings pose the question of where the source of the central bleeding is.

Anatomical studies have demonstrated blood vessels in the intervertebral disk only in children not in adults.[8,41,82,83] The bone can be excluded as a source of bleeding because even completely separated disks only exhibit central bleeding.[7,84]

Nonaxial Loading

With axial loading, the compression indirectly leads to intervertebral disk injury. With nonaxial loading, traction has this effect. The usual type of intervertebral disk injury in a nondegenerative disk is therefore avulsion of the insertions from the inferior and/or superior endplate. However, the form of disk injury is also influenced by the direction of loading. Whereas most cervical spine injuries result from combined motions with a rotational component, the posterior disk injury differs from the lateral injury only in that the posterior longitudinal ligament is involved. For this reason, only anterior and posterior disk injuries should be compared.

According to Unterharnscheidt,[42,74] the vector describing the extension trauma in the sagittal plane –Gx should be designated +Gx in the comparison with flexion trauma.

Extension Trauma (–Gx)

Traction injuries to the disk are often associated with anterior hematoma or avulsion of the anterior longitudinal ligament. These avulsions from the annulus fibrosus of the disk occur easily because the anterior longitudinal ligament inserts into the disk with only a few fibers on the anterior surface of the vertebral body.

Injuries to the anterior longitudinal ligament and the anterior portion of the annulus fibrosus can occur in combination or as isolated injuries. In minor trauma, findings tend to include fine partial separations of the intervertebral disk without involvement of the anterior longitudinal ligament. However, separation and partial rupture of the anterior longitudinal ligament may also occur without associated disk injury.

Table 2.2 lists the spectrum of disk injuries, ranging from fine bleeding in the anterior annulus fibrosus to complete separation of the disk from the bony endplates.

However, anterior disk injuries will not necessarily manifest themselves exclusively as fibrous avulsions even in the absence of degenerative changes (Fig. 2.**16**). As with any bone–tendon interface, either the fibers tear or the bone is avulsed. Because the annulus fibrosus of the disk and not the anterior longitudinal ligament inserts into the margins of the vertebral body, the rupture with a –Gx vector may begin with avulsion of the anterior margin of the vertebra.

Figure 2.**17** shows a typical example in which the rupture continues as a separation of the insertions of

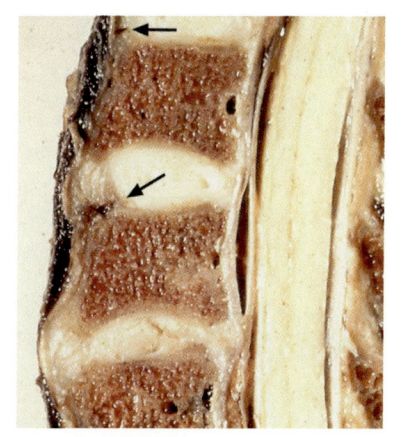

Fig. 2.**16** Typical anterior disruption of the annular fibro-osseous attachment and endplate superiorly with sub-ligamentous hemorrhage deep to the anterior longitudinal ligament (*arrows*).

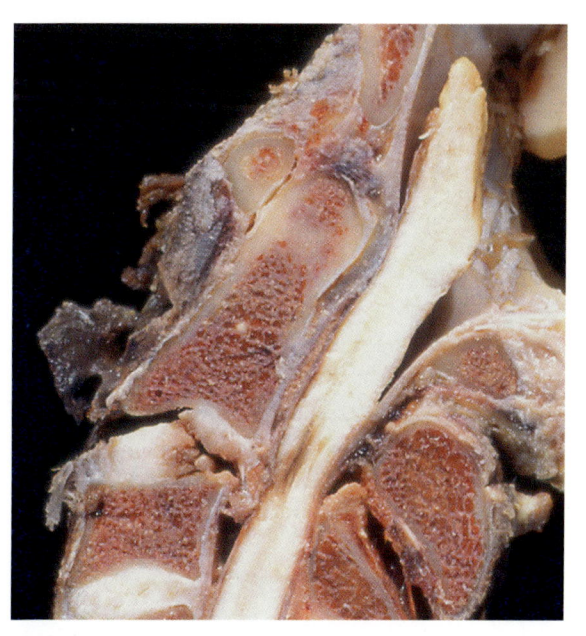

Fig. 2.**17** Hyperextension injury at C2/C3 level showing complete intervertebral disk disruption with hemorrhage in the injured posterior ligaments. Note the cord hemorrhage at this level.

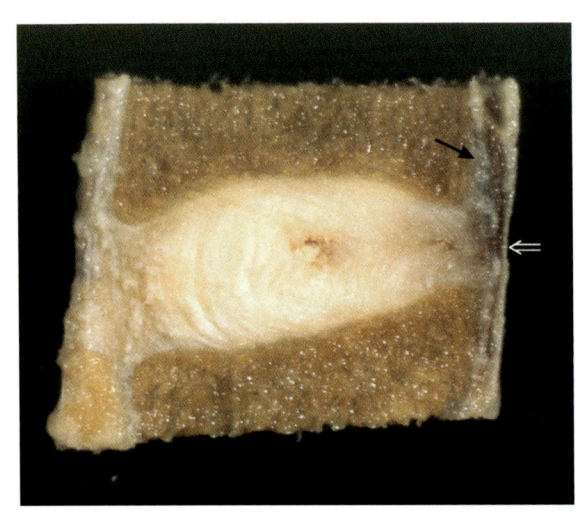

Fig. 2.18 Posterior disruption of an intervertebral disk from the posterior longitudinal ligament with subligamentous hemorrhage appearing as an isolated injury pattern due to a flexing traction strain (*arrows*).

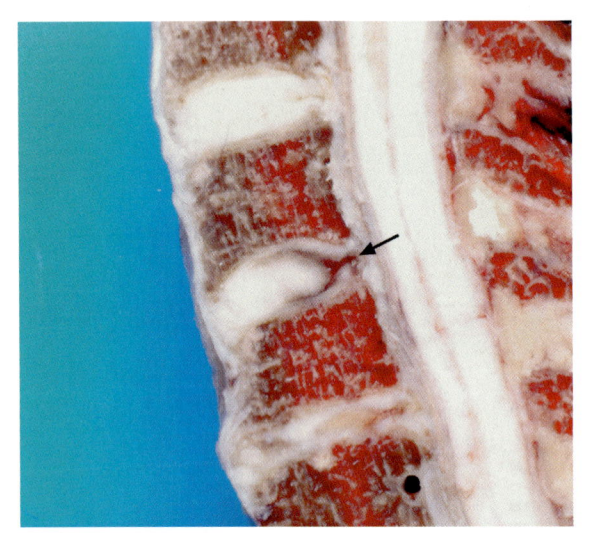

Fig. 2.19 Traumatic hemorrhagic disk ruptures superimposed on preexisting dorsal clefts due to degeneration. Note the partial detachment of the inner annular coat from the nucleus pulposus (*arrow*).

Table 2.2 Staging of traumatic disk separation according to Saternus and coworkers[93]

Phase 1	Hemorrhage within the annulus fibrosus with microtears
Phase 2	Extensive ruptures of bundles of fibers from the annulus fibrosus with secondary cavity bleeding
Phase 3	Partial separation of the intervertebral disk from the inferior and/or superior endplate (circumscribed insertional disruption)
Phase 4	Unilateral separation of the annulus fibrosus >50% or mutually of >25% each
Phase 5	Rupture with separation of the nucleus pulposus or total separation of the intervertebral disk

the annulus fibrosus from the endplate. A special form of this injury is the purely bony separation at the interface between cancellous bone and the inferior or superior endplate. Rarely, the disk will exhibit central bleeding but as a rule it is not involved (see Traction in the section Avulsion Fracture of the Margin of the Vertebra).

Jonsson et al have confirmed the forms of intervertebral disk injury we described.[75] Yet they add a clinically important distinction, and for that reason these studies warrant closer examination. Their traumatic separations of the annulus fibrosus were often associated with bony avulsions. However, we encountered the soft tissue injury far more often than the bony injury in our own study group of approximately 2000 cervical spines examined after fatal trauma. With the exception of bony avulsion of the anterior margin of the vertebra mentioned above, bony avulsions were rare findings in traumatic separation of the intervertebral disk.

One explanation for these differences may lie in the respective examination methods used. These authors used a microtome large-slice technique with cryogenic fixation, which is prone to producing artifacts. In contrast, we used a robust saw technique to produce slices greater than 5 mm. More recently, we have subsequently evaluated the lamellae under fine focus at 5–10 power magnification.

The fixation technique was a problem in that slow cryogenic fixation (–20°C) produced large crystals that interfered with histological examination. However, it was possible to produce high-quality slices for macroscopic evaluation and for radiographic examination.

Rapid cryogenic fixation in liquid nitrogen proved unfavorable. Stresses between the warm core and cooling medium created massive tears in the specimen. For this reason, we have used only formalin fixation for the past 20 years.

Flexion Trauma (+Gx)

The posterior type of disk injury differs from the anterior injury for anatomical reasons. It was described in the context of a special type of trauma, namely suicidal hanging,[57] which involves longitudinal traction on the cervical spine. As traction straightens the cervical spine and pulls it out of its physiological lordosis, it creates tensile stresses especially in the posterior portions of the intervertebral disk and the posterior longitudinal ligament.

In contrast to the anterior longitudinal ligament, the posterior longitudinal ligament and the intervertebral disk are closely interwoven. Yet because the two structures differ in their physical characteristics such as elasticity, plastic deformation, distensibility, and tear strength, traction will produce an avulsion. We can even describe this as a blistering phenomenon.

Minor trauma is present where the two structures are torn apart from each other while each remains intact. However, the intervertebral disk retracts from the posterior longitudinal ligament after separation. Bleeding then occurs into this traumatic defect (Fig. 2.18). Such an injury is not in itself fatal, and in

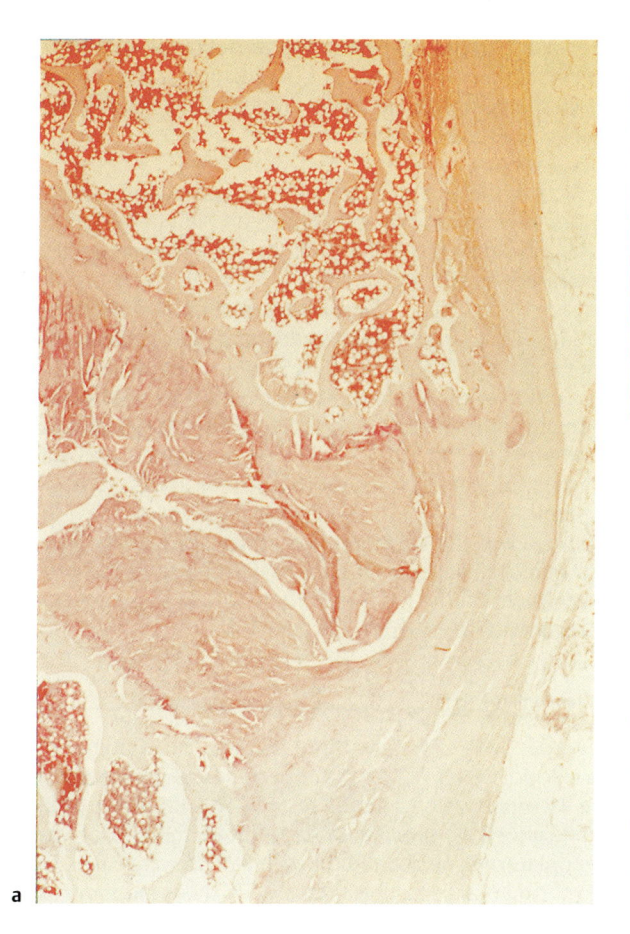

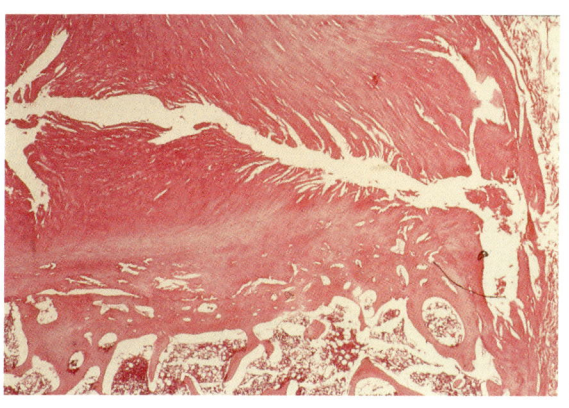

Fig. 2.**20**   **a** Anterior longitudinal ligament thickening due to a vast fibrous proliferation forming the articular capsule of a secondarily formed joint after extensive permeation of the intervertebral disk by clefts. **b** Rarefaction of the anterior longitudinal ligament being the newly formed capsule with distinct spondylotic marginal eminences of a secondarily formed diarthrosis out of the symphyseal juncture of the intervertebral disk.

most cases the hemorrhage will become organized as normal wound healing occurs.

Major trauma differs from minor trauma in that it involves complete separation of the disk from the inferior and superior endplates. Only adolescent intervertebral disks do not exhibit any significant difference between anterior and posterior disk separation. The pattern of injury changes once the lateral clefts appear, and later the posterior clefts. The lateral clefts appear in adolescents with the straightening of the uncovertebral joints,[41,78] whereas our studies have shown that the posterior clefts begin to appear in early adulthood. These clefts later communicate.

As may be expected, lateral disk injuries are most commonly observed with a rotational component. This also applies to combined injuries involving the relatively rare rupture of the ligamenta flava. In a morphological study of over 400 cases of fatal trauma,[7] their proportion was 6.8% with flexion trauma (+Gx), 4% with a –Gx vector, and 9.3% with rotation.

In the presence of posterior clefts, the remaining connections between the annulus fibrosus and the posterior longitudinal ligament tear. Often there will be circumscribed separations of the adjacent portions of the annulus fibrosus from their insertion into the bony endplates. The separated structures then prolapse into the defect.

The principal difference between anterior and posterior injuries is that the posterior clefts tear open or continue to tear in the primary injury. They do not rupture as intact fibers of the annulus fibrosus as in anterior injuries or become avulsed from their insertions.

Powerful loading will cause the clefts to continue to tear in the direction of the envelope of the nucleus pulposus. The propagating clefts do not tear the envelope but usually lead to unilateral separation. Less often, superior and inferior or lateral separation will occur (Fig. 2.**19**), i. e., separation of the nucleus pulposus and its envelope.

Degenerative Disk Pathology

The propagation of the degenerative disk clefts as part of the physiological aging process fundamentally changes the nature of this joint. A symphysis becomes a synovial joint. Kummer refers to the development of a secondary articulation.[85]

The function of the nucleus pulposus again becomes the most important consideration in the analysis of trauma.

In a symphysis, an injury to the anterior or posterior longitudinal ligament is an associated injury that has no immediate functional influence on kinematics. Yet in a synovial joint, it affects the stability of the joint. This is not to say that the muscles and bone are not major joint stabilizers. However, injury to the joint capsule (and the longitudinal ligaments must be regarded as having assumed this function) naturally rep-

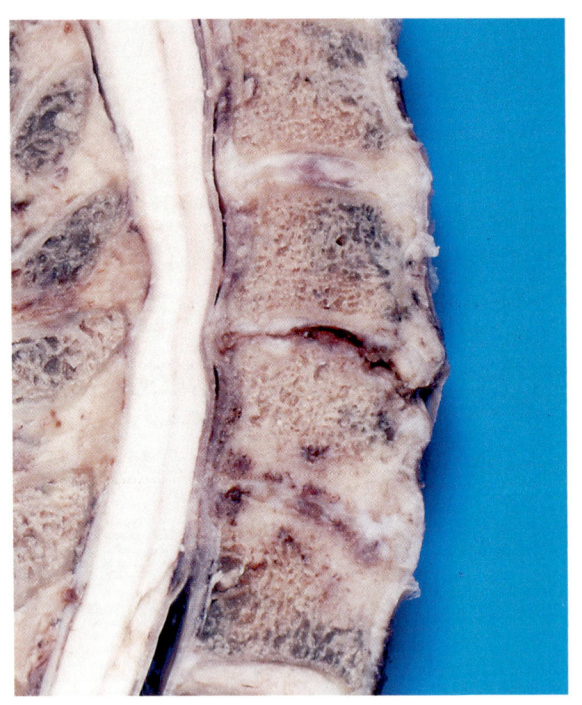

Fig. 2.**21** Extension trauma of a secondary intervertebral articulation with rupture of the anterior longitudinal ligament acting as a functional articular capsule at the level of C4/5.

resents a severe functional impairment. This applies all the more in light of the fact that the spine essentially functions as a chain of linked pairs of mechanical components much in the manner of the linked drive wheels of a steam engine.[86]

The degenerative transformation of the symphysis brought about by the propagating clefts leads to a situation in which the anterior longitudinal ligament must absorb increasing horizontal shear forces. This leads to a compensatory functional response in the bone. According to Schlüter,[87] this includes the development of marginal osteophytes; see also the section Topography of the section Injuries to the Facet Joints and Intervertebral Foramina. This means that the size of the newly formed capsule can vary greatly (Fig. 2.**20a, b**, see p. 27). Therefore, it is possible for strong, tight connective tissue to develop between the marginal osteophytes and the bases of the vertebrae. This tissue may be extremely sturdy. Conversely, a rarefied degenerative anterior longitudinal ligament will be the point of least resistance for a –Gx vector (Fig. 2.**21**).

Vertebral Injury

Compression Fracture

Biomechanics

Compression of the cervical spine as a system of linked pairs of articulating components occurs in two phases,[86,88] a compressive impact and an excursion. Tension banding, in which the musculature and ligaments under tension act as a bowstring construction is only able to prevent axial deviation under compression up to a certain point, which varies between individuals.[15,89,90]

Part of the energy is absorbed by attenuating structures like the intervertebral disks and joints by means of plastic and elastic deformation. The vertebral bodies themselves are well adapted to axial compression stresses (Pauwels' *Causal Histogenesis*).[15,91] Accordingly, MRI examination can demonstrate a post-traumatic edema occurring at threshold stress levels.

Compression tends to involve excursion with compression and traction aspects (Fig. 2.**22**). In spite of this, compression fractures of the cervical spine are not rare, although they are more common in the lumbar spine.

However, the vertebral body does not usually fracture in the shape of an hourglass like a technical test specimen. On the contrary, differences in structure determine the fracture characteristics.

Traumatology

Figures 2.**23**–2.**25** show three characteristic findings in a compression fracture of the vertebral body. Fractures in osteoporosis have not been included. Impressions in the cancellous bone with or without collapse of the endplate are common findings in patients of all ages. In experimental compression tests,[33,92] the impression of the cancellous bone increases the density of the structure, thus reinforcing the fractured vertebral body.

Figure 2.**25** represents traumatic migration of disk material with a central impression of the superior endplate of the body of the collapsed cervical vertebra. Figure 2.**23** shows a fracture of the vertebral body in its dorsal part. This asymmetrical compression injury causes a ventral horizontal shear. The result of this vector is that the inferior endplate breaks above the nucleus pulposus as it cannot be compressed, and the intervertebral disk is ventrally sheared away from the inferior plate. Dorsally it prolapses slightly into the vertebral canal. The nucleus pulposus appears to separate under the initial collapse of the inferior endplate (Phase I, Table 2.**3**). Figure 2.**24** shows a collapse of the endplate combined with cancellous bone fracture and impression of the nucleus pulposus in statu nascendi (Phase II/III, Table 2.**3**).

Assuming the force is incident over a broad area and transmitted via the intervertebral disk, there is no way

Table 2.**3** Traumatic migration of disk material into the cancellous bone

Phase I	Traumatic separation of the envelope of the nucleus pulposus
Phase II	Bending stress on the weaker of the two adjacent endplates
Phase III	Impression of the compression-resistant nucleus pulposus (hydrostatic pressure)
Phase IV	Envelope tears under great stress on the sharp-edged margins and empties

Vertebral Injury | 29

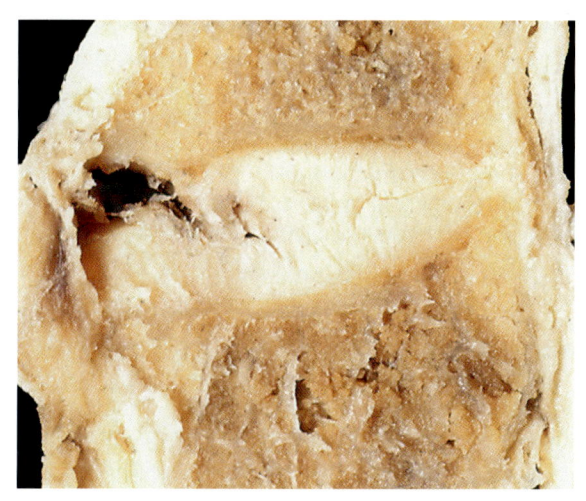

Fig. 2.**22** Avulsion of the annulus fibrosus anteriorly from the endplate of C2 extending into the nucleus pulposus, associated with a compression fracture in the cancellous bone of C3.

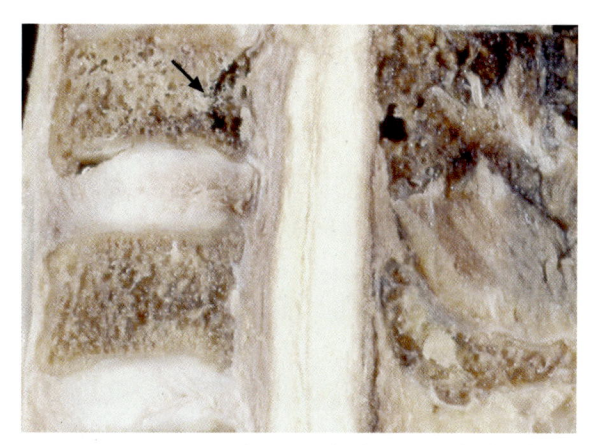

Fig. 2.**23** Compression fracture of inferior vertebral endplate (*arrow*) posteriorly with an anterior horizontal shear/separation of the nucleus pulposus from the cartilaginous endplate (Phase I, see Table 2.**3**).

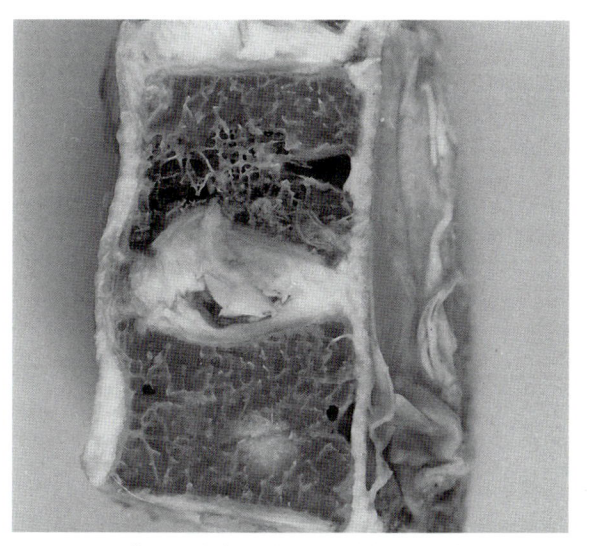

Fig. 2.**24** Collapse of the inferior endplate combined with a cancellous vertebral fracture and impression of the nucleus pulposus in statu nascendi (Phase II/III, see Table 2.**3**).

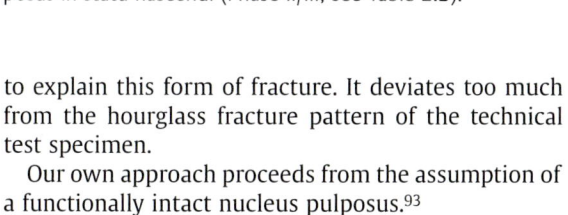

to explain this form of fracture. It deviates too much from the hourglass fracture pattern of the technical test specimen.

Our own approach proceeds from the assumption of a functionally intact nucleus pulposus.[93]

This does not mean that the nucleus pulposus must have the characteristics of a child's or an adolescent's, but it must exhibit clearly distinguishable tissue of high-water content under high pressure. Macroscopic regressive changes that have led to structural alterations may indeed be present.

Two components are of decisive mechanical importance: the intact fibrous envelope of the nucleus pulposus and its higher water content relative to the annulus fibrosis of the adjacent intervertebral disk. This means that the disk may well exhibit lateral and posterior clefts, but no complete clefts through the entire

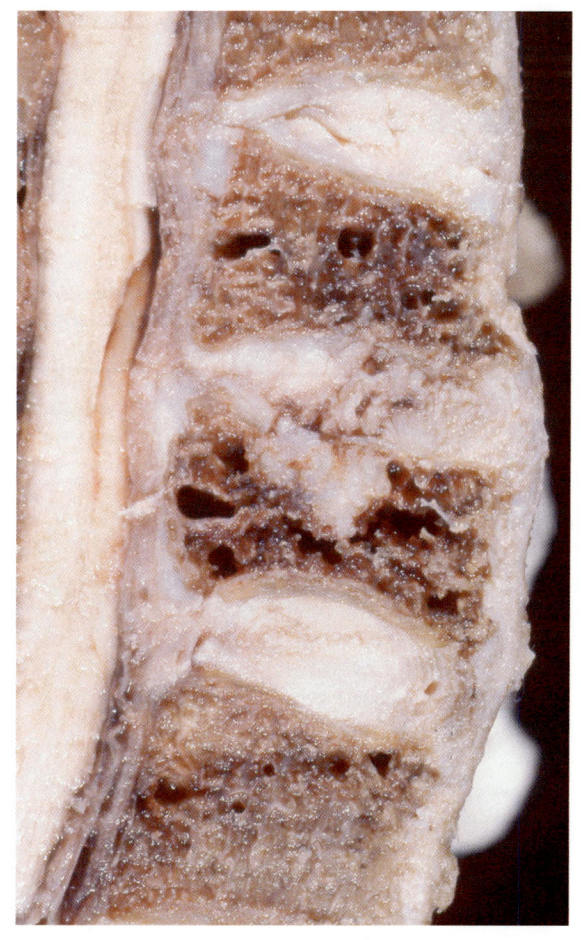

Fig. 2.**25** Intraosseous herniation of nucleus pulposus into the spongy substance of the fractured vertebra (from Saternus et al. 1999).[93]

disk. One possible objection is that there would no longer be any displaced disk material if complete clefts were present. Yet this is not the most important criterion. The fracture follows the mode of disk injury

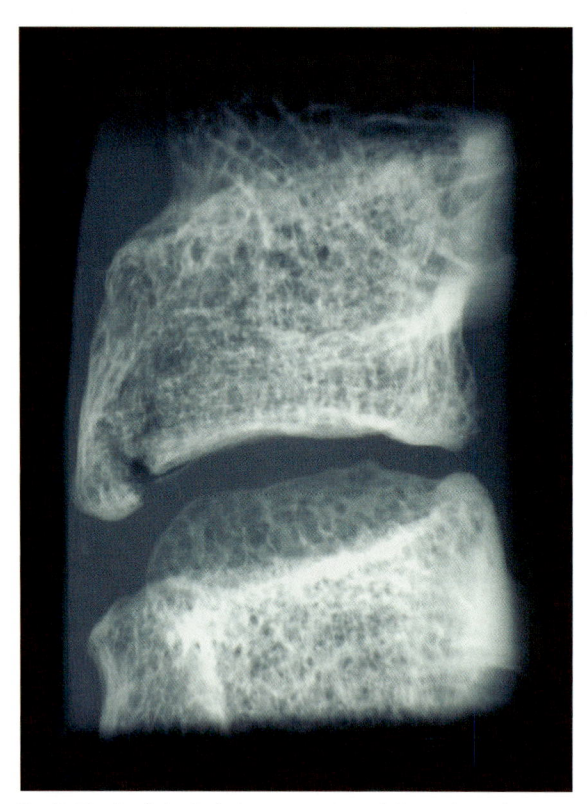

Fig. 2.**26** Radiological demonstration of the V-shaped tear at the anterior lower margin.

A compressive impact that results in avulsion of the inferior margin of the distal cervical vertebra is a sizeable excursion for which an interposed intervertebral disk would be a mechanical impediment. Therefore, the accompanying soft tissue injury must be a separation of the intervertebral disk from the inferior endplate of the affected vertebra. Fig. 2.**23** illustrates such a tear and hematoma beneath the posterior soft tissue.

Traction

Avulsion of the anterior margin of the vertebra or, more precisely, avulsion of its anterior inferior margin, can occur in any cervical vertebra. Yet in our study group, this type of injury was encountered particularly often in the axis. The avulsion can range from a narrow rim of cortical bone (Fig. 2.**16**) to a broad triangular fragment (Fig. 2.**27a,b**). The fracture line courses at 45° to the cancellous trabeculae, which intersect at right angles.

The size of the avulsed wedge is determined by this angle, which has its apex at the level of the convexity of the intervertebral disk (Fig. 2.**27b**).

With the teardrop fracture, the traumatic disk separation is the mechanical precondition for its occurrence, especially with respect to the level of the fracture. Exactly the opposite is true of the avulsion of the anterior margin. The intervertebral disk remains attached to the fragment. This represents a constellation that is not uncommon: Under traction, it is not the insertion (whether of a tendon or intervertebral disk) that separates but the bone that fractures. Strictly speaking, this is not an avulsion of the anterior margin (it is the static element) but an avulsion of the bulk (rest) of the body of the axis except for its anterior margin.

In instances where osteoporotic changes and marginal sclerosis of the endplates are present, the cancellous fracture will not necessarily course at an angle of 45° through the cortex and cancellous bone of the vertebral body. Instead, either a partial separation of the cancellous bone from the inferior endplate will occur or, less often, a complete separation.

described in the section Nonaxial Loading of the Section Injuries to the Intervertebral Disk and Major Longitudinal Ligaments above, a separation with a functionally intact nucleus pulposus.

In summary, this proposed explanation is based on the notion that the nucleus pulposus, under compression in its traumatically displaced envelope, essentially becomes a single incompressible body because of its higher water content. This means that one of the two endplates bends and bursts open under the concentrated stress. The sharp edges of this fracture cut open the nucleus pulposus, which is under increased hydrostatic pressure. In this manner, its liquid gelatinous contents can empty deep into the cancellous bone. Figures 2.**24** and 2.**25** show this finding and also displacement of the portions of the envelope of the nucleus pulposus into the traumatic defect.

Avulsion Fracture of the Margin of the Vertebra

Compression

The typical avulsion of the anterior margin of the vertebral body is the teardrop fracture (Figs. 2.**21**, 2.**26**). This has been widely discussed in the radiological literature. Compressive contact between the superior endplate of the distal vertebra can only occur with axial deviation of the cervical spine in this segment. Therefore, the vector describes anterior flexion compression. This means that the traction side must be the posterior aspect.

Injuries to the Facet Joints and Intervertebral Foramina

Topography

A physiological increase in the angle of inclination of the articular surfaces of the facet joints may be observed as one moves distally down the cervical spine.[85,94–96]

The anterior shear force, a function of the sagittal curvature, the weight of the head, and muscle tension, is absorbed by the facet joints and transmitted via the pedicles to the vertebral bodies.[85,87,94] From a traumatological standpoint, this means that the ability of bony structures to resist horizontal shearing increasingly diminishes as one moves distally.

Schlüter demonstrated in a photoelasticity study that the annulus fibrosus from C2–C3 on down absorbs a large share of the horizontal shear stress.[87] These stu-

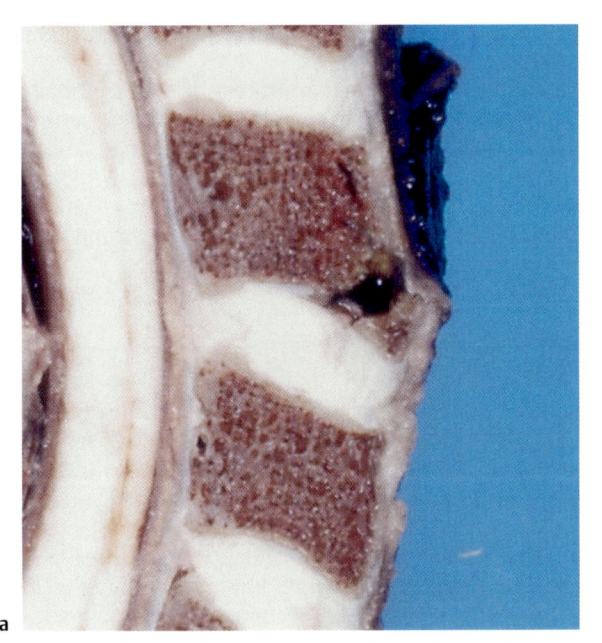

Fig. 2.**27** **Traction injuries. a** Disruption of the anterior margin of a vertebra due to hyperextension appearing as an osseous traction injury. Anteroinferior osseous disruption at an angle of 45° with anterior ligamentous hemorrhage representing an isolated anterior osteo-ligamentous injury. **b** Extreme disruption of the anterior attachment of the vertebra involving the neighboring intervertebral disk in a pediatric cervical spine.

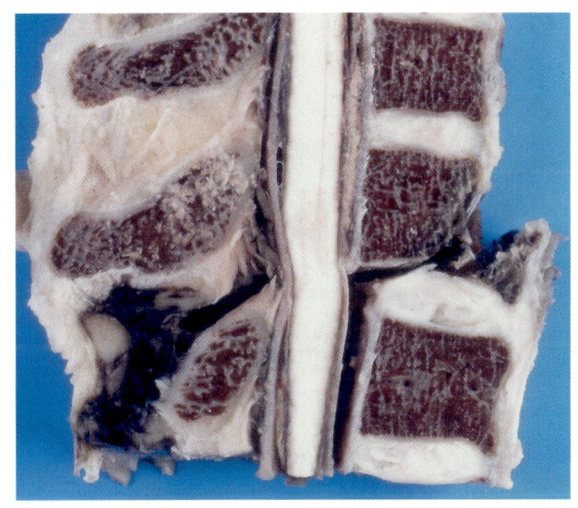

dies show that damage to that structure results in complete remodeling of the segment with development of osteophytes and massive widening of the cortex with a corresponding reduction in the cancellous bone of the vertebral body. As clefts increasingly propagate through the disk with advancing age, obvious signs of increased stresses include sclerosis of the endplates and degenerative remodeling of the facet joints. The consensus in the literature is that these degenerative changes manifest themselves first and most frequently in segments C5–C6 and C6–C7.

Traumatology

Our own comparative radiographic studies of specimens have failed to demonstrate any relation between the degree of degenerative changes, the level of the injury, and the severity of injury to the foramina or facet joints. These findings contradict earlier clinical data.

The time after trauma at which the studies were performed probably does not explain the differing results. On the contrary, there is a disparity between the morphological and clinical findings. This would suggest that post-traumatic edema in the foramina more probably leads to neurological deficits, albeit with a latency period, more so where space is constrained than where it is not. The edema largely escapes diagnostic detection in morphological evaluation. Only bleeding is detected. Bleeding into the foramina occurred in at least 10% of all cases. Bilateral hemorrhaging was far more common than unilateral hemorrhaging. Our studies showed that this occurred more often in segment C6–C7, confirming Emminger's results.[7,97,98]

Figures 2.**28**–2.**30** show such post-traumatic hemorrhaging into the foramina in connection with epidural

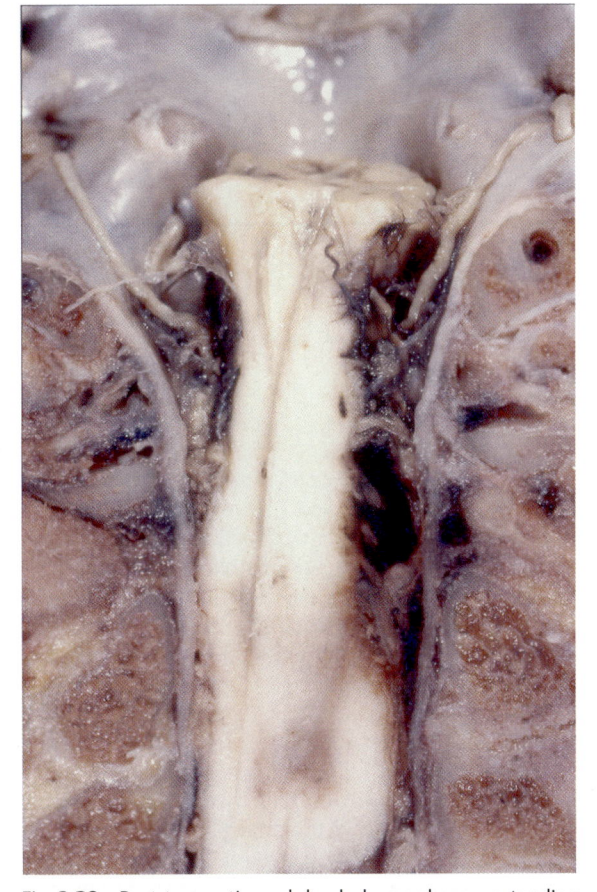

Fig. 2.**28** Post-traumatic subdural hemorrhage extending around the roots injured from their cord attachment.

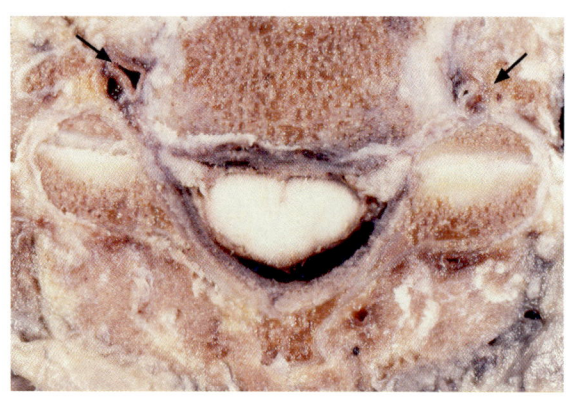

Fig. 2.**29** Transverse cut through the same spine showing the same hemorrhagic features at the level of C3/C4 with intact facet articulations. Vertebral arteries (*arrows*) with distinct differences in their calibers are also noted.

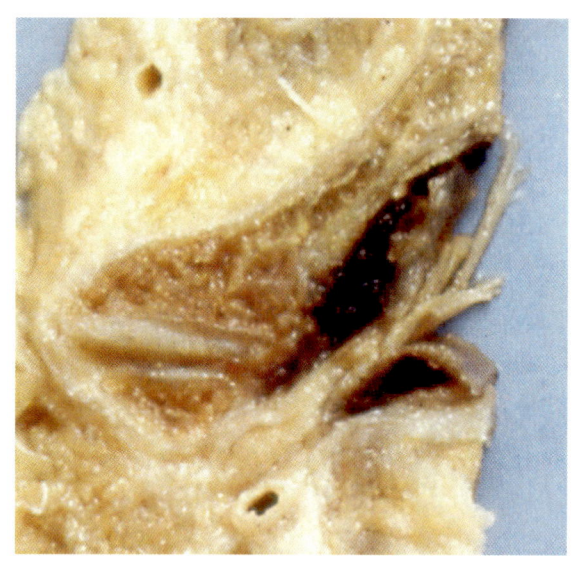

Fig. 2.**30** Slightly lower plane of the transverse section with hemorrhage around the nerve root.

bleeding. Here too, several adjacent segments are typically affected.

Despite the topographic proximity of the foramina to the facet joints, the two structures differ with respect to the incidence and segmental distribution of post-traumatic pathology. The facet joints were often unilaterally injured on the traction side. In many compound motions, the rotational component also plays a role. The unilaterally increased incidence of facet joint injuries in the middle of the cervical spine is indicative of this component. On the whole, the injuries to the facet joints were 17% more common than injuries to the foramina. Figure 2.**31** shows one of the two typical injuries, namely bleeding into the menisci. Zukschwerdt et al regard this injury as the morphological substrate of the spinal block.[99] Often it is associated with capsular bleeding or complete rupture of the joint capsule.

One rare finding proved to be related to prior degenerative pathology, namely traumatic damage to the articular cartilage.[100] This occurs with severe insults whereby the atlanto-occipital and atlanto-axial joints were affected significantly more often that the facet joints.

Fractures of the articular process of the facet joints (Figs. 2.**32**–2.**34**) are not that rare in a clinical setting but are very rare in forensic traumatology (0.5% of all cases). Examples in our own study group are found with two different types of incident forces, namely compression in extension injury and in flexion as a bony avulsion extending in the facet joint.

Spinous Process Fractures

Spinous process fractures in the cervical spine occur in nearly 10% of all cases in forensic studies. In over one quarter of the cases, these fatal trauma cases involve bleeding into and/or tears of the interspinal ligaments and muscles without bony injury.

The predilection of the C6 and C7 spinous processes mentioned in the literature is a regular finding. A bending stress invariably leads to a spinous process fracture. However, the signs of tension in the structure, i.e., traction and compression, change.

Traction is the salient quality in an anterior bending fracture, and compression in extension trauma. In such a case, the bending stress pushes the spinous processes over each other like shingles.[26] The fracture of the spinous process is interrelated with the rupture of the ligamenta flava. However, these strong, elastic structures rarely tear. When they do, the injury takes the form of avulsed insertions.

Conclusion

The major aim of this chapter was to show the spectrum of cranio-cervical injuries from a functional perspective. This approach is based on the physical principle that there is traction on the opposite side every time compression is applied at one location within the components that make up the cervical spine. Coexisting injuries and patterns may be deduced from this principle. This is done by comparison of injuries due to flexion with those due to extension. Ventral compression of the vertebra due to flexion is associated with a corresponding concomitant injury dorsally, on the side of traction. These lesions include rupture of the intraspinal and interspinal muscles, fractures of the spinous processes, and/or insertional rupture of the ligamentum flavum. Unexpectedly the most frequently found injuries included dorsal epidural hemorrhages and traumatic detachments of the posterior longitudinal ligament from its connection with the fibrous ring of the intervertebral disk itself.

There is a high frequency of insertional disruptions within the cervical spine. This type of injury is demonstrated as lesions of bony structures or of soft tissues. Bony disruption of the alar ligaments from the occipital condyles in sagittal fractures of the base of the skull, horizontal fracture of the anterior arch of the atlas, and disruption of the anterior vertebral margin are

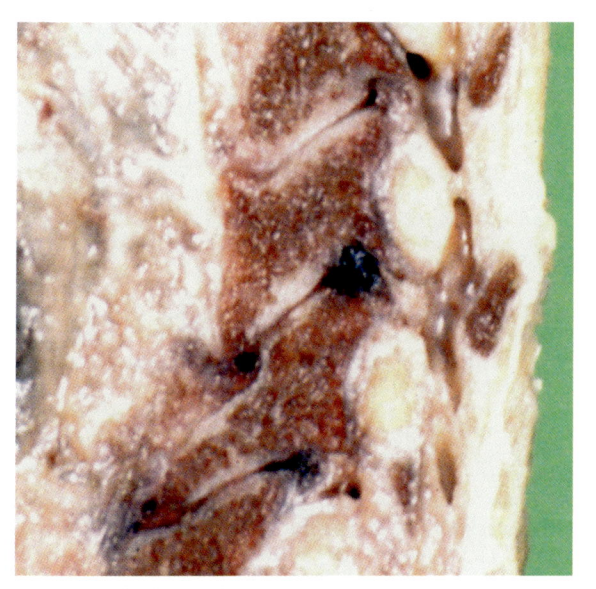

Fig. 2.**31** Bleeding within the meniscus of the vertebral facet joints.

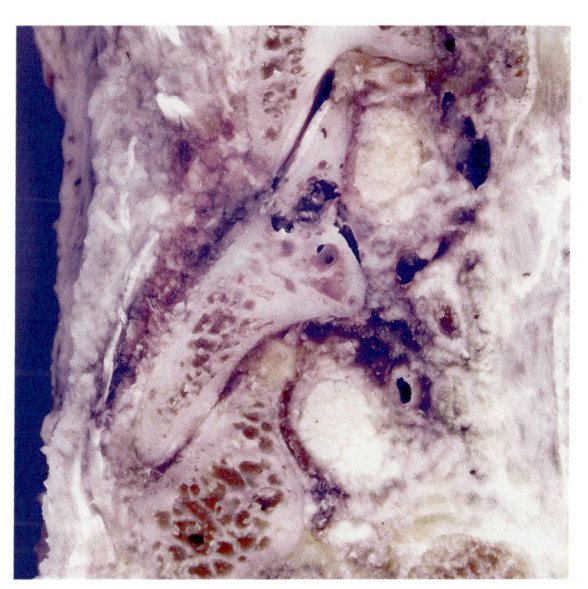

Fig. 2.**33** Fracture of the superior articular processes with hemarthrosis and minor dislocation. Point loading via the lower articular process (*upper part of the figure*) shows commencement of the fracture extending anteriorly across the superior facet process with subperiosteal bleeding anteriorly located.

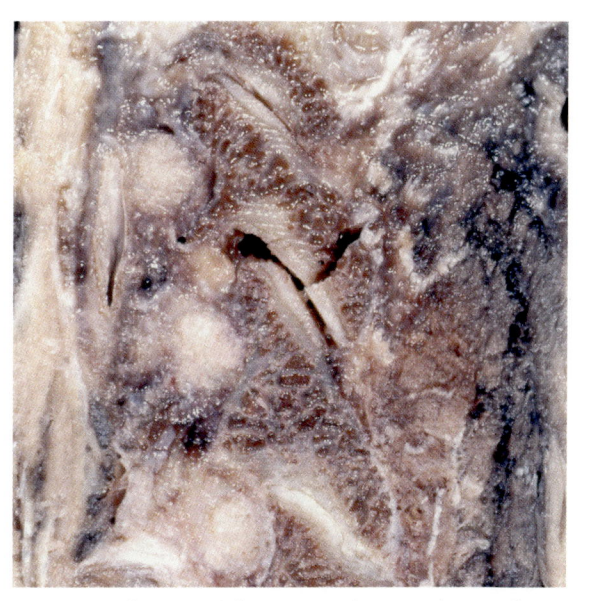

Fig. 2.**34** Inferior articular process fracture due to flexion trauma extending into the facet joint.

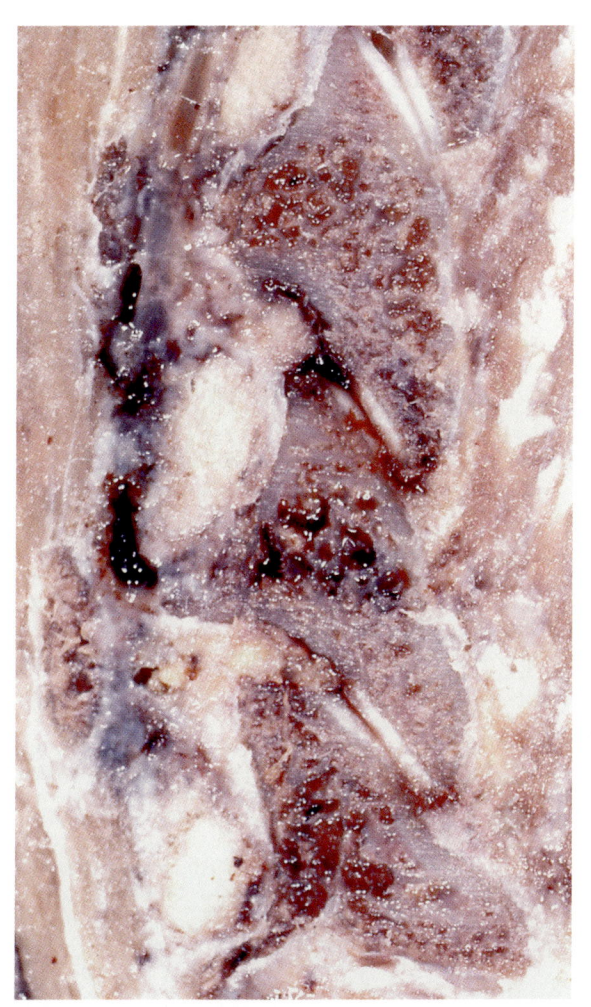

Fig. 2.**32** Multiple facet joints with hemarthrosis, osseous hemorrhage, hemorrhage within the menisci and the intervertebral foramina.

examples of bony injuries. Partial or complete insertional disruption of the fibrous ring from the endplate of a vertebra with no involvement of bony structures represents a frequent finding. Similarly ruptures of the ligamenta flava and the very rare rupture of the transverse ligament of the atlas show further types of insertional disruption.

Primarily, all injuries of ligaments including those of the capsules of the atlanto-occipital joints and of the vertebral arch joints are regarded as being due to traction.

There are reasons why the Jefferson fracture, classified as a burst of the atlas ring with a widespread location due to bending following instability, should not be regarded as a prototype of compression. Conversely, the intraosseous herniation of material from the nucleus pulposus into the spongiosa of a vertebra within the affected segment is due to axial compression.

The relevance of the post-mortem findings gained by detailed study of spines after real accidents stresses the fact that a clinical diagnosis of the described lesions can only be made using modern imaging techniques. This subject is covered in the following chapter.

References

1. Bell C. Surgical observations. *Middlesex Hospital J.* 1817;4:469.
2. Schliack VH, Schaefer P. Hypoglossus und Accessoriuslähmung bei einer Fraktur des Condylus occipitalis. *Nervenarzt.* 1965;36:362–364.
3. Spencer JA, Yeakley JW, Kaufman HH. Fracture of the occipital condyle. *Neurosurgery.* 1984;15:101–103.
4. Wackenheim A. *Roentgendiagnosis of the craniovertebral region.* Berlin Heidelberg New York: Springer Verlag; 1974.
5. Alker GJ, Oh YS, Leslie EV. High cervical spine and craniocervical junction injuries in fatal traffic accidents: A radiological study. *Orthop Clin North Am.* 1978;9:1003–1010.
6. Miltner E, Kallieris D, Schmidt G, Müller M. Verletzungen der Schädelbasiscondylen bei tödlichen Straßenverkehrsunfällen. *Z Rechtsmed.* 1990;103:523–528.
7. Saternus KS. Die Verletzungen von Halswirbelsäule und von Halsweichteilen. In: *Die Wirbelsäule in Forschung und Praxis.* Vol. 84. Stuttgart: Hippokrates Verlag; 1979.
8. Töndury G, Theiler K. Entwicklungsgeschichte und Fehlbildungen der Wirbelsäule. In: *Die Wirbelsäule in Forschung und Praxis.* Vol. 98. Stuttgart: Hippokrates Verlag; 1990.
9. Voigt GE, Sköld G. Ring fractures of the base of the skull. *J Trauma.* 1974;14:494–505.
10. Caroli E, Rocchi G, Ramundo Orlando E, Delfini R. Occipital condyle fractures: report of five cases and literature review. *Eur Spine J.* 2005;14:487–492.
11. Cirak B, Akpinar G, Palaoglu S. Traumatic occipital condyle fractures. *Neurosurg Rev.* 2000;23:161–164
12. Leone A, Cesare A, Colosimo C, Lauro L, Puca A, Marano P. Occipital condylar fractures: A review. *Radiology.* 2000; 216:635–644.
13. Momjian S, Dehdashti AR, Kehrli P, May D, Rilliet B. Occipital condyle fractures in children. Case report and review of the literature. *Pediatr Neurosurg.* 2003;38:265–270.
14. Saternus KS. Bruchformen des Condylus occipitalis. *Z Rechtsmed.* 1987;99:95–108.
15. Kummer B. *Biomechanik.* Cologne: Ärzte-Verlag; 2005.
16. Anderson PA, Montesano PX. Morphology and treatment of occipital condyle fractures. *Spine.* 1988;13:731–736.
17. Tuli S, Tator CH, Fehlings MG, Mackay M. Occipital condyle fractures. *Neurosurg.* 1997;41:368–376.
18. Dvorak J, Hayek I, Zehnden R. CT-functional diagnostics of the rotatory instability of upper cervical spine. II. An evaluation on healthy adults and patients with suspected instability. *Spine.* 1987;12:726–731.
19. Dvorak J, Schneider E, Soldinger P, Rahn B. Biomechanics of the cranio-cervical region: the alar and transverse ligaments. *J Orthop Res.* 1988;6:452–461.
20. Dvorak J, Sandler A. Strategie bei Weichteilverletzungen der HWS. In: Kügelgen B, ed. *Distorsion der Halswirbelsäule. Neuroorthopädie 6.* Berlin Heidelberg New York: Springer Verlag; 1995:53–67.
21. Pfirrmann CWA, Binkert CA, Zanetti M, Boos N, Hodler J. MR morphology of alar ligaments and occipito-atlantoaxial joints. Study in 50 asymptomatic subjects. *Radiology.* 2001;218:133–137.
22. Thrun C. *Morphologie und Traumatologie der Ligamenta alaria* [inaugural dissertation]. Göttingen: Universität Göttingen; 1990.
23. Krmpotic-Nemanic J, Keros P. Funktionale Bedeutung der Adaptation des Dens axis beim Menschen. *Ver Anat Ges.* 1973;67:393–397.
24. Dvorak J, Panjabi MM. The functional anatomy of the alar ligaments. *Spine.* 1987;12:183–189.
25. Saternus KS, Thrun C. Zur Traumatologie der Ligamenta alaria. *Akt Traumatol.* 1987;17:214–218.
26. Hinz P. *Die Verletzung der Halswirbelsäule durch Schleuderung und Abknickung.* Stuttgart: Hippokrates Verlag; 1970.
27. Deliganis AV, Baxter AB, Hanson JA, et al. Radiologic spectrum of craniocervical distraction injuries. *RadioGraphics.* 2000;20:237–250.
28. Unterharnscheidt F. Pathological and neuropathological findings in rhesus monkeys subjected to – Gx and +Gx indirect impact acceleration. In: Sances A, Thomas DJ, Ewing CL, Larson SJ, Unterharnscheidt F, eds. *Mechanisms of Head and Spine Trauma.* Goshen, New York: Aloray Inc; 1986:565–664.
29. Voigt GE. Zur Mechanik der Ringbrüche der Schädelbasis und der Verletzungen der oberen Halswirbelsäule. *Arch Orthop Unfallchir.* 1962;54:598–611.
30. White AA, Panjabi MM. *Clinical biomechanics of the spine.* Philadelphia, Toronto: Lippincott Company; 1978.
31. Fielding JW, van Cochran GB, Lawsing JF, Hohl M. Tears of the transverse ligament of the atlas, a clinical and biomechanical study. *J Bone Joint Surg.* 1974;56-A:1683–1691.
32. Krantz P. Isolated disruption of the transverse ligament of the atlas: An injury easily overlooked at post-mortem examination. *Injury.* 1980;12:168–170.
33. Plaue R. Das Frakturverhalten von Brust- und Lendenwirbelkörpern. *Z Orthop.* 1972;110:159–166.
34. Imhof H, Fuchsjager M. Traumatic injuries: imaging of spinal injuries. *Eur Radiol.* 2002;12:1262–1272.
35. Lustrin ES, Karaks SP, Ortiz AO, et al. Pediatric cervical spine: normal anatomy, variants, and trauma. *RadioGraphics.* 2003;23:539–560.
36. Torklus D, Gehle W. *Die Obere Halswirbelsäule.* 2nd edn. Stuttgart: Thieme; 1975.
37. Töndury G, Tillmann B. Atlas und Axis P 234 – 239. In: Tillmann B, Töndury G, eds. *Anatomie des Menschen (Rauber/Kopsch) B I Bewegungs-apparat.* 2nd edn. Stuttgart: Thieme; 1998.
38. Aufdermaur M. Regressive Veränderungen der Wirbelbogengelenke und ihre Folgezustände. In: *Die Wirbelsäule in Forschung und Praxis.* Vol. 87. Stuttgart: Hippokrates Verlag; 1981:83–89.
39. Aufdermaur M. Wirbelsäulenverletzungen. In: Doerr W, Seifert G, eds. *Spezielle Pathologische Anatomie, Pathologie der Gelenke und Weichteiltumoren.* Berlin Heidelberg New York: Springer Verlag; 1984:1175–1236.
40. Saternus KS, Paul E. Bruchformen des Atlas II. Frakturen des Arcus anterior et posterior. *Beitr gerichtl Med.* 1985;43:69–81.
41. Töndury G. *Entwicklungsgeschichte und Fehlbildungen der Wirbelsäule.* Stuttgart: Hippokrates Verlag; 1958.
42. Unterharnscheidt F. Neuropathology of rhesus monkeys undergoing – Gx impact acceleration. In: Ewing CL, Thomas DJ, Sances A, Larson SJ, eds. *Impact injury of the head and spine.* Springfield (Ill): Charles C Thomas; 1983:94–176.
43. Jefferson G. Fracture of the atlas vertebra. *Brit J Surg.* 1920;7:407–422.
44. Jefferson G. Fracture of the first cervical vertebra. *Brit Med J.* 1927;2:153–157.
45. Teo EC, Ng HW. Analytical static stress analysis of first cervical vertebra (atlas). *Ann Acad Med Singapore.* 2000;29:503–509.
46. Urban Ch. *Modellversuche zur Atlasfraktur bei exzentrisch-rotatorischer Krafteinleitung* [inaugural dissertation]. Göttingen: Universität Göttingen; 1990.
47. Wagner Ch. *Modellversuche zur Atlasfraktur bei ante, retro- und lateral-flektierter sowie axialer Krafteinleitung* [inaugural dissertation]. Berlin: Universität Berlin (FU); 1988.
48. Koebke J. Morphological and functional studies on the odontoid process of the human axis. *Anat Embryol.* 1979;155:197–208.
49. Abel MS, Teague JH. Unilateral lateral mass compression fractures of the axis. *Skeletal Radiol.* 1979;4:92–98.
50. Schmitt HP, Gladisch R. Multiple Frakturen des Atlas mit zweizeitiger tödlicher Vertebralisthrombose nach Schleuder-

trauma der Halswirbelsäule. *Arch Orthop Unfall Chir.* 1977;87:235–244.
51. Ludolff. Fraktur der linken Massa lateralis des Atlas. *Z. Elektrother.* 1906;93.
52. Barker EG, Krumpelman J, Long JM. Isolated fracture of the medial portion of the lateral mass of the atlas. A previously undescribed entity. *Am J Roentgenol.* 1976;126:1053–1958.
53. Günter Müller KH. Eine seltene Atlasfraktur (Berstungsfraktur Typ Jefferson). *Fortschr Röntgenstr.* 1980;132:468–469.
54. Hipp E, Keyl W. Frakturen an Atlas und Axis. *Fortschr Med.* 1963;81:589–596.
55. Saternus KS. Bruchformen des Atlas. I. Frakturen der Massa lateralis. *Beitr gerichtl Med.* 1985;43:63–68.
56. Marlin AE, Williams GR, Lee JF. Jefferson fractures in children. Case report. *J Neurosurg.* 1983;58:277–279.
57. Saternus KS. Verletzungen der Halswirbelsäule beim Suizid durch Erhängen. *Z Rechtsmed.* 1978;81:299–308.
58. Sköld G. Fracture of the Arches of the Atlas: A Study of Their Causation. *Z Rechtsmed.* 1983;90:247–258.
59. Braakman R, Penning L. *Injuries of the cervical spine.* Amsterdam, London, Princeton: Experta Medica; 1971.
60. Anderson LD, D'Alonzo RT. Fractures of the odontoid process of the axis. *J Bone Jt Surg.* 1974;56A:1663–1674.
61. Saternus KS, Koebke J. Verletzungen der oberen HWS. In: Wolff HD, ed. *Die Sonderstellung des Kopfgelenksbereichs.* Berlin Heidelberg New York: Springer Verlag; 1988:117–128.
62. Paul E. *Über das Bruchverhalten des Dens axis bei ventralflektierter Krafteinleitung. Modellversuche an zwei Formen mit unterschiedlicher Winkelstellung des Dens axis* [inaugural dissertation]. Köln:Universität Köln; 1985.
63. Voigt HD. *Modellversuche zur Axisfraktur. Der Einfluß der Mm. atlanto-occipitalis et axialis posterior auf den Axisfrakturtyp bei ventralflektierter Krafteinleitung* [inaugural dissertation]. Berlin: Universität Berlin (FU); 1988.
64. Saternus KS. Verletzungen der Occipito-Atlanto-Axis-Region. *Z Orthop.* 1981;119:662–664.
65. Wood-Jones F. The ideal lesion produced by judical hanging. *Lancet I.* 1913:53.
66. Finnegan MA, McDonald H. Hangman's fracture in an infant. *Can Med Assoc J.* 1982;127:1001–1002.
67. McGrory BE, Fenichel GM. Hangman's fracture subsequent to shaking in an infant. *Ann Neurol.* 1977;2:82.
68. Schneider RC, Livingston KE, Cave AJE, Hamilton G. Hangman's fracture of the cervical spine. *J Neurosurg.* 1965;22:141–154.
69. Williams TG. Hangman's fracture. *J Bone Joint Surg Br.* 1975;57:82–88.
70. Götz W, Bertagnoli R, Herken R. Struktur und Zusammensetzung der extrazellulären Matrix normaler menschlicher Nuclei pulposi. In: Wilke HJ, Claes LE, eds. *Die traumatische und degenerative Bandscheibe.* Berlin Heidelberg New York: Springer Verlag; 1999:3–15.
71. Brashear R, Venters GC, Preston ET. Fractures of the neural arch of the axis. *J Bone Joint Surg Am.* 1975;57:879–887.
72. Seljeskog EL, Chou SN. Spectrum of the Hangman's fracture. *J Neurosurg.* 1976;45:3–8.
73. Sköld G. Fracture of the Neural Arch and Odontoid Process of the Axis: A Study of Their Causation. *Z Rechtsmed.* 1978;82:89–103.
74. Unterharnscheidt F. Pathologie des Nervensystems. Traumatologie von Hirn und Rückenmark. Traumatische Schäden des Gehirns (forensische Pathologie). In: Doerr W, Seifert G, Uehlinger E, eds. *Spezielle pathologische Anatomie.* Vol. 13, VI B. Berlin Heidelberg New York: Springer Verlag; 1993.
75. Jonsson H, Bring G, Rauschning W, Sahlstedt B. Hidden cervical spine injuries in traffic accident victims with skull fractures. *J Spin Disord.* 1991;4(3):251–263.
76. Kathrein A, Daniaux H, Rabl W, Freund M, Beck E. Pathomorphologie der verletzten zervikalen Bandscheibe. *H Unfallchirurg.* 1999;271:145–156.
77. Unterharnscheidt F. Pathologie des Nervensystems. In: Doerr W, Seifert G, Uehlinger E, eds. *Spezielle pathologische Anatomie.* Vol. 13/VII. Berlin Heidelberg New York: Springer Verlag; 1992.
78. Ecklin U. *Die Altersveränderungen der Halswirbelsäule.* Berlin Heidelberg New York: Springer Verlag; 1960.
79. Götz W, Kasper M, Miosge N, Colin Hughes R. Detection and distribution of the carbohydrate bindung protein galectin-3 in human notochord, intervertebral disc and chordoma. *Differentiation.* 1997;62:149–157.
80. Tillmann B, Rudert M. Funktionelle Anatomie des Discus intervertebralis. In: Schmitt E, Lorenz R, eds. *Die Bandscheibe und ihre Erkrankungen.* Stuttgart: Enke Verlag; 1996:1–7.
81. Junghanns H. Wirbelsäule. In: Bürkle de la Camp, ed. *Handbuch der gesamten Unfallheilkunde.* Vol. 2. Stuttgart: Enke Verlag; 1966.
82. Christ B. Formmerkmale, Lagebeziehungen und Entwicklung der oberen HWS. In: Graf-Baumann, T, Lohse-Busch H, eds. *Weichteildistorsionen der Oberen Halswirbelsäule.* Berlin Heidelberg New York: Springer Verlag; 1997:3–38.
83. Rudert M, Tilmann B. Detection of lymph and blood vessels in the human intervertebral disc by histochemical and immunhistochemical methods. *Ann Ant.* 1993;175:237–242.
84. Saternus KS. Halsweichteil-, Wirbelsäulen- und Rückenmarksverletzungen bei Unfalltodesfällen – Die Bandscheibenverletzung. *Hefte Unfallheilk.* 1978;132:297–302.
85. Kummer B. Biomechanik der Wirbelgelenke. In: Meinecke FW, ed. *Die Wirbelbogengelenke ausschließlich der Okzipito-Zervikalregion. Die Wirbelsäule in Forschung und Praxis.* Vol. 87. Stuttgart: Hippokrates Verlag; 1981:29–34.
86. Kubein-Meesenburg D, Nägerl H. Biomechanische Prinzipien der Gelenkmechanik.. In: Saternus KS, Bonte W, eds. *Forensiche Osteologie.* Lübeck: Schmidt-Römhild Verlag; 1995:27–92.
87. Schlüter K. *Form und Struktur des normalen und des pathologisch veränderten Wirbels.* Stuttgart: Hippokrates Verlag; 1965.
88. Ziffer D, Henn R. Das Verhalten der Halswirbelsäule in Verbindung mit der Schädelbasis und der oberen Brustwirbelsäule bei schlagartiger Druckbeanspruchung (Stütze auf unnachgiebige Hindernisse – Stahlplatten) und bei schlagartiger Zugbeanspruchung (Zerreißung). *Zentralbl Verkehrsmed.* 1967;13:193–217.
89. Slijper EJ. Comparative biologic-anatomical investigations on the vertebral column and spinal musculature of mammals. *Verh Kon Ned Akad v Wetensch Afd Nat Kde.* 1946;2(Sect D42).
90. Strasser. 1908. Cited by: Kummer B. *Bauprinzipien des Säugerskelettes.* Stuttgart: Thieme; 1959.
91. Pauwels F. Die Bedeutung der Bauprinzipien des Stütz- und Bewegungsapparates für die Beanspruchung der Röhrenknochen. In: Pauwels F, ed. *Gesammelte Abhandlungen zur funktionellen Anatomie des Bewegungsapparates.* Berlin Heidelberg New York: Springer Verlag; 1965.
92. Plaue R. Experimentelle Untersuchungen zur funktionellen Wirbelbruchbehandlung. *Monatsschr Unfallheilk.* 1972;6:395–402.
93. Saternus KS, Kernbach-Wighton G, Moritz JD. Typen der Bandscheibenverletzung. In: Wilke HJ, Claes LE, eds. *Die traumatische und degenerative Bandscheibe.* Berlin Heidelberg New York: Springer Verlag; 1999.
94. Kummer B. Welchen Beitrag leisten die Wirbelbogengelenke zur Tragfunktion der Wirbelsäule? In: Hackenbroch MM, Refior HJ, Jäger M, eds. *Biomechanik der Wirbelsäule.* Stuttgart: Thieme; 1983:19–24.
95. Putz R. Anatomie der Halswirbelsäule. In: Moorahrend U, ed. *Die Beschleunigungsverletzung der Halswirbelsäule.* Stuttgart: Fischer; 1993:1–12.
96. Veleanu C, Grün U, Diaconescu M, Cocota E. Structural peculiarities of the thoracic spine. *Acta Anat.* 1972;82:97–107.
97. Emminger E. Die Gelenkdisci an der Wirbelsäule (eine mögliche Erklärung wirbelsäulenabhängiger Schmerzzustände). *Hefte Unfallheilk.* 1955;48:142–148.
98. Emminger E. Pathologisch-anatomische Befunde bei frischen Halswirbelsäulenverletzungen. *Verh Dtsch Orthop Ges.* 1968;54:282–293.
99. Zukschwerdt L, Emminger E, Biedermann F, Zettel H. *Wirbelgelenk und Bandscheibe.* 2. Aufl. Stuttgart: Hippokrates; 1960.
100. Saternus KS, Eckardt U. Knorpelverletzungen der Kopf- und Wirbelbogengelenke. *Aktuel Traumatol.* 1995;2:43–50.

3 Optimizing the Imaging Options

B. Tins and V. N. Cassar-Pullicino

Introduction

Spinal injuries are potentially devastating for the patient and pose a challenge for the clinicians involved in patient care. They require a conjoined approach of several clinical specialties. Imaging plays an important role in establishing the diagnosis, giving a prognosis, aiding treatment, and in the further follow-up of spinal injury patients. The imaging approach will vary with the clinical scenario. An unconscious polytraumatized patient with head, thoracic, and abdominal injuries will probably undergo multi-detector row CT of head, neck, thorax, abdomen, and pelvis with dedicated reconstructions of the spine.[1–4] On the other hand a patient who could be classed as "walking wounded" with minor trauma and perhaps some neck ache will probably be assessed according to the guidelines of the Canadian C-spine rule (Tabs. 3.**1**–3.**3**, p. 46) to establish whether any imaging investigation is indicated.[1,5]

The guiding principle for any assessment of the spine is to diagnose or exclude **significant** spinal injury utilizing the imaging modalities available in a cost-effective manner while keeping the radiation dose to the patient as low as possible. Missing a significant spinal injury can have disastrous consequences with neurological deterioration reported in as many as 10 to 50% of missed spinal injuries.[6–9] Earlier studies on patients with significant spinal injuries found that in between 4.6% and 10.5% of patients significant spinal injuries were initially missed.[6–9] This emphasizes the importance of a diligent approach to the diagnosis of spinal injuries. The role of the radiologist does not commence with image interpretation but before that by helping to determine an optimized imaging strategy for a given clinical scenario.

Frequently the radiologist will be asked to establish whether a spinal injury is present but he or she might also be asked specific questions as for example the state of a particular nerve root or the extent of cord damage (Figs. 3.**1**, 3.**2**). The imaging approach will vary in these circumstances and the radiologist needs to be aware of the advantages and disadvantages of the various imaging modalities in different phases of patient work-up and treatment. This subject is reviewed fairly regularly in the radiological and trauma care literature and this chapter tries to distill the recent trends for the reader.[10–13]

This chapter does not offer a dogmatic, overly prescriptive view on imaging of spinal injuries. Any approach will depend on local facilities, philosophy, and expertise.

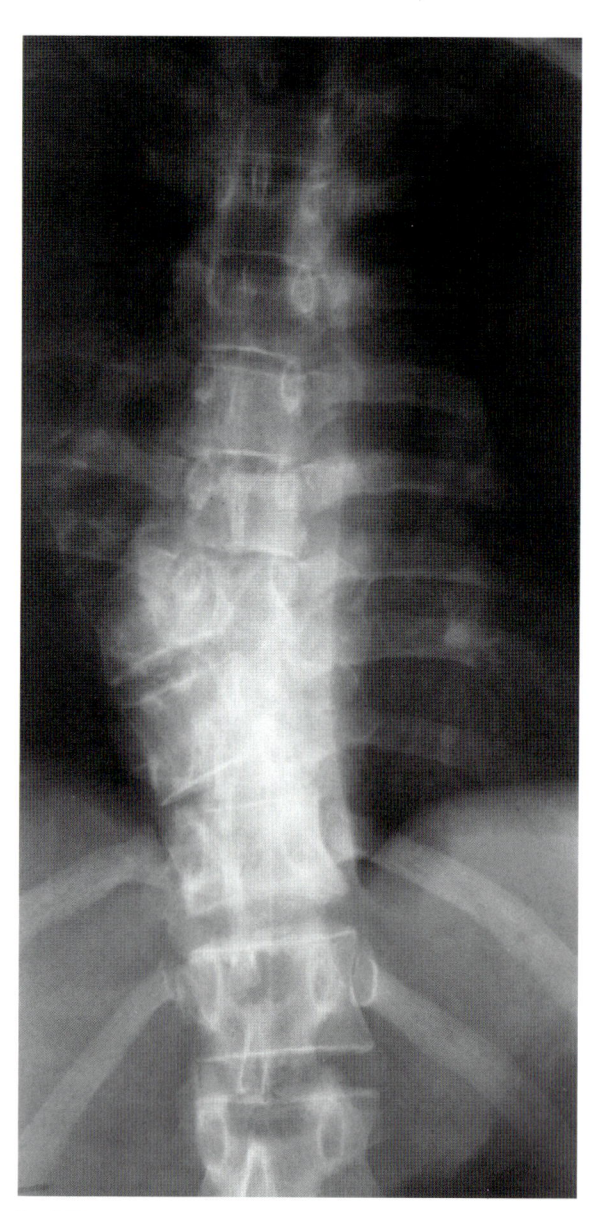

Fig. 3.**1 a**

Introduction

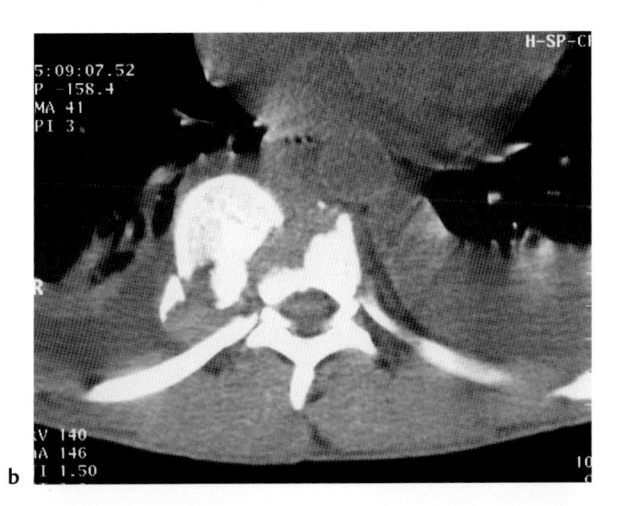

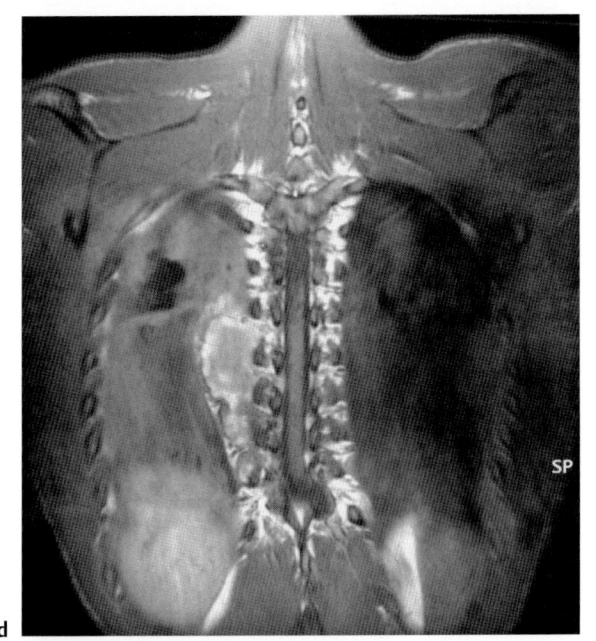

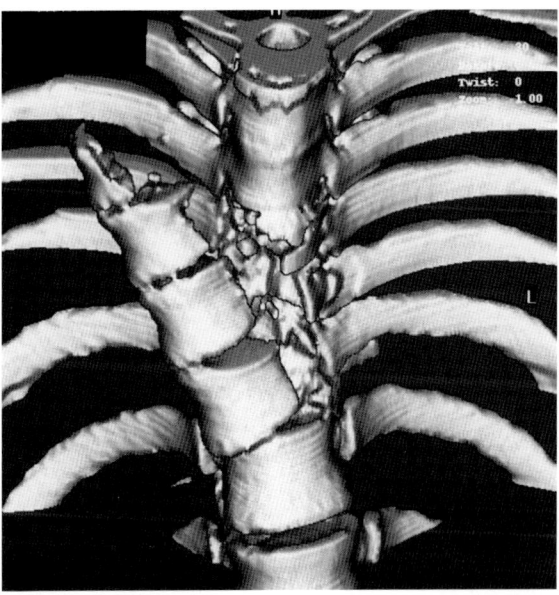

Fig. 3.1 **24-year-old male patient after a motorbike accident.** Neurologically intact! A radiograph demonstrates a grossly displaced segment of the lower thoracic spine (**a**). CT demonstrates shearing off of the anterior part of the vertebral body with preservation of the spinal canal (**b**). This is well demonstrated on surface-shaded reconstructions (**c**). Coronal MRI demonstrates the intact spinal cord (**d**). Imaging confirmation of an intact spinal canal and cord resulted in conservative treatment only with an uneventful recovery.

Fig. 3.2 **21-year-old male, road traffic accident.** Right-sided C7 and C8 weakness. A lateral radiograph (**a**) demonstrates a C7 fracture (*arrows*) but the injury and its extent are difficult to appreciate. MRI (**b**) demonstrates a burst fracture of C7 and spinal cord edema.

Fig. 3.**2c–f** ▷

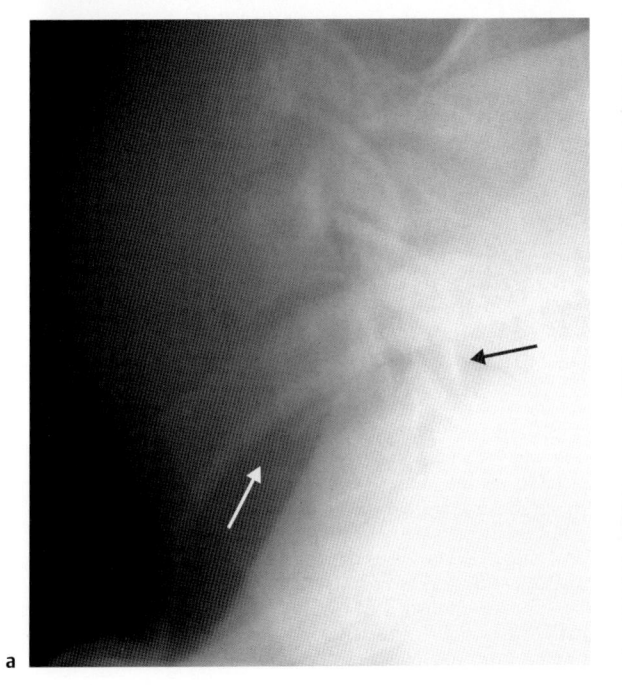

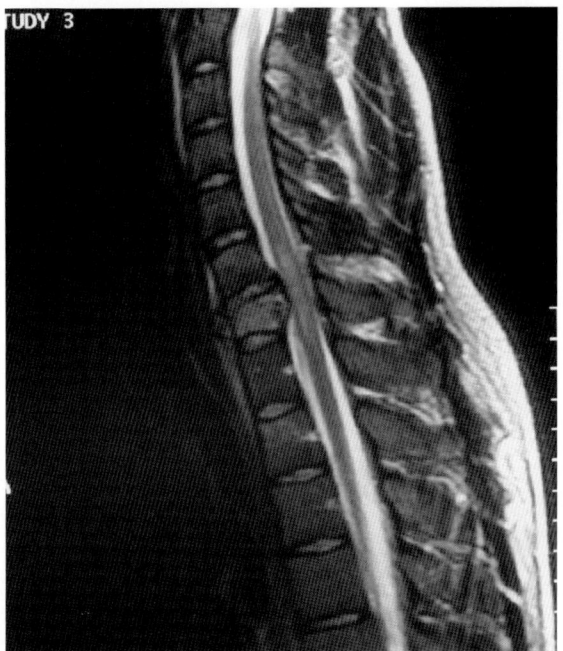

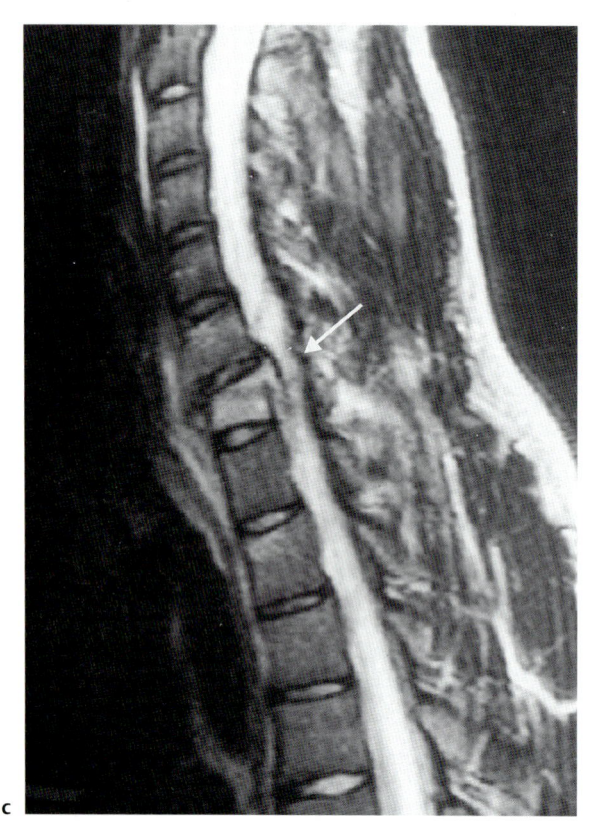

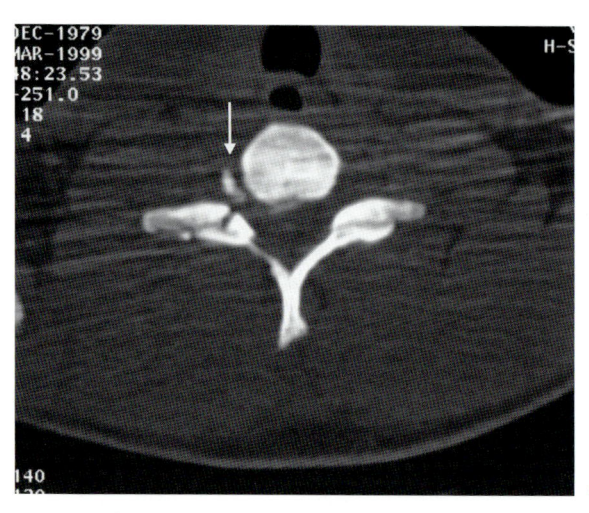

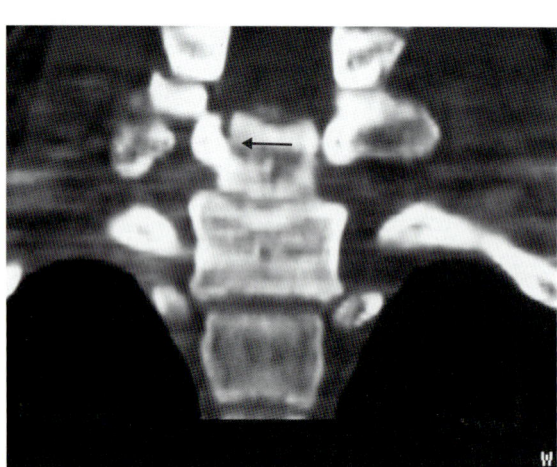

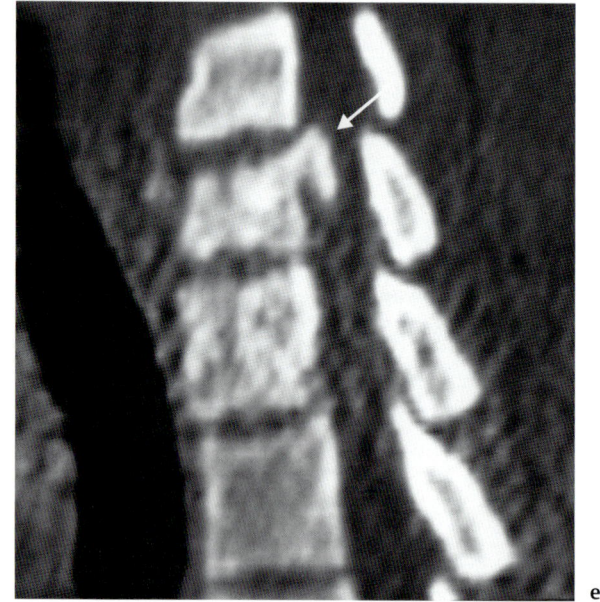

Fig. 3.**2c–f** The right paramedian plane (**c**) demonstrates a bone fragment protruding into the spinal canal (*arrow*) but no further cord compromise. Axial CT (**d**) and CT reconstructions (**e, f**) show this fragment to be in the intervertebral foramen (*arrows*). This was difficult to appreciate on MR and underlines the complementary nature of CT and MR imaging.

Imaging Modalities

Radiography was traditionally the mainstay of imaging examinations performed for spinal injuries work-up. Unfortunately, this imaging modality is neither particularly sensitive nor specific. Particularly in the imaging of cervical spine injuries the unreliable nature of radiographs for the diagnosis or exclusion of significant injuries has been well documented. It is now accepted that about 10–20% of **significant** cervical spine injuries are missed with radiographs.[6,14–16] Suboptimal radiographs and errors in image interpretation account for a large number of these but some injuries are missed even in retrospect as they are not visible on the initial radiographs (Fig. 3.**3**).[6–9,14,15,17–19] Compared to

Fig. 3.**3 20-year-old male**. He was ejected from his vehicle during a high-speed traffic accident. Radiographs were taken, no injury was seen and he was discharged from hospital. Two weeks later he presented to a GP for persisting numbness and weakness of his lower limbs. A lateral radiograph (**a**) demonstrates anterior subluxation of C7 (*arrows*). This injury is easily (and was initially) missed if the cervicothoracic junction is not included on the view. The lateral view of the thoracic spine (**b**) demonstrates mild wedging of upper thoracic vertebrae (*arrows*) but they are not well visualized. T1W (**c**) and T2W (**d**) MR images demonstrate the complete disruption of the ligamentous structures at the C7/T1 level (*arrows*) and infraction of the superior endplates of C7, T1–T5 (*arrowheads*). Post-traumatic cord signal change. Only mild soft tissue swelling 2 weeks after the injury.

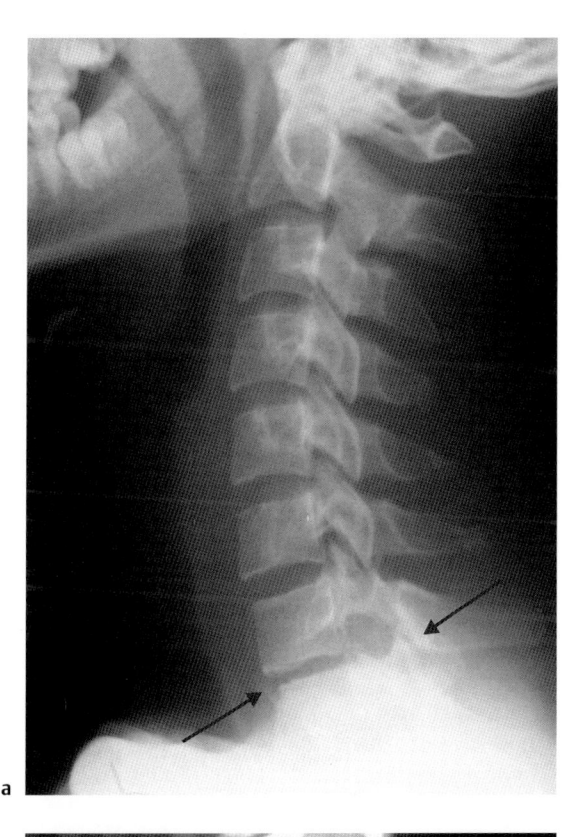

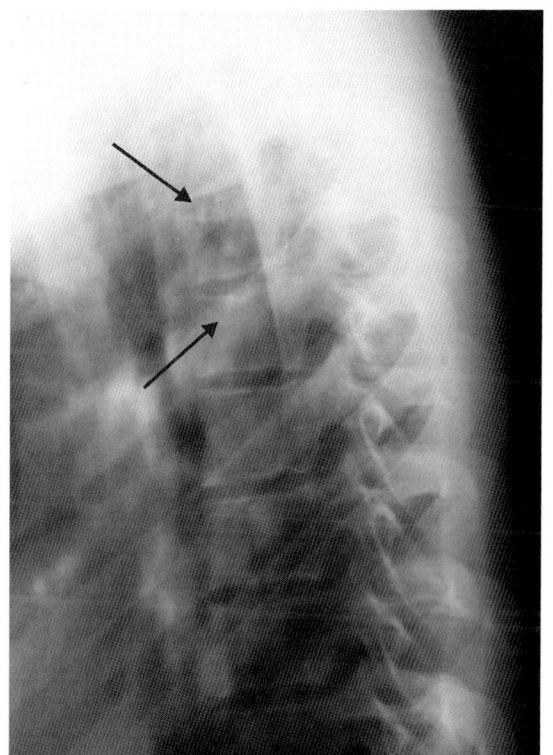

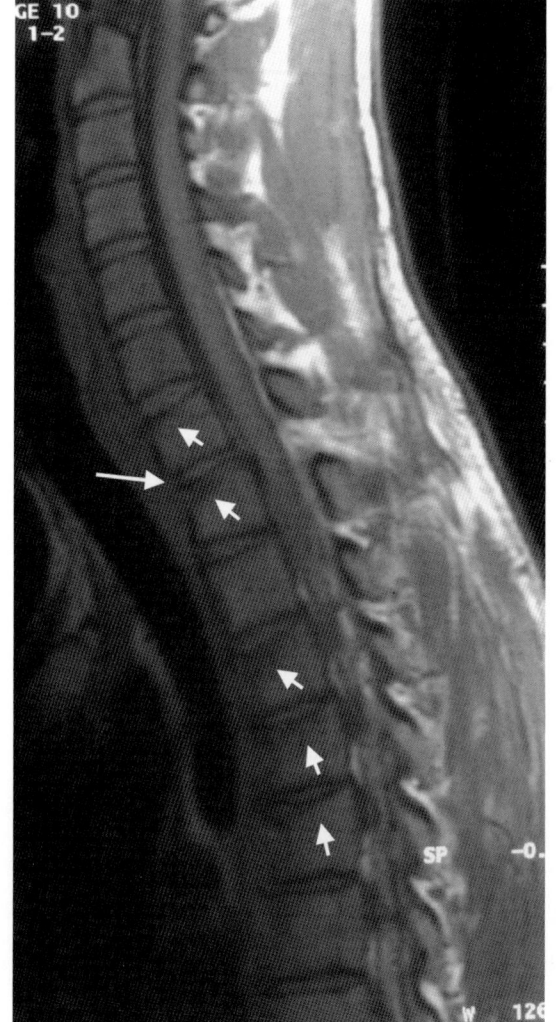

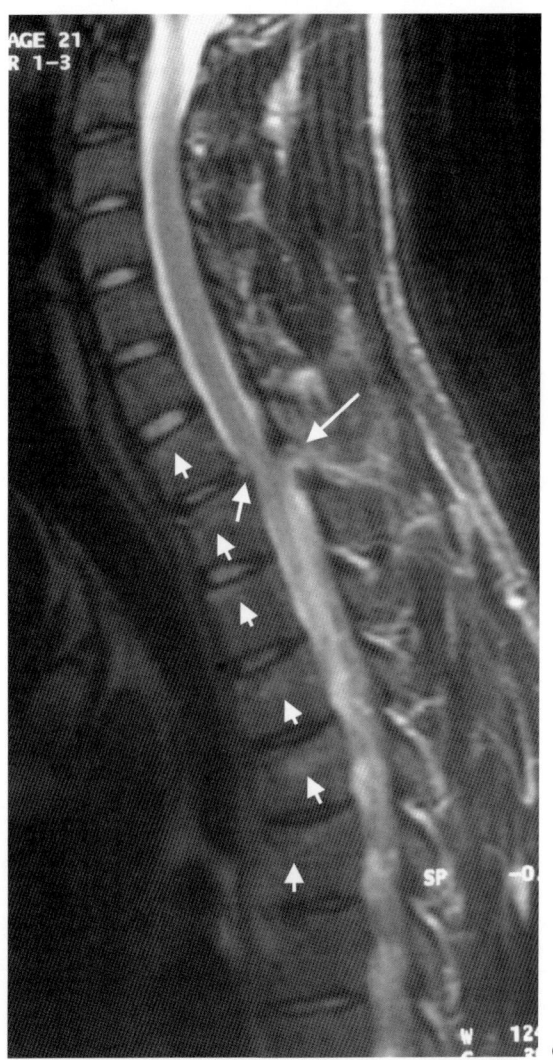

Imaging Modalities

CT, the diagnostic performance of radiographs is relatively poor in the cervical as well as the remainder of the spine.[23–28] About 10–20% of significant injuries of the cervical spine are missed radiographically when compared with CT, but the absolute number of missed injuries is even higher and most studies quote a number of around 60%.[16,20,29–32] For single detector row CT, conventional rather than helical acquisition was found to be more sensitive[33] while more recently multi-detector row CT was found to be superior in fracture detection to single-slice CT with its increased speed and z-axis resolution.[34]

MRI is particularly useful in diagnosing soft tissue spinal injuries including the spinal cord, and injuries to vertebral bodies by demonstrating marrow edema (Fig. 3.**4**). Injuries to cortical bone are not well depicted unless there is displacement (Figs. 3.**5**, 3.**6**). MRI is cumbersome for immobile patients and patients needing close medical supervision. It is also much more time consuming than radiographs and CT. Imaging protocols have to be tailored for specific areas unlike CT where the new generation scanners can image almost the entire body in less than a minute. Recently multi-detector row CT (MD-CT) has been increasingly advocated for C spine clearance also in obtunded patients.[35,36]

Flexion and extension views of the spine have been studied for cervical spine clearance of obtunded and alert patients. In alert patients there is no role for this technique in the acute phase due to muscle spasm.[37,38] However, they are useful for delayed imaging for persistent complaints at about two weeks after an injury when the initial radiographs are normal.[38–42] Their use in obtunded patients is controversial. There is no supportive literature (and no role) for the use of flexion/extension views in the acute diagnosis of lumbar or thoracic spinal injuries.

Pros and Cons

Radiography is universally available, familiar to doctors of all specialties and experience level and can be performed in the trauma room. It can be difficult though to obtain images of adequate quality, the interpretation requires skill and experience (more than often appreciated), soft tissue trauma is often missed (unless associated with significant bony malalignment or soft tissue swelling), and bone trauma is also frequently missed. The upper cervicocranial junction and the upper thoracic spine are notoriously difficult to image (Figs. 3.**3**, 3.**7**).[6,14–16,20–28,43] CT is much more sensitive in depicting bone trauma when compared to radiographs and allows for better assessment of the extent and nature of the bone trauma (Fig. 3.**2**). Two-dimensional reformatted images of the spine can be the by-product of CT imaging of head, thorax, abdomen, and pelvis when cranial and visceral injuries are suspected.[4,23–28,43] If the C-spine is included in such cases, the entire spine is imaged making radiographs of the spine unnecessary.[2,43] Nevertheless, regardless of the technical protocol, CT can miss bony injuries and has been found to perform poorly in the assessment of spinous or paraspinous soft tissues.[28,29,39,44–53]

More recently MD-CT has been examined as the sole imaging modality for clearance of the cervical spine in obtunded trauma patients.[35,36] It was found that MD-CT did not miss *unstable* injuries in either study. Other studies looked at using only MD-CT for clearance of the cervical spine for patients presenting without motor deficit.[54] Obtunded patients who were moving all their limbs on admission were assessed.[55] It was suggested that CT is sufficient to clear the cervical spine with regard to unstable injuries in these patients. The number of ligamentous injuries in these studies was low. A recent review of the literature on assessing the cervical spine in obtunded trauma patients[56] also makes this point and specifically cites a risk of missing about 0.5% of unstable cervical spine injuries in obtunded trauma patients. MD-CT does not image ligamentous injuries directly and relies on secondary signs such as alignment, extent and location of soft tissue swelling, and nature and location of bony injuries to draw conclusions about stability. Another interesting point raised in this review is the relative higher frequency of ligament injuries needing surgical treatment in the MRI and fluoroscopy based studies when compared to CT of the cervical spine. This suggests that CT does miss ligamentous injuries that would receive surgical treatment if imaged and diagnosed with MRI. The good clinical outcome of these limited CT-based studies suggests that despite no treatment ligamentous injuries that would normally be treated surgically do heal without neurologic sequelae.

A further diagnostic concern in the obtunded patient not addressed by any imaging modality except MRI, is spinal cord injury without radiographic or CT abnormalities. If the patient is admitted to a center whose treatment policy includes the administration of steroids, then this type of injury must be diagnosed early. However the limited studies of CT-based assessment of the cervical spine in obtunded patients do not suggest a worse outcome.

Unless there is a reason to image the entire spine, CT examinations are usually limited to a specific area for radiation protection concerns. Noncontiguous spinal injuries are surprisingly common and are seen in up to 50% of patients (Figs. 3.**5**–3.**7**). They are easily missed if the entire spine is not imaged in a patient with an acute spinal injury.[2,16,57–60]

MRI does not utilize ionizing radiation. As long as there is no contraindication, there is no detrimental effect to the patient. MRI is excellent for the imaging of soft tissue injuries but relatively poor in the depiction of bony injuries (Fig. 3.**6**).[29,39,44–53,61] This is true particularly for injury to the posterior elements where one study found a sensitivity of MRI compared to CT of only 11.5%.[45] The exception is the imaging of bone compression injuries without cortical disruption where marrow edema sensitive sequences frequently find bony injuries not appreciated on radiographs or CT.[57] MRI is of prognostic value in the assessment of spinal and spinal cord injuries.[62–64] In general though it is not the first line of investigation as it is expensive, access is

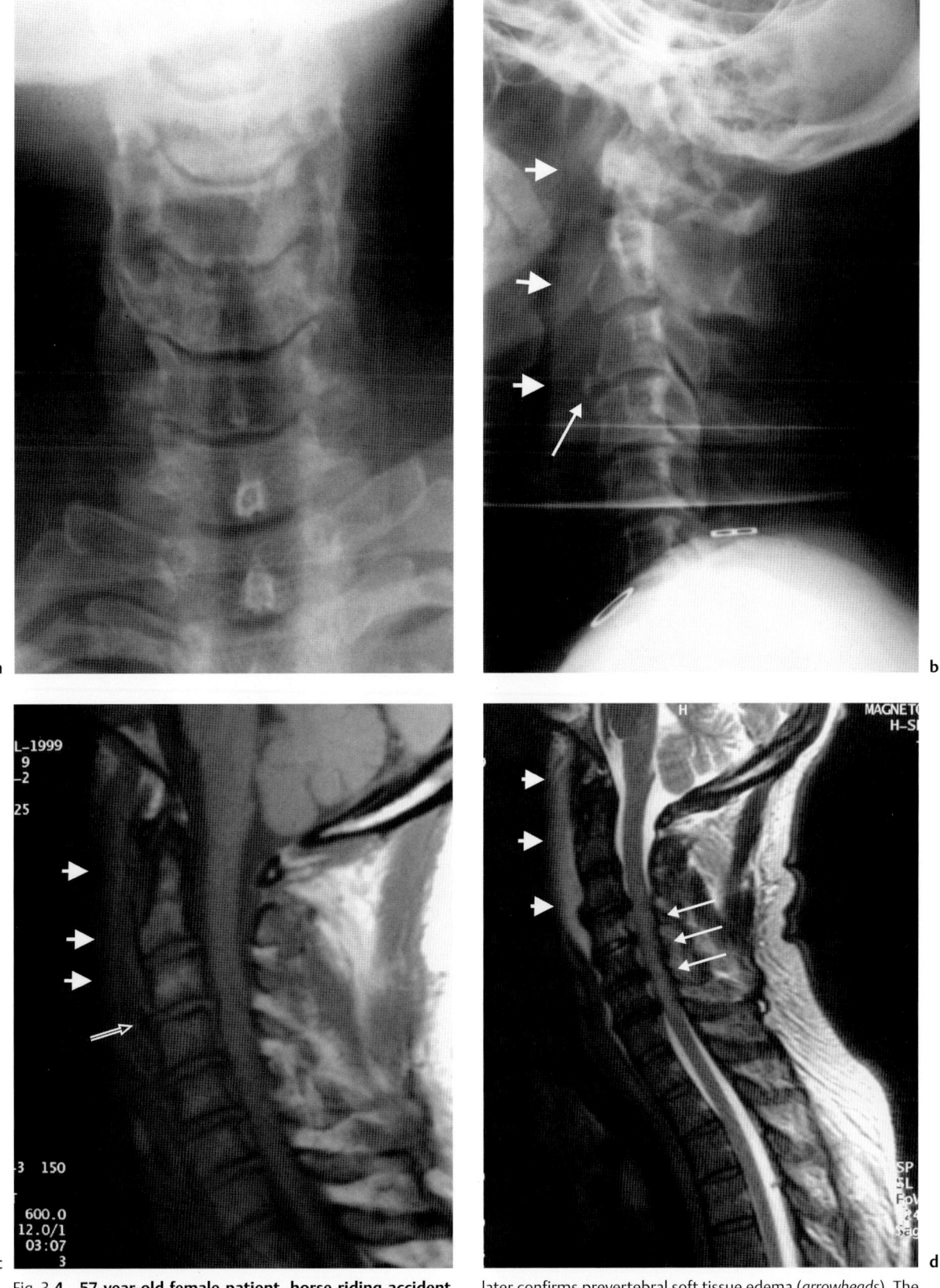

Fig. 3.4 **57-year-old female patient, horse riding accident.** Weakness of all extremities, difficulty with bladder and bowel control. Radiographs of the cervical spine (**a**, **b**) demonstrate chronic spondylotic change with prevertebral soft tissue swelling (*arrowheads*) and an avulsed osteophyte (*arrow*) of the anteroinferior corner of C3. MRI in T1W (**c**) and T2W (**d**) one day later confirms prevertebral soft tissue edema (*arrowheads*). The avulsed osteophyte is visible (*arrow*) but difficult to appreciate compared to the radiograph. Multi-level high signal change of the spinal cord is seen (*open arrow*) but no disruption of the spinal column. Diagnosis: central cord syndrome after trauma in a degenerate spine.

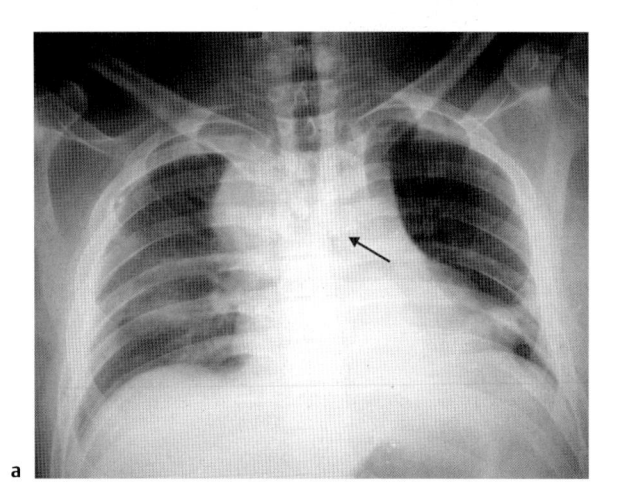

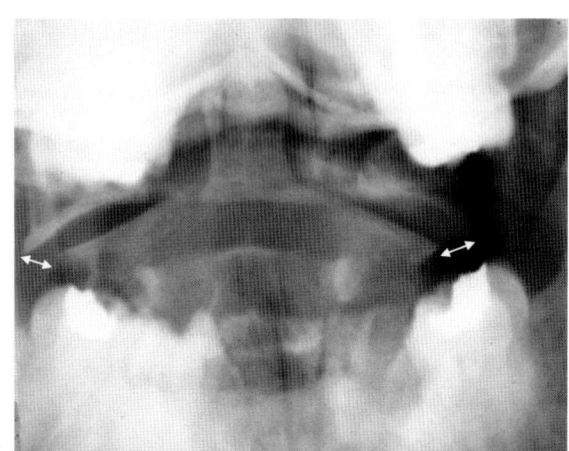

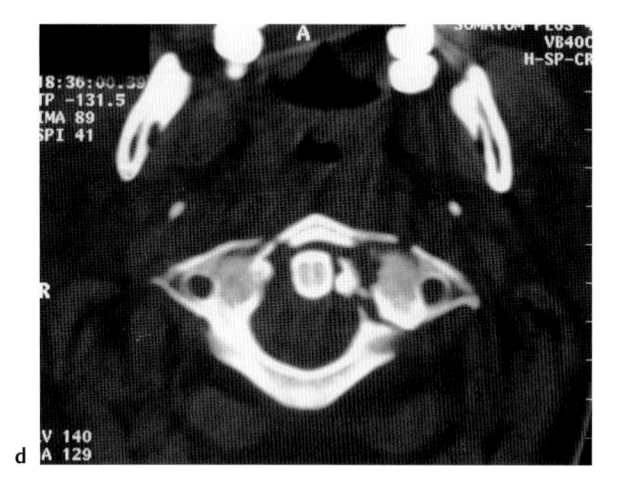

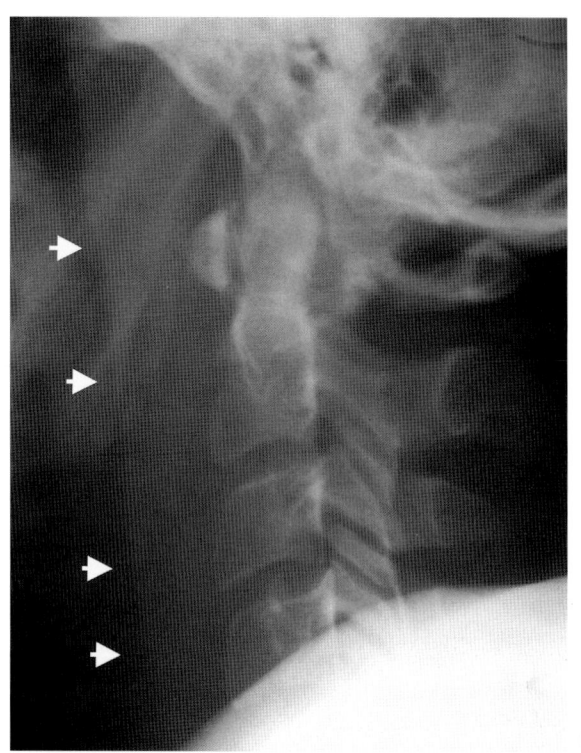

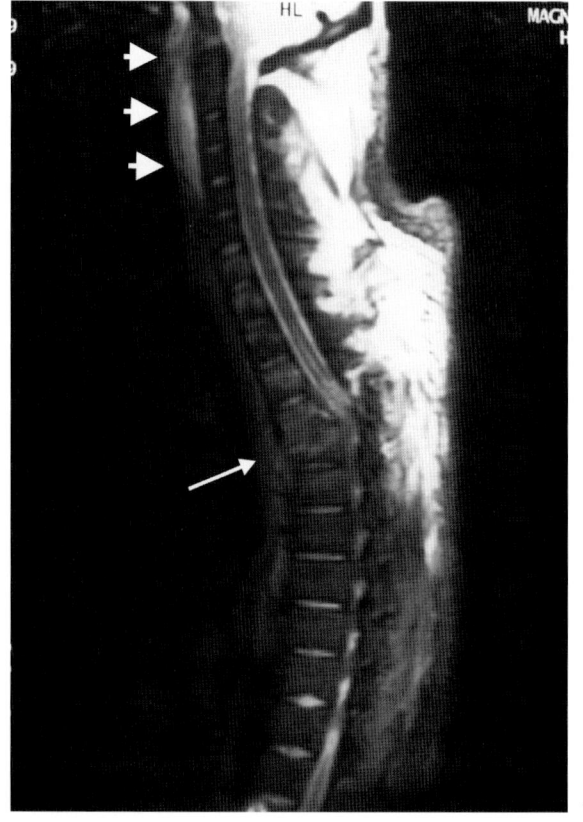

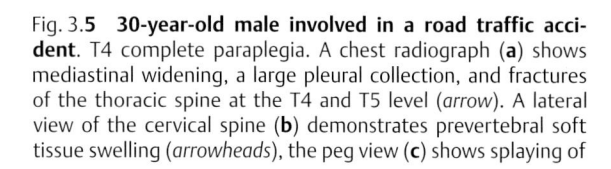

Fig. 3.5 **30-year-old male involved in a road traffic accident.** T4 complete paraplegia. A chest radiograph (**a**) shows mediastinal widening, a large pleural collection, and fractures of the thoracic spine at the T4 and T5 level (*arrow*). A lateral view of the cervical spine (**b**) demonstrates prevertebral soft tissue swelling (*arrowheads*), the peg view (**c**) shows splaying of the atlas (*double arrows*). CT confirms the complex fracture of the atlas (**d**). The C1 fracture was difficult to appreciate on MRI (**e**), but soft tissue edema and hemorrhage (*arrowheads*) indicate an upper cervical injury in addition to the T4 and T5 vertebral body fractures (*arrow*). Bone marrow edema indicating further infraction in multiple further vertebrae.

Imaging Modalities | 43

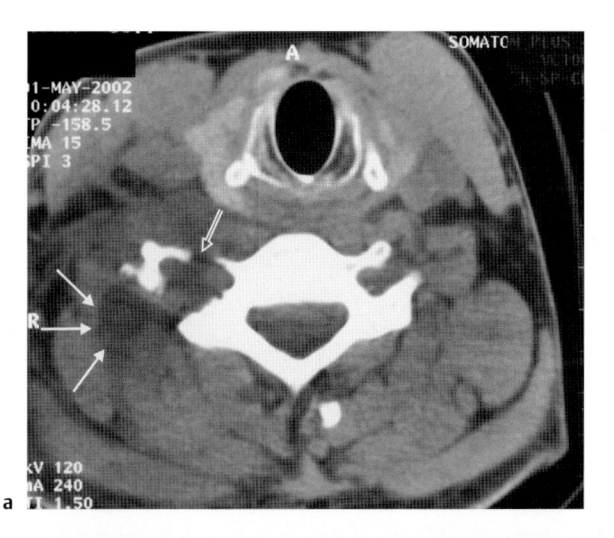

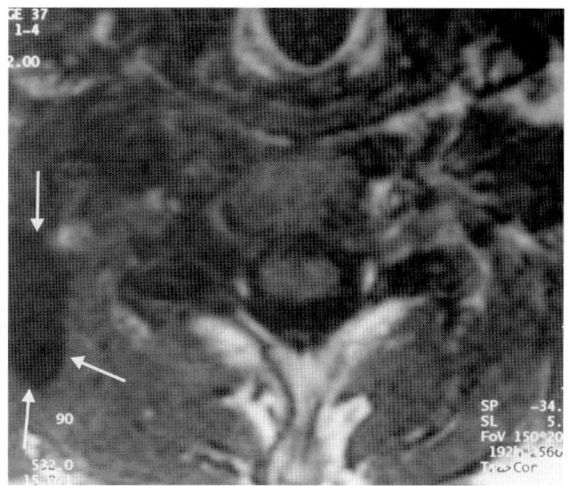

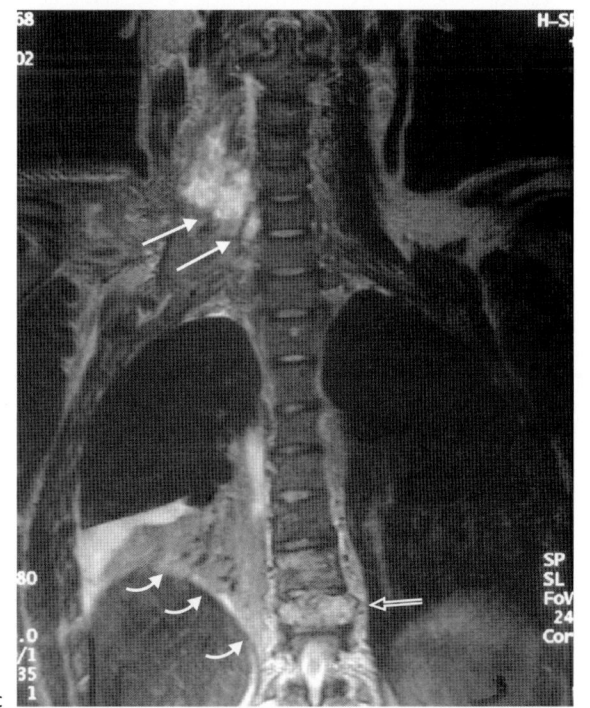

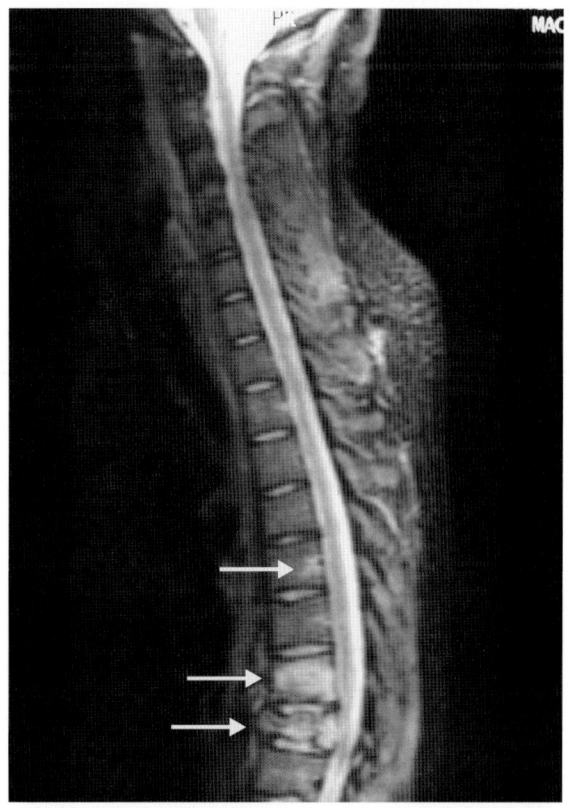

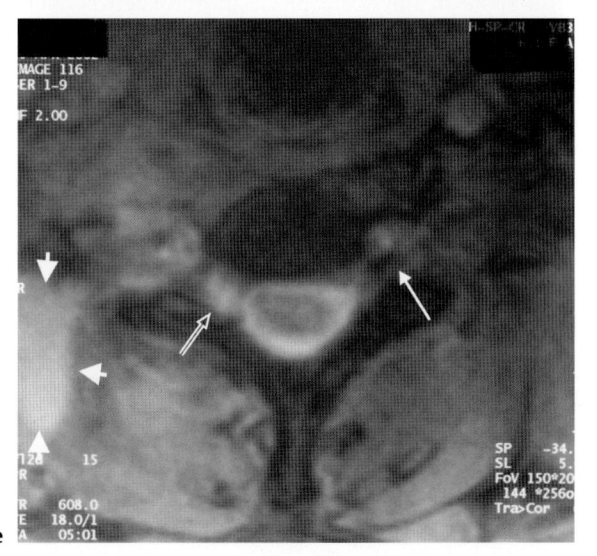

Fig. 3.6 **33-year-old male involved in a road traffic accident with signs of right brachial plexus injury.** A right-sided transverse process fracture of C6 was well demonstrated on CT (**a**; *open arrow*) but difficult to appreciate on MRI (**b**). The vertebral artery was proven to be intact. Low attenuation/signal areas signify CSF leakage after nerve root injury (*arrows* in **a**, **b**). Multiple nerve roots were affected. This is best appreciated on coronal MR images (**c**), which are best suited to imaging the brachial plexus (*arrows*). These demonstrate a further crush fracture of the T8 vertebral body (*open arrow*) and marrow edema in T7, right basal lung consolidation (*curved arrows*) and right-sided pleural collection. A sagittal STIR MR image of the spine (**d**) confirms the structural integrity of the cervical spine and spinal cord with lower thoracic fractures (*arrows*). An axial MR image (**e**) of the C7/T1 intervertebral foramen demonstrates the nerve root on the left (*arrow*) and the absence of the nerve root on the right (*open arrow*) and adjacent CSF collection (*arrowheads*). This case demonstrates the association of brachial plexus injuries with spinal injuries.

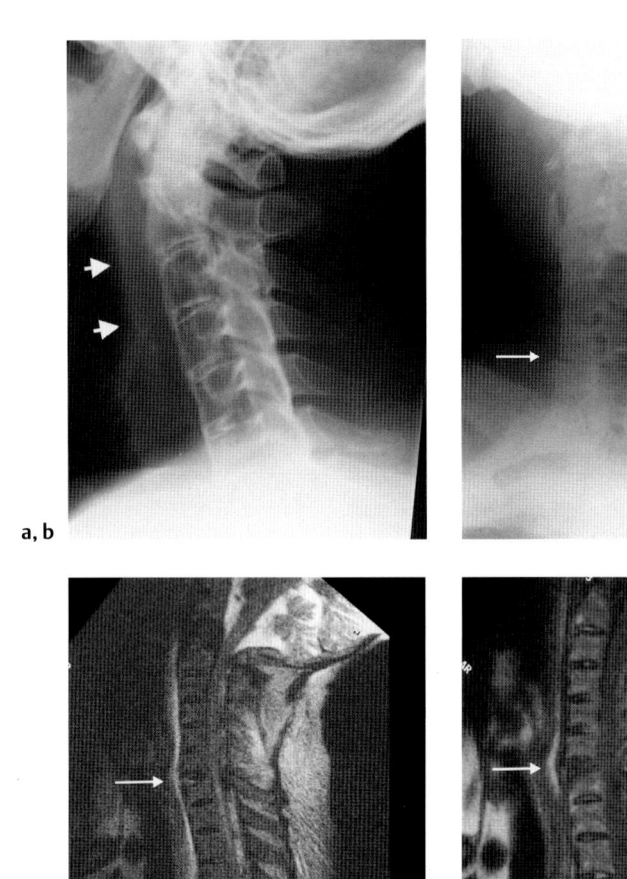

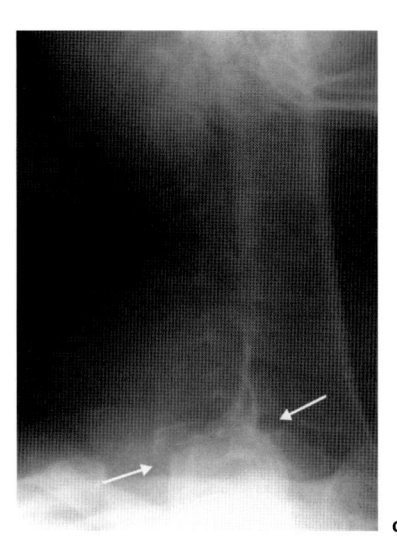

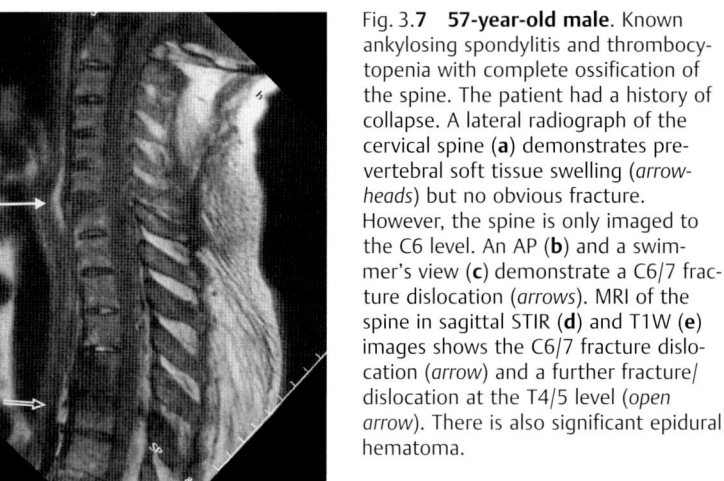

Fig. 3.7 **57-year-old male.** Known ankylosing spondylitis and thrombocytopenia with complete ossification of the spine. The patient had a history of collapse. A lateral radiograph of the cervical spine (**a**) demonstrates prevertebral soft tissue swelling (*arrowheads*) but no obvious fracture. However, the spine is only imaged to the C6 level. An AP (**b**) and a swimmer's view (**c**) demonstrate a C6/7 fracture dislocation (*arrows*). MRI of the spine in sagittal STIR (**d**) and T1W (**e**) images shows the C6/7 fracture dislocation (*arrow*) and a further fracture/dislocation at the T4/5 level (*open arrow*). There is also significant epidural hematoma.

limited, and the examination of severely traumatized patients or any patient needing close medical supervision is logistically demanding. On the other hand, early exclusion of unstable spine trauma can greatly facilitate further diagnostic and therapeutic planning and nursing care. Usually the role of MRI lies in the exact determination of the extent of spinal injuries initially diagnosed by other imaging methods. Here it is particularly valuable in defining the extent and severity of soft tissue (i.e. ligament and spinal cord) injuries and in identifying bone marrow edema (indicating bone trauma) in other areas of the spine (Figs. 3.5–3.8).[57] Cases of neurological deficits with no explanatory imaging evidence have been described[48,49] though usually MRI imaging will reveal a spinal cord abnormality (Fig. 3.4).[16,39,44,46,48,49,51,52,65] Some patients, however, do have contraindications for MRI imaging, for example cardiac pacemakers, intracranial surgical clips or cochlear implants. CT and in some cases CT myelography might be of help here as well as flexion/extension views of the cervical spine.

Fluoroscopic flexion and extension views of the cervical spine in the acute phase in obtunded patients seem to be able to exclude significant local instability when performed by experienced clinicians in a dedicated setup.[56,66,67] Some authors disagree with this view[68–70] but the key to success seems to be a dedicated setup and clarity about the aim of this examination. Despite suggestions to the contrary, this type of study should not be performed as radiographs in flexion and extension, and does not exclude all injuries but merely aims at excluding significant instability. As pointed out in a recent commentary[72] the studies performed suffer also from small numbers.[63] This makes a meaningful assessment of complication rates difficult. Logistically this examination is easier to perform than MRI. However, it cannot demonstrate cord compression by a dorsal disk herniation and cannot exclude or diagnose a cord injury. Hence, its usefulness for patient management is limited and it is potentially detrimental to the spinal cord. An excellent review of the literature concluded that as yet there is no clear evidence to

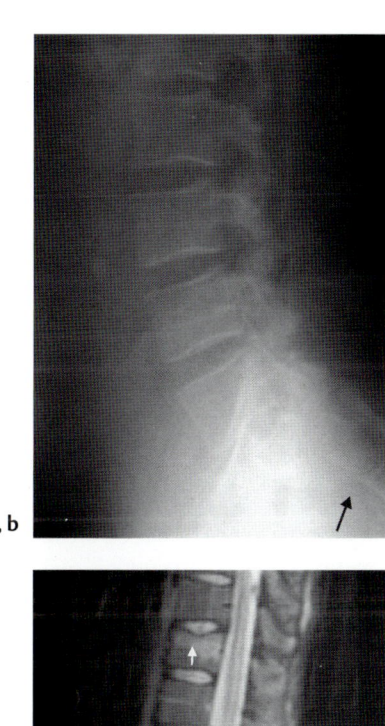

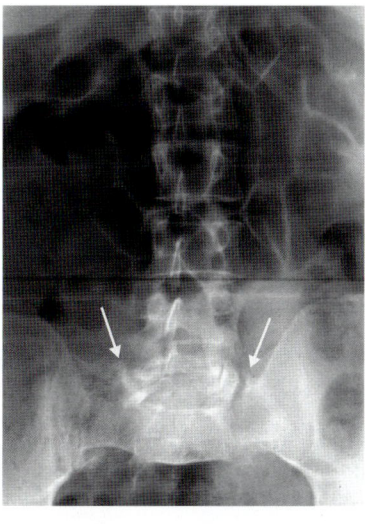

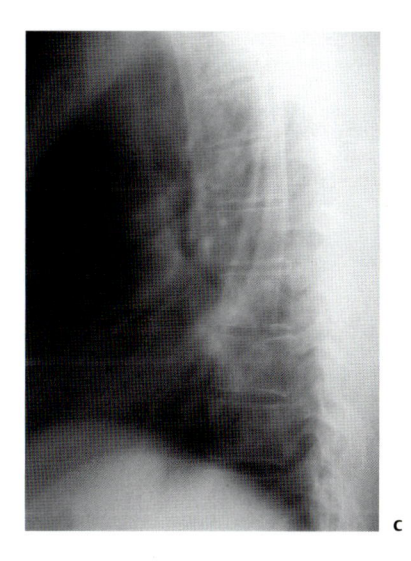

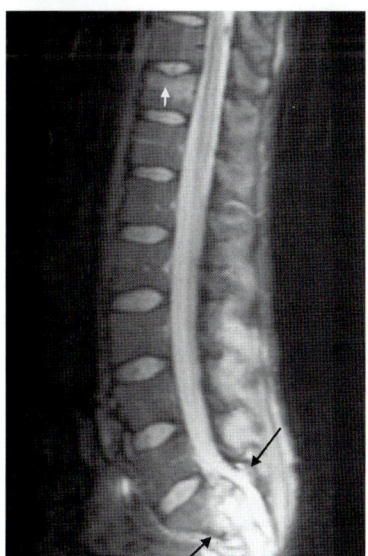

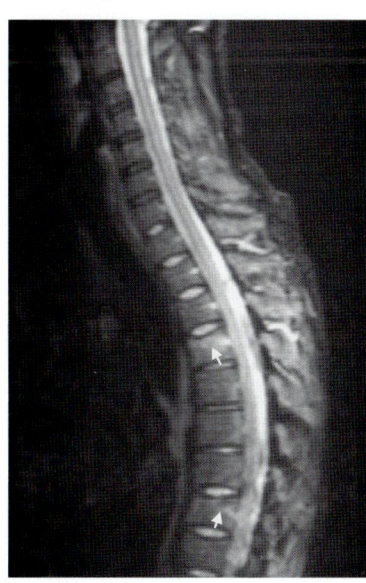

Fig. 3.8 **37-year-old male**. Motorbike accident. Radiographs (**a**, **b**) demonstrate a severe sacral fracture (*arrows*). Subtle endplate changes in the thoracic spine (**c**) are difficult to appreciate on the radiograph. MRI (**d**, **e**) demonstrates the sacral fracture (*arrow*) and several noncontiguous thoracic fractures (*small arrows*). Sacral fractures have a known association with injuries in other areas of the spine.

either favor dynamic fluoroscopy or MRI of the cervical spine to assess stability in obtunded patients. The authors suggest that the inherent advantages of MRI favor this examination where available.[56]

Imaging Approaches and Dilemmas

As the facts presented so far show, the biggest problem in the imaging of spinal injury patients is the choice of the appropriate imaging modality in the different stages of patient care.

If a spinal injury is identified by any one imaging modality, further imaging with other modalities is often indicated to complement or offset the specific constraints of the modality initially employed. For the clinician in charge of the patient, prognostic information is of particular importance. Older classification systems of spinal injuries such as the Holdsworth and the Louis classification were based on radiographic findings.[73] Newer classification systems such as the AO classification and partly the Denis classification are based on radiographic as well as CT findings.[73] However, there remain significant shortcomings, and a new classification system based on the combination of all imaging modalities appears necessary.[74] Some authors even promote MRI as the modality of choice for the imaging of the thoracic and lumbar spine and as the basis for trauma classification.[75,76] The problem of inter- and intraobserver variation remains, however[27,75], and this stresses the importance of close cooperation between the clinician in charge and the radiologist. Presently there is work underway to establish a classification system for the thoracolumbar spine combining the mechanism of trauma and the imaging and clinical findings, aiming at aiding communication between doctors and providing a more objective basis for treatment decisions.[77] The rationale and relevance of classification systems in spinal trauma are dealt with further in Chapter 4.

Table 3.1 Canadian C-spine rule (for low- and high-risk factors see Tabs. 3.2 and 3.3); this rule applies only to adult, alert (Glasgow coma scale 15), and stable patients

It is safe to assess active rotation of neck 45° left and right in the absence of a high-risk factor and in the presence of any low-risk factor
No radiograph necessary if patient able to rotate neck
Radiograph necessary: if high risk factor, or no low risk factor, or not able to rotate

Table 3.2 Canadian C-spine rule: high-risk factors mandating radiography

Age ≥ 65 years
Fall from ≥ 1 m/5 stairs
Axial load to head, e. g., diving
Motor vehicle collision (MVC) speed > 100 km/h, rollover, ejection
Motorized recreational vehicles
Bicycle collision
Paresthesia in extremities

Table 3.3 Canadian C-spine rule: low-risk factors; presence of any one of these factors allows safe assessment of range of motion in the absence of high-risk factors

Simple rear end MVC (excludes: being pushed into oncoming traffic, hit by bus/large truck/rollover, hit by high-speed vehicle)
Sitting position in emergency department
Ambulatory at any time
Delayed onset of neck pain (i. e., not immediate)
Absence of midline C spine tenderness

If trauma classification of spinal injuries requires CT and MR imaging[64,74–77] and radiographic imaging frequently misses significant injuries when compared to CT and MRI, is there still a role for radiographs or should they be replaced with cross-sectional imaging? If there is indication for CT of the vital organs the spine is covered apart from the cervical spine which is often included in the imaging protocol in these cases.[4,43,78–81] However, the vast majority of patients attending a hospital after trauma will not fall into this category and the appropriate choice of imaging protocol is difficult. A liberal policy towards CT imaging incurs high financial cost and also carries significant radiation exposure of the population.[82,83] Some authors have tried to define high-risk criteria necessitating CT rather than radiographs for imaging of the cervical spine.[16,60,84,85] Others suggest using CT for any patient with possible cervical spine injury.[54,55,78,86] CT of the cervical spine increases the radiation dose to the thyroid gland more than 14-fold which in patients with a borderline indication needs to be justified.[82] However, the groups implementing the Canadian C-spine rule used radiographs prospectively as the first line of investigation supplemented by other imaging modalities as needed, with excellent results missing only one unstable injury in 16 000 patients.[1,5] The NEXUS study came to a similar conclusion, as long as technically adequate films were obtained. A 3-view radiographic series is an appropriate first line of investigation for most patients with blunt trauma.[18] While the Canadian C-spine rule proved to be diagnostically superior to the NEXUS criteria, NEXUS included pediatric patients, while the Canadian C-spine rule was only applied to and validated for adult patients. However, the NEXUS study and a review of the literature suggest that a similar approach as taken for the Canadian C-spine rule with clinical assessment first, followed by radiographs for not obviously severely injured patients seems to be safe.[11,87]

A recently recommended algorithm for evaluating the spine after trauma produced by the Spine Trauma Group still suggests an imaging approach based on initial radiographic assessment.[88] A paper is quoted stating that a 3-view radiographic series of the cervical spine can detect up to 99 % of injuries.[14] While this seems unduly sensitive in the light of many recent CT-based studies, it should be noted that the Canadian C spine rule and the NEXUS study achieved similar good results based on primary radiographic screening and for low-risk patients there is no consensus whether to image primarily with radiographs or CT of the cervical spine.[89] However France et al[88] go on to advise that "any patient with neck pain or tenderness despite negative, but adequate, plain radiographs should have cervical CT." This in effect should result in a CT scan in virtually every one of these patients.

In the alert adult without certain high-risk factors (Tab. 3.2) and with at least one low-risk factor (Tab. 3.3), the cervical spine can be assessed clinically (Tab. 3.1) to determine whether further imaging is indicated.[1,5]

The Canadian C spine rule specifically excluded patients older than 65 years and this age group is at higher risk for cervical spine fractures than the younger adult population. A recent study determined predictors of cervical spine fractures following blunt trauma.[90] Unsurprisingly focal neurologic deficit, severe head injury, high-energy and moderate-energy mechanism all significantly increased the risk of a fracture. However 11 % of elderly patients with C spine fractures sustained the injuries after falls from the standing or sitting position and 7 of these 11 patients had no neurologic deficit, head injury, loss of consciousness, or other associated injuries. These injuries would potentially be missed if imaging were only performed in the high-risk group of patients.

However, no such criteria exist for the diagnosis of injuries to the thoracic or lumbar spine which can initially be asymptomatic in patients with a history of high-energy trauma.[24,25,27,28] For this reason some authors suggest CT of the thoracolumbar spine instead of radiographs in all cases of high-energy trauma regardless of the clinical presentation,[24] or in patients with transverse process fractures on radiographs.[25] Since only half of transverse or spinous process fractures are diagnosed with radiographs and these injuries are frequently associated with further severe injuries not visualized with radiography[23,26], the use of CT instead of radiographs has definite diagnostic and prognostic[77] benefits.

It has to be emphasized that a "watchful waiting" approach is not suitable for potential spinal injury patients. The exclusion of a spinal injury at an early stage is important to avoid potential complications arising from the otherwise necessary precautions. Immobilization on a spinal board will after a few hours lead to back pain and tenderness even in otherwise healthy subjects making clinical assessment difficult. Prolonged immobilization increases the financial cost of patient care, makes patient handling more difficult and can cause medical complications such as respiratory compromise, increase in intracranial pressure, pain in the cranial area, and if vigorously applied can even be the cause of neurological deterioration for some patients (e.g., for ankylosing spondylitis patients).[91-95] Where possible, clinical clearance of the spine before hospital admission avoids these complications, and results in a reduction of the number of imaging examinations performed.[92] This requires a set of protocols and well-trained medical personnel.[91-93,96]

Specific Scenarios and Technical Considerations

Some specific clinical problems demand a specific imaging approach. If for example after blunt spinal trauma, clinically a focal nerve root trauma is diagnosed and MRI does not convincingly demonstrate an abnormality, CT is required to look for a bony fragment in the spinal canal or intervertebral foramen. If bony trauma to the vertebral bodies near the course of the vertebral arteries is demonstrated, the patency and status of the vertebral arteries needs to be established (Fig. 3.**9**). If radiographs and CT of the spine are normal but there is neurological deficit, MRI is required. Similarly, apparently isolated injuries to a single nerve root or for example parts of the brachial plexus are often associated with further spinal injuries and even if locally no spinal injury is seen the whole spine should be examined for further injuries.[97] Patients with ossification of the spine such as in ankylosing spondylitis are prone to spine fracture and even after minor trauma there should be a liberal approach towards further imaging (especially MRI) to enable early treatment and prevent the complications of untreated spinal fractures. In addition there is an increased risk of significant hemorrhage in ankylosing spondylitis due to the fracture through cancellous bone (Fig. 3.**7**). Ossification of the posterior longitudinal ligament also deserves special attention as the cervical spinal canal is often significantly narrowed and even minor trauma can lead to spinal cord injury without radiographic abnormality (SCIWORA) type injuries only appreciated on MRI.[44,48] The same is true for patients with marked degenerative change of the cervical spine or a habitually narrow spinal canal (see Fig. 3.**4**). Penetrating injuries to the spine are another group of injuries deserving special attention (Fig. 3.**10**). While still relatively rare in western Europe,[98] in the USA spinal injuries due to violence are almost as common as those due to road traffic accidents and these are mainly due to stabbings and shootings (Fig. 3.**11**).[99] While the spine is most likely mechanically stable there can be significant soft tissue and vascular trauma and even introduction of a foreign body into the spinal canal without a radiographic abnormality.[99,100] Of particular concern are gun shot injuries from military weapons. The high velocity and fragmenting ammunition can cause extensive soft tissue trauma and can lead to spinal cord trauma solely due to shock waves without direct cord trauma.[90,101] Overlooked foreign bodies are also a source of recurrent infection which can be difficult to localize in paraplegic patients and can cause direct cord or nerve root compression (Fig. 3.**10**).[99,101,102] These are usually readily identified by CT or MR imaging, and MR imaging is particularly useful for identifying soft tissue and cord trauma as in stabbing injuries (Fig. 3.**11**).[102]

In every patient with a proven spinal injury the whole spine should be imaged with cross-sectional imaging to look for further injuries.[2,16,57-60]

Technical considerations will to an extent depend on the equipment and expertise available. Nevertheless, there are a few "rules of thumb" that are important to keep in mind when imaging injuries of the spine.

For imaging of the cervical spine, a radiographic approach should consist of a 3-view series (anteriorposterior, lateral, and dens axis view). This can be amended by further views but there is no proven benefit in routinely performing larger series.[14,15,103] However, trauma oblique views can increase diagnostic confidence; if findings on the 3-view series are equivocal or image quality is insufficient, cross-sectional imaging and therefore usually CT, are indicated.[1,5]

The most important question facing the radiologist is whether to accept the limited performance of cervical spine radiographs when compared to CT. If a test is consistently shown to be poor why persist with it? On the other hand there is a radiation risk and also cost and availability issues. Furthermore the large Canadian C spine rule and the NEXUS study have achieved very good results based on primary radiographic screening for injuries. Some subgroups, such as the elderly with the increased risk of injury after any given trauma mechanism and frequently pre-existing degenerative changes, might benefit from primary assessment by CT; to date, however, there is no defining study on this subject.

CT of the cervical spine should include the skull base and should be extended caudally to the T4 level since injuries of the craniocervical junction[19,29,59] and the upper thoracic spine are notoriously difficult to diagnose with radiographs and are otherwise easily missed (Figs. 3.**3**, 3.**5**, 3.**7**).[28,60]

The imaging parameters of the CT protocol used are also important. Generally, it has been shown that thinner resolution results in better fracture detection.[19,34] For single-slice CT it has been shown that conventional

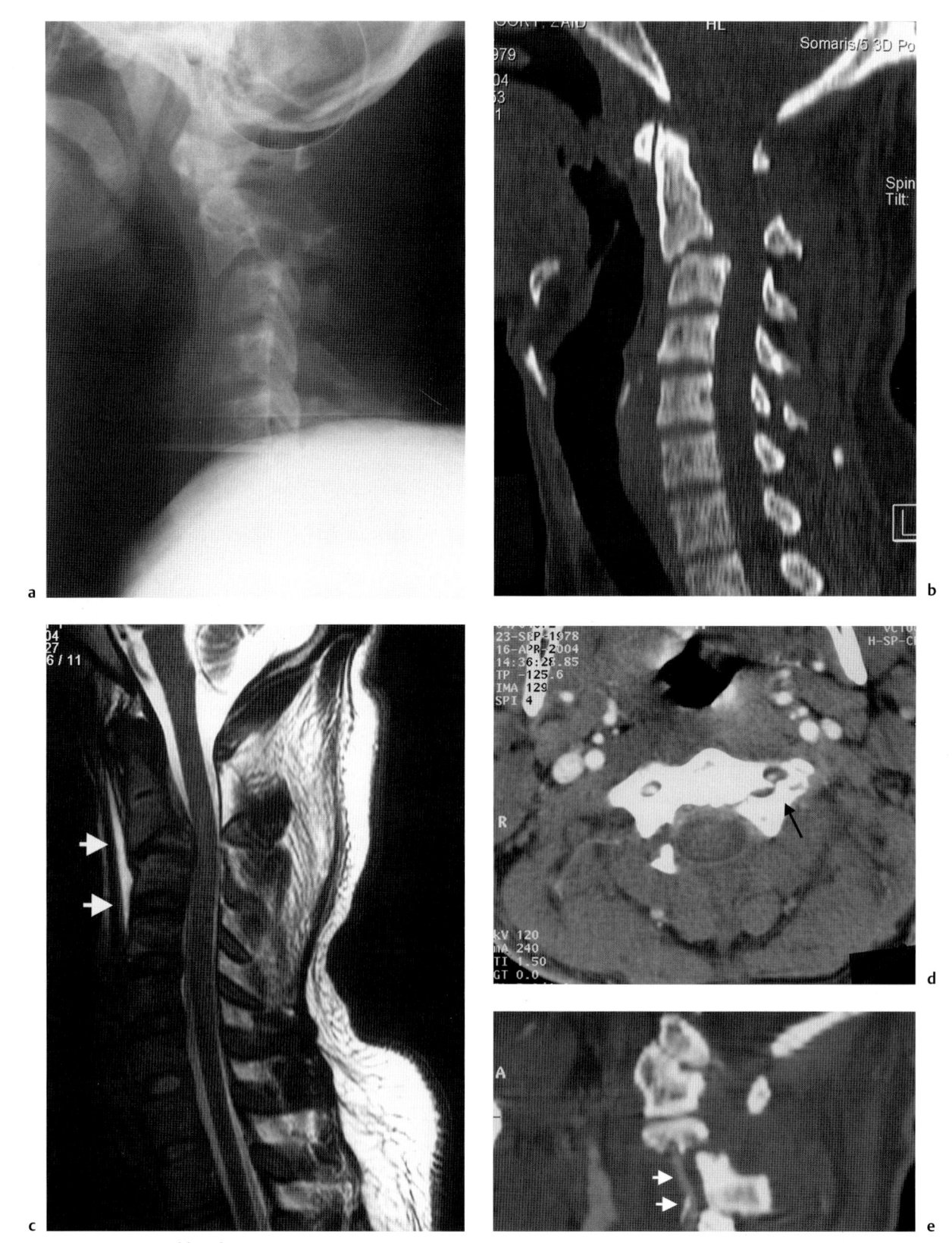

Fig. 3.**9** **25-year-old male**. Passenger in a van involved in a road traffic accident. After the accident transient right-sided paralysis. Lateral radiograph (**a**) and CT reconstruction (**b**) of the cervical spine show fracture dislocation of C2 vertebra on C3. Soft tissue swelling is only appreciated on MRI (*arrowheads* in **c**), with mild impingement of the spinal cord. CT (**d**) demonstrates also the involvement of the foramen transversarium (*arrow*), contrast-enhanced CT with reconstruction (**e**) confirmed patency and integrity of the left vertebral artery (*arrowheads*).

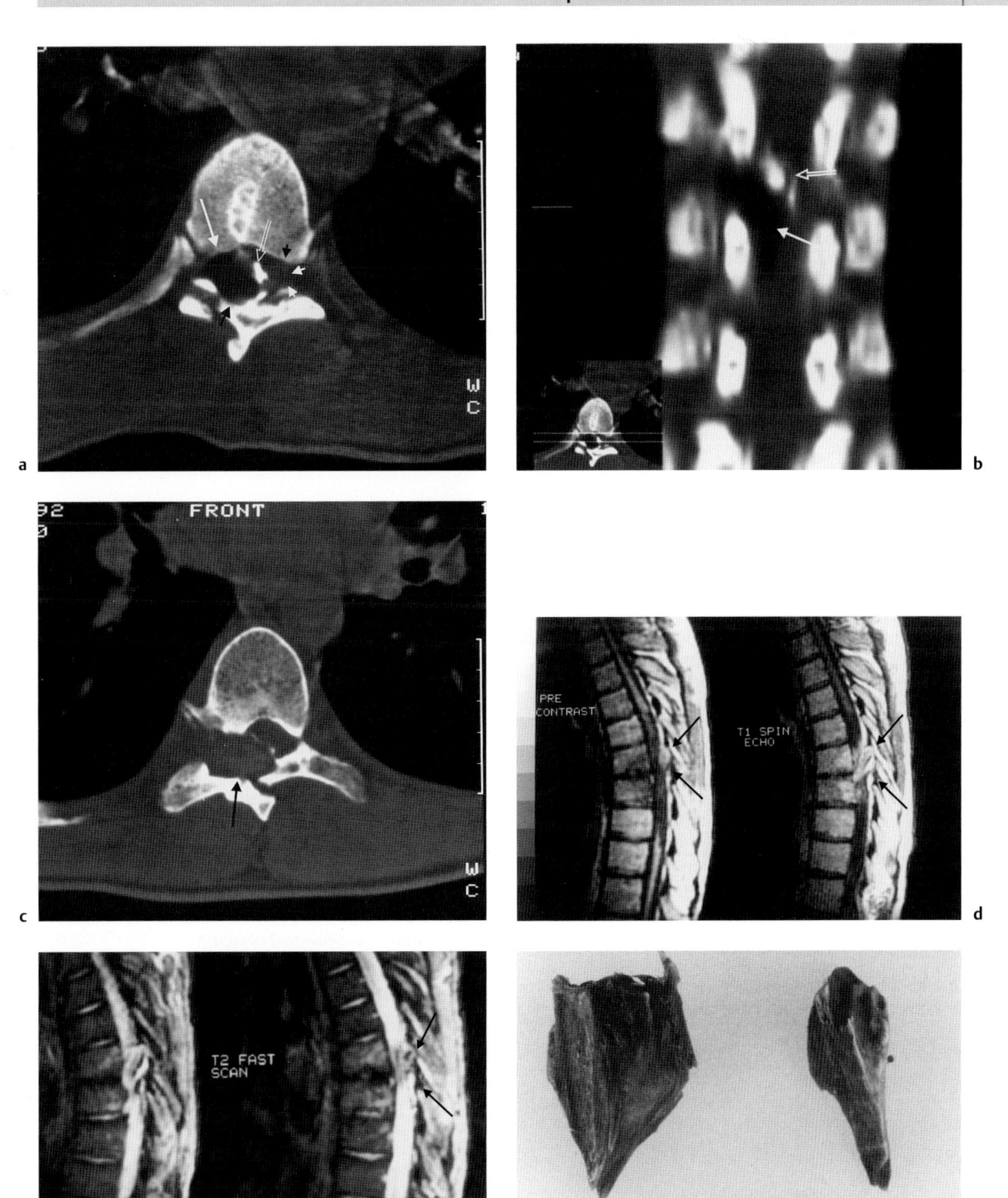

Fig. 3.**10** **20-year-old male**. Ejected from a car during a road traffic accident and impaled on a wooden post with immediate paraplegia. CT (**a**) with coronal reconstruction (**b**) after the accident demonstrates a low attenuation area within the spinal canal of the thoracic spine (*arrows*) with an adjacent bone fragment (*open arrow*) and compression of the spinal cord (*arrowheads*). This was assumed to be air. Subsequently recurrent infections, until further CT (**c**) and MRI imaging (**d**, **e**) pre and post i. v. gadolinium administration diagnosed a now higher CT attenuation foreign body within the spinal canal (*arrow*) with adjacent edema and contrast enhancement in MRI (*arrows*). This was surgically removed and confirmed to be a piece of wood (**f**). Dry wood has very low attenuation values on CT and can be mistaken for gas. With time the wood becomes saturated with fluid and assumes higher attenuation values.

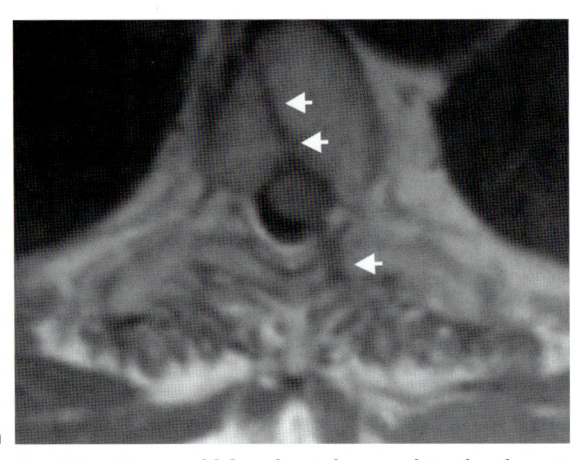

Fig. 3.**11** **30-year-old female, stab wound to the thoracic spine.** Brown–Sequard lesion. T1W (**a**) and T2W (**b**) MR images demonstrate the knife track, traversing the posterior elements and the spinal cord into the vertebral body (*arrowheads*).

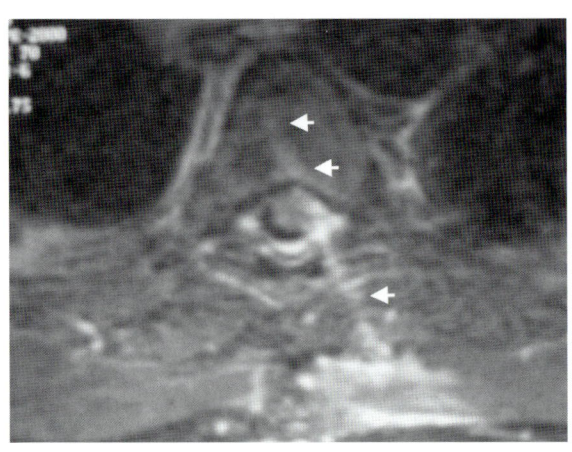

image acquisition instead of helical acquisition results in better image quality for the axial images.[33] However, the quality of sagittal and coronal reconstructions suffers with conventional protocols and the imaging time is also increased. Multi-detector row CT (MD-CT) can easily achieve high spatial resolution in all three planes, image a large area, and still be fast. However, in the increasingly common scenario of head, cervical spine, and body imaging with CT in a trauma patient, the imaging protocol is usually not optimized for imaging of the spine, and thicker slices are used even in MD-CT applications. This results in some loss of image quality compared with dedicated protocols but has been found to still produce diagnostic images.[4]

MRI of the spine usually uses sagittal planes amended by axial planes where necessary. Generally speaking, STIR or T2 fat sat type sequences are particularly useful for demonstrating bone marrow and soft tissue trauma, the anterior longitudinal ligament is best appreciated on sagittal T1W sequences, the posterior longitudinal ligament on (fat sat) T2W and hemorrhage (especially intramedullary) on gradient-echo T2W images (Fig. 3.**3**).[48] Newer MRI scanners with multiple coil elements enable whole spine imaging without time consuming repositioning and might in the future increase the use of MRI earlier in the patients work-up.

An Approach to Imaging of Spinal Injuries

With the lack of conclusive evidence, differences in equipment availability and expertise and the infinitely variable trauma mechanisms, there can be no prescriptive approach to the imaging of possible spinal injuries. Nevertheless, in this chapter the authors give their personal opinion on how to approach the imaging of spinal injuries in the light of the current evidence and trends.

For the assessment of the cervical spine in adults the Canadian C-spine rule should be applied where possible (see Tabs. 3.**1**–3.**3**).[1,5] This rule for stable, alert, adult patients either allows clearance of the cervical spine on clinical grounds or suggests further imaging with radiographs. If radiographs are obtained and are not completely normal, there is probably an indication for further, cross-sectional imaging. In the elderly there might well be a role for primary CT of the cervical spine if there is any suspicion of an injury; radiation exposure is less of a risk with a more limited life expectancy. In the pediatric age group the NEXUS criteria might be of help though they have poor specificity in this age group.[87] CT is probably not helpful in children under the age of 5.[104]

In patients with decreased consciousness or suspected significant head or body trauma the threshold to perform cross-sectional imaging (usually CT) of the cervical spine should be low. In patients who undergo CT of head, thorax, abdomen, and pelvis anyway, this should be extended to include the cervical spine. The entire spine can then be assessed on the reformatted images.

If after negative radiographs and CT there is still doubt about a ligamentous injury, supervised flexion/extension views with fluoroscopy might be of use in some circumstances. However, this is a potentially risky procedure. The demonstration of stability does not exclude surgically treatable cord compression and where possible MRI should be preferred.

The assessment of the thoracic and lumbar spine should be made along similar lines with assessment of the patient, the trauma mechanism, and local symptoms. If there is a high index of suspicion, i.e., high-energy trauma, CT of thorax and abdomen is often indicated anyway; if not, radiographs of good quality and completely normal, should be reassuring but do not guarantee the absence of a significant injury. If in doubt further imaging is advised and if possible MRI is particularly useful in these circumstances as it allows imaging of the entire spine without a radiation penalty.

Table 3.4 Type of injury versus suitability of imaging modality to image the injury; radiographs means a three-view series with further views if felt necessary, CT means helical acquisition with reconstructions in three planes

Modality	Injury	Radiographs	CT	MRI	Flexion/extension views
Stability/instability		+	++	+++	++
Fracture	Skull base	−+	+++	−+	−
	Vertebral body	+	++	++	−+
	Posterior elements	+	+++	−+	−+
Malalignment	Vertebrae	++	++	++	+
	Facet joints	+	+++	++	+
	Posterior elements	+	+++	−+	+
Soft tissue injury without malalignment	Paraspinal	−+	+	+++	−+
	Ligaments	−+	+	+++	++
	Disk	−+	+	+++	−+
	Cord	−	−+	+++	−
	Neural/plexus	−	+	+++	−
Canal or intervertebral foramen encroachment	By soft tissue	−	−+	+++	−+
	Bony	−+	+++	++	−+
Concomitant spinal injury		+	++	+++	−
Others	Cervicothoracic junction	−+	++	++	−+
	Associated nonspinal injury	−+	+++	+	−
	Vascular injury	−	+	++	−
	Penetrating injury	−+	++	++	−

− not at all suitable; −+ poorly suitable; + suitable; ++ well suitable; +++ very suitable and the modality of choice

MRI of the entire spine is advocated in every patient with proven spinal cord injury. It is debatable whether all patients with intact neurology and a spinal injury require MRI. At the level of the proven injury MRI can add diagnostic and prognostic information. Imaging of the entire spine frequently reveals additional injuries. Although usually these do not need specific treatment they are often relevant for the further nonoperative treatment (mobilization). They also provide a baseline for the long-term follow-up of spinal injury patients and problems arising later. This examination is usually carried out after the treatment of life-threatening or further disabling injuries.

The authors' preferences for the choice of imaging modality for selected specific indications are depicted in Table 3.4. Again it has to be stressed that technically good images are the starting point of any assessment. However, the most common cause for missed injuries is "user error," the incorrect appreciation of signs of spinal injuries in the clinical and imaging examination. The early involvement of a radiologist plays a vital role in the accurate diagnosis of spinal injuries. Even if the radiologist is involved in the acute phase of imaging immediately after the admission of the patient, a secondary survey of all findings in a suitable (calm) environment is very important to avoid missing significant injuries.

Conclusion

Imaging of spinal injuries requires close cooperation between the clinician in charge and the radiologist to optimize the use of resources to achieve a diagnostic imaging protocol tailored for each patient. This will often be achieved by following an established protocol with adaptations as required for the individual needs of the patient. Currently, the Canadian C-spine rule offers an evidence-based approach to imaging for injuries of the cervical spine in a subgroup of patients. Evidence for the remainder of the spine is sketchier. Careful clinical evaluation should always be the starting point.

References

1. Stiell IG, Clement CM, McKnight RD, et al. The Canadian C-spine rule versus the NEXUS low-risk criteria in patients with trauma. *N Engl J Med.* 2003;349:2510–2518.
2. Bensch FV, Kiuru MJ, Koivikko MP, Koskinen SK. Spine fractures in falling accidents: analysis of multidetector CT findings. *Eur Radiol.* 2004;14:618–624.
3. Wintermark M, Poletti PA, Becker CD, Schnyder P. Traumatic injuries: organization and ergonomics of imaging in the emergency environment. *Eur Radiol.* 2002;12:959–968.
4. Roos JE, Hilfiker P, Platz A, et al. MDCT in emergency radiology: is a standardized chest or abdominal protocol sufficient for evaluation of thoracic and lumbar spine trauma? *AJR Am J Roentgenol.* 2004;183:959–968.
5. Stiell IG, Wells GA, Vandemheen KL, et al. The Canadian C-spine rule for radiography in alert and stable trauma patients. *Jama.* 2001;286:1841–1848.

6. Reid DC, Henderson R, Saboe L, Miller JD. Etiology and clinical course of missed spine fractures. *J Trauma*. 1987;27:980–986.
7. Poonnoose PM, Ravichandran G, McClelland MR. Missed and mismanaged injuries of the spinal cord. *J Trauma*. 2002;53: 314–320.
8. Gerrelts BD, Petersen EU, Mabry J, Petersen SR. Delayed diagnosis of cervical spine injuries. *J Trauma*. 1991;31:1622–1626.
9. Davis JW, Phreaner DL, Hoyt DB, Mackersie RC. The etiology of missed cervical spine injuries. *J Trauma*. 1993;34:342–346.
10. Sengupta DK. Neglected spinal injuries. *Clin Orthop Relat Res*. 2005;93–103.
11. Slack SE, Clancy MJ. Clearing the cervical spine of paediatric trauma patients. *Emerg Med J*. 2004;21:189–193.
12. Tins BJ, Cassar-Pullicino VN. Imaging of acute cervical spine injuries: review and outlook. *Clin Radiol*. 2004;59:865–880.
13. Cassar-Pullicino VN. Spinal injury: optimising the imaging options. *Eur J Radiol*. 2002;42:85–91.
14. MacDonald RL, Schwartz ML, Mirich D, Sharkey PW, Nelson WR. Diagnosis of cervical spine injury in motor vehicle crash victims: how many X-rays are enough? *J Trauma*. 1990;30: 392–397.
15. Vandemark RM. Radiology of the cervical spine in trauma patients: practice pitfalls and recommendations for improving efficiency and communication. *AJR Am J Roentgenol*. 1990; 155:465–472.
16. Diaz JJ, Jr., Gillman C, Morris JA, Jr., May AK, Carrillo YM, Guy J. Are five-view plain films of the cervical spine unreliable? A prospective evaluation in blunt trauma patients with altered mental status. *J Trauma*. 2003;55:658–663; discussion 663–654.
17. Ross SE, Schwab CW, David ET, Delong WG, Born CT. Clearing the cervical spine: initial radiologic evaluation. *J Trauma*. 1987; 27:1055–1060.
18. Mower WR, Hoffman JR, Pollack CV, Jr., Zucker MI, Browne BJ, Wolfson AB. Use of plain radiography to screen for cervical spine injuries. *Ann Emerg Med*. 2001;38:1–7.
19. Link TM, Schuierer G, Hufendiek A, Horch C, Peters PE. Substantial head trauma: value of routine CT examination of the cervicocranium. *Radiology*. 1995;196:741–745.
20. Woodring JH, Lee C. Limitations of cervical radiography in the evaluation of acute cervical trauma. *J Trauma*. 1993;34:32–39.
21. Blacksin MF, Lee HJ. Frequency and significance of fractures of the upper cervical spine detected by CT in patients with severe neck trauma. *AJR Am J Roentgenol*. 1995;165:1201–1204.
22. Borock EC, Gabram SG, Jacobs LM, Murphy MA. A prospective analysis of a two-year experience using computed tomography as an adjunct for cervical spine clearance. *J Trauma*. 1991;31:1001–1005; discussion 1005–1006.
23. Hauser CJ, Visvikis G, Hinrichs C, et al. Prospective validation of computed tomographic screening of the thoracolumbar spine in trauma. *J Trauma*. 2003;55:228–234; discussion 234–225.
24. Gestring ML, Gracias VH, Feliciano MA, et al. Evaluation of the lower spine after blunt trauma using abdominal computed tomographic scanning supplemented with lateral scanograms. *J Trauma*. 2002;53:9–14.
25. Krueger MA, Green DA, Hoyt D, Garfin SR. Overlooked spine injuries associated with lumbar transverse process fractures. *Clin Orthop*. 1996;191–195.
26. Patten RM, Gunberg SR, Brandenburger DK. Frequency and importance of transverse process fractures in the lumbar vertebrae at helical abdominal CT in patients with trauma. *Radiology*. 2000;215:831–834.
27. Wintermark M, Mouhsine E, Theumann N, et al. Thoracolumbar spine fractures in patients who have sustained severe trauma: depiction with multi-detector row CT. *Radiology*. 2003;227:681–689.
28. van Beek EJ, Been HD, Ponsen KK, Maas M. Upper thoracic spinal fractures in trauma patients – a diagnostic pitfall. *Injury*. 2000;31:219–223.
29. Schenarts PJ, Diaz J, Kaiser C, Carrillo Y, Eddy V, Morris JA, Jr. Prospective comparison of admission computed tomographic scan and plain films of the upper cervical spine in trauma patients with altered mental status. *J Trauma*. 2001;51:663–668; discussion 668–669.
30. Schroder RJ, Vogl T, Hidajat N, et al. [Comparison of the diagnostic value of CT and MRI in injuries of the cervical vertebrae]. *Aktuelle Radiol*. 1995;5:197–202.
31. Woodring JH, Lee C. The role and limitations of computed tomographic scanning in the evaluation of cervical trauma. *J Trauma*. 1992;33:698–708.
32. Edwards MJ, Frankema SP, Kruit MC, Bode PJ, Breslau PJ, van Vugt AB. Routine cervical spine radiography for trauma victims: Does everybody need it? *J Trauma*. 2001;50:529–534.
33. Link TM, Meier N, Rummeny EJ, et al. Artificial spine fractures: detection with helical and conventional CT. *Radiology*. 1996; 198:515–519.
34. Obenauer S, Alamo L, Herold T, Funke M, Kopka L, Grabbe E. Imaging skeletal anatomy of injured cervical spine specimens: comparison of single-slice vs multi-slice helical CT. *Eur Radiol*. 2002;12:2107–2111.
35. Brohi K, Healy M, Fotheringham T, et al. Helical computed tomographic scanning for the evaluation of the cervical spine in the unconscious, intubated trauma patient. *J Trauma*. 2005;58:897–901.
36. Hogan GJ, Mirvis SE, Shanmuganathan K, Scalea TM. Exclusion of unstable cervical spine injury in obtunded patients with blunt trauma: is MR imaging needed when multi-detector row CT findings are normal? *Radiology*. 2005;237:106–113.
37. Insko EK, Gracias VH, Gupta R, Goettler CE, Gaieski DF, Dalinka MK. Utility of flexion and extension radiographs of the cervical spine in the acute evaluation of blunt trauma. *J Trauma*. 2002; 53:426–429.
38. Pollack CV, Jr., Hendey GW, Martin DR, Hoffman JR, Mower WR. Use of flexion–extension radiographs of the cervical spine in blunt trauma. *Ann Emerg Med*. 2001;38:8–11.
39. Frank JB, Lim CK, Flynn JM, Dormans JP. The efficacy of magnetic resonance imaging in pediatric cervical spine clearance. *Spine*. 2002;27:1176–1179.
40. Brady WJ, Moghtader J, Cutcher D, Exline C, Young J. ED use of flexion–extension cervical spine radiography in the evaluation of blunt trauma. *Am J Emerg Med*. 1999;17:504–508.
41. Ralston ME, Chung K, Barnes PD, Emans JB, Schutzman SA. Role of flexion–extension radiographs in blunt pediatric cervical spine injury. *Acad Emerg Med*. 2001;8:237–245.
42. Dwek JR, Chung CB. Radiography of cervical spine injury in children: are flexion–extension radiographs useful for acute trauma? *AJR Am J Roentgenol*. 2000;174:1617–1619.
43. Brown CV, Antevil JL, Sise MJ, Sack DI. Spiral computed tomography for the diagnosis of cervical, thoracic, and lumbar spine fractures: its time has come. *J Trauma*. 2005;58:890–895; discussion 895–896.
44. Koyanagi I, Iwasaki Y, Hida K, Akino M, Imamura H, Abe H. Acute cervical cord injury without fracture or dislocation of the spinal column. *J Neurosurg*. 2000;93:15–20.
45. Klein GR, Vaccaro AR, Albert TJ, et al. Efficacy of magnetic resonance imaging in the evaluation of posterior cervical spine fractures. *Spine*. 1999;24:771–774.
46. Katzberg RW, Benedetti PF, Drake CM, et al. Acute cervical spine injuries: prospective MR imaging assessment at a level 1 trauma center. *Radiology*. 1999;213:203–212.
47. Stabler A, Eck J, Penning R, et al. Cervical spine: postmortem assessment of accident injuries – comparison of radiographic, MR imaging, anatomic, and pathologic findings. *Radiology*. 2001;221:340–346.
48. Keiper MD, Zimmerman RA, Bilaniuk LT. MRI in the assessment of the supportive soft tissues of the cervical spine in acute trauma in children. *Neuroradiology*. 1998;40:359–363.
49. Dickman CA, Zabramski JM, Hadley MN, Rekate HL, Sonntag VK. Pediatric spinal cord injury without radiographic abnormalities: report of 26 cases and review of the literature. *J Spinal Disord*. 1991;4:296–305.
50. D'Alise MD, Benzel EC, Hart BL. Magnetic resonance imaging evaluation of the cervical spine in the comatose or obtunded trauma patient. *J Neurosurg*. 1999;91:54–59.
51. Benzel EC, Hart BL, Ball PA, Baldwin NG, Orrison WW, Espinosa MC. Magnetic resonance imaging for the evaluation of patients with occult cervical spine injury. *J Neurosurg*. 1996;85:824–829.

52. Grabb PA, Pang D. Magnetic resonance imaging in the evaluation of spinal cord injury without radiographic abnormality in children. *Neurosurgery*. 1994;35:406–414; discussion 414.
53. Silberstein M, Tress BM, Hennessy O. Prevertebral swelling in cervical spine injury: identification of ligament injury with magnetic resonance imaging. *Clin Radiol*. 1992;46:318–323.
54. Sanchez B, Waxman K, Jones T, Conner S, Chung R, Becerra S. Cervical spine clearance in blunt trauma: evaluation of a computed tomography-based protocol. *J Trauma*. 2005;59:179–183.
55. Schuster R, Waxman K, Sanchez B, et al. Magnetic resonance imaging is not needed to clear cervical spines in blunt trauma patients with normal computed tomographic results and no motor deficits. *Arch Surg*. 2005;140:762–766.
56. Sliker CW, Mirvis SE, Shanmuganathan K. Assessing cervical spine stability in obtunded blunt trauma patients: review of medical literature. *Radiology*. 2005;234:733–739.
57. Qaiyum M, Tyrrell PN, McCall IW, Cassar-Pullicino VN. MRI detection of unsuspected vertebral injury in acute spinal trauma: incidence and significance. *Skeletal Radiol*. 2001;30:299–304.
58. Shear P, Hugenholtz H, Richard MT, et al. Multiple noncontiguous fractures of the cervical spine. *J Trauma*. 1988;28:655–659.
59. Lee C, Rogers LF, Woodring JH, Goldstein SJ, Kim KS. Fractures of the craniovertebral junction associated with other fractures of the spine: overlooked entity? *AJNR Am J Neuroradiol*. 1984;5:775–781.
60. Hanson JA, Blackmore CC, Mann FA, Wilson AJ. Cervical spine injury: a clinical decision rule to identify high-risk patients for helical CT screening. *AJR Am J Roentgenol*. 2000;174:713–717.
61. Beggs I, Addison J. Posterior vertebral rim fractures. *Br J Radiol*. 1998;71:567–572.
62. Silberstein M, Tress BM, Hennessy O. Prediction of neurologic outcome in acute spinal cord injury: the role of CT and MR. *AJNR Am J Neuroradiol*. 1992;13:1597–1608.
63. Flanders AE, Schaefer DM, Doan HT, Mishkin MM, Gonzalez CF, Northrup BE. Acute cervical spine trauma: correlation of MR imaging findings with degree of neurologic deficit. *Radiology*. 1990;177:25–33.
64. Oner FC, van Gils AP, Faber JA, Dhert WJ, Verbout AJ. Some complications of common treatment schemes of thoracolumbar spine fractures can be predicted with magnetic resonance imaging: prospective study of 53 patients with 71 fractures. *Spine*. 2002;27:629–636.
65. Hendey GW, Wolfson AB, Mower WR, Hoffman JR. Spinal cord injury without radiographic abnormality: results of the National Emergency X-Radiography Utilization Study in blunt cervical trauma. *J Trauma*. 2002;53:1–4.
66. Brooks RA, Willett KM. Evaluation of the Oxford protocol for total spinal clearance in the unconscious trauma patient. *J Trauma*. 2001;50:862–867.
67. Sees DW, Rodriguez Cruz LR, Flaherty SF, Ciceri DP. The use of bedside fluoroscopy to evaluate the cervical spine in obtunded trauma patients. *J Trauma*. 1998;45:768–771.
68. Anglen J, Metzler M, Bunn P, Griffiths H. Flexion and extension views are not cost-effective in a cervical spine clearance protocol for obtunded trauma patients. *J Trauma*. 2002;52:54–59.
69. Bolinger B, Shartz M, Marion D. Bedside fluoroscopic flexion and extension cervical spine radiographs for clearance of the cervical spine in comatose trauma patients. *J Trauma*. 2004;56:132–136.
70. Freedman I, van Gelderen D, Cooper DJ, et al. Cervical spine assessment in the unconscious trauma patient: a major trauma service's experience with passive flexion–extension radiography. *J Trauma*. 2005;58:1183–1188.
71. Dormans JP. Evaluation of children with suspected cervical spine injury. *Instr Course Lect*. 2002;51:401–410.
72. Harrison JL, Ostlere SJ. Diagnosing purely ligamentous injuries of the cervical spine in the unconscious trauma patient. *Br J Radiol*. 2004;77:276–278.
73. Leibl T, Funke M, Dresing K, Grabbe E. [Instability of spinal fractures – therapeutic relevance of different classifications]. *Rofo Fortschr Geb Rontgenstr Neuen Bildgeb Verfahr*. 1999;170:174–180.
74. Petersilge CA, Pathria MN, Emery SE, Masaryk TJ. Thoracolumbar burst fractures: evaluation with MR imaging. *Radiology*. 1995;194:49–54.
75. Oner FC, Ramos LM, Simmermacher RK, et al. Classification of thoracic and lumbar spine fractures: problems of reproducibility. A study of 53 patients using CT and MRI. *Eur Spine J*. 2002;11:235–245.
76. Oner FC, van Gils AP, Dhert WJ, Verbout AJ. MRI findings of thoracolumbar spine fractures: a categorisation based on MRI examinations of 100 fractures. *Skeletal Radiol*. 1999;28:433–443.
77. Lee JY, Vaccaro AR, Lim MR, et al. Thoracolumbar injury classification and severity score: a new paradigm for the treatment of thoracolumbar spine trauma. *J Orthop Sci*. 2005;10:671–675.
78. Berne JD, Velmahos GC, El-Tawil Q, et al. Value of complete cervical helical computed tomographic scanning in identifying cervical spine injury in the unevaluable blunt trauma patient with multiple injuries: a prospective study. *J Trauma*. 1999;47:896–902; discussion 902–893.
79. Nunez DB, Jr., Zuluaga A, Fuentes-Bernardo DA, Rivas LA, Becerra JL. Cervical spine trauma: how much more do we learn by routinely using helical CT? *Radiographics*. 1996;16:1307–1318; discussion 1318–1321.
80. Nunez DB, Jr., Quencer RM. The role of helical CT in the assessment of cervical spine injuries. *AJR Am J Roentgenol*. 1998;171:951–957.
81. Ptak T, Kihiczak D, Lawrason N, et al. Screening for cervical spine trauma with helical CT: experience with 676 cases. *Emergency Radiology*. 2001;8:315–319.
82. Rybicki F, Nawfel RD, Judy PF, et al. Skin and Thyroid Dosimetry in Cervical Spine Screening: Two Methods for Evaluation and a Comparison Between a Helical CT and Radiographic Trauma Series. *Am J Roentgenol*. 2002;179:933–937.
83. Berrington de Gonzalez A, Darby S. Risk of cancer from diagnostic X-rays: estimates for the UK and 14 other countries. *Lancet*. 2004;363:345–351.
84. Blackmore CC, Ramsey SD, Mann FA, Deyo RA. Cervical spine screening with CT in trauma patients: a cost-effectiveness analysis. *Radiology*. 1999;212:117–125.
85. Blackmore CC, Emerson SS, Mann FA, Koepsell TD. Cervical spine imaging in patients with trauma: determination of fracture risk to optimize use. *Radiology*. 1999;211:759–765.
86. Griffen MM, Frykberg ER, Kerwin AJ, et al. Radiographic clearance of blunt cervical spine injury: plain radiograph or computed tomography scan? *J Trauma*. 2003;55:222–226; discussion 226–227.
87. Viccellio P, Simon H, Pressman BD, Shah MN, Mower WR, Hoffman JR. A prospective multicenter study of cervical spine injury in children. *Pediatrics*. 2001;108:E20.
88. France JC, Bono CM, Vaccaro AR. Initial radiographic evaluation of the spine after trauma: when, what, where, and how to image the acutely traumatized spine. *J Orthop Trauma*. 2005;19:640–649.
89. Holmes JF, Akkinepalli R. Computed tomography versus plain radiography to screen for cervical spine injury: a meta-analysis. *J Trauma*. 2005;58:902–905.
90. Bub LD, Blackmore CC, Mann FA, Lomoschitz FM. Cervical spine fractures in patients 65 years and older: a clinical prediction rule for blunt trauma. *Radiology*. 2005;234:143–149.
91. Stroh G, Braude D. Can an out-of-hospital cervical spine clearance protocol identify all patients with injuries? An argument for selective immobilization. *Ann Emerg Med*. 2001;37:609–615.
92. Domeier RM, Swor RA, Evans RW, et al. Multicenter prospective validation of prehospital clinical spinal clearance criteria. *J Trauma*. 2002;53:744–750.
93. Domeier RM. Indications for prehospital spinal immobilization. National Association of EMS Physicians Standards and Clinical Practice Committee. *Prehosp Emerg Care*. 1999;3:251–253.
94. Hauswald M, Ong G, Tandberg D, Omar Z. Out-of-hospital spinal immobilization: its effect on neurologic injury. *Acad Emerg Med*. 1998;5:214–219.

95. Podolsky SM, Hoffman JR, Pietrafesa CA. Neurologic complications following immobilization of cervical spine fracture in a patient with ankylosing spondylitis. *Ann Emerg Med.* 1983;12:578–580.
96. Domeier RM, Evans RW, Swor RA, et al. The reliability of prehospital clinical evaluation for potential spinal injury is not affected by the mechanism of injury. *Prehosp Emerg Care.* 1999;3:332–337.
97. Webb JC, Munshi P, Saifuddin A, Birch R. The prevalence of spinal trauma associated with brachial plexus injuries. *Injury.* 2002;33:587–590.
98. Connell RA, Graham CA, Munro PT. Is spinal immobilisation necessary for all patients sustaining isolated penetrating trauma? *Injury.* 2003;34:912–914.
99. Waters RL, Sie IH. Spinal cord injuries from gunshot wounds to the spine. *Clin Orthop.* 2003:120–125.
100. Apfelbaum JD, Cantrill SV, Waldman N. Unstable cervical spine without spinal cord injury in penetrating neck trauma. *Am J Emerg Med.* 2000;18:55–57.
101. Heary RF, Vaccaro AR, Mesa JJ, Balderston RA. Thoracolumbar infections in penetrating injuries to the spine. *Orthop Clin North Am.* 1996;27:69–81.
102. Moyed S, Shanmuganathan K, Mirvis SE, Bethel A, Rothman M. MR imaging of penetrating spinal trauma. *AJR Am J Roentgenol.* 1999;173:1387–1391.
103. Freemyer B, Knopp R, Piche J, Wales L, Williams J. Comparison of five-view and three-view cervical spine series in the evaluation of patients with cervical trauma. *Ann Emerg Med.* 1989;18:818–821.
104. Hernandez JA, Chupik C, Swischuk LE. Cervical spine trauma in children under 5 years: productivity of CT. *Emerg Radiol.* 2004;10:176–178.

4 Classification: Rationale and Relevance

F. C. Oner

Why Classify?

Fracture classification schemes have commonly been used in surgical practice. Most surgeons consider them necessary tools as a conceptual framework for diagnosis and treatment. Furthermore, these schemes are used as communication systems with regard to the relative severity of the injuries and the potential results of different treatment options. However, these schemes have been gradually introduced into the field without a proper discussion of their meanings and consequences. During the last decade the usefulness of these schemes has been a matter of intense debate. In a controversial editorial in the *Journal of Bone and Joint Surgery* in 1993, Albert Burstein asked in conjunction with two other articles in the same issue: "Fracture classification systems: Do they work and are they useful?"[3] As a scientist outside the field of surgical practice, he observed:

"Fracture classification systems are, in effect, tools. The purpose of the tool is to help the surgeon to choose an appropriate method of treatment for each and every fracture occurring in a particular anatomical region. The classification tool should not only suggest a method of treatment; it should also provide the surgeon with a reasonably precise estimation of the outcome of that treatment. Generally, we think of an orthopedic tool as working if it produces the same desired results, time after time, in the hands of anyone who is likely to use it. Thus, each practitioner should produce the same classification every time the same patient data are reviewed (intraobserver reliability or repeatability), and different practitioners should agree on the classification of the data for a particular patient (interobserver reliability)... To use this tool before its workability has been proved is inappropriate... Any classification scheme, be it nominal, ordinal, or scalar, should be proved to be a workable tool before it is used in a discriminatory or predictive manner...Once the tool has been shown to be functional, the next step in the process is to prove that it is useful. This step requires clinical studies in which the classification has been used as the basis for the choice of treatment."

The discussion of the value of such classification schemes began as a result of an evaluation of the Neer classification system for proximal humerus fractures, which proved to be a very unreliable scheme despite its widespread acceptance and use since 1970! If the orthopedic community has failed in the proper evaluation of something as relatively simple as fractures of the proximal humerus, what are clinicians to think of classification schemes for complex injuries of a compound structure such as the spine?

Classification of Thoracolumbar Spine Fractures

There has indeed been a great deal of controversy concerning the classification of fractures of the thoracolumbar spine. A plausible classification of these injuries was only possible after reliable imaging of the spine with proper radiographs became available on a large scale. After the first attempts at classification by Böhler in 1929, many authors recognized the difficulty of a comprehensive classification.[2] The main difficulty lies in the fact that: (a) unlike the fractures of long bones, the pattern of spine fractures may be progressive, evolving into an increasing deformity even after apparent union of the fractured spine; and (b) fractures of the spine represent complex injuries of a structure composed of parts each with a different susceptibility to injury and different healing potentials. Böhler recognized five types of injury:
1. Compression fracture with vertebral body injury.
2. Flexion-distraction injuries with anterior injury due to compression fracture and posterior injury due to distraction.
3. Extension fractures with injury to the anterior and posterior longitudinal ligaments and posterior arch injuries.
4. Shear fractures.
5. Torsion injuries.

The following efforts of Watson-Jones and Nicoll were more directed towards defining instability patterns so that the classification could be used as a predictive tool and a guide for treatment.[29,18] Watson-Jones was the first who introduced the concept of "instability." He recognized the importance of ligamentous injuries for the stability of the spinal column. Nicoll,[18] on the basis of a study of 166 fractures and fracture-dislocations in 152 miners during the period 1939–1945, classified the fractures on an anatomical basis into four main types:
- Anterior wedge fracture.
- Lateral wedge fracture.
- Fracture-dislocation.
- Isolated fracture of the neural arch.

Recognizing the role of different structures in the generation of different patterns of fractures, he pointed out four different structures involved: the vertebral body, the disk, the intervertebral joints, and the interspinous ligament. He called the disk the fulcrum of the motion segment. He also referred to the importance of differentiating between stable and un-

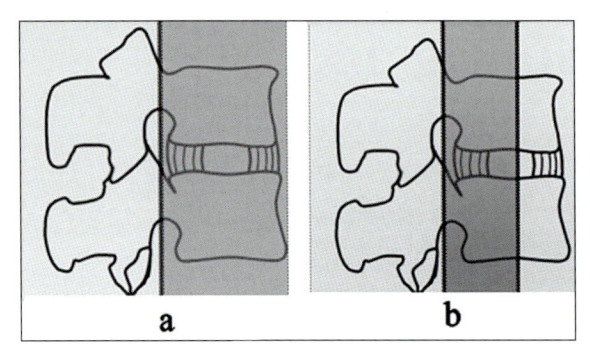

Fig. 4.1 **a** The two columns of Holdsworth. **b** The three columns of Denis.

stable varieties and the danger of increasing neurology or increasing deformity of unstable injuries.

Holdsworth tried to capture the problem of stability in the columnar spine.[8] He tried to abstract the vertebral stability with an architectonic two-column concept (Fig. 4.**1a**). This concept has been influential ever since. His anterior column consisted of the vertebral bodies and the intervertebral disk. He called the posterior column the "posterior ligament complex" consisting of the facet joints, the intraspinous and supraspinous ligaments, and the ligamenta flava. In his theory the integrity of this posterior column is crucial for the stability of the spine. He called all injury patterns with an intact posterior column stable. He classified injuries into six groups:
- Anterior wedge compression.
- Dislocation.
- Fracture/dislocation by rotation.
- Extension injury.
- Burst fractures.
- Shear fractures.

He was the first to introduce the concept of the "burst fracture," which he described as a result of compression force rupturing one of the endplates and forcing the disk into the body of the vertebra causing it to burst out. Although the concept of Holdsworth remained influential throughout the 1960s and 1970s, it was severely criticized from the outset. Kelly and Whitesides demonstrated that bony fragments retropulsed from the body in burst fractures, which gave them a high potential for instability.[9] Roberts and Curtiss were the first to point to the late progression of deformities in the burst fractures, with possible neurological consequences.[26] Roy-Camille and Demeulenaer emphasized in that context the role of their *segment moyen*, formed by the posterior part of the disk, annulus fibrosus, and the posterior longitudinal ligament, together with the pedicles and the facet joints.[27] Louis tried to elaborate the spinal column concept with the introduction of a three-column architecture of the spine.[14]

The Three-Column CT Era

The introduction of computed tomography (CT) in the second half of the 1970s for spinal fractures provided new insight into the fine structural details of these injuries. The possibility of imaging the spine in transverse sections drew attention to the comminution of fractures and canal encroachment, which would not even have been suspected with traditional radiographs. These CT findings had a large impact on the thinking concerning a new classification system, based on the more accurate description of the extent and place of injury now possible. McAfee et al, in their extensive studies showed the indispensability of computed tomography for an exact description of the injuries.[16] Efforts in this direction in the early 1980s culminated in the three-column concept of Denis, which has become the dominant classification system (Fig. 4.**1b**).[4]

Denis classified fractures into four types (Fig. 4.**2**):
- **Compression fractures**: Failure under compression of the anterior column. The middle column is intact.
- **Burst fractures**: Failure of anterior and middle columns under axial loads.
- **Seat-belt injuries**: Failure of both the posterior and middle columns under tension forces generated by flexion and distraction.
- **Fracture dislocations**: Failure of all columns under compression, tension, rotation or shear.

Denis also introduced the concept of different degrees of instability:
- Instability of the first degree is a mechanical instability with risk of progressive kyphosis.
- Instability of the second degree is a neurological instability.
- Instability of the third degree is both a mechanical and a neurological instability. Fracture/dislocations and unstable burst fractures are in this category.

Although this classification was a refinement of the understanding of the nature of these injuries, it was amenable to many simplifications and led to some confusion that still exists. As usual this scheme was also introduced without a proper analysis of reproducibility or predictive power. Although Denis emphasized that his columns are formed by osseous and nonosseous structures, no attempt has been made to further the diagnosis of nonosseous injuries. The three-column concept was reduced to what is visible with transverse CT images. It has been simplified and reduced to a simple rule of thumb, which states that any injury to two of the three columns, as seen on CT (bony injury), make the spine unstable. Further, an intact middle column has been seen as a guarantee of stability, although Denis mentioned some of these lesions as being first-degree unstable. Also the differentiation between first, second, and third degree instability has been lost, leading to a vague, poorly defined and alarming instability concept, which has remained dominant during the past two decades.

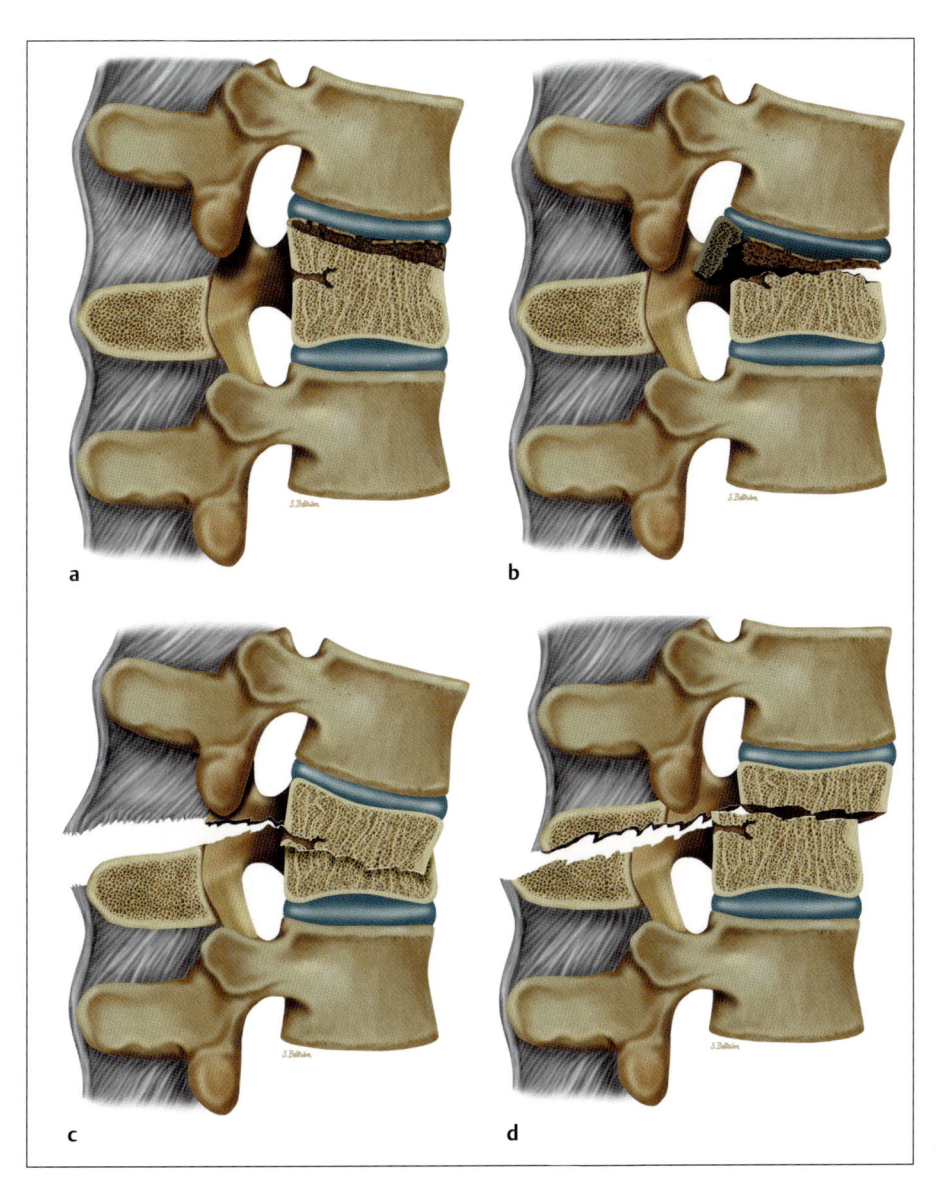

Fig. 4.2 **Denis classification.** **a** Compression; **b** Burst; **c** Seat-belt; **d** Fracture-dislocation.

Despite its widespread acceptance there has been criticism of the Denis classification and attempts have been made to modify it from the beginning. Ferguson and Allen called the columns a poor semantic choice because these tissues do not anatomically or biomechanically resemble a column.[6] They argued: "the term, although appealing for its verbal ring, is anatomically and biomechanically incorrect." They suggested a mechanistic classification instead, according to a presumed mechanism of injury deduced from the patterns of tissue failure. McAfee et al suggested a division of the burst fractures as stable and unstable.[16] Finally, Farcy et al modified the Denis classification to include both bone and soft tissue injuries in each of the three columns of a motion segment.[5] They developed a scheme of instability graded from 1 to 6, with injuries greater than or equal to grade 3 being unstable. But they also failed to develop diagnostic means to make the distinction between bone and soft tissue injuries.

The Load-Sharing Classification

Dissatisfaction with these vague concepts led to attempts to define some specific questions disturbing the practitioners. One of the most remarkable attempts was the load-sharing classification proposed by McCormak et al in 1994.[17] This scheme is a specific elaboration of the Denis system with a specific problem in mind. The authors were disturbed by the high rate of failure of posterior fixation in their patients with some types of fractures, and searched for factors predictive of this failure. Their conclusion was that the degree of comminution of the vertebral body together with the apposition of fragments and the degree of deformity correction were factors predictive of the failure of posterior fixation. The authors developed a system of rating as follows:

A: Comminution of the vertebral body: little (1), more (2), gross (3 points).

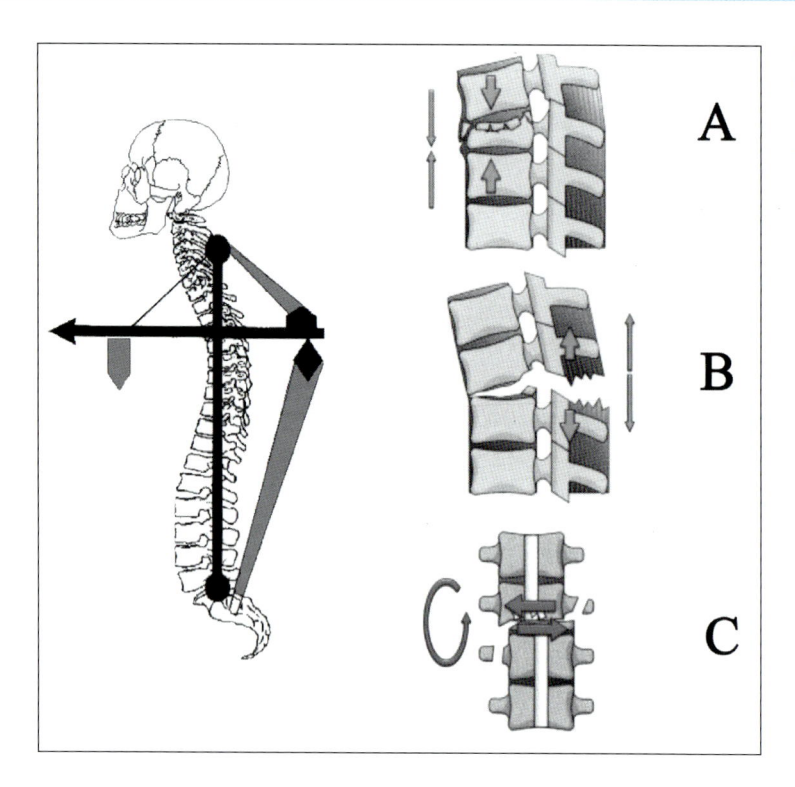

Fig. 4.3 **Comprehensive classification (AO) is based on the crane model.** Type A: caused predominantly by compression; Type B: transverse disruption; Type C: rotation or translation.

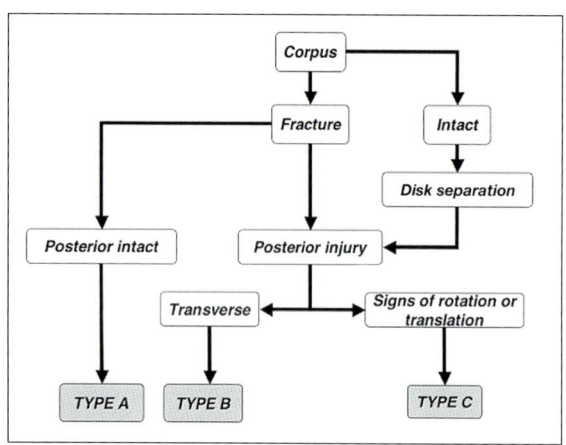

Fig. 4.4 Flow diagram for determining the type level of the AO classification.

B: Apposition of fragments: minimal (1), spread (2), wide (3 points).
C: Deformity correction: little (1), more (2), most (3 points).

They observed that, in their series of 28 patients, all 10 cases with a screw fracture had a sum of 7 or more points, and no patient with a sum of 6 or less points had a screw fracture.

The AO (Comprehensive) Classification

The classification scheme of the AO group is a culmination of efforts of many practitioners over a 10-year period.[15] This scheme is primarily based upon the pathomorphological characteristics of the injuries and is based on the mechanical model of a crane. Three main categories with a common injury pattern, classified as types, are formed (Fig. 4.3):
Type A: Vertebral body compression.
Type B: Anterior and posterior element injury with distraction.
Type C: Anterior and posterior element injury with rotation or translation.

The authors abandoned the three-column concept and went back to the two-column concept of Holdsworth, i.e., an anterior column consisting of the vertebral body and the disk, and a posterior complex. They also depended on the mechanistic classification of Ferguson and Allen for identification of common denominators of the types: type A injuries represent compression forces, type B tensile forces, and type C axial torque or shear (Fig. 4.4). A biomechanical study showed a good relation between this type categorization of the scheme and the resulting mechanical instability in a cadaveric fracture model.[11] For further subclassification, the authors used the common AO 3–3-3 grid. Subclassification of the type B and C injuries essentially follows the subclassification of type A injuries (Fig. 4.5).

Type A injuries: Injuries caused mainly by axial compression causing predominantly injury to the anterior elements (vertebral body and disk). There is no or insignificant injury to the tension band function of the posterior column. The subclasses of type A:
A1: **Impaction fractures.** The deformation of the vertebral body is due to compression (plastic deformation) of the cancellous bone rather than fragmentation.
A1.1: Endplate impaction with minor wedging up to 5°.
A1.2: Wedge impaction with loss of anterior vertebral height resulting in an angulation of more than 5°.

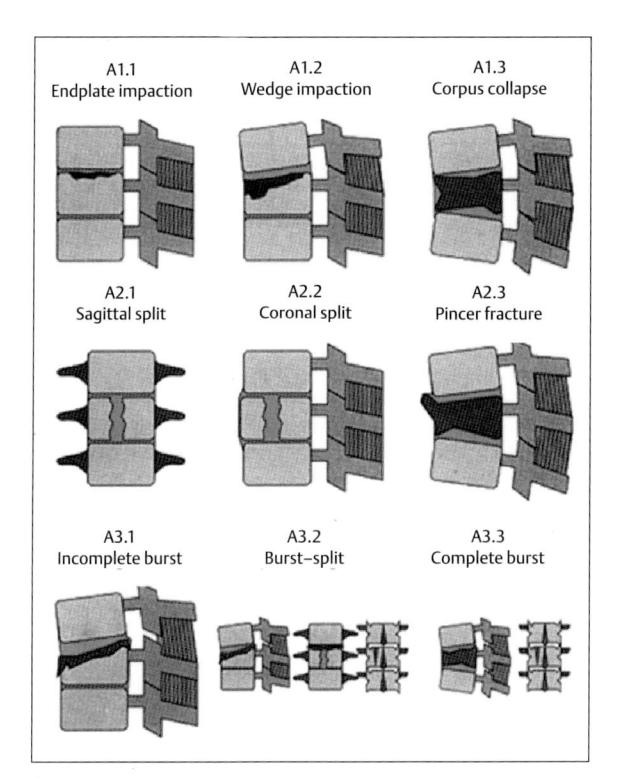

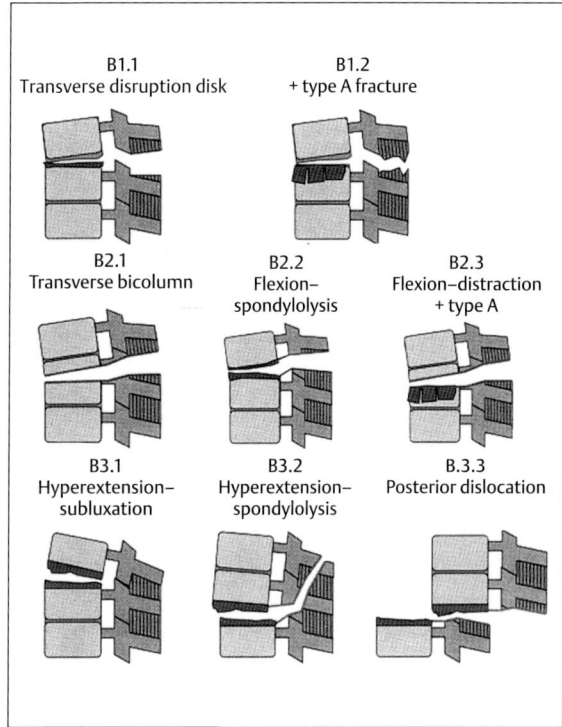

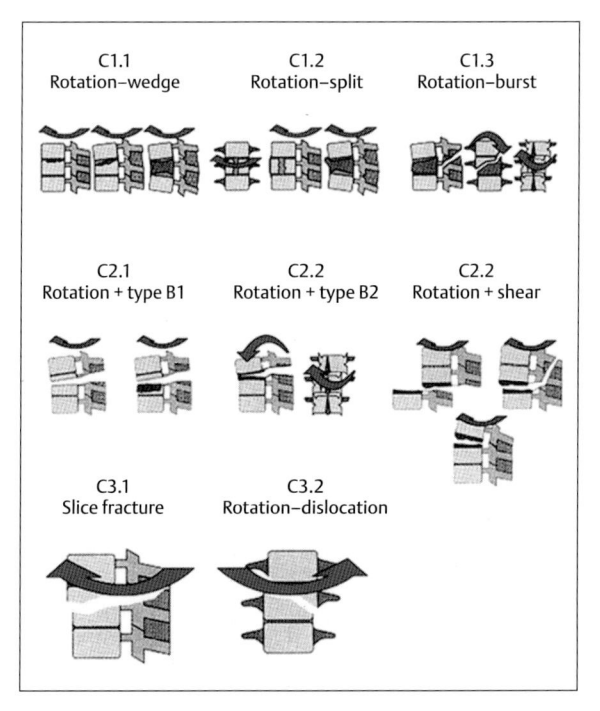

Fig. 4.5 Subclassifications of the main AO types.

A1.3: Vertebral body collapse. Symmetrical loss of vertebral body such as observed in osteoporotic spines without significant extrusion of fragments.
A2: **Split fractures.** The vertebral body is split in the coronal or sagittal plane with dislocation of fragments and filling of the defect with disk material.
A2.1: Sagittal split fractures.
A2.2: Coronal split fractures.
A2.3: Pincer fracture, in which the central part of the body is crushed and filled with disk material.
A3: **Burst fractures** with fragments of posterior wall extruding into the canal.
A3.1: Incomplete burst fractures. Burst of the upper or lower half of the body.
A3.2: Burst-split fracture. Burst of one-half of the vertebra and split of the rest.
A3.3: Complete burst fracture. Entire body is burst.

Type B injuries: The main criterion is a transverse disruption of one or both spinal columns leading to failure of the tension band. The subclasses of type B:
- **B1:** Posterior disruption predominantly ligamentous.
- **B1.1:** Associated with transverse disruption of the disk.
- **B1.2:** Associated with type A fracture of the vertebral body.
- **B2:** Posterior disruption predominantly osseous.
- **B2.1:** Transverse bicolumn fracture.
- **B2.2:** Posterior disruption predominantly osseous with transverse disruption of the disk.
- **B2.3:** Posterior disruption predominantly osseous associated with type A fracture of the vertebral body.
- **B3:** Anterior disruption through the disk.
- **B3.1:** Hyperextension–subluxation.
- **B3.2:** Hyperextension–spondylolysis.
- **B3.3:** Posterior dislocation.

Type C injuries: Anterior and posterior element injuries with rotation or translation. Two-column injury with rotational and/or translational displacement. Subtypes:
- **C1:** Type A with rotation.
- **C1.1:** Rotation + wedge fracture.
- **C1.2:** Rotation + split fracture.
- **C1.3:** Rotation + burst fracture.
- **C2:** Type B with rotation.
- **C2.1:** Rotation + type B1.
- **C2.2:** Rotation + type B2.
- **C2.3:** Rotation + type B3.
- **C3:** Rotational shear injuries.
- **C3.1:** Slice fracture.
- **C3.2:** Rotation–dislocation.

This classification represents a taxonomic beauty in that each and every injury can be fitted to a certain category in ever-expanding detail. But one should not forget that the dream of a taxonomist might be the nightmare of a practitioner. Although conceptually sound, the *apparent* complexity frightened many practitioners and obstructed the diffusion of the basic ideas behind this sophisticated scheme.

Influence of Imaging Modality

Although all authors have been emphasizing the importance of soft-tissue injury and included these in their classification schemes, there were no clinical or radiological means to detect them with conventional means. The introduction of MRI offered the possibility of directly imaging all structures involved. Some early studies showed ligamentous involvement, which would be unsuspected on radiographs and CT scans.[25] Two cadaver studies in the 1990s showed excellent correlation between MRI findings and anatomical sections. Kliewer et al showed in a cadaver study good correlation between MR images and anatomical sections of acute spinal ligament disruption.[10] In a similar study, Oner et al reported perfect correlation between MRI images and anatomical sections of injuries to the disks and vertebral bodies.[20] These studies established MRI as a highly accurate modality for determining injury patterns and described the MRI features of the different structures involved. In their 1996 review article concerning the role of imaging in the diagnosis and management of thoracolumbar fractures, Saifuddin et al concluded that any future classification of thoracolumbar injuries should include MRI findings, allowing for an assessment of the disko-ligamentous element of the injury as well as of the bony element.[28] Oner et al have categorized the MRI findings of thoracolumbar spine fractures in a prospective study of 100 fractures (Fig. 4.**6**). Categorizing all possibly relevant structures (ALL, PLL, PLC, endplate, disk, and vertebral body), they found a wide variation of injury patterns in most cases unsuspected on conventional radiograms and CT scans.[21] The clinical relevance of these findings is not in every case evident. In the follow-up of 53 of these patients some interesting correlations with the final clinical and radiological results were reported.[23] An unfavorable outcome in the conservative group was related to the progression of kyphosis, which in most cases was predictable with the use of trauma MRI findings concerning the endplate comminution and vertebral body involvement. In the operatively treated group, recurrence of the kyphotic deformity was predictable by the lesion of the posterior longitudinal ligamentary complex together with endplate comminution and vertebral body involvement as seen on trauma MRI. The same authors also tried to redefine the AO classification using the MRI categorization scheme.[21] Although it seemed possible to define the different types, groups, and subgroups of the AO classification using this scheme, the authors concluded that this classification does not capture all the variations in the parameters defined. Using their criteria based on MRI findings, they found that 28 fractures had to be reallocated, 16 of them being major shifts between Type A and Type B. Since the advent of the AO classification and the following MRI studies, more attention has been paid to the injuries of the posterior ligamentous complex. Leferink et al reported that at least in 30% of their cases, PLC injuries went undetected with conventional methods.[12] Lee et al compared MRI with peroperative findings of PLC injuries and found that the fat-suppressed T2W sagittal sequence of MRI was a highly sensitive, specific, and accurate method for evaluating posterior ligament complex injury.[13]

Another point, which was insufficiently addressed in existing schemes, was the fate of the intervertebral disk. Changes in the disk space were frequently observed and were incriminated for progressive or recurrent kyphosis. Although it was assumed that this represented a process similar to the degenerative disk disease, Oner et al showed that in the majority of the cases the disks did not resemble degenerative disk disease patterns.[19] On the basis of a MRI study of 63 patients at a minimum of 18 months post-trauma, a classification scheme of the post-traumatic disk types was developed. They con-

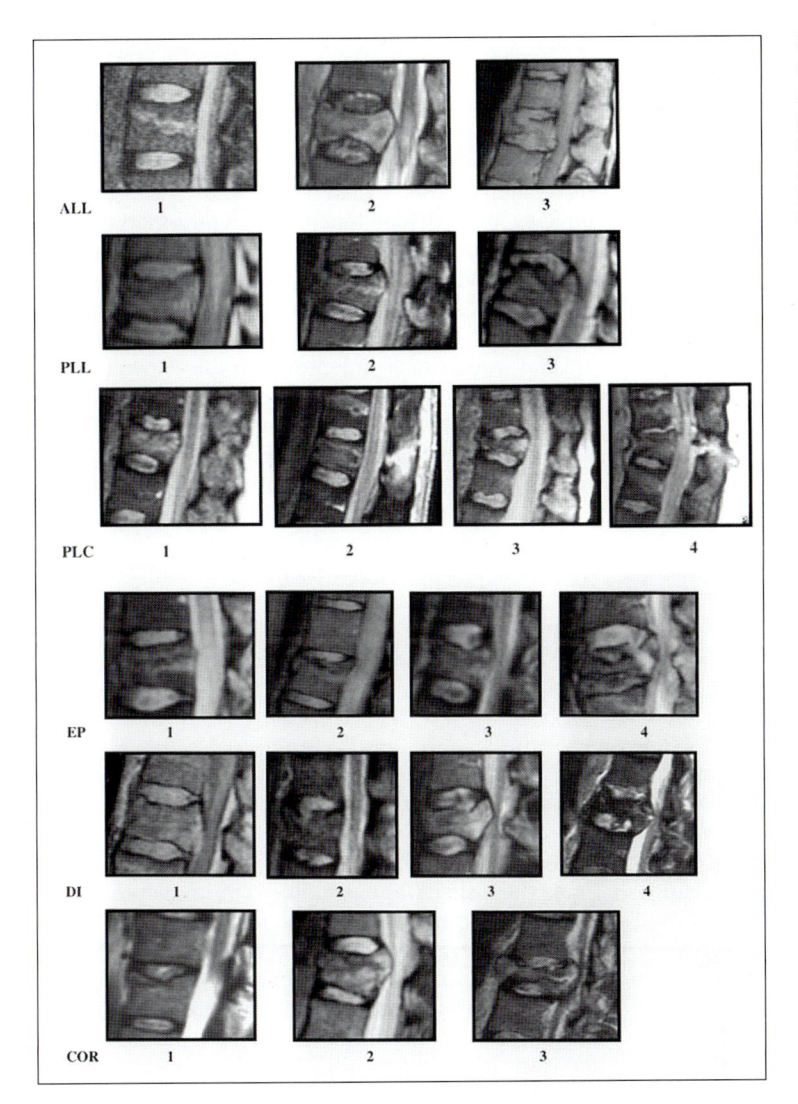

Fig. 4.6 **Categorization scheme developed by Oner et al for MR images.** ALL: anterior longitudinal ligament; PLL: posterior longitudinal ligament; PLC: posterior ligamentary complex; EP: endplate; DI: disk; COR: corpus (vertebral body). (Reprinted with permission from Springer Verlag GmbH.[21])

cluded that the majority of the disks showed predominantly morphological changes with no change in signal intensity. Some disk types were associated with progressive kyphosis in the conservatively treated patients. In the operatively treated patients recurrent kyphosis seemed to have resulted from the creeping of the disk in the central depression of the bony endplate rather than from disk degeneration.

Although these studies established MRI as a highly sensitive imaging modality capable of detecting all kinds of injury to a fractured spine, they do not yet provide answers to some of the essential problems of creating meaningful classification schemes.

Problems of Reproducibility

One of the main purposes of classification systems is to create a common language for use between the investigators of the field. This requires an acceptable degree of interobserver agreement on the main distinctions of a scheme. Also, each investigator or clinician should be able to reproduce the same classification on different occasions, i. e., the scheme should also have reasonable intraobserver repeatability. Both have been problematic with fracture classification systems in general. To understand these problems, we should first discuss what a fracture classification scheme actually does.[24]

A classification system is based upon a presumption about an underlying common characteristic of the subsets of a domain. In the case of a fracture classification system this is based upon the presumption that the interaction of various forces with the parts of a living organism involved create some basic observable patterns. The main difficulty of all fracture classification schemes lies in the innumerable variables involved in a traumatic lesion. The classification has to presuppose an all or none result of some of the interactions. A classification scheme tries to compress the available information into reproducible categories without loss of information content, which means that it is an *algorithmic compression process*. It is then inevitable that two kinds of problems arise with categorization schemes. Either there is a loss of information content in favor of simplicity and thus higher reproducibility, or a loss of simplicity and reproducibility in favor of higher fidelity to the information content. Changes in the information content, for example as a result of novel technology may have different effects on these two different strategies.

The most commonly used classification systems during the last decade, the Denis scheme and the AO (comprehensive) classification, have been introduced without proper studies of their reproducibility. Studies later performed by independent groups raised serious concerns about the reproducibility issues.

Blauth et al conducted a multi-center study to assess the interobserver reliability of the AO classification system using the radiographs of 14 fractures of the lumbar spine.[1] The radiographs and CT scans were reviewed in 22 hospitals experienced with spinal trauma. The mean interobserver agreement for all 14 cases was found to be 67% (41–91%), when only the three main types (A, B, C) were used. The corresponding kappa value, however, of the interobserver reliability showed a coefficient of 0.33 (range 0.30 to 0.35) indicating fair reliability. The reliability decreased by increasing the categories. Oner et al studied the reproducibility of the Denis and AO schemes using radiographs, CT, and MRI in 53 patients.[22] Five observers of varying professions and experience (one general trauma surgeon, one neuroradiologist, one orthopedic spine surgeon, and two orthopedic residents) were involved. They found that the main distinction of the AO system at the primary type level (A/nonA) was fairly reproducible with CTs (κ 0.34). With MRI this reached only moderate levels (κ 0.42). The same was true for type (A, B, C) distinction (CT: κ 0.35; MRI: κ 0.39). Subclassification of type A (groups) yielded higher kappa values corresponding to substantial agreement (CT: κ 0.61; MRI: κ 0.73), which dropped with the A subgroups (CT: κ 0.37; MRI: κ 0.34). Intraobserver kappa values between CT and MRI readings were A/nonA 0.45, for type 0.41, for A group 0.76, and for A subgroup 0.47.

The agreement was in general better with the Denis classification (CT type κ: 0.60; CT whole classification κ 0.45, MRI type: κ 0.52; MRI whole classification 0.39) but the variance was higher due to the difficulties of determining the proper categories for some injury patterns.

Thus, the AO scheme seems to choose fidelity to the information content by providing categories for all kinds of possible injury patterns. This leads inevitably to an increase in the complexity of the scheme but also provides a means for classification in accordance with increasing information content following novel technology. However, although the AO scheme recognizes the difference in injuries with or without transverse plane soft-tissue involvement, the means to make this distinction reliable were not sufficiently explored. The classification presupposes that the posterior ligamentary complex is either injured or not although the authors recognize that transient forms do exist. However mechanically sound this distinction may be, in reality one observes varying *degrees* of involvement of the posterior ligamentary complex. It is not clear which MRI findings are indicative of *mechanically significant* failure of the tension band system.

The Denis classification was based on the, for that time, novel technology of transverse CT images and represents a strategy of simplification. Refinement of the imaging technology in the form of CT-MPR and MR imaging proved that much of the information from these new modalities is difficult to integrate into this scheme. Much of the ligamentous involvement of the posterior column cannot be accounted for in the scheme. As a result, either injury patterns with or without posterior ligamentous complex involvement are grouped together into categories based upon the patterns of bony involvement, or injury patterns with posterior ligamentous complex involvement are assigned to higher categories constituting an overestimation of the severity. In the study of Oner et al, the more experienced observer assigned more often these injuries to higher categories, leading to a marked variance in the results. This type of confusion may have contributed in the past to the widely different results of conservative treatment strategies reported in the literature.

The Concept of Stability

This continuing effort to classify spinal fractures reflects the difficulties encountered in prediction of the stability of these injuries. Stability has been a major issue in spine surgery in general, but it has been poorly defined and has led to different interpretations. Biomechanicians and clinicians tried to develop a reproducible stability concept. Nicoll defined the stability of the spine as a condition in which there is no increased deformity or neurological deficit over time.[18] Whitesides called a spine unstable if deformity progressively leads to increasing neurological compromise.[31] Denis' "degrees of instability" added to the confusion. White and Panjabi devised the most comprehensive definition:[30]

"Clinical instability is defined as a loss in the ability of the spine under physiologic loads to maintain relationships between vertebrae in such a way that there is neither damage nor subsequent irritation to the spinal cord or nerve roots. In addition there is no development of incapacitating deformity or pain due to structural changes."

From this discussion we can conclude that a meaningful categorization of the stability of the spine is supposed to address different *kinds* of stability in place of different *degrees*. A surgeon confronted with a patient with a spinal fracture has the task of evaluating three *kinds* of stability:

- Immediate mechanical stability.
- Neurological stability.
- Long-term stability.

Any classification system or biomechanical concept should be able to provide the surgeon with reliable predictions about these different *kinds of stability*.

Do We Need Any Classification at All?

Following the criticism of Burstein and the disappointing results of reproducibility studies, there has been a growing skepticism among the scholars and practitioners concerning all efforts of classification in traumatology. The ever-increasing precision of our imaging technology has led some to take the view that a precise description of the injury patterns in spinal injury would be sufficient.[7] So the question arises whether we need any classification system at all. To answer this question we need to think about the efforts undertaken during the last century to develop classification schemes.[24]

Every classification scheme is actually a pattern recognition process. Which patterns are observable is also dependent on our level of knowledge and the technological means at our disposal. On the other hand, the recognition of different injury patterns only makes sense if it helps us to predict the final outcome better than a simple chance distribution. Recognition of some patterns of injury does not necessarily lead to a better understanding of the prognosis. Only when a relation can be shown between the observed patterns and certain outcome parameters can we speak of their prognostic significance. A classification scheme is actually a mental construct or a model of a complex phenomenon that is supposed to inform us about the severity of the injury and the possible consequences. This information should finally provide us with a reasonable estimation of the outcome of different treatment modalities. Creation of an abstract mental construct of a complex phenomenon is a complicated process. Two possible strategies can be used for this purpose:

One is the "top-down" strategy, which tries to recognize the patterns in some images of the injury and construct from there a mental picture of the *essence* of the injury. This strategy has led, for thoracolumbar spine fractures, to the creation of the architectonic concept of " spinal columns," which is supposed to provide information about the state of the lower-level structures, the components of the injured spine. This conceptualization, developed by Holdsworth in 1963, and based upon the descriptive classification schemes of Böhler and Nicoll, has been highly influential in shaping the approach to these injuries.[8] Many variations on this theme have been developed, following different strategies of refinements of the "columns" or by adding more columns to the scheme. However, one should never forget that these columns are mental constructs and do not correspond directly to any anatomical or biomechanical entity. This strategy is an "idealistic deduction," which carries the danger of reification of the mental construct. The "column" becomes a "thing" that is superimposed on reality in order to understand it. The result of this is that the mental construct, which has to be produced and reproduced each time by an observer in order to understand the injury, becomes a necessary component of the classification scheme. But reproduction of a mental construct is a highly subjective process, which makes the whole enterprise quite unstable and unreliable. In other words, one is never sure what others reconstruct in their minds as "columns," this being highly dependent on the personal experience of the observer with this mental construct in particular and mental abstractions in general. Besides, this deductive strategy leads to a certain rigidity of the whole enterprise, in that revision of the scheme to make it more congruent with novel information from new observations, for example as a result of a new imaging technology or substantial changes in injury patterns, requires the addition of new mental constructs, new columns, to the schemes. In short this strategy is not easily "evolvable" in accordance with new data.

Another strategy may be a "bottom-up" inductive process. In such a process, data are gathered about the states of individual clinical and radiological parameters. Then these data are used to investigate the prognostic significance of these individual parameters alone and in combination with each other. This process finally yields an information space of the various parameters together with their prognostic significance and their interparametric relations. At this stage, one can search in this particular information space for possible patterns in order to construct an abstract mental picture of the whole phenomenon through an algorithmic compression process. That means one can look for an abbreviated representation of all relevant observations in a shorthand formula. Meaningful patterns are probably to be found in this information space rather than in the sole space of imaging. Such a strategy would yield an "evolvable" pattern recognition process in which the changes in the information space, the congruence of the shorthand formulas, can be continuously tested and increased.

The development of the highly elaborate AO classification scheme has apparently been a mixture of these two strategies. Although there is emphasis on a detailed analysis of the component parts of an injured spine, the designers were still under the influence of a "top-down" strategy, which actually requires a pre-existent mental concept in order to make sense of these detailed analyses of the component parts. Besides, there is no analysis of the prognostic significance of these observed patterns and no clear strategy concerning the evolution of the scheme when new data are acquired.

Although Burstein's argument has been a valuable contribution to the discussion of uncritical development and use of classification schemes in orthopedics,[3] his "crude materialistic" approach to the problem can lead to a devaluation of all attempts to create mental tools in order to understand and to exchange information about phenomena encountered in orthopedic practice. Burstein compares fracture classification schemes to "appliances and tools" manufactured to perform a task efficiently. Hence, he argues that an orthopedic tool (a classification scheme) works only if it produces the same desired results, time after time, in the hands of anyone who is likely to use it. Therefore, "to use this tool before its workability is proved is inappropriate." Only if the tool has been shown to be functional, according to Burstein, can one go on to the next step of proving that it is useful in clinical studies in which the classification has been used as the basis for the choice of treatment. This is a serious confusion of levels of abstraction. A mental tool is in no ways comparable to a "manufactured" tool, which is the material result of a deliberate design process to perform a specific task. In sharp contrast, a mental tool, in this sense, is an iconic representation process, which involves the active creation of a mental image based on the sensory data of a complex observed reality. A mental picture is not a photographic picture but an active creation. Although the human mind is very competent in producing these mental images of complex observed phenomena in order to navigate in the dangerous world around him/her, it is very well known that this process is always an approximation strongly biased by the purposes of the subject. The consequence of this is: (a) this process cannot be perfectly repeatable by the same observer because it involves an active creation each time, under slightly different circumstances; and (b) the workability (repeatability) of the mental image is not separable from its usefulness (predictive power) because human minds do not create mental imagery of complex phenomena without a purpose. Another point is that these mental images are also "social constructs," created in an environment of incessant communication with other minds by way of this kind of symbolic imagery. This means that any classification scheme is also a "cultural" product, which is created in a social process of many interactions between different agents with various historical backgrounds. This introduces another important "noise" into the whole system, which makes a perfect interobserver repeatability impossible. Disregarding these aspects of classification systems in orthopedic practice, as is done by Burstein, would raise unrealistic expectations and can eventually undermine all the collective efforts for the creation of predictive tools. The most important property of a classification scheme is not its repeatability and usefulness, defined once and forever, but its capacity to evolve into forms with increasing repeatability and increasing predictive power during an active process of assessment, reassessment, and refinement by as many participants of the field as possible.

Our aim should be to create a "bottom-up" strategy in order to develop an "evolvable" process of thoracolumbar spine fracture classification, which can lead to an increasing predictive power of our mental pictures of these injuries with an increasing repeatability. Even highly sophisticated and detailed images such as those obtained with modern CT and MRI constitutes only a subset of the vast space of all things knowable about a patient with a broken spine. The choice for this particular subset is only justified if it in some way relates to a future event, such as final deformity, patient satisfaction etc., which may be interesting for our purposes of predicting the final outcome. A real understanding of a phenomenon, which is necessary for the development of a predictive tool, requires further conceptualization, i.e., a classification scheme. An abstract conceptualization is the creation of a model. From this particular subset of observational data, that is imaging findings and some clinical parameters such as age, sex, neurological status, etc., it is possible to create a limited number of models. These models can then be tested for their repeatability and their predictive power in order to find the best model with the available data. It is better to use an existing elaborate scheme, such as the AO classification, as a starting point for the development of a model. "Tinkering" may be a better strategy than the development of a whole new scheme.

Such a "bottom-up" strategy, of course, requires a vast amount of raw data in order to create schemes with the requested qualifications. Only multi-center prospective studies with standardized data acquisition protocols can achieve this. This should be seen as the real challenge for the practitioners of the field.

Meanwhile, we should not forget that there are no simple algorithms providing us with simple answers. Classification schemes are only mental tools, which may help us to make better "educated guesses" about the prognosis of our individual patients. No classification scheme is a substitute for sound clinical judgment and treatment protocols based solely on classification schemes may lead to dangerous oversimplifications. We should accept that we have only certain statistical truths for the subject, that we can only make predictions to a certain level of reliability at the moment, that our means of pattern recognition in spinal injury are not highly developed, that we will probably disagree from time to time, and that we all make less then accurate decisions quite often. But we should not lose sight of one concrete joint aim: to develop instruments of communication and education, which can assure that a larger number of surgeons make the right decisions more often so that our patients will suffer less disability and will be less unhappy.

References

1. Blauth M, Bastian L, Knop C, Lange U, Tusch G. Interobserverreliabilität bei der Klassifikation von thorakolumbalen Wirbelsäulenverletzungen. *Orthopäde*. 1999;28(8):662–681.
2. Böhler L. *Die Technik der Knochenbruchbehandlung im Frieden und im Kriege*. Vienna, Austria: Wilhelm Maudrich Verlag; 1929.
3. Burstein AH. Fracture classification systems: Do they work and are they useful? *J Bone Joint Surg*. 1993;75-A:1743–1744.
4. Denis F. The three-column spine and its significance in the classification of acute thoracolumbar spinal injuries. *Spine*. 1983;8:817–831.
5. Farcy JPC, Weidenbaum M, Glassman SD. Sagittal index in management of thoracolumbar burst fractures. *Spine*. 1990;15:958–965.
6. Ferguson RL, Allen BL. A mechanistic classification of thoracolumbar spine fractures. *Clin Orthop*. 1984;189:77–88.
7. Flanders AE. Imaging of thoracolumbar injury. American Academy of Orthopedic Surgeons, 66th annual meeting. Instructional Course Lecture 365:1999.
8. Holdsworth FW. Fractures, dislocations and fracture-dislocations of the spine. *J Bone Joint Surg*. 1963;45-B:6–20.

9. Kelly RP, Whitesides TE. Treatment of lumbodorsal fracture-dislocations. *Ann Surg.* 1968;167:705–717.
10. Kliewer MA, Gray L, Paver J, Richardson WD, Vogler JB, McElhaney JH, Myers BS. Acute spinal ligament disruption: MR imaging with anatomic correlation. *J Mag Resonan Imaging.* 1993; 3:855–861.
11. Lange U, Bastian L, Knop C, Blauth M. Stabilitätsverhalten verschiedener Verletzungen der thoracolumbalen Wirbelsäule. Eine biomechanische Studie. *Ned Tijd Traum.* Supplement 1998. Proceedings of the 3rd European Traumatology Congress; Amsterdam: 110.
12. Leferink VJM, Veldhuis EFM, Zimmerman KW, ten Vergert EM, ten Duis HJ. Classificational problems in ligamentary distraction type vertebral fractures: 30% of all B-type fractures are initially unrecognized. *Eur Spine J.* 2002;11:246–250.
13. Lee HM, Kim HS, Kim DJ, Suk KS, Park JO, Kim NH. Reliability of magnetic resonance imaging in detecting posterior ligament complex injury in thoracolumbar spinal fractures. *Spine.* 2000;25:2079–2084.
14. Louis R. Les theories de l'instabilité. *Rev Chir Orthop.* 1977;63: 423–425.
15. Magerl F, Aebi M, Gertzbein SD, Harms J, Nazarian S. A comprehensive classification of thoracic and lumbar injuries. *Eur Spine J.* 1994;3:184–201.
16. McAfee PC, Yuan HA, Frederickson BE, Lubicky JP. The value of computed tomography in thoracolumbar fracture. *J Bone Joint Surg.* 1983;65-A:461–473.
17. McCormack T, Karaikovic E, Gaines RW. The load-sharing classification of spine fractures. *Spine.* 1994; 19:1741–1744.
18. Nicoll EA. Fractures of the dorsolumbar spine. *J Bone Joint Surg.* 1949;31-B:376–394.
19. Oner FC, vd Rijt RHH, Ramos LMP, Dhert WJA, Verbout AJ. Changes in the disc space after thoracolumbar spine fractures. *J Bone Joint Surg.* 1998;80-B:833–839.
20. Oner FC, vd Rijt RHH, Ramos LMP, Groen GJ, Dhert WJA, Verbout AJ. Correlation of MR images of disc injuries with anatomic sections in experimental thoracolumbar spine fractures. *Eur Spine J.* 1999;8:194–198.
21. Oner FC, van Gils AP, Dhert WJ, Verbout AJ. MRI findings of thoracolumbar spine fractures: a categorisation based on MRI examinations of 100 fractures. *Skeletal Radiol.* 1999;28(8):433–443.
22. Oner FC, Ramos LMP, Simmermacher RKJ, Kingma PTD, Diekerhof CH, Dhert WJA, Verbout AJ. Classification of thoracic and lumbar spine fractures: problems of reproducibility. A study of 53 patients using CT and MRI. *Eur Spine J.* 2002; 11(3):235–245.
23. Oner FC, van Gils APG, Faber JAJ, Dhert WJA, Verbout AJ. Some complications of common treatment schemes of thoracolumbar spine fractures can be predicted with magnetic resonance imaging. Prospective study of 53 patients with 71 fractures. *Spine.* 2002;27:629–636.
24. Oner FC. *Thoracolumbar spine fractures: diagnostic and prognostic parameters* [Thesis]. University of Utrecht; 1999. ISBN: 90-393-2245-7. Available at: http://www.library.uu.nl/digiarchief/dip/diss/1885237/inhoud.htm. Accessed August 5, 2005.
25. Petersilge CA, Pathria MN, Emery SE, Masaryk TJ. Thoracolumbar burst fractures: Evaluation with MR imaging. *Radiology.* 1995;194(1):49–54.
26. Roberts JB, Curtiss PH. Stability of the thoracic and lumbar spine in traumatic paraplegia following fracture or fracture-dislocation. *J Bone Joint Surg.* 1970;52-A:115–130.
27. Roy-Camille R, Demeulenaer C. Osteosynthese du rachis dorsal, lombaire et lombosacre par plaques metalliques vissées dans les pedicles vertebraux et les apophyses articulaires. *Presse Med.* 1970;78:1447–1448.
28. Saifuddin A, Noordeen H, Taylor BA, Bayley I. The role of imaging in the diagnosis and management of thoracolumbar burst fractures: current concepts and a review of the literature. *Skeletal Radiol.* 1996;25:603–613.
29. Watson-Jones R. *Fractures and Joint Injuries.* 3rd edn. Edinburgh: E. & S. Livingstone Ltd; 1943.
30. White AA, Panjabi MM. *Clinical biomechanics of spine.* Philadelphia: Lippincott; 1978.
31. Whitesides TE. Traumatic kyphosis of the thoracolumbar spine. Clin Orthop. 1977;128:79–92.

5 Malalignment: Signs and Significance

J. H. Harris, Jr

Introduction

Malalignment, for the purpose of this chapter, shall be defined as "the displacement of one cervical vertebra, or vertebral component, from its normal position with respect to adjacent vertebrae or components."

Gross clinical malalignment is obvious and should not present a diagnostic problem. Minor cervical malalignment, however, may be radiographically subtle and, if not recognized, may lead to devastating neurological consequences. It is important to recognize congenital and positional (physiological) malalignment for what they are in order to avoid performing other unnecessary imaging procedures when possible, to expedite patient care, and prevent unnecessary patient radiation. Even in this age of readily available multi-detector CT (MDCT), conventional radiography remains commonly the initial imaging examination of the cervical spine in patients who are not severely injured. It is in this circumstance that relatively minor, but clinically significant, cervical malalignment could go unrecognized. Should that occur, the patient could be denied a definitive CT examination. It is for these reasons, that in each case shown in this chapter, the initial imaging study was conventional radiography.

This discussion is limited to the cervical spine in order to provide as many examples of congenital, physiological or positional, and traumatic malalignment as possible in the space allotted (see also Table 5.1).

The unusual format of this chapter is a reflection of the chapter title "Malalignment: Signs and Significance."

Table 5.1 Radiographic signs of malalignment

Cervicocranium (occiput–C2 interspace)

Antero-posterior projection

Rotation and lateral tilt (C1–C2)
    Physiological
        —positioning
        —atlanto-axial rotary displacement (torticollis)
    Pathological
        —atlanto-axial rotary fixation
        —atlanto-axial rotary subluxation
        —atlanto-axial rotary dislocation

Lateral displacement of dens
    —type II or III dens fracture

Bilateral lateral displacement, lateral masses, C1
    —Jefferson bursting fracture

Lateral projection

Anterior translation with or without rotation
    —physiological pseudosubluxation, C2 on C3, children to age 8 years
    —type II or III dens fracture
    —traumatic (TS) or atypical traumatic spondylolisthesis (ATS)

Anterior rotation
    —physiological pseudosubluxation, C2, children to age 8 years
    —TS and ATS

Lower cervical spine (C3–C7)

Antero-posterior projection

Rotation
    Physiological
        —positioning
        —spinous processes progressively further displaced from the mid-line at each successive higher level
    Pathological
        —unilateral interfacetal dislocation (UID)/unilateral interfacetal fracture-dislocation(UIFD—spinous processes displaced from the mid-line at level of the injury and above
        —pediculaminar fracture-separation—rotation of articular mass in the lateral column

Table 5.1 (Continued)

    Focal widening of interspinous space
        —anterior subluxation (hyperflexion sprain)

    Bilateral displacement of hemivertebra
        —burst (bursting, axial loading) fracture

    Disruption of lateral column
        —pillar fracture
        —pedicolaminar fracture-separation, types I–IV

Lateral projection

Flexion
    Physiological
        —reversal of cervical lordosis
        —military (chin-on-chest) position
        —Philadelphia collar
    Pathological
        —focal hyper-kyphotic angulation—anterior subluxation (AS) (hyper flexion sprain)
Anterior translation (horizontal forward movement)
    —AS
    —UID (<50% AP diameter of vertebral body)
    —bilateral interfacetal dislocation (BID) (>50% AP diameter, vertebral body)

Anterior rotation
    —AS

Anterior translation and rotation
    —AS

Fanning (focal widening of interspinal distance)
    —AS
    —UID
Extension
    —Hyperextension dislocation
        —abnormally wide intervertebral disk space, usually anteriorly > posteriorly
        —avulsion of ring apophysis, adolescent

Extension and rotation
    —PLF-S—rotation of separated articular mass

Normal Alignment

Cerviocranium (Occiput–C2–C3 Interspace)

Anteroposterior (open-mouth) radiograph (Fig. 5.1): Optimally, the open-mouth radiograph should include the occipito-atlantal articulations. The following observations constitute normal alignment:

- The dens should be equidistant from the lateral masses of C1.
- The medial and lateral margins of the atlanto-axial facets should be on the same medial and lateral vertical (parasagittal) planes.
- The bifid spinous process of C2 should be in the midsagittal plane of the dens and the space between the maxillary central incisor teeth when present.

Lateral radiograph: The lateral radiograph of the cervical spine, or of the cervicocranium, must include the basion (the midsagittal plane of the anterior margin of the foramen magnum).

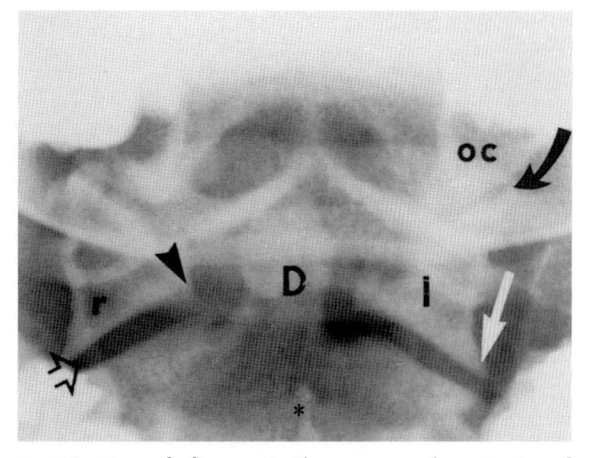

Fig. 5.1 **Normal alignment.** The open-mouth projection of the cervicocranium shows the atlanto-axial articulation (*open arrow*), the dens (D) equidistant from the lateral masses (r, l) of C1, the medial (*arrowhead*) and lateral (*arrow*) margins of C1 superimposed on their counterparts of C2, and the bifid spinous process of C2 (*asterisk*) in the mid-saggital plane, the occipito-atlantal joint space (*curved arrow*), and the occipital condyles (OC).

5 Malalignment: Signs and Significance

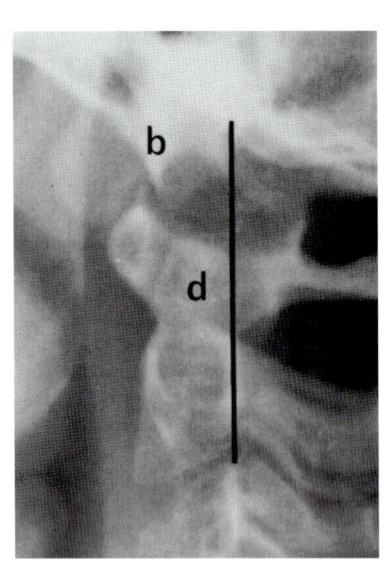

Fig. 5.2 **Normal alignment**. The lateral radiograph of the cervicocranium shows the basion (b), the posterior axial line (*solid black line*), and dens (d).

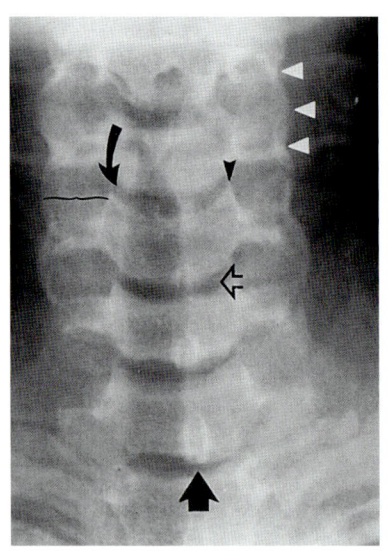

Fig. 5.4 **Normal alignment**. Anteroposterior radiograph of the lower cervical spine shows the spinous processes in the mid-line (*arrow*); parallel endplates and uniform disk spaces (*open arrow*); uncinate processes (*arrowhead*) on the same parasagittal plane with uniform uncovertebral (Luschka) joint spaces (*curved arrow*); lateral column (*curved black line*) appearing as a solid column of bone with smoothly undulating lateral margin (*white arrowheads*).

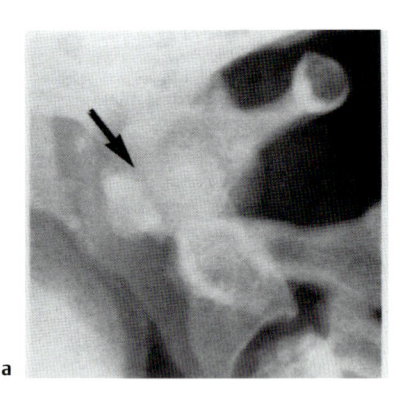

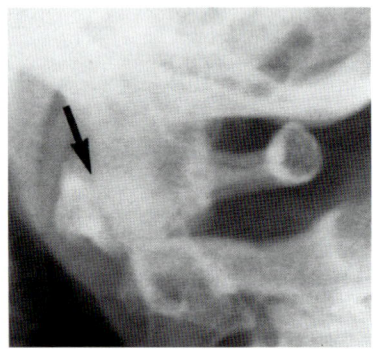

Fig. 5.3 **Normal alignment**. The anterior AADI (*arrow*) is normally maintained at 3.0 mm in flexion **a** and extension **b** by the intact transverse atlantal ligament.

- The basion must be within 12 mm of the posterior axial line (Fig. 5.2).[2,3]
- The dens may be posteriorly angulated as much as 36°.[4]
- In adults, the anterior atlanto-dental interval (AADI) should not exceed 3.0 mm in neutral, flexion, and extension (Fig. 5.3),[5] and in infants and young children should not exceed 6.0 mm.[6]

- The spino-laminar line of C1 and C2 should fall on the lordotic arch of the imaginary posterior spinal line extending from the opisthion to the spino-laminar line of C3.
- The anterior margin of the inferior endplate of C2 may normally lie slightly anterior to the anterior margin of the superior endplate of C3; the contiguous posterior margins are on the same plane.
- The C2–C3 apophyseal joints should be posterior to the axis body.

Lower Cervical Spine (C3–C7)

Anteroposterior radiograph (Fig. 5.4): From the mid-sagittal plane laterally, the following constitute normal alignment:
- Spinous process in the mid-line.
- When visible, vertebral endplates parallel and intervertebral disk-spaces uniform.
- Uncinate processes on same parasagittal plane.
- Luschka (uncovertebral) joints should be on the same parasagittal plane, and the joint spaces of similar width.
- The following normal observations apply to the lateral column, which is defined as the seemingly solid, vertically oriented area of bone between the uncovertebral joints and the lateral margin of the cervical spine:
  - Apophyseal joint spaces should not be visible.
  - The lateral margins should be intact and smoothly undulating.

Malalignment

Lateral radiograph (Fig. 5.5): Normal alignment is established by the following:
- The traditional lordotic curves connecting (1) the anterior cortex of the vertebral bodies, (2) their posterior cortices, (3) the spinolaminar lines, and (4) the posterior cortical margins of the articulating masses.
- Intervertebral disk spaces should be of similar width.
- Articular masses must be posterior to the vertebral bodies, the apophyseal (facet, interfacetal) joints of similar width; adjacent facets must be congruent and the contiguous posteroinferior margins of each apophyseal joint must be on the same vertical plane.
- Anterior displacement (malalignment) less than 3.5 mm of one cervical vertebral body with respect to the subjacent vertebra is normal.

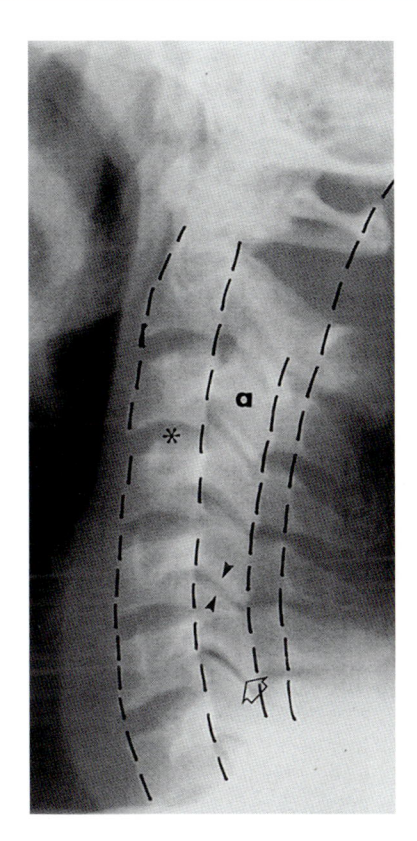

Fig. 5.5 **Normal alignment.** Lateral radiograph of the lower cervical spine showing the four lordotic curves; intervertebral spaces (*asterisk*) of uniform width; articular masses (a) and apophyseal (facet, interfacetal) joints (*open arrow*) posterior to the vertebral body; congruous contiguous facets (*arrowheads*) and joint spaces of uniform width.

Malalignment

Case 1

This 7-year-old boy hurt his neck while wrestling with a friend. He had neither localized physical nor neurological signs or symptoms.

Signs of Malalignment

The initial lateral radiograph (Fig. 5.6a) was considered normal and lateral flexion (Fig. 5.6b) and extension (Fig. 5.6c) radiographs were also obtained.

Figure 5.6a shows a neutral lateral radiograph of the cervicocranium. (1) The anterior inferior corner of the body of C2 (*arrowhead*) is slightly anteriorly translated with respect to the body of C3. (2) The anterior atlantodental interval (AADI) (*open arrow*) appears too wide.

Figure 5.6b shows a lateral flexion radiograph of the cervicocranium. (1) The anterior inferior corner of C2 (*arrowhead*) is slightly more anteriorly translated than in Figure 5.6a. (2) The AADI (*open arrow*) appears too wide.

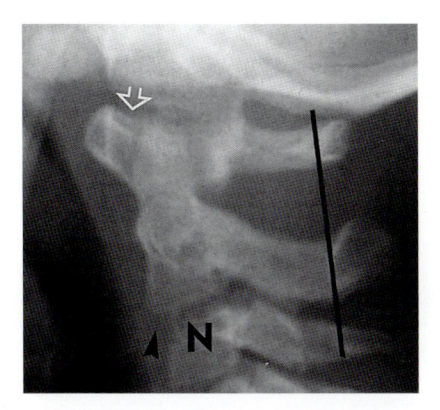

Fig. 5.6a

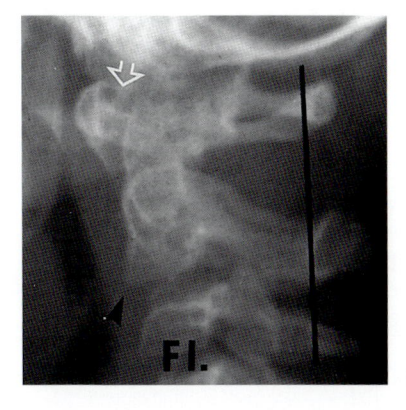

Fig. 5.6b

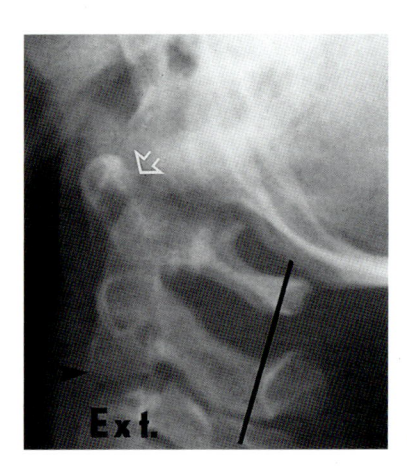

Fig. 5.6c

Figure 5.6c shows a lateral extension radiograph of the cervicocranium. (1) The anterior inferior corner of C2 (*arrowhead*) is normally aligned with respect to the body of C3. (2) The AADI (*open arrow*) is not as wide as on either Figures 5.6a or 5.6b

Significance

All the signs of malalignment relative to C2 and C3 shown on Figures 5.6a and 5.6b and reversed in Figure 5.6c represent physiological pseudosubluxation of C2 on C3. That these changes represent pseudosubluxation of C2 on C3 is proven by the relationship of the spinolaminar line of C2 to the posterior spinal line that connects the spinolaminar lines of C1 and C3 (*dark line*). In the neutral position, the spinolaminar line of C2 will normally be on (Fig. 5.6a), or slightly anterior to the posterior spinal line; in flexion (Fig. 5.6b), slightly anterior to; and in extension (Fig. 5.6c), posterior to the posterior spinal line. Physiological pseudosubluxation of C2 on C3 occurs in approximately 24% of children to age 7.

The AADI normally, in children, is approximately 4 mm in width and rarely exceeds 6 mm and may change with flexion and extension. This is due to the physiological laxity of the transverse atlantal ligament in children.

The signs of malalignment shown in this case are all physiological and have no clinical significance.

Suggested Reading:
Swischuk LE. *Imaging of the Cervical Spine in Children.* Berlin: Springer; 2001:20–22.
Harris JH Jr, Mirvis SE. *The Radiology of Acute Cervical Spine Trauma.* 3rd ed. Baltimore, MD: Williams and Wilkins; 1996:15–19.

Case 2

This 29-year-old woman sustained a pelvic ring disruption in a motor vehicle crash. She was brought to the emergency department on a backboard with a cervical collar in place. Although she had no complaints referable to her cervical spine, the cervical spine was examined radiographically because of the major distracting pelvic injury. The open-mouth view (Fig. 5.7) was obtained with the patient on the board. The margin of a circular defect (*arrowheads*) in the board obscures the spinous process of C2.

Signs of Malalignment

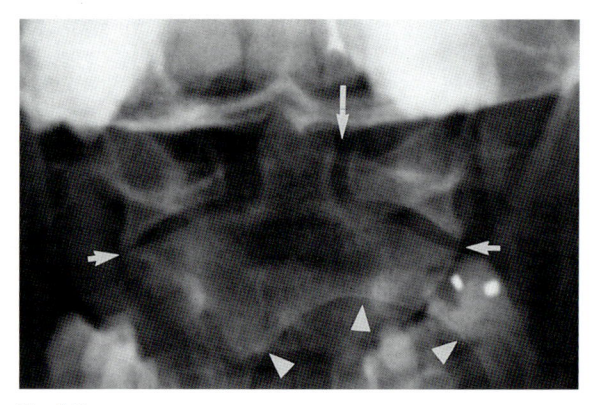

Fig. 5.7

Figure 5.7 shows an open-mouth view that was obtained with the patient on the backboard. The margin of a circular defect (*arrowheads*) in the board obscures the spinous process of C2. (1) The left lateral atlantodental interval (ADI) (*long arrow*) is narrower than the right.

Significance

Because the margins of the inferior facets of the lateral masses of C1 are superimposed on the lateral margins of the superior facets of C2 (*short arrows*), the C1–C2 relationship is anatomic. The asymmetry of the lateral ADIs represents the normal variance in the transverse diameter of the lateral masses of C1. Thus, the asymmetric lateral atlantodental intervals are normal and represent neither rotation of C1 with respect to C2 nor a Jefferson bursting fracture.

Case 3

This 29-year-old woman complained of mild, non-localized neck pain, without posterior mid-line tenderness, following a low-speed motor vehicle accident.

Signs of Malalignment

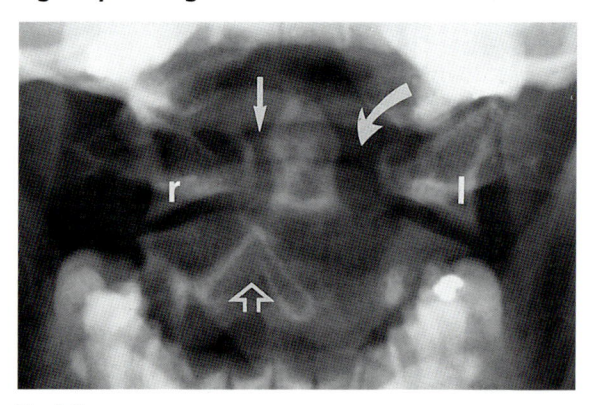

Fig. 5.8

Figure 5.**8** shows an open-mouth radiograph of the cervicocranium. (1) The spinous process of C2 (*open arrow*) is rotated off the mid-line to the patient's right side. (2) The lateral masses of C2 have each shifted to the patient's left side. (3) The right lateral mass of C1(r) has a greater transverse diameter than that of the left. (4) The right lateral atlantodental interval (ADI) (*white arrow*) is narrower than the left (*curved arrow*). (5) The left (l) lateral mass of C1 is truncated.

Significance

All the findings described above indicate rotation of the patient's head to the left side. During rotation to the left, the right lateral mass of C1 rotates anteriorly becoming wider in transverse diameter and the right ADI becomes narrow. Conversely, the left lateral mass of C1 rotates posteriorly becoming truncated and its ADI widens. During rotation to the left, C1 also tilts to the left with respect to C2 as indicated by each lateral mass of C1 being offset to the left with respect to the superior facets of C2. During rotation to the left, C2 also rotates to the left and its spinous process is reciprocally displaced in the opposite direction.

Thus, the malalignment could be all positional. Had the patient awakened with a stiff neck and the head rotated to the left, the malalignment described above would indicate torticollis ("wry neck," atlanto-axial rotatory displacement). Identical findings are present in patients with old, nontreated torticollis (atlanto-axial rotatory fixation).

Suggested Reading:
Harris JH Jr, Mirvis SE. *Radiology of Acute Cervical Spine Trauma.* 3rd ed. Baltimore: Williams and Wilkins; 1996:31–38, 458–462.

Case 4

This adult man was involved in a motor vehicle crash.

Signs of Malalignment

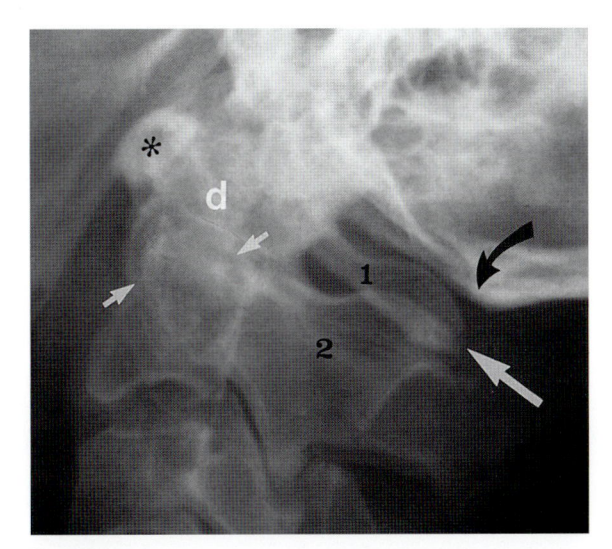

Fig. 5.**9a**

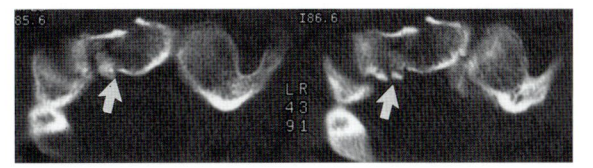

Fig. 5.**9b**

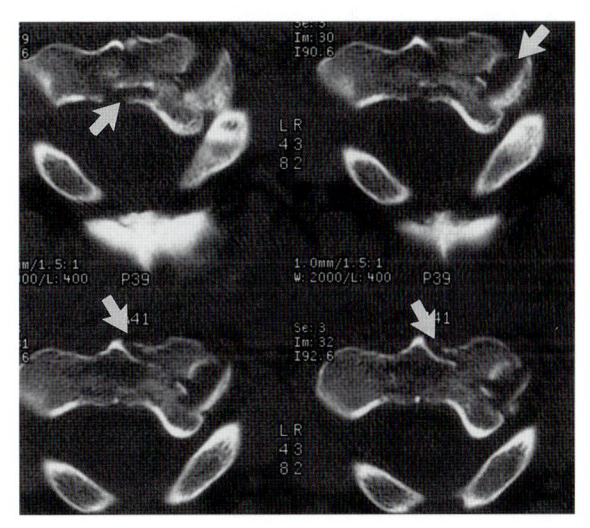

Fig. 5.**9c**

Figure 5.**9a** shows a lateral radiograph of the cervical spine. (1) The posterior elements of C2 (2) and the posterior arch of C1 (1) are hypoplastic and the posterior arch of C1 is unfused (*long arrow*). (2) The opisthion (*curved arrow*) lies anterior to the spinolaminar line. (3) The anterior tubercle of C1 (*asterisk*) is anteriorly displaced with respect to the body of C2. (4) The dens (d) is anteriorly displaced with respect to the axis body. (5) The axis ring is disrupted (*short arrows*).

Significance

The signs of malalignment relative to the configuration of the posterior arch of C1 and the posterior elements of C2 are congenital and of no clinical significance.

The position of the tip of the posterior arch of C1 and of the opisthion, the anterior displacement of the anterior tubercle of C1 and of the dens with respect to the axis body coupled with disruption of the axis ring indicate a low (Type III) dens fracture caused by hyperflexion. The appearance of the axis body is sometimes also referred to as the "fat axis body."

Axial CT images (Figs. 5.**9b** and 5.**9c**) confirm the comminuted displaced fracture through the base of the dens extending into the axis body (*arrows*).

Suggested Reading:
Harris JH Jr, Mirvis SE. *The Radiology of Acute Cervical Spine Trauma.* 3rd ed. Baltimore: Williams and Wilkins; 1996:429–458.

Rogers LF. *Radiology of Skeletal Trauma.* 3rd ed. New York: Churchill Livingston; 2001:408–411.

Case 5

This adult woman was involved in a major motor vehicle crash. She was found unconscious and was intubated at the scene.

Signs of Malalignment

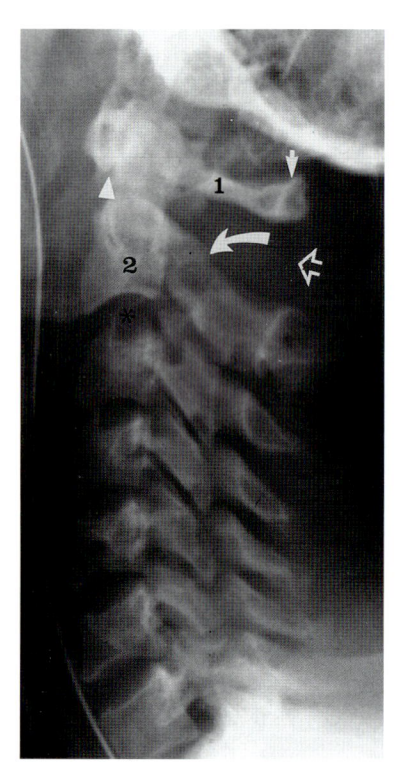

Fig. 5.**10**

Figure 5.**10** shows a cross-table lateral radiograph of the cervical spine. (1) The spinolaminar line of C1 (*short arrow*) is anterior to the posterior spinal line. (2) The anterior atlantodental interval (AADI) (*arrowhead*) is normally maintained. (3) The posterior arch of C1 (1) is rotated slightly anterosuperiorly resulting in (4) widening of the C1–C2 interspinous space (*open arrow*). (5) The second intervertebral disk space is abnormally wide (*asterisk*). (6) The body of C2 (2) is slightly rotated and displaced anteriorly. (7) The pars interarticularis of C2 is disrupted (*curved arrow*).

Significance

Anterior displacement of the spinolaminar line of C1 with respect to the posterior spinal line can occur with an acute tear of the transverse atlantal ligament, a displaced type II or III dens fracture, or traumatic spondylolisthesis. The normal AADI excludes an acute traumatic tear of the transverse atlantal ligament. The intact anterior and posterior cortex of the dens and the intact axis ring exclude a type II or III dens fracture.

Increased vertical height of the second disk space associated with anterior rotation and displacement of the axis body indicates an Effendi type II traumatic spondylolisthesis, which is indicated by disruption of the pars interarticularis of C2.

Suggested Reading:

Harris JH Jr, Mirvis SE. *The Radiology of Acute Cervical Spine Trauma.* 3rd ed. Baltimore: Williams and Wilkins; 1996:377–391.

White AA, Panjabi MM. *Clinical Biomechanics of the Spine.* 2nd ed. Philadelphia: Lippincott Williams and Wilkins; 1990:208–215.

Case 6

This 13-year-old boy injured his neck while tumbling in a gym class. He had no neurological signs and his neck pain was generalized and not severe. After the neutral lateral radiograph (Fig. 5.**11a**) was interpreted, the lateral flexion view (Fig. 5.**11b**) was obtained. With superimposition of the neutral and flexed lateral projections, all visualized cervical segments remain in identical alignment.

Signs of Malalignment

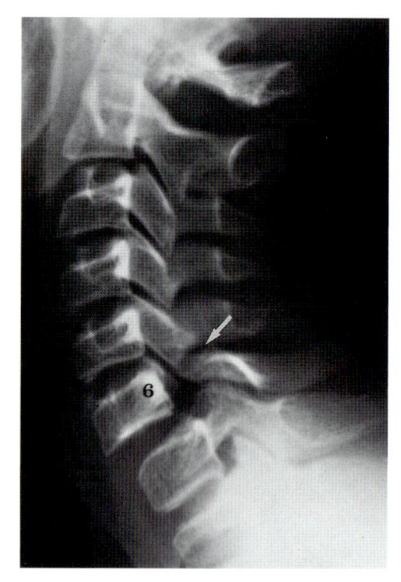

Fig. 5.**11 a**

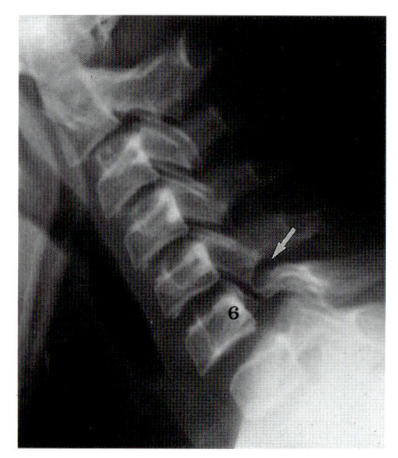

Fig. 5.**11 b**

Malalignment

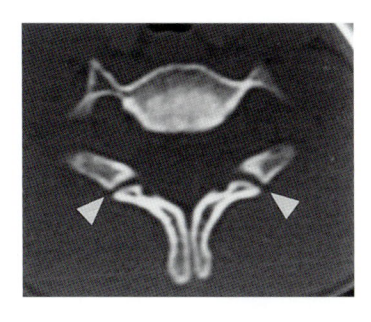

Fig. 5.11 c

Figures 5.**11a** and 5.**11b** show lateral radiographs of the cervical spine. (1) The body of C6 (6) is anteriorly translated with respect to that of C7. (2) There is a defect (*arrow*) in the pars interarticularis of C6. Figure 5.**11c** shows axial CT image of C6. (1) The axial CT image shows a bilateral pars interarticularis defect of C6 (*arrowheads*).

Significance

The smoothly corticated margins of the bilateral pars defect indicate a congenital spondylolytic defect. The anterior translation of C6 indicates congenital spondylolisthesis. The tumbling injury has no significance relative to the congenital defect.

Case 7

This 23-year-old man complained of mild, diffuse neck pain following a motor vehicle collision in which he suffered a fracture-dislocation of his left ankle. A Philadelphia-type cervical collar was applied at the scene. The initial lateral cervical spine radiograph was taken with the collar in place.

Signs of Malalignment

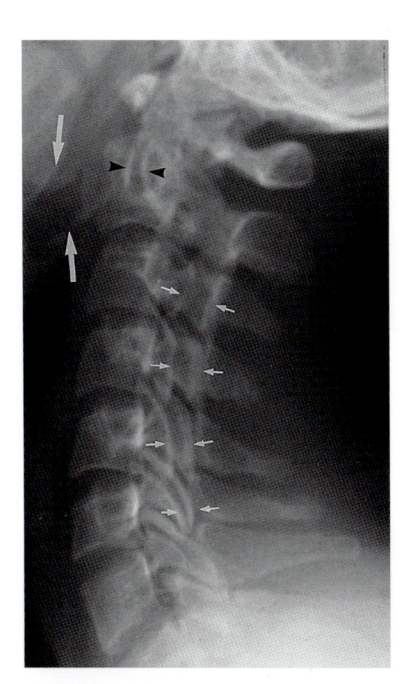

Fig. 5.**12a**

Figure 5.**12a** shows an initial lateral radiograph of the cervical spine. (1) The articular masses of the lower cervical vertebrae are progressively out of superimposition from C7 through C2 (*small arrows*). (2) The anterior margins of the axis rings (*arrowheads*) are not superimposed. (3) Rotation of the head is indicated by lack of superimposition of the ascending mandibular rami (*arrows*).

Because of the patient's minimal neck symptoms, the cervical collar was removed and the neck examined clinically. The patient had a pain-free range of motion and no localized tenderness. The lateral cervical spine radiograph was repeated without the collar (Fig. 5.**12b**) and shows the visualized cervical vertebrae to be anatomically aligned and intact.

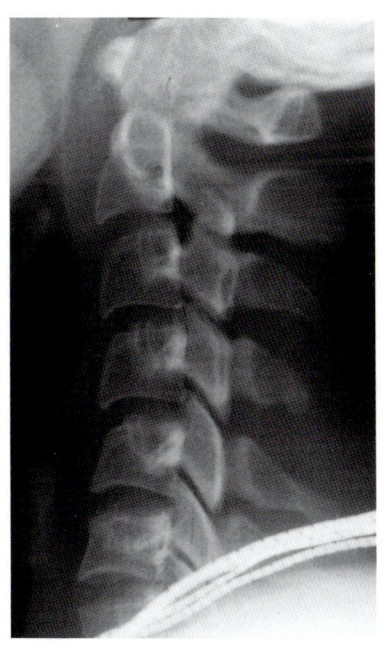

Fig. 5.**12b**

Significance

All the changes of malalignment shown on Figure 5.**12a** are physiological and due to improper positioning secondary to the presence of the collar.

Suggested Reading:

Harris JH Jr, Mirvis SE. *The Radiology of Acute Cervical Spine*. 3rd ed. Baltimore: Williams and Wilkins; 1996:58–61.

Case 8

This 15-year-old male sustained a "stinger" of his left arm while attempting to tackle another football player. A Philadelphia-type collar was applied at the field.

Signs of Malalignment

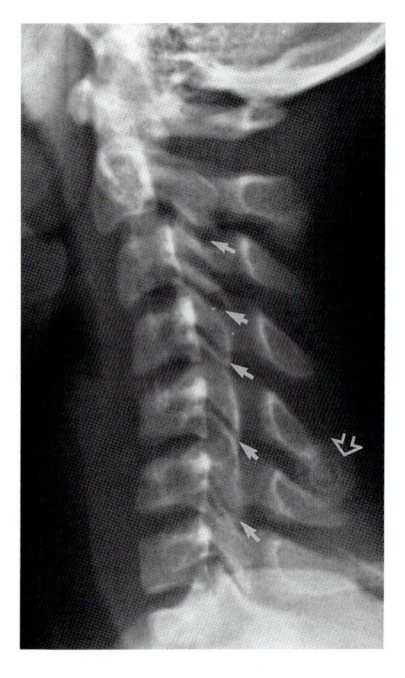

Fig. 5.13

Figure 5.13 shows a supine lateral radiograph of the cervical spine. (1) Reversal of the normal cervical lordosis from C5 through C1.

Significance

The lateral radiograph shows no sign of subluxation, dislocation, or fracture. The reversal of the normal cervical lordotic curve is smooth, continuous, and progressively greater from C5 through the upper cervical segments. Widening of the apophyseal joint spaces (*arrows*) increases physiologically progressively from C5 through the upper segments. A collar snap (*open arrow*) is visible. The back of the hard collar, being taller than the front, forces the head and cervical spine into minor hyperflexion. Therefore, the significance of the malalignment as shown in Figure 5.13 is physiological and of no clinical significance.

Case 9

This adult male was the seat-belted passenger in a car that had stopped at an intersection. The stopped car was rear-ended by a second automobile. The patient's head and neck were thrown into hyperextension and rebound hyperflexion. The patient complained of pain and tenderness in the region of the mid-cervical spinous processes but denied neurological signs or symptoms.

Signs of Malalignment

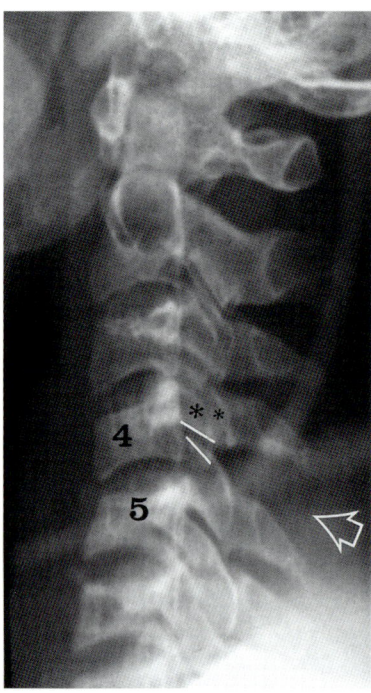

Fig. 5.14a

Figure 5.14a shows a lateral radiograph of the cervical spine. (1) Hyperkyphotic angulation at C4–5. (2) Widening ("fanning") of the C4–5 interspinous and interlaminar spaces (*open arrow*). (3) Superoanterior rotation of the articular masses of C4 (*asterisk*) with respect to those of C5. (4) Incongruity of the contiguous facets of C4–C5 (*white lines*).

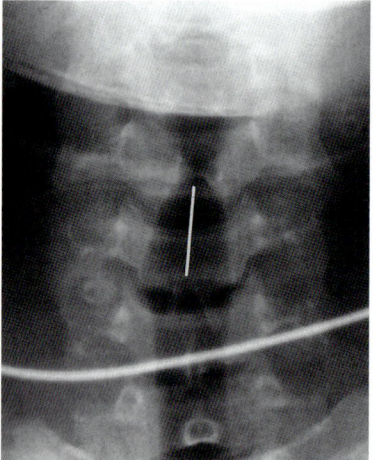

Fig. 5.14b

Figure 5.14b shows an anteroposterior radiograph of the cervical spine. (1) Widening of the C4–5 interspace (*white line*).

Significance

All of the signs of malalignment shown in Figures 5.14a and 5.14b indicate disruption of the posterior ligament complex, due to the hyperflexion mechanism of injury, which is pathognomonic of anterior subluxation (hyperflexion sprain).

Suggested Reading:

Harris JH Jr, Mirvis SE. *The Radiology of Acute Cervical Spine Trauma*. 3rd ed. Baltimore: Williams and Wilkins; 1996:245–270.

White AA, Panjabi MM. *Clinical Biomechanics of the Spine*. 2nd ed. Philadelphia: Lippincott Williams and Wilkins; 1990:229–235.

Gunzburg R, Szpalski M. *Whiplash Injuries*. Philadelphia: Lippincott-Ravin Publishers; 1998.

Case 10

This adolescent boy struck his head on the bottom of a swimming pool after diving. He experienced severe pain in his neck and had greater neurological deficits in the upper extremities than in the lower (acute central cervical spinal cord syndrome).

Signs of Malalignment

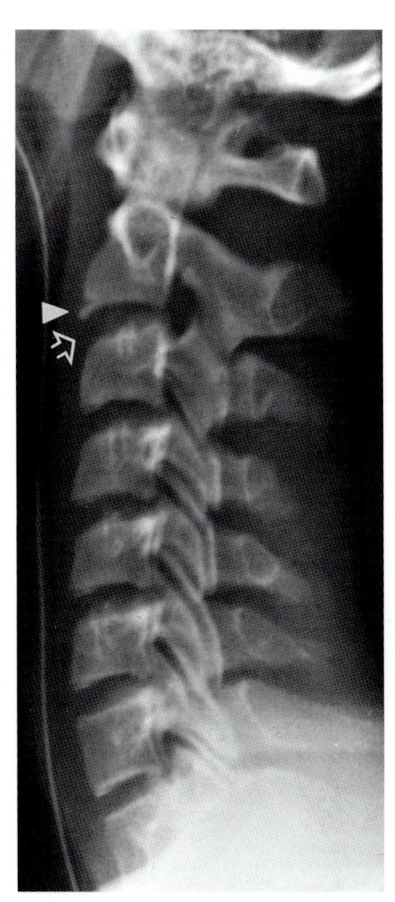

Fig. 5.**15**

Figure 5.**15** shows a cross-table lateral radiograph of the cervical spine. (1) The C2 ring apophysis (*arrowhead*) is displaced anteroinferiorly. (2) The second intervertebral disk space is widened anteriorly (*open arrow*).

Significance

The signs described above indicate a hyperextension injury, specifically hyperextension dislocation. In this example of hyperextension dislocation, the intact anterior Sharpy's fibers of the annulus fibrosis caused avulsion of the incompletely fused ring apophysis. Anterior widening of the disk space indicates the disk was, at least, partially torn during the hyperextension mechanism of injury. Retropulsion of the intervertebral disk compressing the cervical cord resulted in the acute central cervical cord syndrome. The degree of cervical cord damage in this adolescent was less than occurs in the classic hyperextension dislocation of adults (see Case 11).

Suggested Reading:
Please see Case 11.

Case 11

This adult male was involved in a major motor vehicle collision during which his head struck the steering wheel and his head was then thrown into severe hyperextension. When seen in the emergency department, he had lacerations on his face and nose and physical signs of the acute central cervical spinal cord syndrome (i. e., simply put, neurological changes greater in the upper than the lower extremities).

Signs of Malalignment

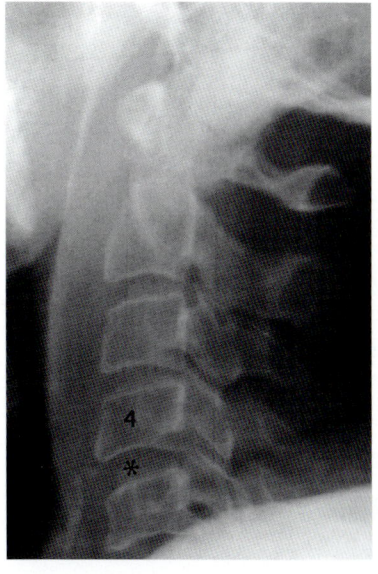

Fig. 5.**16**

Figure 5.**16** shows a cross-table lateral radiograph of the cervical spine. (1) Widened C4–5 disk space (*asterisk*) greater anteriorly than posteriorly with widened pre-vertebral soft-tissue space.

Significance

The significance of the malalignment described above is that it indicates a hyperextension injury of the lower (C3–C7) cervical spine. This malalignment, in conjunction with the facial injury, the signs of acute central cervical cord syndrome, and the diffuse prevertebral soft tissue swelling are pathognomonic of the specific injury hyperextension dislocation.

Suggested Reading:
Harris JH Jr, Mirvis SE. *The Radiology of Acute Cervical Spine Trauma*. 3rd ed. Baltimore: Williams and Wilkins; 1996:391–402.

Case 12

This workman fell from the second floor of a construction site striking the right side of his face and head on the ground. He complained of severe pain in his neck, primarily on the left side, which was aggravated by limited cervical motion. He had no neurological signs or symptoms.

Signs of Malalignment

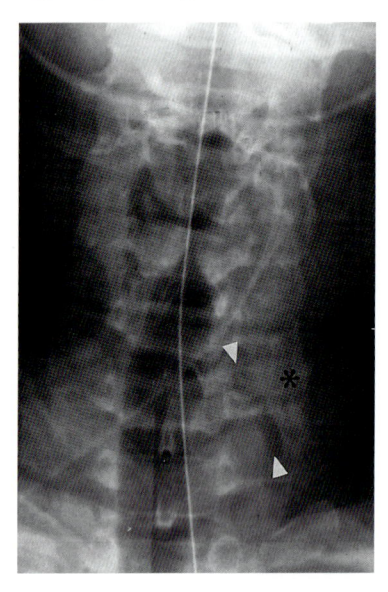

Fig. 5.**17a**

Figure 5.**17a** shows an anteroposterior radiograph of the cervical spine. (1) The cervical spine is bowed to the patient's left side. (2) The left lateral mass of C6 (*asterisk*) is laterally displaced disrupting the normal undulating margin of the left lateral column. (3) An oblique lucent defect (*arrowheads*) is present between the lateral mass and the body of C6.

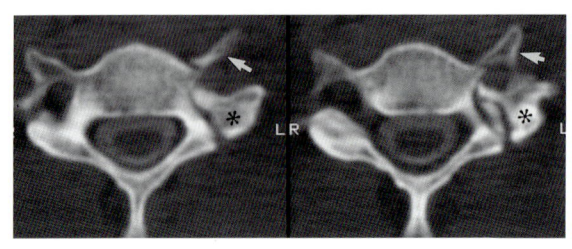

Fig. 5.**17b**

Figure 5.**17b** shows axial CT images of C6. (1) The left lateral mass of C6 (*asterisk*) is laterally displaced. (2) The anterior margin of the left C6 transverse process (*arrows*) is anteromedially displaced as the result of a fracture at its base.

Significance

Lateral displacement of the left lateral mass of C6 secondary to the comminuted fracture oriented in the parasagittal plane and without a transverse fracture of either the adjacent pedicle or lamina indicates the fracture is limited to the articular mass (pillar). The malalignment shown in Figures 5.**17a** and 5.**17b** is classic for the uncommon "pillar" fracture which is the result of a combined hyperextension and rotation mechanism of injury. Because of the involvement of the foramen transversarium, multi-planar CT (MPCT), MRI, or catheter angiography of the left vertebral artery is recommended today.

Suggested Reading:
Harris JH Jr, Mirvis SE. *The Radiology of Acute Cervical Spine Trauma*. 3rd ed. Baltimore: Williams and Wilkins; 1996:320–329.
Rogers LF. *The Radiology of Skeletal Trauma*. 3rd ed. New York: Churchill Livingston; 2001:441–442.

Case 13

This adult male was the driver of a truck that rolled into a ditch. The patient complained of severe neck pain but had no neurological signs or symptoms.

Signs of Malalignment

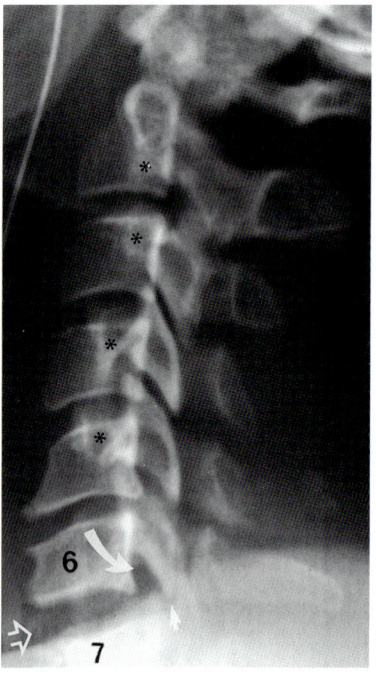

Fig. 5.**18a**

Figure 5.**18a** shows a cross-table lateral radiograph of the cervical spine. (1) The C6–7 disk space is abnormally wide (*open arrow*). (2) One of the articular masses of C6 (*arrow*) lies anterior to its C7 counterpart. (3) There is an empty space ("naked facet") beneath the malaligned articular mass of C6 (*curved arrow*). (4) The body of C6 is anteriorly translated with respect to that of C7 by less than 50%. (5) The articular masses (*asterisk*) above C6 on one side are superimposed upon the vertebral bodies.

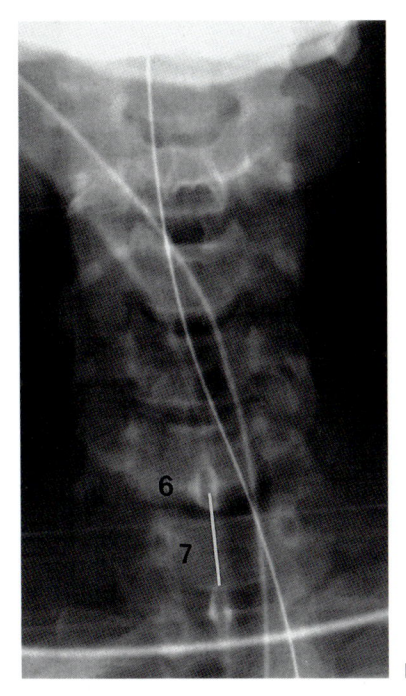

Fig. 5.**18 b**

Figure 5.**18b** shows an anteroposterior radiograph of the cervical spine. (1) The C6–7 interspinous distance is approximately twice normal (*white line*). (2) The spinous process of C6 is rotated off the mid-line to the patient's right side. (3) The right C6–7 articular masses are severely distracted.

Significance

The signs of malalignment seen on both the lateral and anteroposterior radiographs indicate a simultaneous hyperflexion and rotation mechanism of injury resulting in unilateral interfacetal dislocation (UID). Typically, UID (the "locked facet") is considered to be mechanically and neurologically stable. This patient underwent a posterior fusion of C6–7 and returned to his work as a truck driver.

Suggested Reading:

Harris JH Jr, Mirvis SE. *The Radiology of Acute Cervical Spine Trauma.* 3rd ed. Baltimore: Williams and Wilkins; 1996:290–308.
White AA, Panjabi MM. *Clinical Biomechanics of the Spine.* 2nd ed. Philadelphia: Lippincott Williams and Wilkins; 1990:220–224.

Case 14

This 54-year-old man was involved in a motor vehicle collision. He complained of severe pain in his neck and but had no neurological signs or symptoms.

Signs of Malalignment

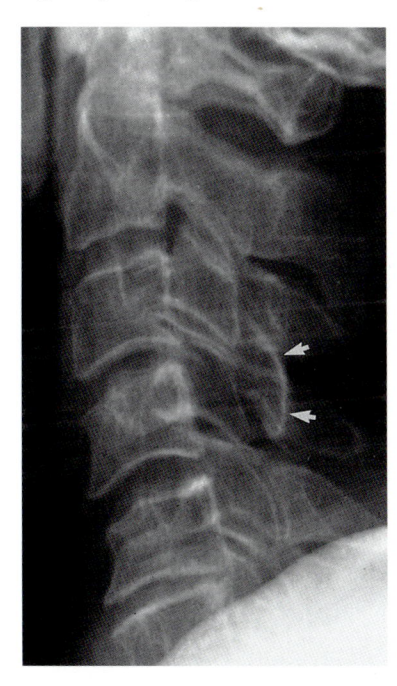

Fig. 5.**19 a**

Figure 5.**19a** shows a cross-table lateral radiograph of the cervical spine. (1) One of the articular masses of C4 (*arrows*) is posteriorly displaced.

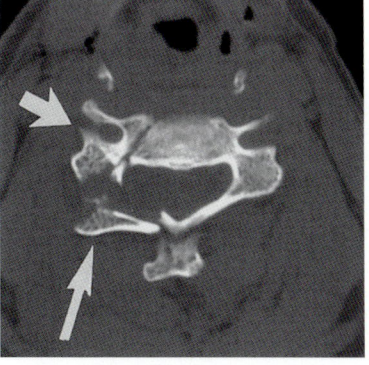

Fig. 5.**19 b**

Figure 5.**19b** shows an axial CT image of C4. (1) The right articular mass and transverse process (*large arrow*) are laterally displaced secondary to fractures of the vertebral pedicle and the right lamina. (2) The right lamina (*long arrow*) constitutes a separate fragment by virtue of anterior and posterior fractures.

Significance

Posterior displacement of an articular mass, with or without rotation, indicates that the articular mass has become a free-floating fragment, which can only be accomplished as the result of an ipsilateral pedicle and laminar fracture as shown in Figure 5.**19b**. Posterior displacement of an articular mass, with or without rotation, is pathognomonic of pedicolaminar fracture-separation.

Suggested Reading:
Harris JH Jr, Mirvis SE. *The Radiology of Acute Cervical Spine Trauma.* 3rd ed. Baltimore: Williams and Wilkins; 1996:321–339.
Louis R, Louis CA, Aswad R. Extension Injuries of the Lower Cervical Spine. In: Clark CR, ed. *The Cervical Spine.* 3rd ed. Philadelphia: Lippincott-Ravin; 1998:476–477.

Case 15

This 15-year-old male struck his head on the bottom of the swimming pool while diving. He complained of severe neck pain, aggravated by attempted movement, but had no neurological signs of symptoms. A hard cervical collar was applied at the scene.

Signs of Malalignment

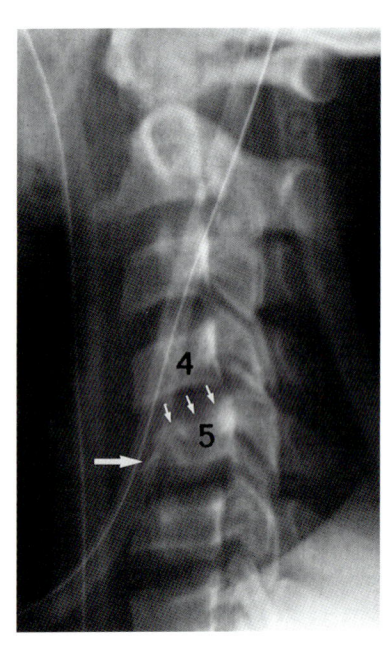

Fig. 5.**20a**

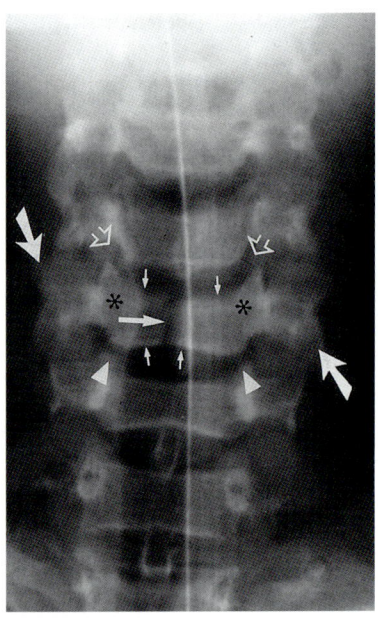

Fig. 5.**20b**

Figure 5.**20a** shows a lateral radiograph of the cervical spine. (1) Slight hyperkyphotic angulation of the C4–5 level. (2) The superior endplate of C5 is impacted and angulated (*small arrows*). (3) A fracture involves the anteroinferior aspect of the body of C5 (*long arrow*).

Figure 5.**20b** shows an anteroposterior radiograph of the cervical spine. (1) The superior endplate of C5 is bowed inferiorly (*small arrows*), and (2) the inferior endplate of C5 is bowed superiorly (*small arrows*). (3) A vertical fracture extends through the body of C5 (*long arrow*). (4) Each hemi-vertebra of C5 (*asterisk*) is laterally displaced, and (5) the articular masses of C5 are laterally displaced and rotated disrupting the normal contour of each lateral column (*oblique arrows*). (6) The C4–5 Luschka joint spaces are abnormally wide (*open arrows*). (7) The C5–6 Luschka joint spaces are abnormally narrowed (*arrowheads*).

Significance

Although hyperkyphotic angulation is present at the C4–5 level, the relationship of the C4–5 articular masses and the corresponding interfacetal joints is normal. The normal interspinous and interlaminar distances indicate the posterior ligament complex to be intact. These observations exclude anterior subluxation (hyperflexion sprain).

Indirect signs of fracture of the superior endplate and primary signs of fracture of the inferior endplate of C5, the vertical fracture through the body of C5 with lateral displacement of each hemi-vertebra of C5 with a resultant change in the C4–5 and C5–6 Luschka joints all indicate a burst (bursting, axial loading) fracture of the lower cervical (C5).

Suggested Reading:
Harris JH Jr, Mirvis SE. *The Radiology of Acute Cervical Spine Trauma.* 3rd ed. Baltimore: Williams and Wilkins; 1996:345–358.
Aebi M, Benzel EC. Cervical Spine Burst Fractures. In: Clark CR, ed. *The Cervical Spine.* 3rd ed. Lippincott-Ravin; 1998:465–467.

Malalignment

Case 16

This adult man, who was involved in a major motor vehicle collision, complained of severe, diffuse neck pain, but had no neurological deficits.

Signs of Malalignment

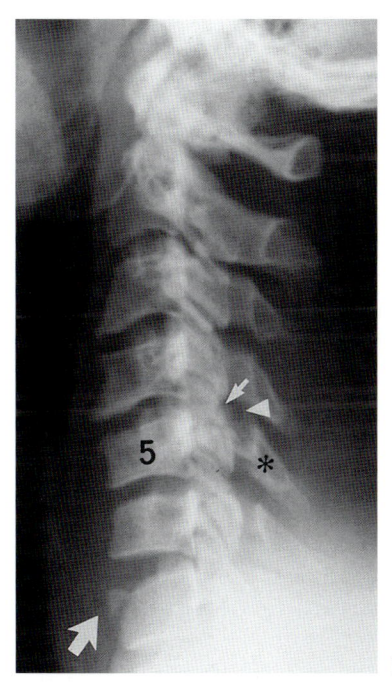

Fig. 5.21 a

Figure 5.**21a** shows a lateral radiograph of the cervical spine. (1) Simple wedge compression fracture of C7 (*arrow*). (2) The articular masses of C5 are indistinct and there is disruption of the cortex at the junction of one superior facet and it contiguous posterior cortical margin (*small arrow*). (3) The C5 laminar cortex is disrupted (*arrowhead*) and the fragments of the lamina are malaligned (*asterisk*).

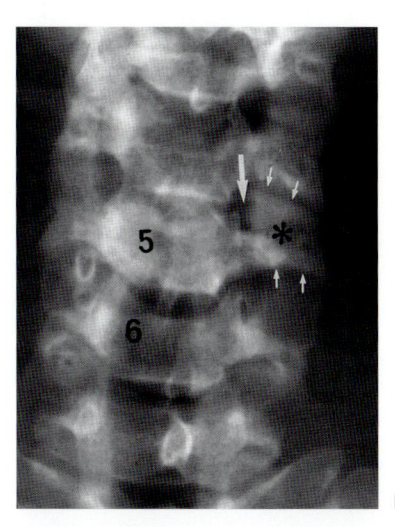

Fig. 5.**21 b**

Figure 5.**21b** shows an anteroposterior radiograph of the cervical spine. (1) The left articular mass of C5 (*asterisk*) is rotated anteriorly making its superior and inferior facets (*small arrows*) visible and; (2) the left articular mass of C5 is laterally displaced. (3) A vertical lucent defect (*long arrow*) is present between the body and the left articular mass of C5. (4) The left lateral column is malaligned from C5 through C6.

Significance

The wedge compression fracture of C7 is obvious and is typically of minor clinical significance. What is not so obvious and could be easily overlooked given the C7 fracture, and which is clinically significant, are the signs of malalignment at the C5 level shown on both the lateral and anteroposterior radiographs. These indicate a pediculaminar fracture-separation.

This case was chosen to emphasize the importance of searching for another, possibly subtle injury, co-existing with a radiographically obvious injury.

Suggested Reading:
Rogers LF. *The Radiology of Skeletal Trauma*. 3rd ed. New York: Churchill Livingston; 2001:526.

Case 17

This 32-year-old woman was the occupant of the front passenger seat of an automobile involved in a low-velocity "T-bone" motor vehicle collision. The passenger-side airbag inflated, striking the patient in the chest, face, and neck.

Signs of Malalignment

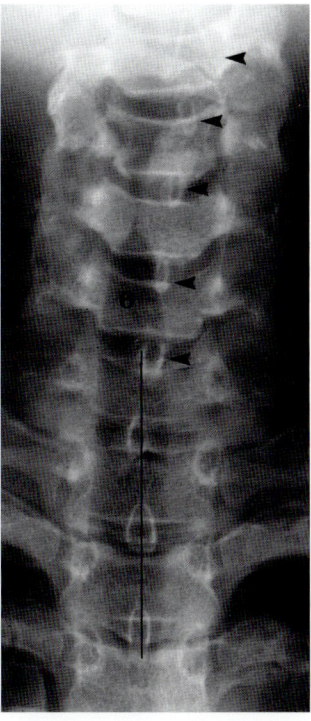

Fig. 5.**22a**

Figure 5.**22a** shows an anteroposterior radiograph of the cervical spine. (1) The spinous processes from C6

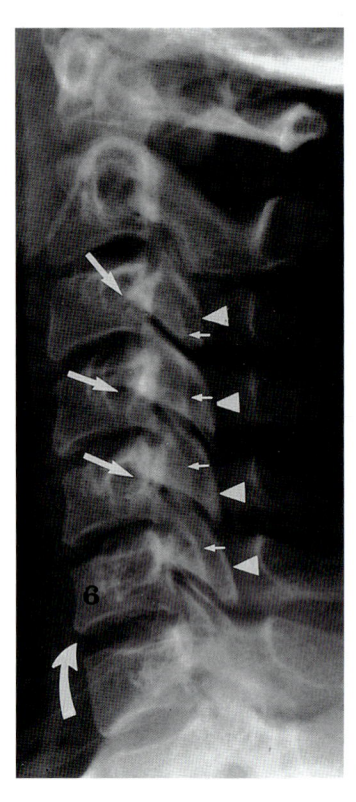

Fig. 5.**22b**

and above (*arrowheads*) are displaced to the patient's left side.

Figure 5.**22b** shows a lateral radiograph of the cervical spine. (1) The articular masses on one side from C6 rostrally (*small arrows*) are rotated anteriorly. (2) Interfacetal joints (*long arrows*) are superimposed on vertebral bodies. (3) The opposite side articular masses from C6 rostrally (*arrowheads*) remain in anatomical relationship to the vertebral bodies. (4) Very minimal anterior translation of C6 on C7 (*curved arrow*).

Significance

Displacement of the spinous processes off the mid-line to the patient's left side on the anteroposterior projection (Fig. 5.**22a**) and superimposition of the interfacetal joints on the intervertebral bodies as seen on the lateral projection (Fig. 5.**22b**) both indicate rotation. Minor, but definite anterior translation of C6 on C7 indicates hyperflexion. Combined hyperflexion and rotation are the mechanism of injury of unilateral interfacetal dislocation (UID). Rotation of the spinous processes from the mid-line and malalignment of the articular masses are diagnostically significant and should add significance to the minimal anterior translation of C6 with respect to C7. Because the radiographic examination shown was interpreted as "negative," CT was not obtained. The patient was treated with analgesics and a soft collar because of persistent neck pain. One week following the motor vehicle collision, while walking in her home, the patient's legs buckled under her and she collapsed onto the floor. Subsequent radiographs of the cervical spine demonstrated a frank unilateral interfacetal fracture-dislocation. The patient remains paraplegic.

Although, as previously stated (Case 13), UID is generally considered to be the "locked" vertebra and, therefore, mechanically stable. The pathophysiology of UID requires complete disruption of the articular capsule on the dislocated side and partial disruption on the contralateral side. Some authors have stressed the importance of the articular capsules as being the key ligamentous component to cervical stability.[1-3] The marked difference in outcome of the patient shown in Case 13 who had a frank UID that was recognized and promptly treated and this patient with a radiographically subtle UID that was not recognized and treated, emphasizes the potential instability of the "locked" vertebra.

Suggested Reading:

Harris JH Jr, Mirvis SE. *The Radiology of Acute Cervical Spine Trauma*. 3rd ed. Baltimore: Williams and Wilkins; 1996:290–308.

Rah AD, Errico TJ. Classification of Lower Cervical Fractures and Dislocations. In: Clark CR. *The Cervical Spine*. 3rd ed. Philadelphia: Lippincott-Ravin; 1998: 452–453.

Acknowledgement

The author freely acknowledges, and with sincere appreciation, that without the secretarial support of Mary Ann Henderson, Administrative Assistant III, and the photographic talent of Dan Klepac, Photographer III, both of the Department of Radiology at The University of Texas Medical School at Houston, this chapter would not exist.

Figures 5.**1**–5.**5** reprinted from *Eur J Radiol*, 2002, Vol. 42. J.H. Harris, Malalignment: signs and significance, pp. 92–99, with permission from Elsevier.

References

1. Scher AT. Anterior cervical subluxation: an unstable position. *AJR*. 1979;133:275–280.
2. Taylor J, Twomey L. Acute injuries to the cervical joints—an autopsy study on neck strain. *Spine*. 1933;18:1115–1122.
3. Jonsson H, Bring G, Rauschning W, Sahlstedt B. Hidden cervical spine injuries in traffic accident victims with skull fractures. *J Spinal Disord*. 1991;4:251–263.

6 Vertebral Injuries: Detection and Implications

R. H. Daffner and S. D. Daffner

Introduction

The indications and imaging options for evaluating patients with suspected vertebral trauma have been discussed in earlier chapters. Once a decision is made that imaging is indicated, radiography will generally be the first study performed. It should be noted, however, that the approach to screening for suspected vertebral trauma has undergone a dramatic and sometimes controversial transition.[1–5] Newer imaging options include the use of a low-dose digital radiography unit (Lodox Systems North America, South Lyon, MI) developed in South Africa and magnetic resonance imaging (MRI).[6–8] In many large medical centers within the United States, multi-detector computed tomography (MDCT) is replacing conventional radiography for evaluation of suspected cervical injury.[9,10] CT has been shown to detect more fractures than radiography, in a faster and more cost-efficient manner.[1,11–15] Furthermore, our experience in our trauma center with a large trauma patient population, as well as that of other investigators has indicated that the incidence of noncontiguous, multi-level vertebral injuries is approximately 20 %.[7,16,17] Therefore, once a decision has been made to perform imaging on any segment of the vertebral column for suspected injury, the *entire* spinal column should be examined. Although at the present time, radiography is the procedure of choice for the thoracic and lumbar regions, the Harvard group at Massachusetts General Hospital report success with MDCT.[2]

This chapter will cover five areas: indicators of high risk for injury; mechanisms of injury and their imaging "fingerprints"; the ABCS or imaging "footprints" of injury; the determination of stability following injury; and the significance of injuries. The key to understanding this approach lies in the authors' premise that all injuries due to a particular mechanism produce the same imaging changes regardless of the location. Thus, a burst fracture of the cervical region looks identical to that in the thoracic and lumbar regions (Fig. 6.1). Furthermore, it is necessary for the reader to understand that while many of the principles discussed here are illustrated using radiographs, the same abnormalities may be seen on CT or even MR images.

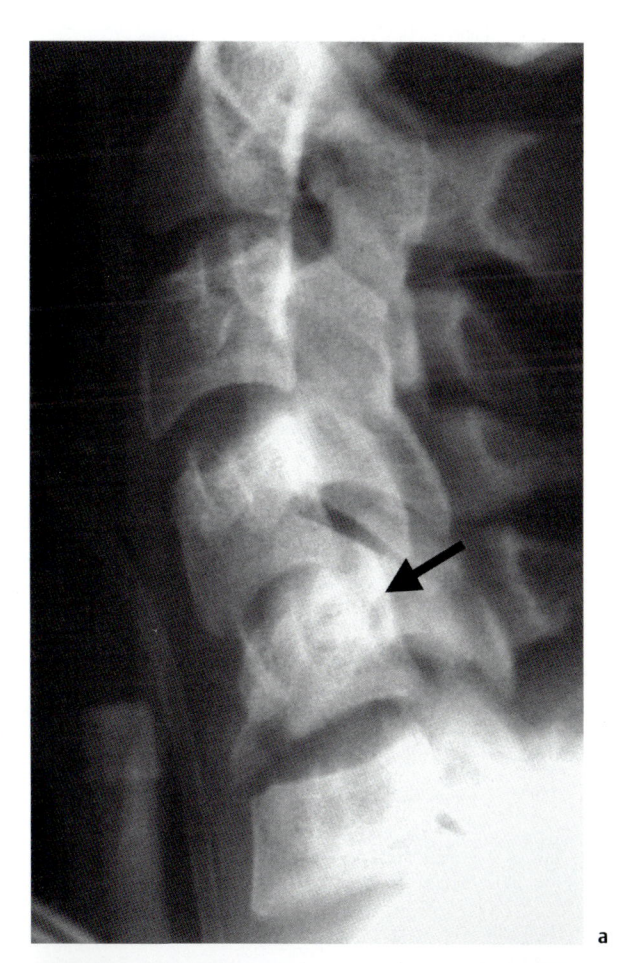

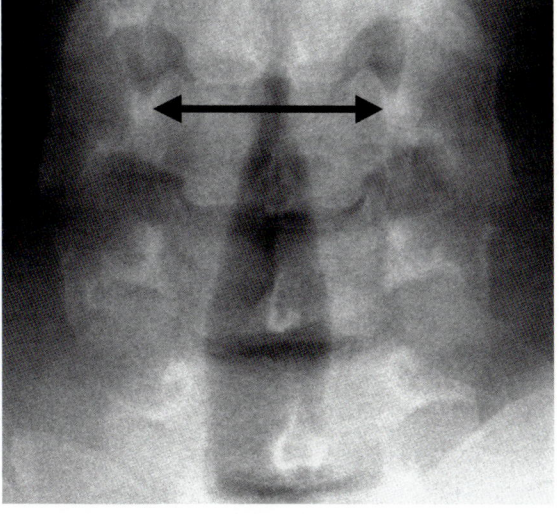

Fig. 6.1 **Burst fractures showing similarity between levels**. **a–c**: C5; **d–f**: L1. **a** Lateral radiograph shows kyphotic angulation, fragmentation of the body, and posterior displacement of the posterior vertebral line (*arrow*) of C5. The C4 disk space is narrowed. **b** Frontal radiograph shows wide interpedicle distance of C5 (*double arrow*).

Fig. 6.1 c–f ▷

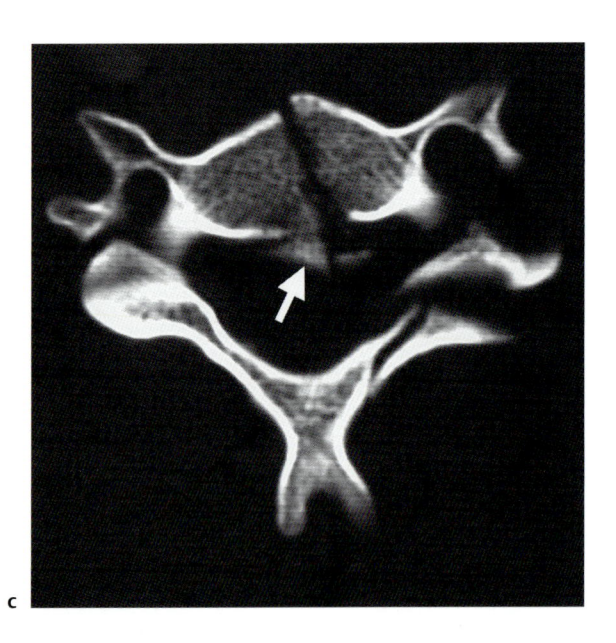

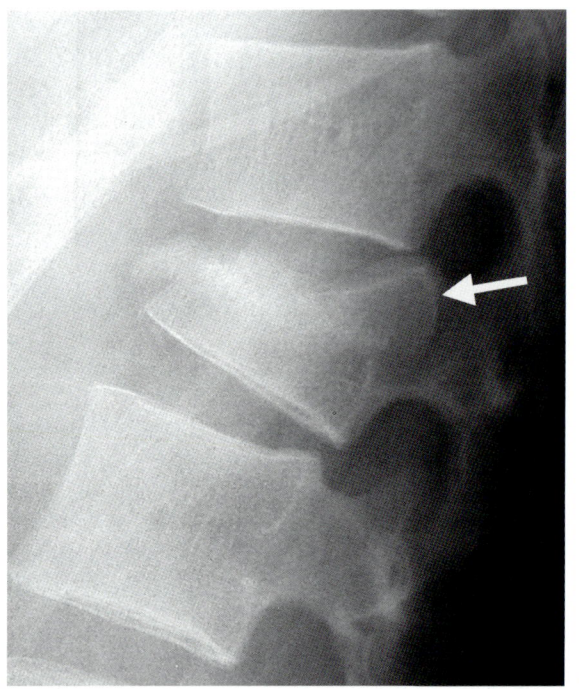

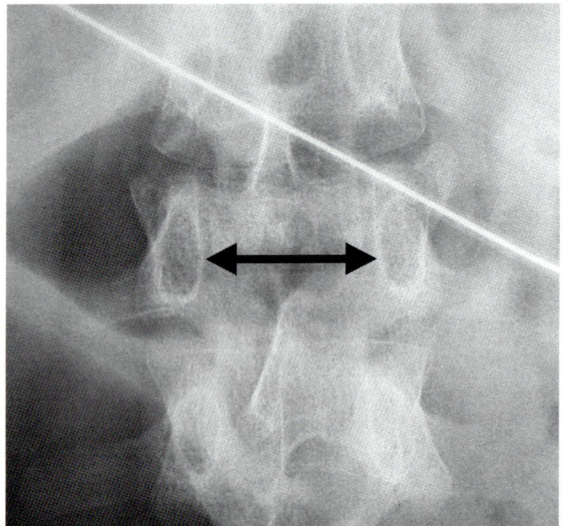

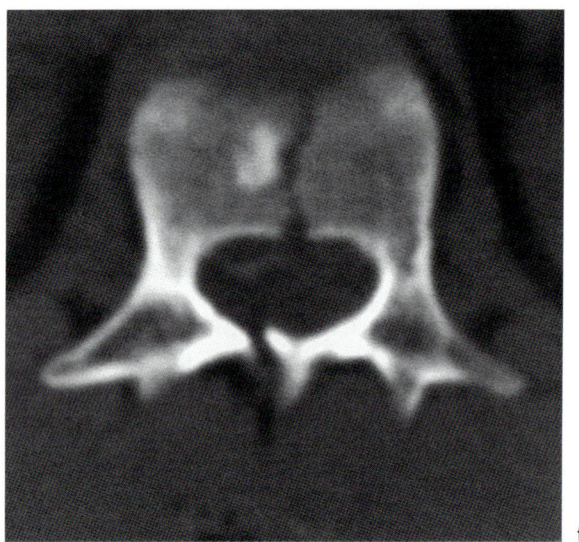

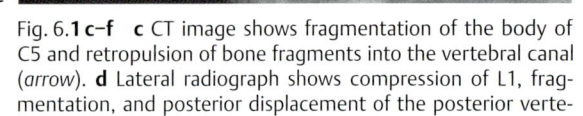

Fig. 6.1 c–f **c** CT image shows fragmentation of the body of C5 and retropulsion of bone fragments into the vertebral canal (*arrow*). **d** Lateral radiograph shows compression of L1, fragmentation, and posterior displacement of the posterior vertebral body line (*arrow*). Note the narrow T12 disk space. **e** Frontal radiograph shows wide interpedicle distance of L1 (*double arrow*). **f** CT image shows sagittal cleavage of L1. Note the displaced bone fragment in the vertebral canal.

Indicators of High Risk for Injury

No subject has generated more controversy in clinical and radiology circles within the past decade as that of indications for imaging for suspected trauma. In many large medical centers the indications are dictated by trauma protocols. This has led to unnecessary imaging of many patients, with consequent exposure to radiation. Concerns with overuse of radiography and CT as well as attempts at cost-containment have led a number of investigators to assess the indications for imaging in trauma patients. Vandemark, in 1990, published a set of 10 high-risk criteria for indicating the necessity of imaging for possible cervical injury.[18] These included high velocity blunt trauma; the presence of multiple fractures; cervical pain, spasm or deformity; altered mental status (of any etiology); drowning or diving accident; a fall of 3 m (10 ft) or greater; any head or facial injury; presence of thoracic and/or lumbar fractures; rigid vertebral disease (ankylosing spondylitis, DISH); and paresthesias or burning in extremities. Blackmore and colleagues investigated fracture risk factors to optimize the use of imaging.[19] Ten years later, Hanson and colleagues added mechanism parameters to the clinical findings for determining indications for CT scanning of the cervical spine in trauma patients.[20] These included any high-speed crash, defined at over 60 kph (35 mph), or a death at the crash scene. Stiell and colleagues added age over 65 years; crash at over 100 kph or with a rollover or ejection of victims; crash involving motorized recreational vehicles (snowmobiles, wave runners, "quad runners"); or bicycle collision.[21] If any of these was present, they recommended radiography.

Two studies looked at low-risk criteria. The first was the National Emergency X-radiography Utilization Study (NEXUS) which identified five criteria that could be used to determine low risk of cervical injury: normal alertness; absence of intoxication; no mid-line cervical tenderness; no painful distracting injuries; and no focal neurological deficits.[22,23] Finally, the Canadian group led by Stiell defined additional low risk factors: simple rear-end collision (no rollover, vehicles not pushed into oncoming traffic, not due to being hit by a bus, large truck, or high speed vehicle); and four clinical criteria (patient ambulatory at any time following the crash, patient in sitting position in emergency department, delayed onset of neck pain, and absence of mid-line cervical tenderness).[21] If these factors were present, they asked the patient to move the neck in flexion, extension, and lateral rotation of 45° to each side.[21]

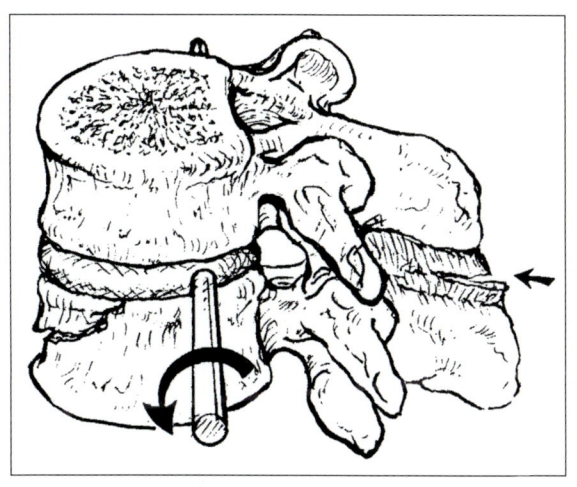

Fig. 6.2 **Drawing showing mechanism of flexion.** Forward flexion (*curved arrow*) with the posterior third of the disk space as the fulcrum produces anterior compression. Further force produces posterior distraction (*straight arrow*).

Mechanisms of Injury and Their Imaging "Fingerprints"

There are many classifications of vertebral injuries in the medical literature. The authors prefer a simple approach in which there are four main injury mechanisms: flexion, extension, rotary, and shearing. Each of these primary mechanisms may be combined, particularly as the result of secondary impacts that occur, such as when an individual is thrown from a motor vehicle. With the exception of extension injuries, axial loading is frequently a component to the injury. Most important, however, is the fact that when an injury occurs, it produces a series of indelible radiographic changes that allow the informed observer to tell not only the mechanism of the injury, but also to alert him or her to look for subtle findings that represent the full extent of that injury. We call these changes the radiological "fingerprints."

Flexion injuries are the most frequent types to be encountered in patients who have suffered vertebral trauma. The common thread of all flexion injuries is that forward bending occurs through a fulcrum centered on the posterior third of the intervertebral disks. This produces anterior compression and posterior distraction (Fig. 6.2). This mechanism produces four distinct subtypes of injury: simple, burst, distraction, and dislocation. *Simple* injuries produce compression of the superior or inferior vertebral endplates of the involved vertebrae. The posterior parts of the vertebral body as well as the posterior elements remain intact. Simple injuries typically produce a

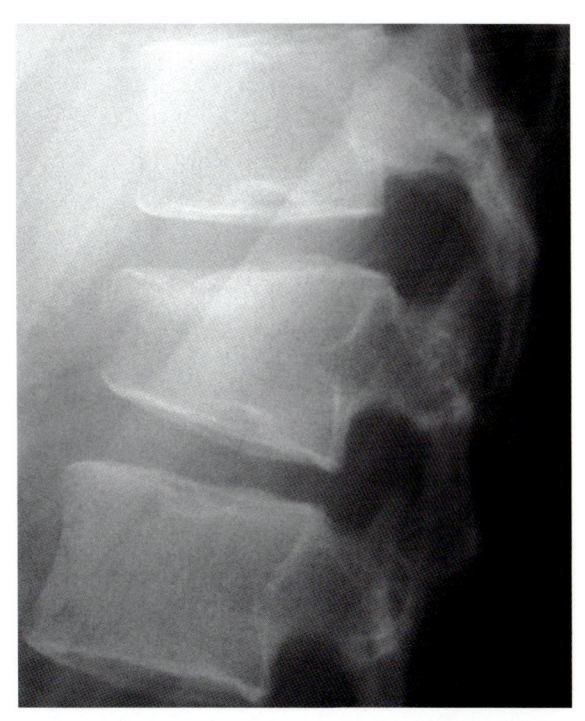

Fig. 6.3 **Simple compression fracture of L1.** Lateral radiograph shows anterior compression without disruption of the posterior vertebral body line.

wedge-shaped vertebra (Fig. 6.3). The disk space above a simple fracture, as with all flexion injuries, is typically narrowed. These injuries rarely produce neurological deficits.

Burst fractures are the result of severe compressive forces that literally explode the vertebra. The vertebral body is comminuted and there is retropulsion of bone fragments that encroach upon the vertebral canal. Typically, the posterior arch of the vertebra is fractured as well. Of particular importance in identifying burst fractures are three radiographic signs: severe compres-

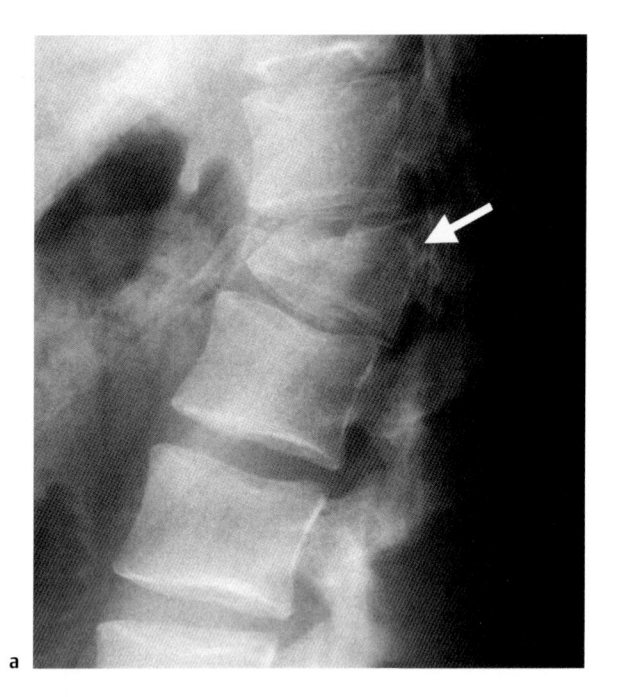

Fig. 6.4 **L1 burst fracture**. **a** Lateral radiograph shows compression, fragmentation, and disruption of the posterior vertebral body line of L1 (*arrow*). **b** Frontal radiograph shows a compressed vertebra and widening of the interpedicle distance of L1 (*double arrow*). **c** CT image through L1 shows comminution and flattening of the posterior vertebral body line. There are bone fragments in the vertebral canal. **d** Sagittal CT reconstruction shows the degree of canal compromise from retropulsed fragments (*arrow*).

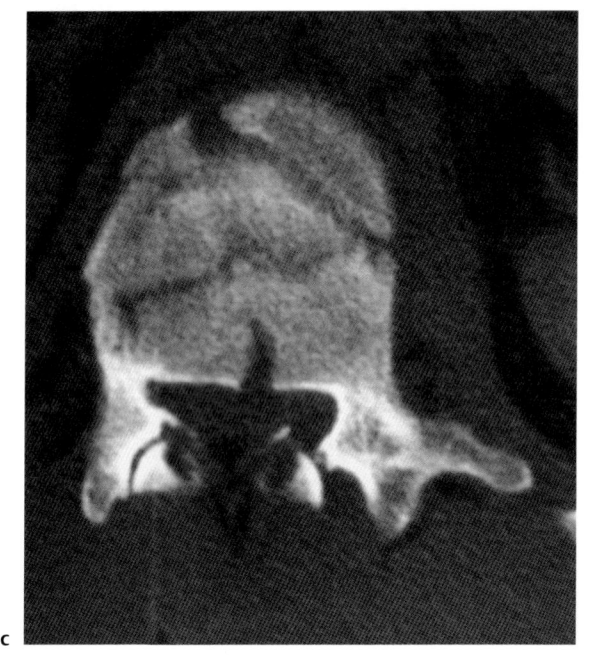

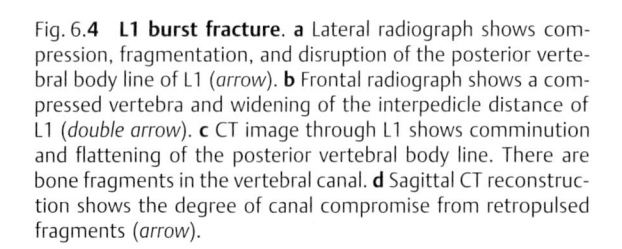

sion of the vertebral body, disruption of the posterior body line, and widening of the interpedicle distance. These features may all be seen in Figures 6.**1** and 6.**4**.

The posterior vertebral body line is a single uninterrupted structure in the cervical and upper thoracic region. In the lower thoracic and lumbar regions, a nutrient vessel interrupts it centrally. At C2, this line should extend cephalad along the posterior aspect of the dens. Any displacement, duplication, angulation, rotation, or absence of this line is abnormal. In a typical

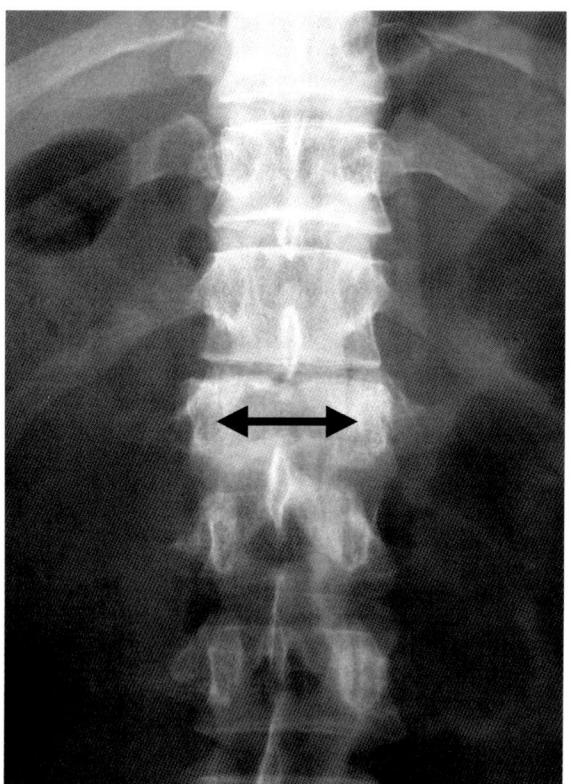

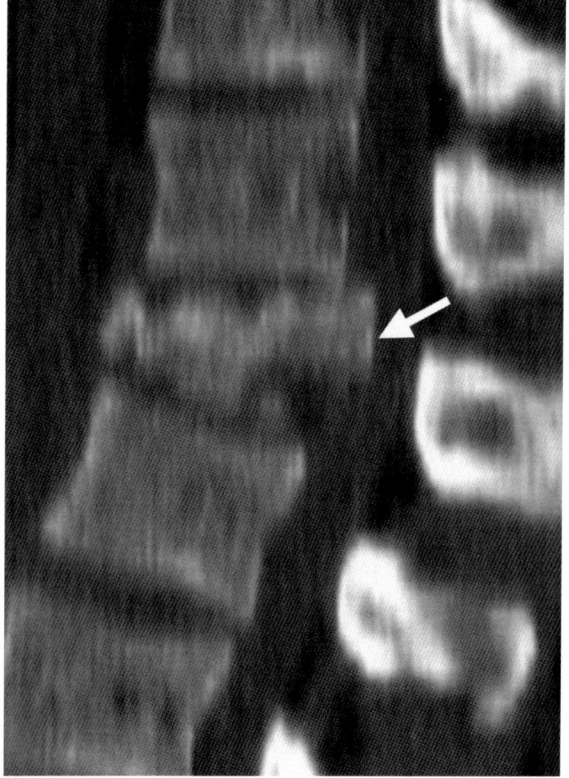

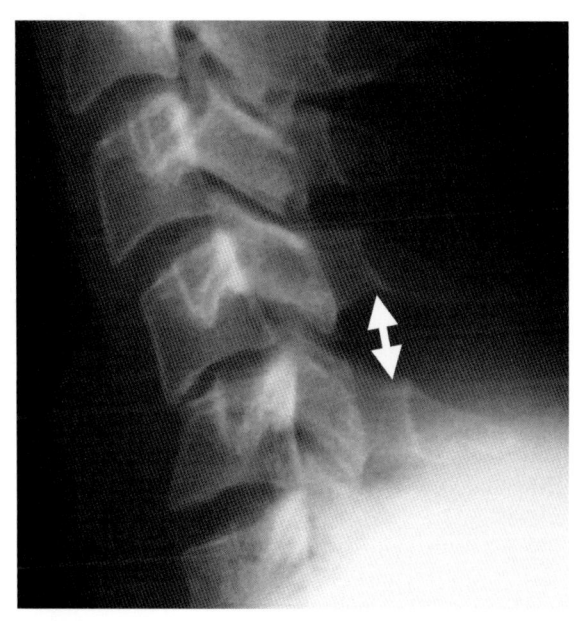

Fig. 6.**6** Hyperflexion sprain C4–5. Note kyphotic angulation and widening of the interlaminar space (*double arrow*).

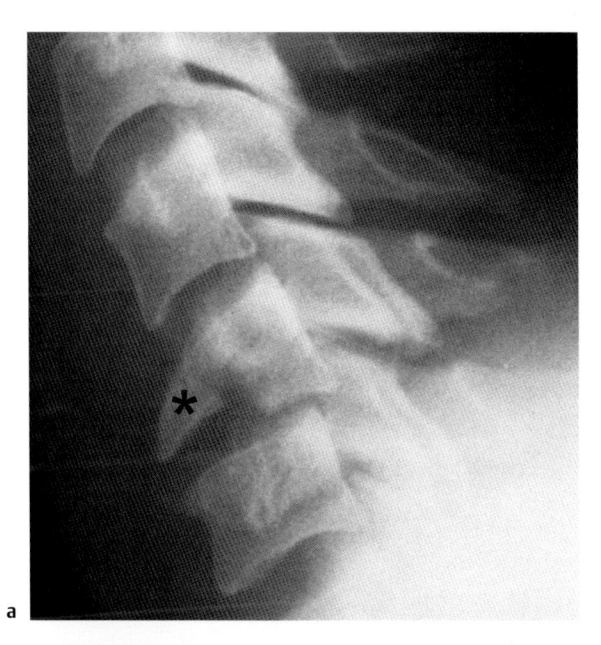

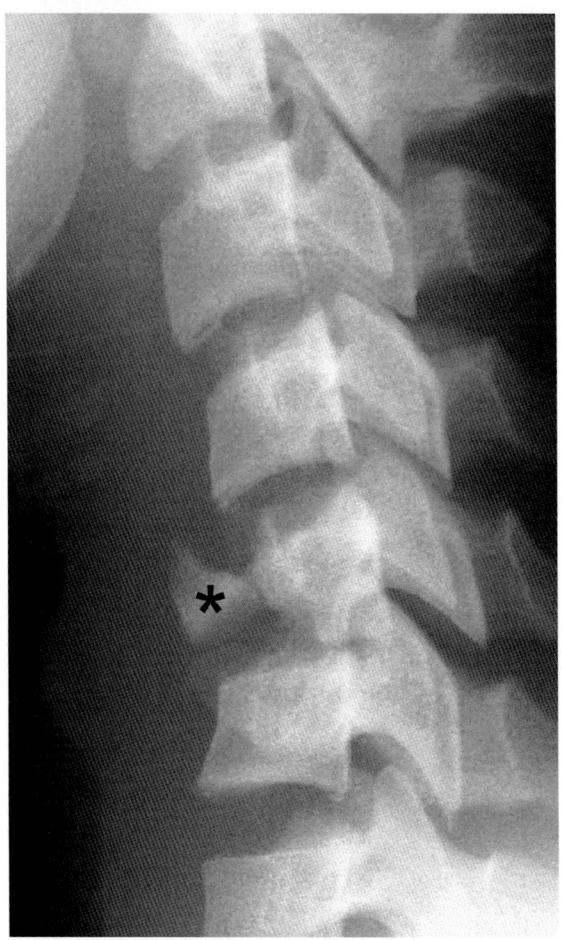

Fig. 6.**5 Flexion "teardrop" injuries in two different patients**. Forward flexion has produced anterior inferior "teardrop" fragments (*). In both instances there is slight retrolisthesis of the vertebral bodies.

burst fracture, there is posterior displacement of this line on lateral radiographs, and this displacement represents the retropulsed bone fragment within the vertebral canal. CT (and/or MRI) will confirm this (Figs. 6.**1**–6.**4**).

The interpedicle distance is measured from the medial sclerotic areas of the pedicles on frontal radiographs. The difference in the distance between two contiguous levels should never exceed 2 mm. Burst fractures, particularly those of the sagittal cleavage variety, widen this space, a finding which may be frequently seen on frontal radiographs (Fig. 6.**4b**). Another manifestation of sagittal cleavage is widening of the facet joints at the involved level(s). The implication of this finding, when encountered on a frontal radiograph, is that the vertebra has been split along the sagittal plane both through the body as well as through the lamina. A variation of the burst fracture is the flexion "teardrop" injury in the cervical spine. In this variant, a triangular fragment of bone is displaced from the anteroinferior margin of the vertebral body. There is slight retrolisthesis of the remainder of the body (Fig. 6.**5**). When this finding is associated with evidence of posterior distraction, severe neurological deficits result.

Distraction injuries occur primarily in two varieties. The first is primarily a ligamentous and soft tissue type of injury. In the cervical region, this is referred to as the hyperflexion sprain. If fractures occur in association with this injury, they are usually small avulsion fractures. In this injury, the posterior ligaments are torn as well as the posterior longitudinal ligament and the posterior third of the intervertebral disks. This produces widening of the interlaminar or interspinous spaces, widening of the facets, and varying degrees of anterolisthesis (Figs. 6.**6**, 6.**7**). Intervertebral disk herniation frequently occurs with distraction injuries.

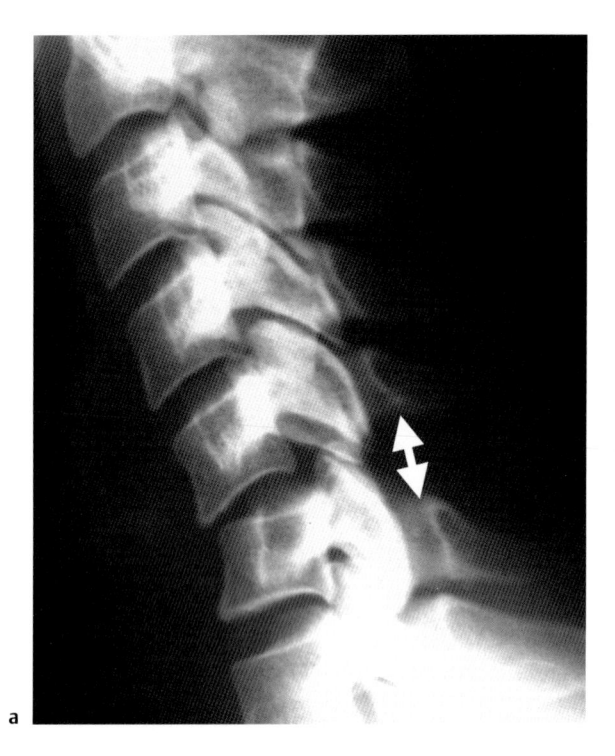

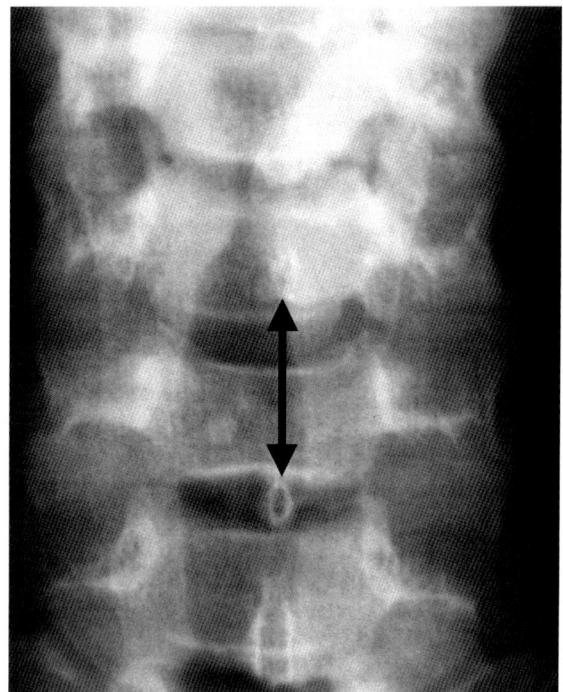

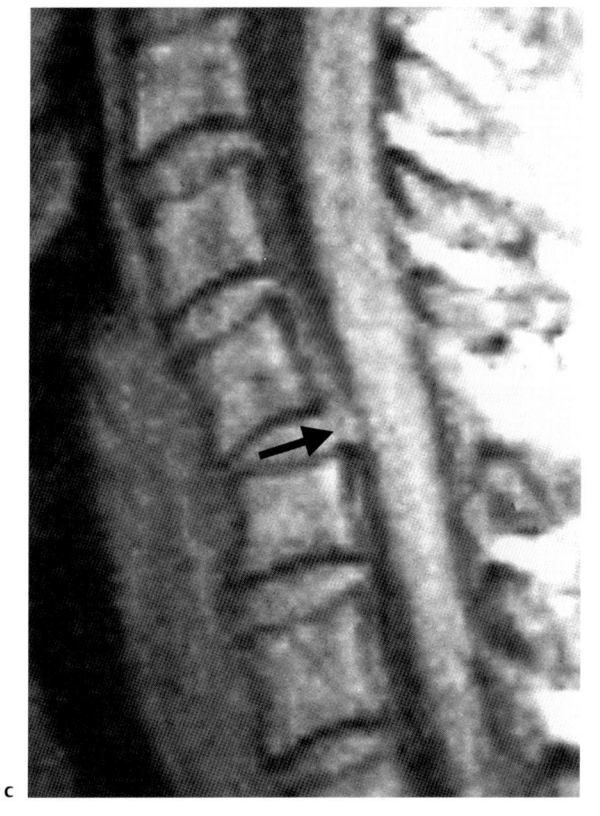

Fig. 6.**7** Hyperflexion sprain C5–C6. **a** Lateral radiograph shows kyphotic angulation, anterolisthesis of C5 on C6, and widening of the interlaminar space (*double arrow*), and facet joints. **b** Frontal view shows widening of the interspinous distance (*double arrow*). **c** Proton density-weighted MR sagittal image shows rupture of the posterior longitudinal ligament and disk herniation at C5–C6 (*arrow*).

A pure distraction-type of injury also occurs in the thoracolumbar region where the findings are similar to those in the cervical region. One feature, however, that is fairly unique in the thoracic and lumbar distraction injuries are the so-called "naked facets" (Fig. 6.**8**).

The second form of distraction injury is one in which there are horizontally oriented fractures through the vertebral body that may continue through the pedicles, articular pillars, laminae, and/or spinous processes. These are better known as the Chance-type injuries and are the result of forward flexion on a lap-type seat-belt (Fig. 6.**9**). While one level appears to be involved from a radiographic standpoint, MRI frequently shows evidence of injury to contiguous

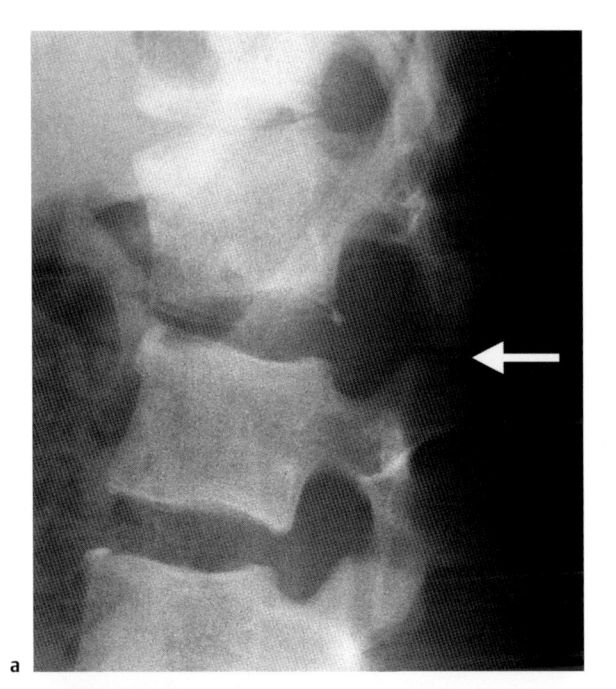

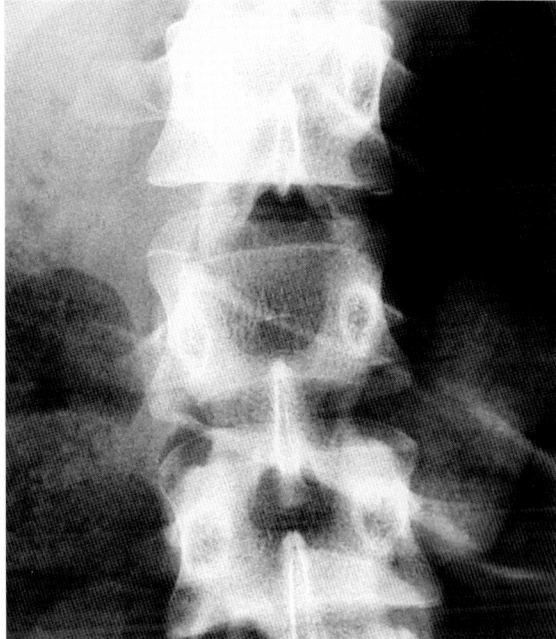

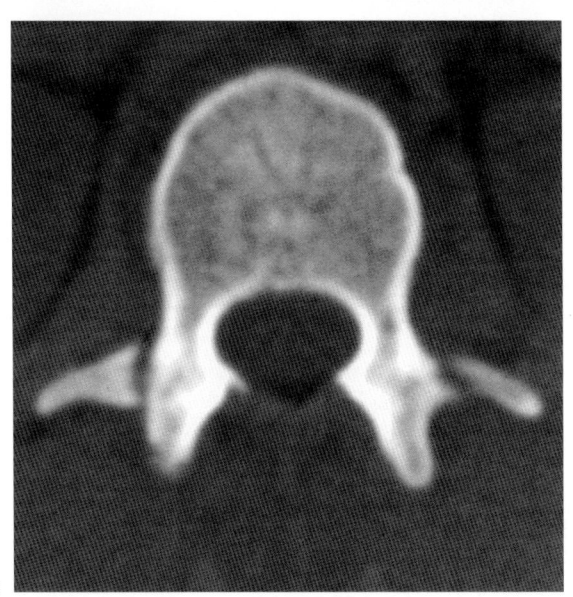

Fig. 6.8 **L1–L2 flexion distraction injury with perched facets. a** Lateral radiograph shows widening of the L1 disk space and perching of the facets of L1 on L2 (*arrow*). There is a small avulsion fragment from the posterior inferior margin of L1, as well. **b** Frontal radiograph shows widening of the interspinous space between L1 and L2 and "naked" facets on the left. **c** CT image through the injury shows absence of posterior elements from the adjoining vertebra and "naked" facets of L1. There are also bilateral transverse process fractures.

levels (Fig. 6.10). Patients with Chance-type fractures frequently suffer abdominal visceral injuries.

Flexion-dislocation injuries are the result of severe distractive forces. These may or may not be associated with fractures. A prime example of this type of injury is a unilateral (Fig. 6.11) or bilateral jumped and locked facet. These injuries frequently produce severe neurological deficits.

The "fingerprints" of flexion injuries are summarized in Table 6.1.

Extension injuries are much more common in the cervical region than in the thoracic and lumbar regions. The reason for this is the greater mobility of the cervical spine. All extension injuries are the result of varying degrees of backward bending where the fulcrum of motion is at the level of the articular pillars.

The radiographic hallmark of extension injuries is *widening* of the intervertebral disk space *below* the level of injury. In the cervical region, widening is frequently accompanied by an avulsion of the anterosuperior lip of the subjacent vertebral body. If the force is severe enough to disrupt the anterior longitudinal ligament and intervertebral disk, retrolisthesis may occur. In the most severe cases, the articular pillars are crushed since they are the fulcrum of motion.

There are three subtypes of extension injury: simple, distraction, and dislocation. A *simple* extension injury is usually nothing more than an avulsion of the anterosuperior portion of a vertebral body with minimal or no widening of the disk space above. This injury usually produces no neurological deficits. The *distraction* injury produces obvious widening of the intervertebral

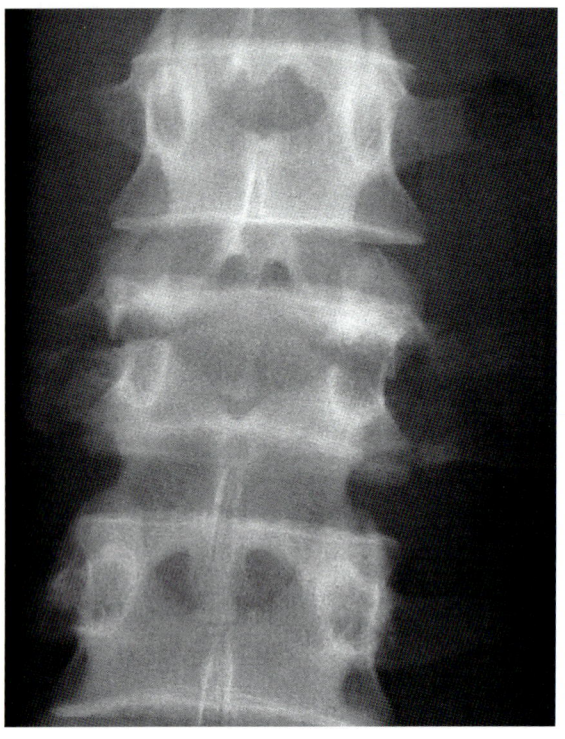

Fig. 6.9 **Chance-type fracture of L3 as a result of a lap belt.**
a Frontal radiograph shows horizontal fractures involving the vertebral body, pedicles, and transverse processes. **b** Lateral radiograph shows fragmentation of the vertebral body and posterior distraction. Note the fractures through the pedicles (*arrow*).

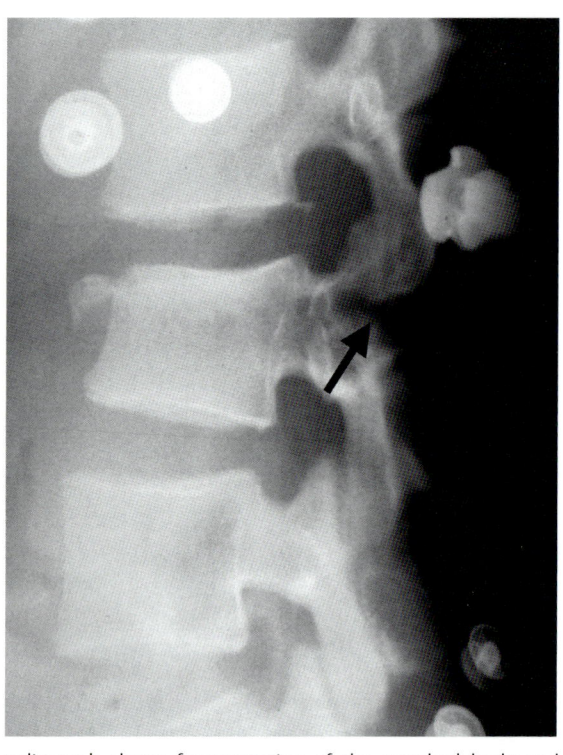

Table 6.1 "Fingerprints" of vertebral injury

Flexion	Compression, fragmentation, burst of vertebral bodies "Teardrop" fragments Anterolisthesis Disrupted posterior vertebral body line Wide interlaminar (interspinous) space Locked facets Narrow disk space **above** involved vertebra
Extension	Wide disk space **below** involved vertebra Triangular avulsion fracture anteriorly Retrolisthesis Neural arch and/or pillar fracture Anterolisthesis with **normal** interlaminar space and spinolaminar line
Rotary	Rotation Dislocation Disrupted posterior vertebral body line Facet and/or pillar fracture or dislocation Transverse process and/or rib fracture Spinous process fracture Rotary array of fragments on CT
Shearing	"Windswept" appearance Lateral distraction Lateral dislocation Transverse process and/or rib fracture Linear "windswept" array of fragments on CT

disk space with or without an avulsion fracture of the subjacent vertebra. The most common type of these injuries is the "hangman's" fracture of C2 (Fig. 6.12). A more severe type of distraction injury is the so-called hyperextension sprain (Fig. 6.13). This variant occurs most commonly in elderly individuals who have suffered an injury to the chin. Hyperextension sprains produce widening of the intervertebral disk space and retrolisthesis (Fig. 6.13). These patients have severe neurological deficits, usually a central cord syndrome, whereas those with a hangman's fracture usually suffer no neurological deficits (unless the injury occurred during a judicial hanging).

A wide disk space is never a normal finding. The finding of a wide disk, particularly in older individuals with degenerative changes of the spine, should always raise one's suspicion that an extension sprain has occurred. Extension *dislocations* are, fortunately, rare. These are severely disruptive injuries that surprisingly often result in *anterolisthesis,* crushed articular pillars, and no disruption in the spinolaminar line. It is this last feature, which distinguishes the extension fracture dislocation from the more common flexion injury.

Extension injuries in the thoracic and lumbar areas are infrequent. In most instances, they occur in individuals with rigid spine disease (ankylosing spondyl-

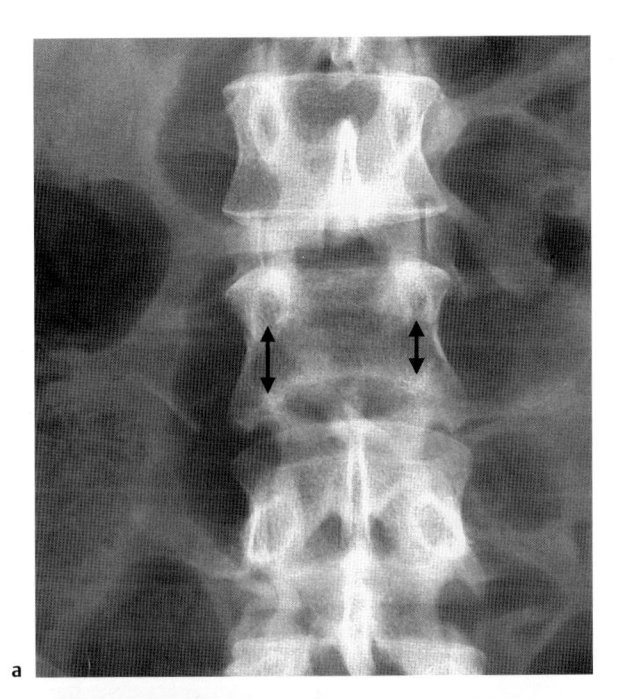

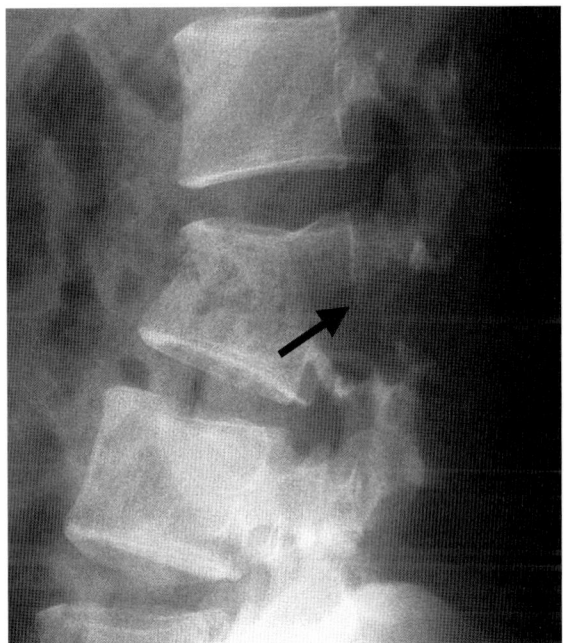

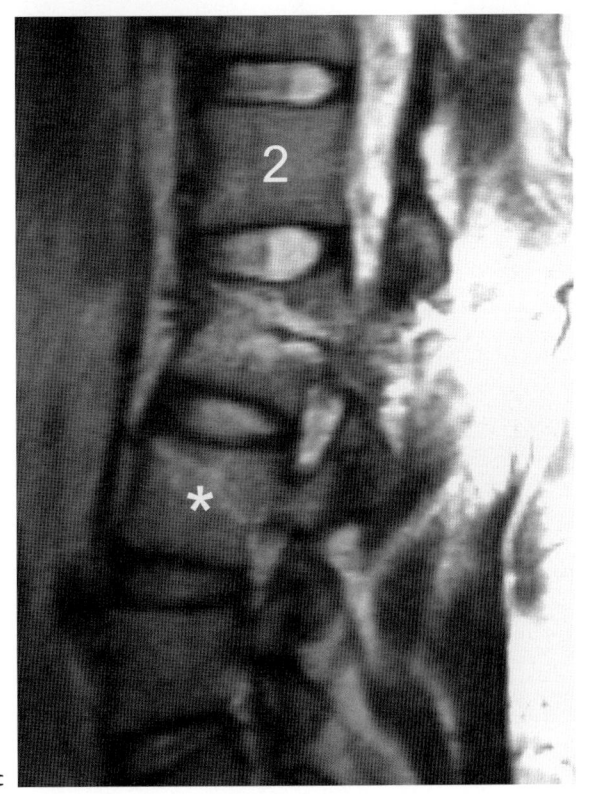

Fig. 6.**10 Chance-type fracture of L3 with adjacent injury. a** Frontal radiograph shows widening of the interspinous space and fractures through the vertebral body, lamina, pedicles, and transverse processes of L3. Note the wide separation of the fragments from the pedicles (*double arrows*). **b** Lateral radiograph shows anterior compression and posterior distraction of L3. Note the angulation in the upper portion of the posterior vertebral body line (*arrow*). **c** T2W sagittal MR image shows the fracture line and surrounding edema in L3. There is increased signal in L4 (*) indicating occult injury at that level also. Radiographs and CT of L4 were normal.

itis or DISH) (Fig. 6.**14**). The "fingerprints" of extension injuries are summarized in Table 6.**1**.

Rotary injuries occur primarily in two areas. The less severe of these occur at the craniocervical junction in the form of either rotary subluxation or fixation of C1 on C2. The more severe rotary injuries occur at the thoracolumbar junction as the result of torsional forces combined with axial loading. The typical mechanism is that of the victim having suffered a severe blow in the shoulder region that produces axial loading while rotation has occurred in the lower torso. We most frequently encounter this type of injury in patients who have been thrown from motor vehicles and strike a solid object after being ejected. As the result of these forces, the vertebra is literally pulverized. This is the most severe form of vertebral injury and almost always produces severe neurological deficits. The typical imaging findings of these injuries include dislocation and rotation of fragments. The posterior vertebral body line is usually disrupted. A common manifestation of this

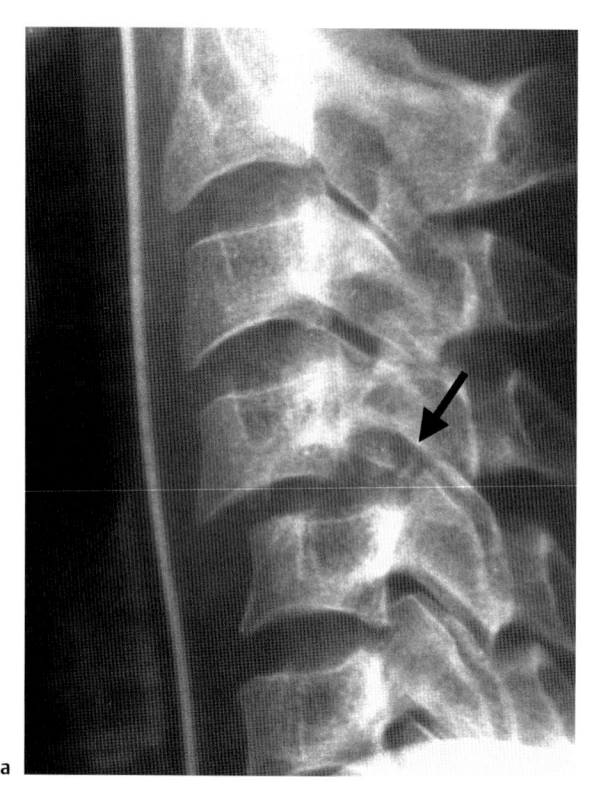

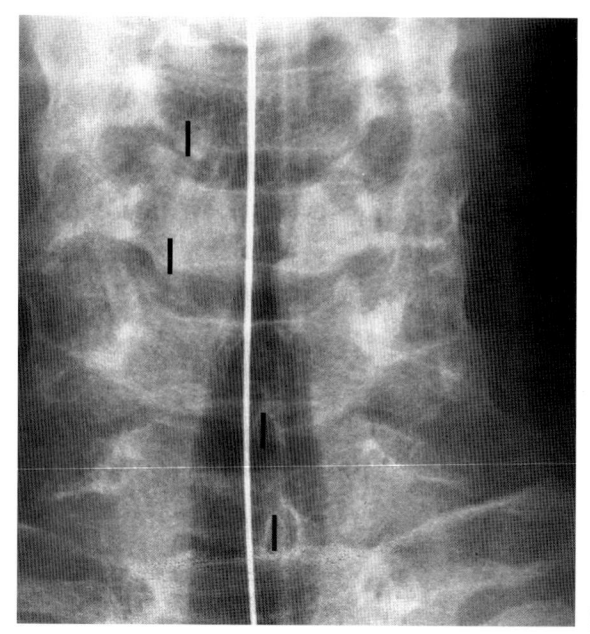

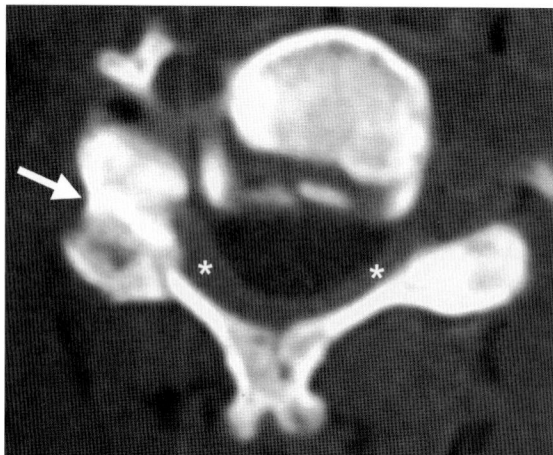

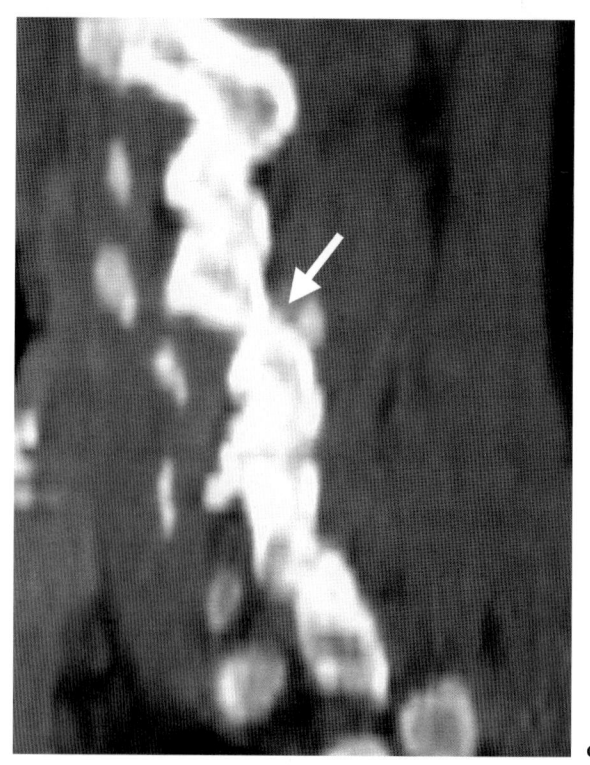

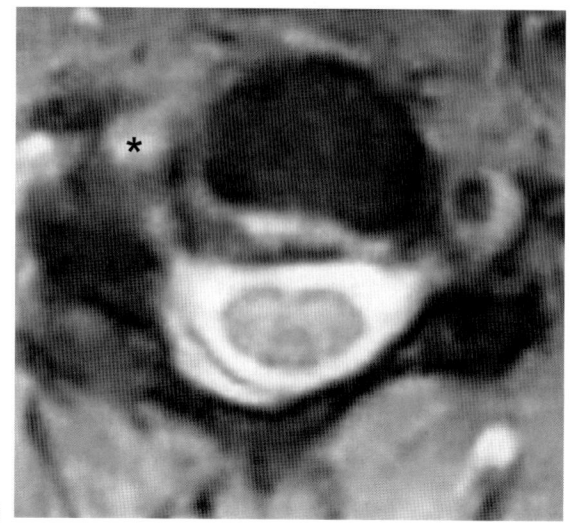

Fig. 6.11 **Unilateral jumped and locked facet at C4–C5 on the right. a** Lateral radiograph shows anterolisthesis of C4 on C5. The pillars of C5 and below superimpose; those of C4 and above are duplicated. The point of locking is demonstrated (*arrow*). **b** Frontal radiograph shows widening of the interspinous distance and rotation of the spinous processes of C3 and C4 to the right (I), the side of locking. The other spinous processes are in the mid-line. **c** CT image through the injury level shows the point of locking on the right (*arrow*) as well as anterolisthesis of C4 on C5. There is an epidural hematoma posteriorly (*). **d** Sagittal reconstructed CT image through the pillars on the right show the point of locking (*arrow*) as well as a fracture of the superior facet of C5. **e** Fat-saturated T2W image through the injury level shows lack of the normal flow void in the right vertebral artery (*). Compare this with the left side. Vertebral artery occlusion is a frequent complication of this type of injury.

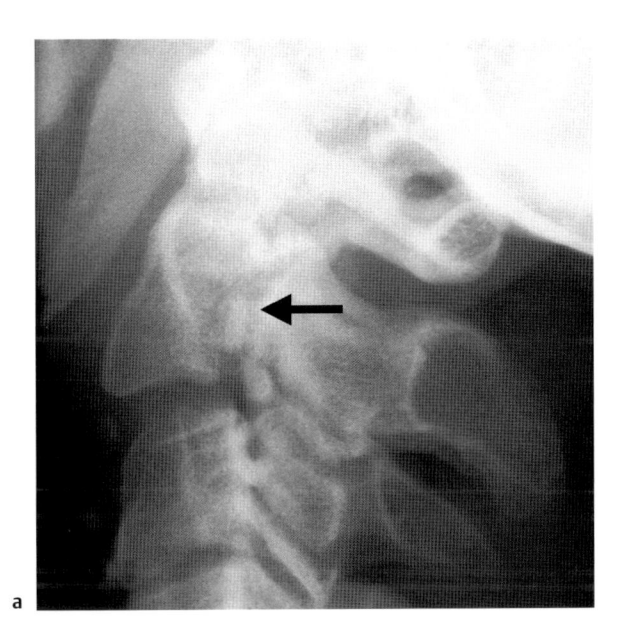

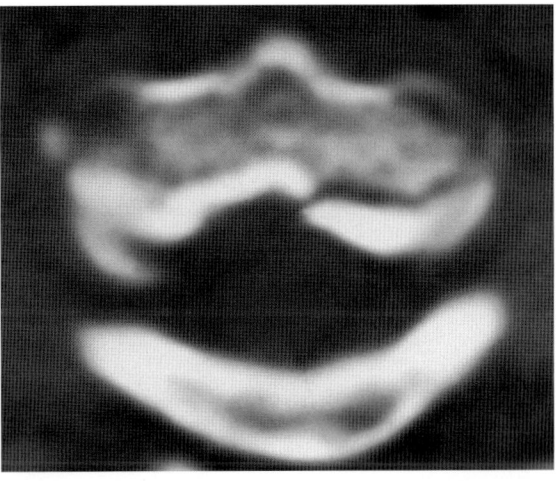

Fig. 6.**12** **Hangman's fracture of C2. a** Lateral radiograph shows a fracture through the posterior body of C2 (*arrow*). The C2 disk space is slightly widened. **b** CT image shows the fracture extending across the posterior body of C2.

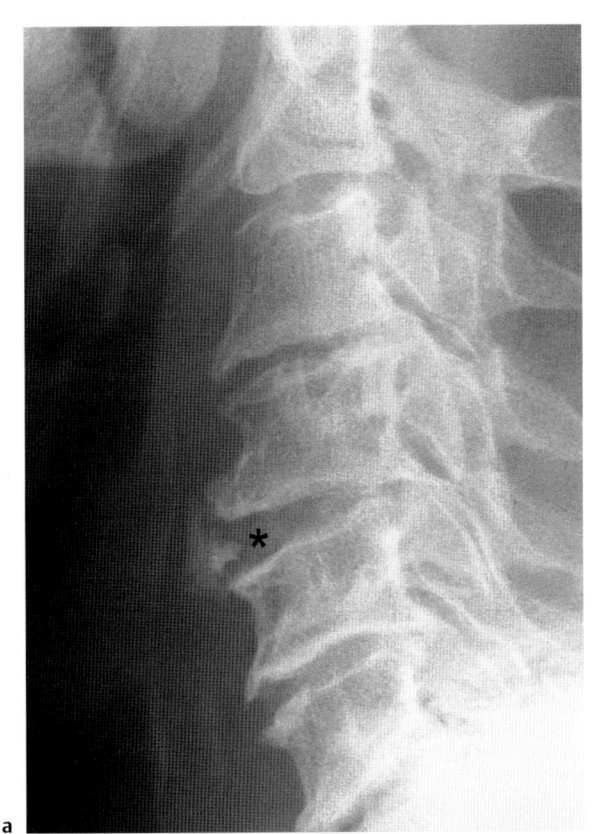

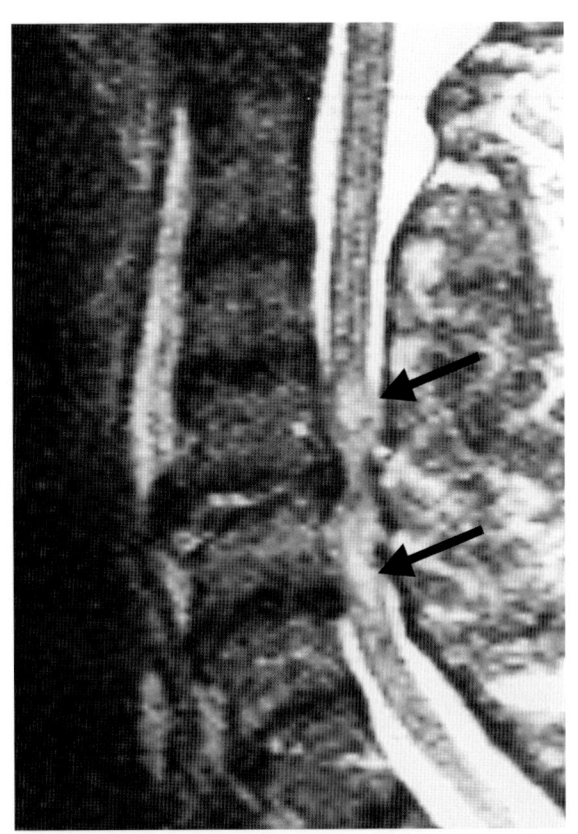

Fig. 6.**13** **Hyperextension sprain C4. a** Lateral radiograph shows widening of the C4 disk space (*), slight retrolisthesis of C4 on C5 and an avulsed bone fragment from the inferior margin of C4. **b** T2W sagittal image shows spinal stenosis, edema in the spinal cord at C4 and C5 (*arrows*) and edema in the C5 disk space and prevertebral soft tissues. The patient had a central cord syndrome.

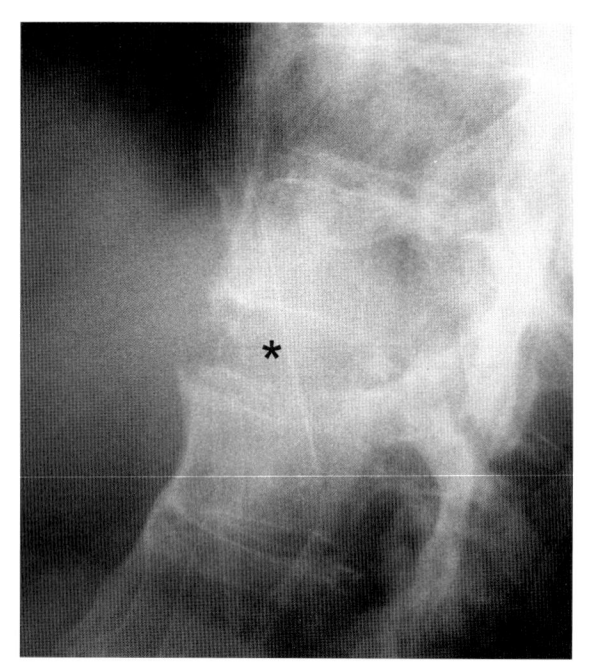

injury is the avulsion of a large triangular fragment from the anterosuperior margin of the subjacent vertebra (Fig. 6.**15**). In addition, fractures of the transverse processes and/or ribs frequently occur. Facet fractures and dislocations also typically occur as the result of the severe rotary forces applied to them. On the CT examination, the findings are also characteristic and consist of severe fragmentation with a *concentric* distribution of the fragments. The pattern of disruption of the facet joints that accompany these injuries can frequently allow one to tell whether the rotary force occurred to the right or to the left (Fig. 6.**15**).

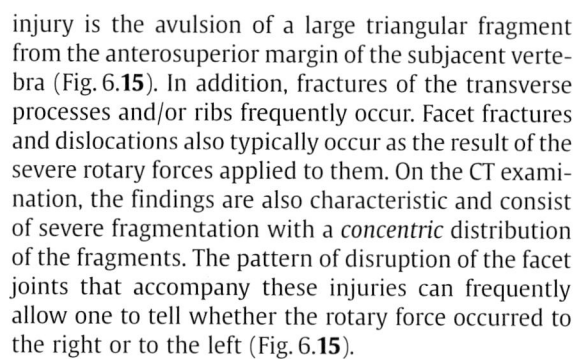

It is extremely important to recognize the rotary mechanism and to distinguish such injuries from burst fractures because the treatment of each is significantly different. The operative treatment of a burst fracture provides stabilization along the plane of flexion and extension. Rotary injuries require that the treatment be directed not only to the flexion component of the injury but also to the rotary component. Failure to recognize the rotary nature of the injury may result in failure of the surgical construct. The "fingerprints" of the rotary injury are summarized in Table 6.**1**.

Shearing injuries are produced by horizontal or obliquely directed forces in which axial loading is gener-

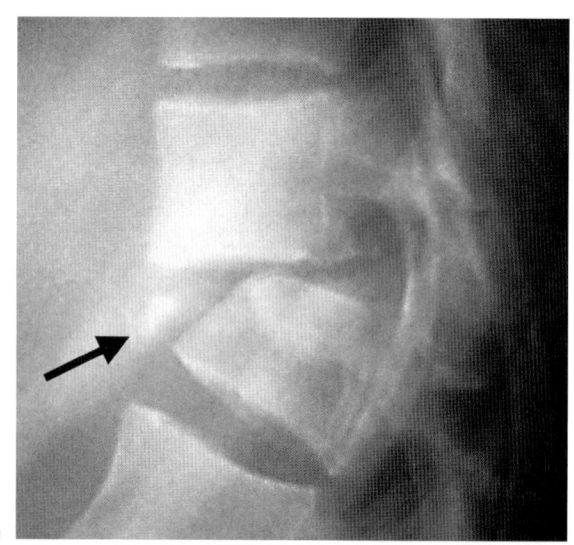

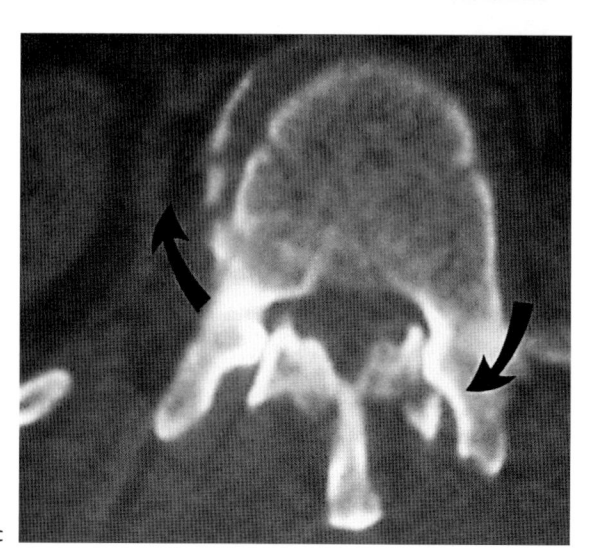

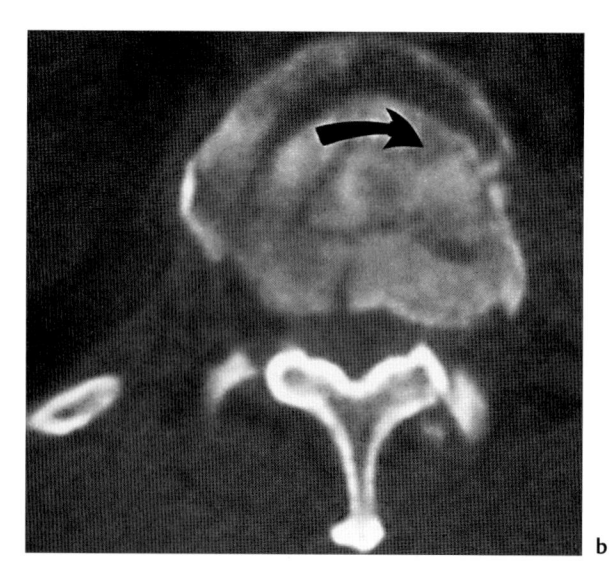

Fig. 6.**14** **Hyperextension injury at T11–T12 in a patient with DISH.** Note the wide disk space (*). Compare this figure with Figure 6.**13a**.

Fig. 6.**15** **Rotary ("grinding") injury at T12–L1. a** Lateral radiograph shows anterolisthesis of T12 on L1. There is a small-avulsed fragment from the anterior superior margin of L1 (*arrow*). **b** CT image shows a concentric distribution to the fracture fragments. *Arrow* indicates the direction of rotation that occurred. **c** CT image slightly lower shows disruption of the facet joints. *Arrows* indicate direction of rotation with the right facet displaced anteriorly and the left facet displaced posteriorly.

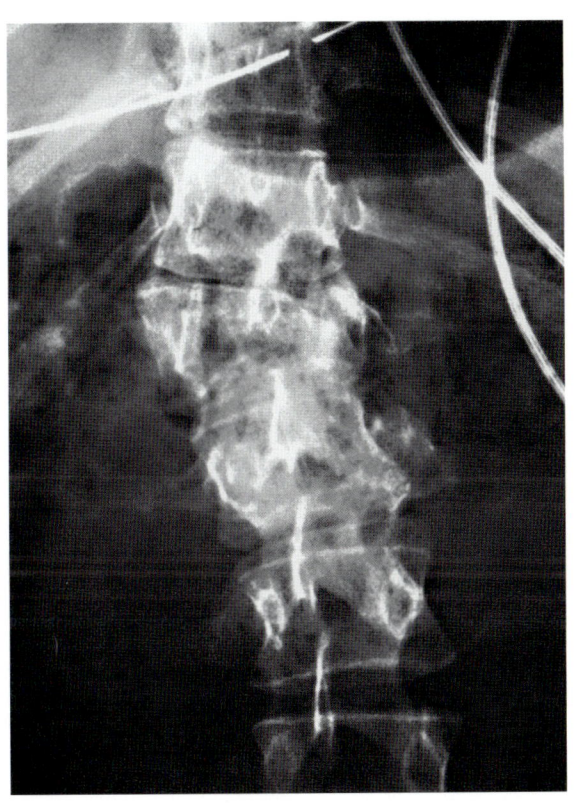

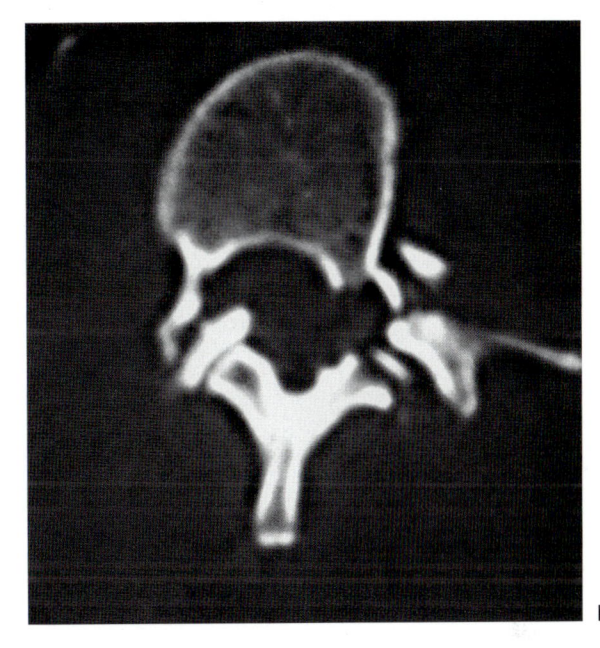

Fig. 6.**16** **Shearing injury. a** Frontal radiograph shows a "windswept" appearance at the thoracolumbar junction. Note the severe disruption of L1 and transverse process fractures at multiple levels. **b** CT image through the level of injury shows a "windswept" appearance to the vertebra as well as multiple fracture fragments.

ally not a factor. In the typical mechanism, the lower portion of the body is fixed. The vertebral column absorbs the horizontal or oblique forces and moves with it. Typically this occurs also when patients are ejected from a motor vehicle or when struck by a large, solid object. On occasion, shearing injuries are also combined with rotary forces as the result of secondary impact. Most shearing injuries produce severe neurological compromise.

Shearing injuries occur typically at the thoracolumbar junction. The classic radiographic features are of horizontal or oblique distraction and dislocation. The vertebrae often have a "windswept" appearance (Fig. 6.**16**). Shearing injuries typically also have associated transverse process and/or rib fractures. A CT examination will frequently show the "windswept" appearance as well. Shearing injuries need to be distinguished from burst injuries because the treatment implications are identical to those considered for rotary injuries. The "windswept" appearance usually is characteristic enough to establish the distinction between the two injuries. The "fingerprints" of shearing injuries are listed in Table 6.**1**.

"Footprints" of Vertebral Injury— the ABCS

The previous discussion detailed radiographic findings that helped to distinguish injuries due to various mechanisms. While the "fingerprints" tell you what kind of injury has occurred and helps you to determine the extent of that injury, the "footprints" will lead you to the injury. We prefer a simplified approach referred to as the "ABCS": **A**natomy and **A**lignment abnormalities; **B**ony integrity abnormalities; **C**artilage or joint space abnormalities; **S**oft tissue abnormalities.

A detailed description of vertebral anatomy is beyond the scope of this chapter. However, it is incumbent upon the reader to be thoroughly familiar with not only the anatomy of the vertebral column, but also with the terminology used in describing that anatomy. For this purpose, the reader is referred to the chapter on Anatomical Considerations in Daffner (1996),[16] or to a general anatomical text.

Normal alignment may be ascertained on all radiographs as well as on reconstructed CT and MR images. On the lateral or sagittal views, normal markers of anatomy include the anterior and posterior margins of the vertebral bodies, the junctions of the laminae to form the spinous processes (spinolaminar line), the articular pillars and their facet joints, and the interlaminar or interspinous distance. As mentioned previously, the posterior vertebral body line represents the posterior margin of the vertebra. Under normal circumstances,

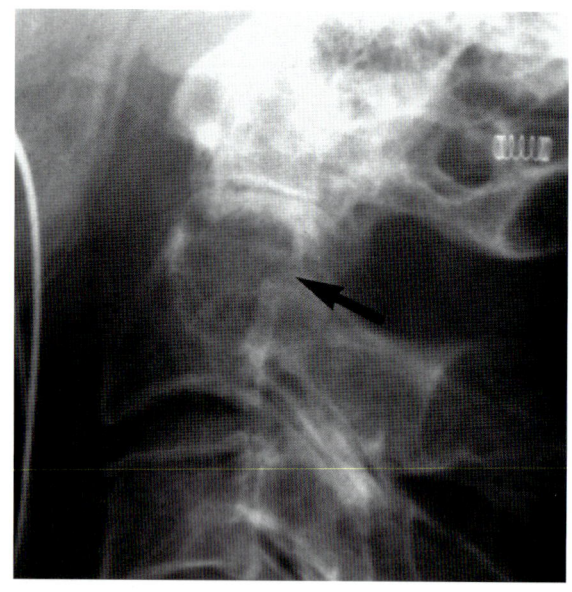

Fig. 6.17 **Disruption of Harris' ring due to a C2 body fracture. a** Lateral radiograph shows a break in the posterior arc of Harris' ring (*arrow*). **b** CT image through C2 shows the fracture as well as an epidural hematoma (*).

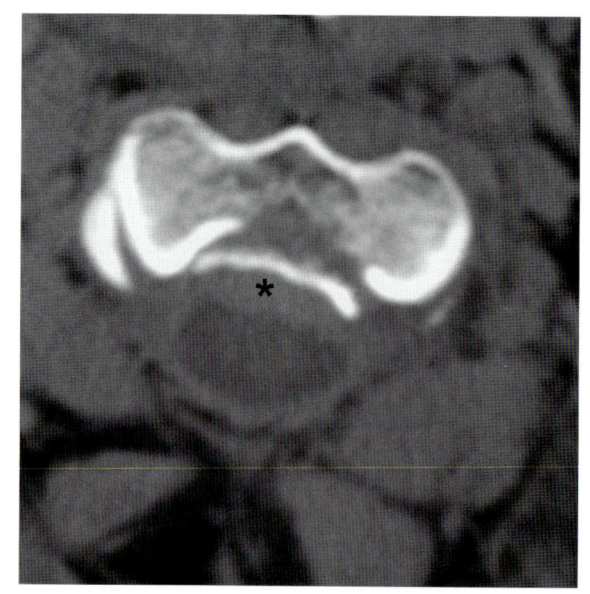

Table 6.2 Anatomy and alignment abnormalities

Disruption of anterior or posterior vertebral body lines
Disruption of spinolaminar line
Jumped and locked facets
Rotation of spinous processes
Wide interpedicle distance
Wide predental space
Wide facet joint
Kyphotic angulation
Loss of lordosis
Torticollis

the line drawn along the anterior or posterior margins of the vertebral bodies should be smooth and uninterrupted. In children, a notable exception known as pseudosubluxation occurs because of the differences in growth rates between various portions of the vertebral column. However, in these individuals, the spinolaminar line is normal. The junction of the laminae with the spinous processes, the articular pillars of the cervical vertebrae, and the articular processes of the thoracic and lumbar vertebrae should be symmetric and should appear like the shingles on a roof (imbrication). Their images should superimpose nearly perfectly. Minor degrees of rotation produce double facet images. However, the change is usually gradual. Abrupt duplication of the images in the cervical region is usually an indication of a unilateral facet lock (Fig. 6.11).

The spaces between the laminae or the spinous processes (the interlaminar or interspinous space) should be symmetric and should not vary by more than 2 mm from adjacent levels.

On the lateral cervical radiograph, there are several additional anatomic considerations, particularly in regard to the relationships at the craniocervical junction. The predental space between the anterior arch of the atlas and the dens should never exceed 3 mm in adults or 5 mm in children.[16] A line drawn along the posterior vertebral body line of C2, extended cephalad along the dens, should be between 6 mm and 12 mm behind the basion (the anterior extent of the foramen magnum). Any deviations from these distances may be a sign of occipitoatlantal disruption. Furthermore, the space between the basion and the tip of the dens should not exceed 12 mm.[24,25]

Another major landmark in the upper cervical spine is known as Harris' ring of C2.[16,26] This ring-like structure is the result of overlap of images of several normal structures: the superior arch represents superior articular facets; the posterior arch represents the posterior vertebral body line; the inferior arch represents a portion of the transverse foramen; and the anterior arch represents the anterior body cortex. Disruption of this ring may frequently be the only manifestation of a fractured C2 (Fig. 6.**17**). Finally, the space between the posterior arch of C1 and the spinous process of C2 should never exceed 18 mm.

On frontal views, three findings deserve mention. The first of these is the interpedicle distance mentioned previously. The second is the interspinous distance between the spinous processes. As previously mentioned, these two measurements should never differ by more than 2 mm from level to level. Finally, duplication of a spinous process image indicates a fracture of that structure.

Alignment abnormalities are summarized in Table 6.**2**. It is important to note that the last three of these findings, kyphotic angulation, loss of lordosis, and torticollis, while extremely common, are never the sole manifestation of an injury. When an injury is present, these findings are usually combined with one or more of the other abnormalities.[16,27]

"Footprints" of Vertebral Injury—the ABCS

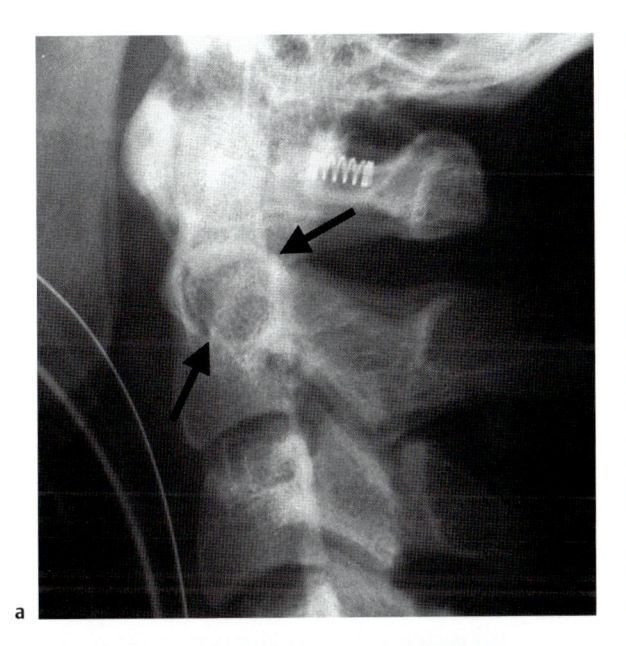

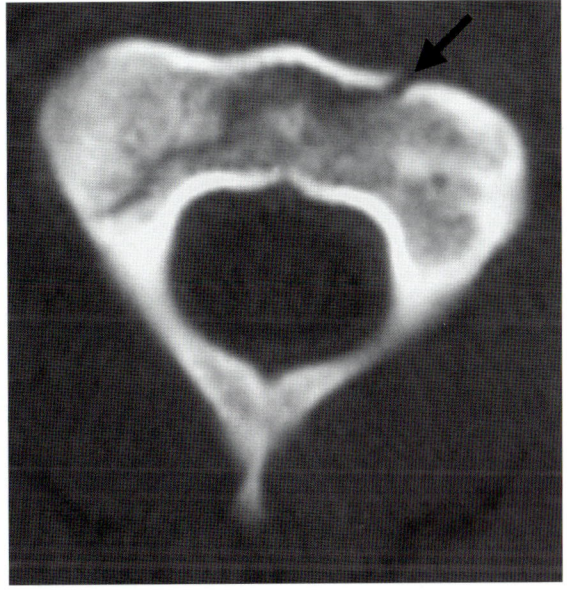

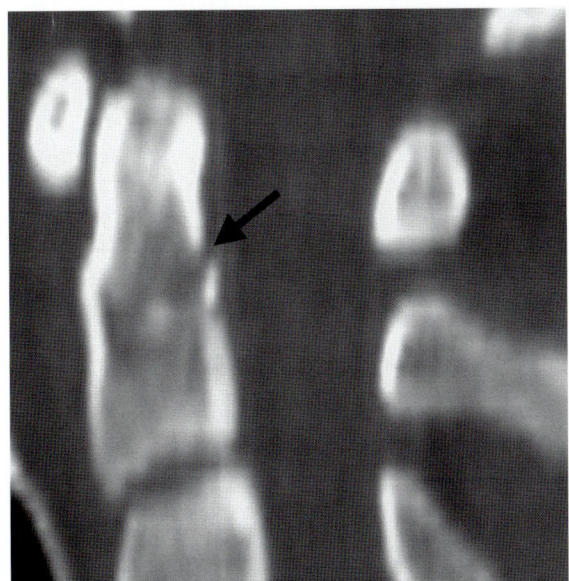

Fig. 6.18 Subtle C2 body fracture. a Lateral radiograph shows disruption of Harris' ring posteriorly and inferiorly (*arrows*). **b** Sagittal CT image shows the fracture to better advantage (*arrow*). **c** Sagittal reconstructed CT image shows the fracture better than the radiograph (*arrow*).

Abnormalities of bony integrity include both direct and indirect signs of fracture. Thoracic and lumbar radiographs are usually adequate for detecting the majority of fractures. In the cervical region, however, CT is much more sensitive in identifying fractures than is radiography (Fig. 6.**18**).[1,2,5,19] For this reason, we rely on a number of radiographic secondary signs that would indicate an injury. Two of these include disruption of Harris' ring and the "fat C2 sign."[28] Fractures of the axis vertebra are extremely common in elderly individuals.[29] In many instances, disruption of Harris' ring may be the only manifestation of such an injury (Fig. 6.**17**). In more severe injuries, other alignment abnormalities such as displacement of the dens or disruption of the spinolaminar line may be in evidence. Smoker and Dolan described another sign that was useful in diagnosing C2 fractures.[28] They made the observation that

Table 6.**3** Bony integrity abnormalities

Obvious fracture
Disrupted "ring" of C2
"Fat" C2 body
Wide interpedicle distance
Disrupted posterior vertebral body line
Disrupted sacral arcuate lines

the anterior-to-posterior width of the body of C2 should be the same as that of C3. Axis fractures frequently result in an increase in the size of the body of C2 on lateral radiographs, which they term the "fat C2 sign." The sign is the result of displacement of fracture fragments. Frequently the posterior arch of the atlas is also displaced anteriorly as is illustrated in Figure 6.**19**. Table 6.**3** summarizes the abnormalities of

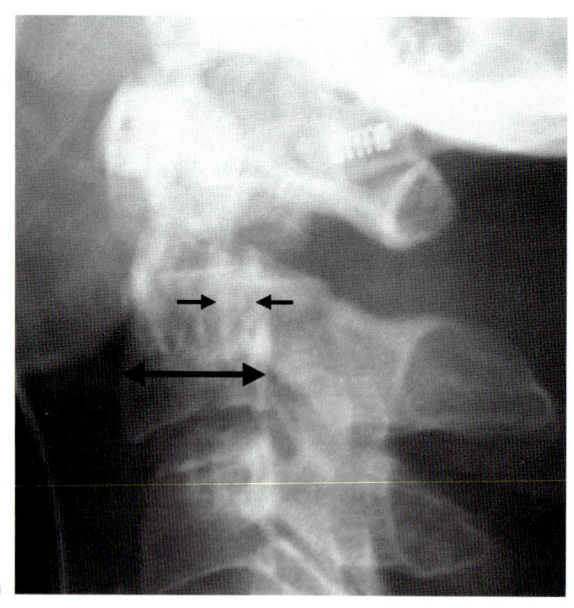

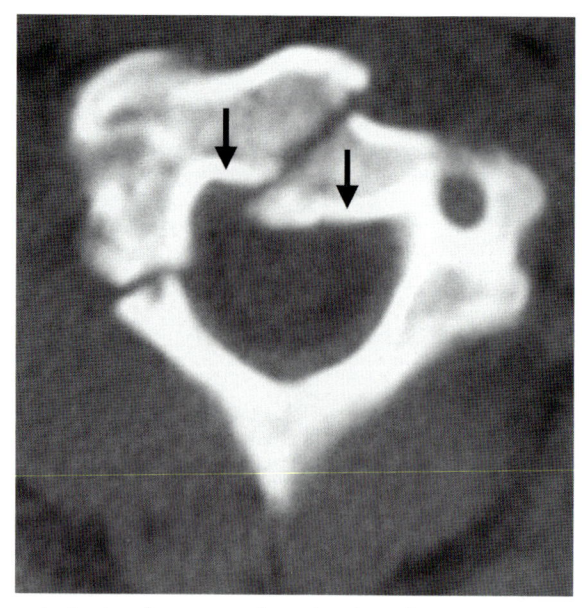

Fig. 6.19 "Fat C2 Sign." a Lateral radiograph shows widening of the body of C2 compared to that of C3 (*double arrow*). There is duplication of the posterior vertebral body line (*short arrows*). b CT image shows an oblique fracture through the body of C2 and a laminar fracture on the right. The right portion of C2 is displaced anteriorly, accounting for the double posterior vertebral body line (*arrows*).

Table 6.4 Cartilage (joint) space abnormalities

Wide predental space (above 3 mm adult, 5 mm child)
Wide or narrow disk space
Wide facet joints
"Naked" facets
Locked facets
Wide interlaminar (interspinous) space
Abnormal occipitoatlantal junction

bony integrity. Note the overlap of some of these signs with abnormalities of alignment. For this reason, we often consider the two categories together.

Abnormalities of the cartilage or joint spaces occur frequently with vertebral injuries. As previously mentioned, flexion injuries usually produce narrowing of the disk space above the level of compression, while extension injuries typically widen the disk space. The narrow disk space is a much less specific sign, since it is a common component of degenerative spondylosis. The common manifestations of flexion injuries include widening of the facet joints and "naked" facets (Figs. 6.4, 6.6). If posterior distraction occurs, the interlaminar distance is frequently increased. Finally, widening of the predental space over 3 mm in an adult or 5 mm in a child is another subtle manifestation of injury. This is most likely to occur in an adult with rheumatoid arthritis or in a child with trisomy 21 (Down's syndrome). When widening of the predental space occurs, there is disruption of the spinolaminar line (Fig. 6.20). Table 6.4 summarizes the abnormalities of the cartilage or joint spaces.

The authors define a fracture as *a soft tissue injury in which a bone is broken*. Injuries to the vertebral column are no exception and produce a number of soft tissue abnormalities, primarily in the cervical region. In some instances, it is the soft tissue changes that direct one's attention to a subtle injury (Fig. 6.21). It should be noted, however, that if CT is used as the primary screening tool for cervical injury, observing the soft tissue abnormalities would take a secondary role. The most important of these soft tissue changes occur at the craniovertebral junction. In this region, retropharyngeal soft tissue width is measured from the anterior-inferior margin of C2 to the pharyngeal air column. This space should never exceed 7 mm in adults or children.[16] Harris has pointed out that the contour of the soft tissue shadows is more important than the width (Fig. 6.21).[30] The reader should be cautioned that there are a large variety of conditions that can cause widening of the retropharyngeal soft tissues that are not the result of cervical injury.[31,32] These include hematoma from any source such as facial fractures or thoracic injuries, infection, vascular transposition, intubation, and crying infants. In a patient who has suffered trauma, the presence of soft tissue swelling and the absence of any evidence of cervical injury should prompt a search for another explanation for the finding.

Another soft tissue finding is widening of the retrotracheal space. This space is measured from the anterior inferior margin of C6 to the posterior margin of the tracheal air column. This space should not exceed 14 mm in a child or 22 mm in an adult. As with the retropharyngeal space, there are other conditions that widen the retrotracheal space. It has been the authors' experience that massive widening of either of these spaces rarely occurs with cervical injury.

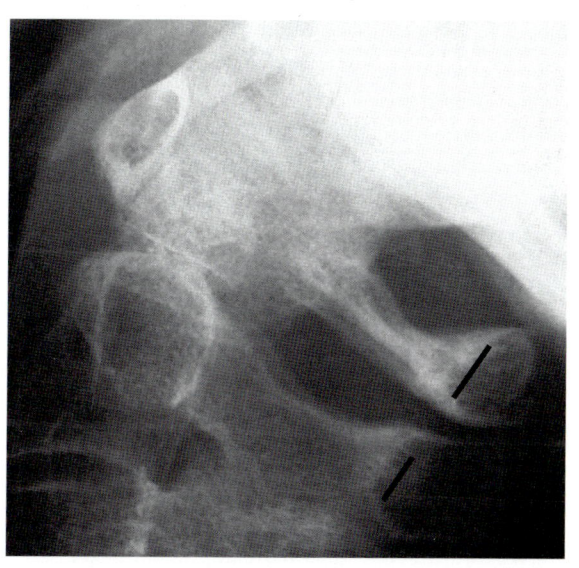

Fig. 6.20 **Wide predental space in rheumatoid arthritis.**
a Lateral radiograph in extension shows normal alignment of the spinolaminar line (l). **b** In flexion there is widening of the predental space (*double arrow*). Note the malalignment of the spinolaminar line (l).

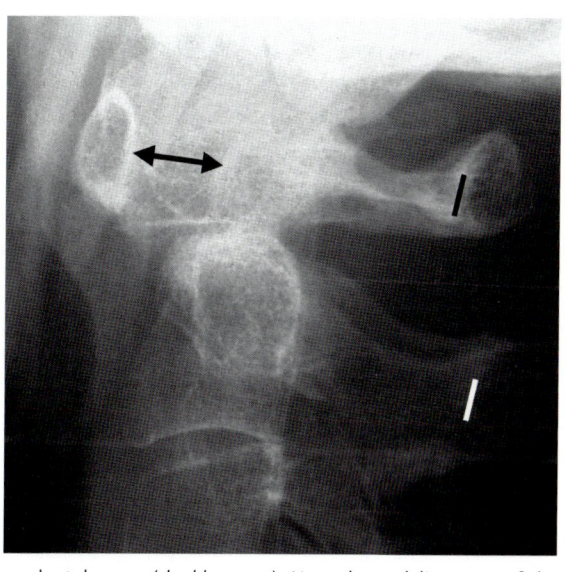

Two other reliable soft tissue changes may be found in the thoracic and lumbar regions respectively with widening of the paraspinous soft tissues in the thoracic spine and loss of the psoas fat stripe in lumbar injuries.[16] Soft tissue abnormalities are summarized in Table 6.5.

While cervical CT has made the diagnosis of cervical injuries easier, there are still many places in the world where this cannot be performed, and physicians must rely upon radiography to do the job. In the above discussion, we have mentioned a large number of signs and findings. The question arises as to exactly how frequently do these signs occur and how reliable are they? In our experience, the most reliable radiographic signs of underlying cervical injury are widening of the interlaminar space and widening of the retropharyngeal space. These findings never occur normally nor are they the sole manifestation of the injury. Loss of lordosis, kyphotic angulation, and tracheal deviation occur in a large number of patients, and may be found in normal people. They, too, never occur as the sole manifestation of injury, and are often combined with one or more of the other findings. The most reliable combination of signs is: widening of the interlaminar space, widening of the facet joint, loss of lordosis, and kyphotic angulation. A narrow disk space and retrolisthesis or slight anterolisthesis are more likely the result of degenerative changes when encountered as isolated findings. A wide disk space, on the other hand, should always suggest an extension injury.[16,27]

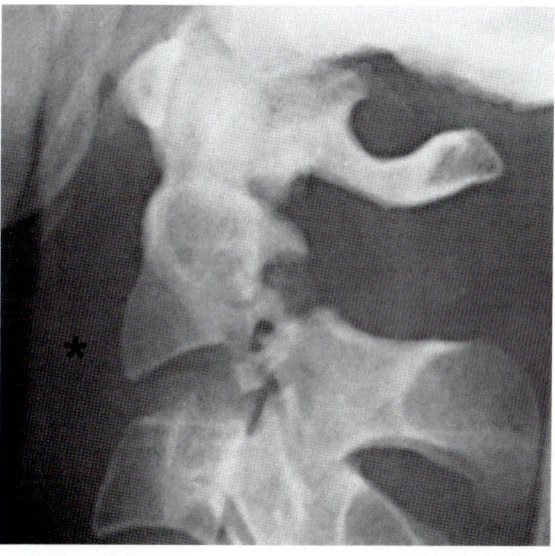

Fig. 6.**21 Wide prevertebral soft tissues in a patient with a hangman's fracture**. Lateral radiograph shows widening of the retropharyngeal soft tissues with anterior bowing (*). Note the wide C2 disk space, fracture line through the neural arch of C2 and the wide interspinous space.

Table 6.5 Soft tissue abnormalities

Wide retropharyngeal space (over 7 mm adult or child)
Wide retrotracheal space (over 22 mm adult, 14 mm child)
Displaced prevertebral fat stripe
Craniocervical soft tissue "mass"
Tracheal or laryngeal deviation
Paraspinal soft tissue "mass"
Loss of psoas stripe

Vertebral Stability Following Trauma

The subject of stability following a vertebral injury is a source of controversy among physicians who treat spine-injured patients. Stability is defined as the ability of the vertebral column to not only maintain support for the head and torso, but also to protect the spinal cord and nerves under normal physiological stress. Stability is dependent not only upon the bones but also upon the posterior third of the intervertebral disks, facet joints, and most important, the ligaments. Unstable injuries by definition are those that have the potential to cause or worsen neurological symptoms or to produce skeletal deformity under normal physiological motion. Most physicians dealing with the spine subscribe to Denis' three-column concept of vertebral stability.[33,34] The anterior column begins at the anterior longitudinal ligament and extends to a vertical line drawn through the junction point of the middle and posterior third of the intervertebral disk. The middle column is that area from this line to the posterior longitudinal ligament, and the posterior column extends from the posterior longitudinal ligament through the supraspinous ligament. Denis was able to show that instability resulted when two contiguous zones were disrupted. Through careful experimentation, he was able to demonstrate that the middle zone—that is, the posterior third of the intervertebral disk and the posterior longitudinal ligament—were the key elements in stability.[33,34]

What, then, are the radiographic signs that would indicate that an unstable condition exists? Five signs have been described, all of which have been illustrated in this chapter.[16,35] These signs include: vertebral displacement (Fig. 6.11), widening of the interlaminar distance (Figs. 6.6, 6.7), widening of the facet joints (Figs. 6.6, 6.7), widening of the interpedicle distance (Fig. 6.4), and disruption of the posterior vertebral body line (Figs. 6.4, 6.15). While many of these signs occur in combination, only one need be present to make a radiographic diagnosis of an unstable injury.

Implications

The imaging of patients with suspected cervical injury has changed dramatically within the past decade. Radiography has been the preferred method for initial evaluation. In the United States, however, CT has been advocated, not only as an adjunct to evaluate patients who have had cervical injury detected by radiographs, but also as the primary method for evaluation.[1–3,5,9] Indeed, CT is the most sensitive means we have for detecting cervical fractures. However, many of those fractures, once detected, need little more than symptomatic and supportive treatment. For this reason, the senior author and colleagues at Allegheny General Hospital reviewed our experience with 1052 cervical injuries encountered in 879 patients over a 15-year period. As the result of this review, we devised a new classification of cervical injuries.[36] In many instances, the designation is determined on whether or not there is radiographic evidence of instability as described above. Injuries that have radiographic and/or CT evidence of instability, are associated with neurological findings, or have the potential to produce neurological findings are categorized as "*major*."[37,38] Those injuries with no evidence of instability, which are not associated with neurological findings, or have no such potential to produce them, are referred to as "*minor*." Minor injuries include such entities as isolated spinous process fracture, simple wedge compression fracture of a vertebral body, isolated transverse process, uncinate process, or articular pillar fracture, isolated fracture of the lateral mass of the atlas, and types I and II occipital condyle fractures.[36] The radiographic and/or CT criteria of a "major" injury are summarized in Table 6.**6**. If none of these findings are present, the injury should be considered to be "minor."

Table 6.**6** Signs of "major" injury

Displacement more than 2 mm in any plane
Wide vertebral body in any plane
Wide interspinous/interlaminar space
Wide facet joint
Disrupted posterior vertebral body line
Wide disk space
Vertebral burst
Locked facets (unilateral or bilateral)
Type III occipital condyle fracture

All other types of fractures may be considered "minor."

Acknowledgement

Figures 6.**1** b, d, e, 6.**6** a, 6.**10** a, b, reprinted from *Eur J Radiol.*, 2002, Vol. 42. R. H. Daffner, S. D. Daffner, Vertebral injuries: detection and implications, pp. 100–16, with permission from Elsevier.

References

1. Nuñez DB Jr, Quencer RM. The role of helical CT in the assessment of cervical spine injuries. *AJR Am J Roentgenol.* 1998;171:951–957.
2. Lawrason JN, Novelline RA, Rhea JT et al. Can CT eliminate the initial portable lateral cervical spine radiograph in the multiple trauma patient? A review of 200 cases. *Emerg Radiol.* 2001;8:272–275.
3. Ptak T, Kihiczak D, Lawrason JN. Screening for cervical spine trauma with helical CT: experience with 676 cases. *Emerg Radiol.* 2001;8:315–319.
4. Schenarts PJ, Diaz J, Kaiser C. Prospective comparison of admission computed tomographic scan and plain films of the upper cervical spine in trauma patients with altered mental status. *J Trauma.* 2001;51:663–669.
5. Barba CA, Taggert J, Morgan AS et al. A new cervical spine clearance protocol using computed tomography. *J Trauma.* 2001;51:652–657.
6. Beningfield S, Potgieter H, Nicol A et al. Report on a new type of trauma full-body digital X-ray machine. *Emerg Radiol.* 2003;10:23–29.

7. Qaiyum M, Tyrrell PNM, McCall IW, Cassar-Pullicino VN. MRI detection of unsuspected vertebral injury in acute spinal trauma: Incidence and significance. *Skeletal Radiol.* 2001;30:299–304.
8. Kihiczak D, Novelline RA, Lawrason JN et al. Should an MR scan be performed routinely after a normal clearance CT scan in the trauma patient? Experience with 59 cases. *Emerg Radiol.* 2001;8:276–278.
9. Li AE, Fishman EK. Cervical spine trauma: evaluation by multidetector CT and three-dimensional volume rendering. *Emerg Radiol.* 2003;10:34–39.
10. Wintermark M, Mouhsine E, Theumann N et al. Thoracolumbar spine fractures in patients who have sustained severe trauma: depiction with multi-detector row CT. *Radiology* 2003;227:681–689.
11. Daffner RH. Cervical radiography for trauma patients: a time-effective technique? *AJR.* 2000;175:1309–1311.
12. Daffner RH. Helical CT of the cervical spine for trauma patients: a time study. *AJR.* 2001;177:677–679.
13. Blackmore CC, Zelman WN, Glick ND. Resource cost analysis of cervical spine trauma radiography. *Radiology.* 2001;220:581–587.
14. Saini S, Seltzer SE, Bramson RT. Technical cost of radiologic examinations: analysis across imaging modalities. *Radiology.* 2000;216:269–272.
15. Saini S, Sharma R, Levine LA et al. Technical cost of CT examinations. *Radiology.* 2001;218:172–175.
16. Daffner RH. *Imaging of Vertebral Trauma.* 2nd ed. Philadelphia, PA: Lippincott-Raven; 1996.
17. Calenoff L, Chessare JW, Rogers LF et al. Multiple level spinal injuries: Importance of early recognition. *AJR.* 1978;130:665–669.
18. Vandemark RM. Radiology of the cervical spine in trauma patients: practice, pitfalls, and recommendations for improving efficiency and communication. *AJR Am J Roentgenol.* 1990;155:465–472.
19. Blackmore CC, Emerson SS, Mann FA, Koepsell TD. Cervical spine imaging in patients with trauma: determination of fracture risk to optimize use. *Radiology.* 1999;211:759–765.
20. Hanson, JA, Blackmore CC, Mann FA, Wilson AJ. Cervical spine injury: a clinical decision rule to identify high-risk patients for helical CT screening. *AJR Am J Roentgenol.* 2000:174:713–717.
21. Stiell IG, Wells GA, Vandemheen KL et al. The Canadian C-spine rule for radiography in alert and stable trauma patients. *JAMA.* 2001;286:1841–1848.
22. Hoffman JR, Mower WR, Wolfson AB et al. Validity of a set of clinical criteria to rule out injury to the cervical spine in patients with blunt trauma. *N Engl J Med.* 2000; 343:94–99.
23. Panacek EA, Mower WR, Holmes JF et al. Test performance of the individual NEXUS low-risk clinical screening criteria for cervical spine injury. *Ann Emerg Med.* 2001;38:22–25.
24. Harris JH, Jr, Carson GC, Wagner LK. Radiologic diagnosis of traumatic occipitovertebral dissociation. 1. Normal occipitovertebral relationships on lateral radiographs of supine subjects. *AJR Am J Roentgenol.* 1994;162:881–886.
25. Harris JH Jr, Carson GC, Wagner LK et al. Radiologic diagnosis of traumatic occipitovertebral dissociation. 2. Comparison of three methods of detecting occipitovertebral relationships on lateral radiographs of supine subjects. *AJR Am J Roentgenol.* 1994;162:887–892.
26. Harris JH Jr, Burke JT, Ray RD et al. Low (type III) odontoid fracture: a new radiographic sign. *Radiology.* 1984;153:353–356.
27. Daffner RH, Verma SV. The significant signs of cervical vertebral trauma: a reassessment. *Appl Radiol.* 1995;24(4):31–35.
28. Smoker WRK, Dolan KD. The "fat" C2: a sign of fracture. *AJNR.* 1987;8:33–38.
29. Daffner RH, Goldberg AL, Evans TC et al. Cervical vertebral injuries in the elderly: a 10-year study. *Emerg Radiol.* 1998;5:38–42.
30. Harris JH Jr. The cervicocranium: its radiographic assessment. *Radiology.* 2001;218:337–351.
31. Daffner RH, Kennedy SL, Fix TJ. The retropharyngeal prevertebral soft tissues revisited. *Emerg Radiol.* 1996;3:247–252.
32. Fix TJ, Daffner RH, Deeb ZL. Carotid transposition: another cause of wide retropharyngeal soft tissues. *AJR Am J Roentgenol.* 1996;167: 1305–1307.
33. Denis F. The three-column spine and its significance in the classification of acute thoracolumbar spinal injuries. *Spine.* 1983;8:817–831.
34. Denis F. Spinal stability as defined by the three-column spine concept in acute spinal trauma. *Clin Orthop Rel Res.* 1984;189:65–76.
35. Gehweiler JA Jr, Daffner RH, Osborne RL Jr. Relative signs of stable and unstable thoracolumbar vertebral trauma. *Skeletal Radiol.* 1981;7:179–183.
36. Daffner RH, Brown RR, Goldberg AL. A new classification for cervical vertebral injuries: influence of CT. *Skeletal Radiol.* 2000;29:125–132.
37. Groves CJ, Cassar-Pullicino VN, Tins BJ, Tyrrell PN, McCall IW. Chance-type flexion-distraction injuries in the thoracolumbar spine: MR imaging characteristics. *Radiology.* 2005;236:601–680.
38. Palmieri F, Cassar-Pullicino VN, Dell'atti C, et al. Uncovertebral joint injury in cervical facet dislocation: the headphones sign. *Eur Radiol.* 2005; Dec 6:1–4 (Epub ahead of print).

7 Neurovascular Injury

M. L. White and G. Y. El-Khoury

Introduction

Neurovascular spinal cord injuries are quite prevalent and in a busy trauma center radiology practice these injuries will be commonly seen. Magnetic resonance imaging (MRI), magnetic resonance angiography (MRA), and computed tomographic angiography (CTA) have greatly facilitated imaging neurovascular injuries. The introduction of MRI revolutionized the evaluation of neurovascular injuries associated with spinal trauma. Magnetic resonance imaging provides a very sensitive in-vivo analysis of the internal status of the spinal cord in trauma patients and MRI findings correlate well with the histopathological changes that occur secondary to acute spinal cord trauma.[1-6] Patient prognosis has also been found to correlate with the MRI findings in spinal cord trauma.

Spinal cord infarcts due to arterial injury from trauma are relatively rare, but it has been shown by imaging that vertebral artery injuries are not an unusual occurrence. Magnetic resonance imaging and magnetic resonance angiography have dramatically facilitated the analysis of vascular injuries, particularly of the vertebral arteries, associated with spinal trauma due to their ability to demonstrate the patency of vessels and the presence of intramural hematomas in cases of dissection.[7,8] In addition, computed tomographic angiography (CTA) can provide information about the presence and extent of arterial injury.[9] The vascular injuries that occur secondary to spinal trauma can lead to brainstem, cerebellar, and cerebral strokes.

Magnetic resonance imaging and MRA techniques are often the preferred procedures of choice for evaluating neurovascular injuries because of their proven accuracy and because they are noninvasive. Magnetic resonance imaging is better than conventional spinal radiography, myelography, and computed tomography with or without myelography for demonstrating the soft tissue injuries that occur in spinal trauma. Computed tomographic angiography has also been demonstrated to be useful for showing arterial injuries associated with spinal trauma. Conventional angiography, however, does remain quite useful for evaluating arterial injuries and several studies have shown that it is overall the best technique for demonstrating arterial injuries secondary to spinal trauma.

MR Imaging/Histopathological Correlation of Acute Spinal Cord Injury

Studies in human and animal models have thoroughly evaluated the pathological changes of traumatic spinal cord injuries.[10-14] Edema, hemorrhage, mechanical axonal disruption, and severing of the nerve roots are the early pathological changes that occur as a result of trauma to the spinal cord.[10-14] Traumatized nerve fibers undergo swelling, fragmentation, and disintegration of both axons and of myelin.[10,14]

Reversible and irreversible traumatic injuries to the spinal cord demonstrate pathophysiological differences.[10] Less severe trauma causes reversible lesions and in these lesions there is mild vascular disturbance, inflammation of a minimal to moderate degree, and petechial hemorrhages that improve over time. Injuries caused by greater forces result in irreversible lesions in which the vascular system to the cord becomes compromised, and hemorrhages in the spinal cord coalesce and increase in extent over time.[10] Inflammation and axonal swelling is seen early in the irreversible lesions and the changes become severe chronically (at 5 days) with extensive central hematomas and marked necrosis of the gray matter.[10]

Hyperacute traumatic spinal cord lesions in human autopsies rarely demonstrate hematomyelia. Hemorrhage usually does not occur in traumatic spinal cord injuries unless the patient survives more than a few hours.[12] True hematomyelia was found in an autopsy series in only one of 123 patients with hyperacute spinal cord injury.[12] The spinal cords were found either to be grossly intact or totally disrupted.[12] However, the mere continuity of the gross specimen does not mean the nerve fibers have not suffered irreversible damage.[12]

The direct effects of the trauma itself are not the only mechanism of injury in spinal cord traumatic injuries. The presence of a secondary mechanism is suggested by the fact that the pathological changes worsen after injury.[13] A secondary vascular mechanism in addition to the effects of the direct trauma likely leads to the development of post-traumatic ischemia and resultant infarction of the spinal cord.[13] The injury to the spinal cord due to post-traumatic ischemia arises from systemic and local effects. Systemic effects of acute spinal cord injury are hypotension and reduced cardiac output while the local effects result in loss of autoregulation and a marked reduction of the microcirculation in both gray and white matter of the injured segment of the spinal cord.[13,15] Oligodendrocyte apoptosis also occurs in the spinal cord after injury and evidence implicates this as a key determinant in the extent of neurological damage and dysfunction.[16]

The MRI findings correlate nicely with the histopathological findings in traumatic spinal cord lesions in animal models.[17–21] Experimentally, however, producing only edematous spinal cord injuries, as are seen in humans, have been difficult.[20] Histopathologically varying degrees of hemorrhage surrounded by edema in the spinal cord is seen in acute traumatic spinal injuries and MRI detects hemorrhage and edema acutely in the spinal cord that is traumatically injured.[17–21] The microscopic abnormalities resulting from the trauma such as inflammation, nerve fiber swelling, nerve fiber tearing, apoptosis, and disintegration are not directly seen by MRI since MRI only provides a macroscopic evaluation of the spinal cord. Less severe injuries have been found to correlate with smaller abnormalities on MRI and more severe lesions have larger MRI abnormalities.[17,18,20]

MRI Features of Spinal Cord Hemorrhage

High-field MRI shows acute spinal cord hemorrhages, proven by pathological correlation, to appear hypointense on T2W images (Fig. 7.**1a**).[20,21] The appearance and detection of blood products at lower field strengths (≤0.5T), has been more variably reported than in series performed at higher field strengths. Acute hemorrhages at 0.5T have been reported to be hyperintense to hypointense on T2W images in the spinal cord.[2,22–24] T2 hypointensity is more likely found in larger hemorrhages imaged at 0.5T.[18] When a hemorrhage imaged at lower field strength appears hyperintense on T2W images the acute blood will have a signal intensity similar to edema making the hemorrhage inseparable from edema. High-field or low-field MRI usually will only show subtle signal intensity changes on T1W images in acute spinal cord hemorrhages and the signal intensity of the hemorrhage will often be isointense to the spinal cord and few cases are found with minimal hypointensity (Fig. 7.**1b**).[6,18,21,22] High-field MRI will demonstrate blood products better than low-field MRI. However, the performance of gradient-echo imaging at lower and higher field strengths will help to detect blood products that may not otherwise be identified (Fig. 7.**1c**).

Spin-echo or fast spin-echo MRI techniques for imaging spinal trauma may be utilized and each technique has different advantages.[25] Spin-echo techniques take longer to perform than fast spin-echo techniques but spin-echo techniques are more sensitive to blood products when compared to fast spin-echo techniques.[25] However, the time saved by performing fast spin-echo MRI is so great that in general fast spin-echo MRI is the preferred technique for T2W spinal imaging. The time saved with fast spin-echo techniques can be spent to significantly increase the resolution of the scan and still have a shorter scan time. The weakness of fast spin-echo techniques for the demonstration of hemorrhage can be overcome by adding a gradient-echo sequence and gradient-echo techniques are more sensitive than spin-echo MRI for detecting hemorrhage anyway.[18,22,25] Unfortunately, the gradient-echo technique by itself is not suitable to be used as the only sequence for imaging spinal cord trauma since it is very poor at demonstrating spinal cord edema.[25]

Table 7.**1** The MRI appearance of hemorrhage at low and high field strength

	Acute		Subacute	
	T2 signal	T1 signal	T2 signal	T1 signal
1.5T	– hypointense	– minimally inhomogeneous – predominantly subtle changes isointense to spinal cord and possibly minimal hypointensity	– hyperintense** rim surrounding central hypointensity	– hyperintense rim surrounding central isointensity
0.5T and less	– hyperintense to hypointense – larger hemorrhages likely to be hypointense	– minimally inhomogeneous – predominantly subtle changes isointense to spinal cord and possibly minimal hypointensity	– hyperintense** rim surrounding central hypointensity	– hyperintense rim surrounding central isointensity

Gradient-echo images will more clearly demonstrate hemorrhages than T1W or T2W images. The hemorrhages will appear hypointense on gradient-echo images in the acute and subacute stages. **The hyperintense rim will form later around the hematoma on the T2W images compared to the T1W images.

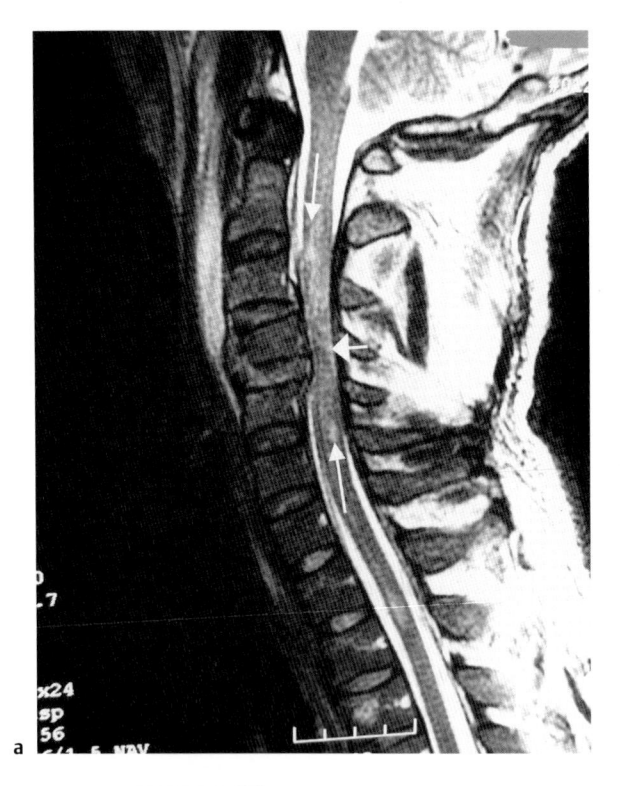

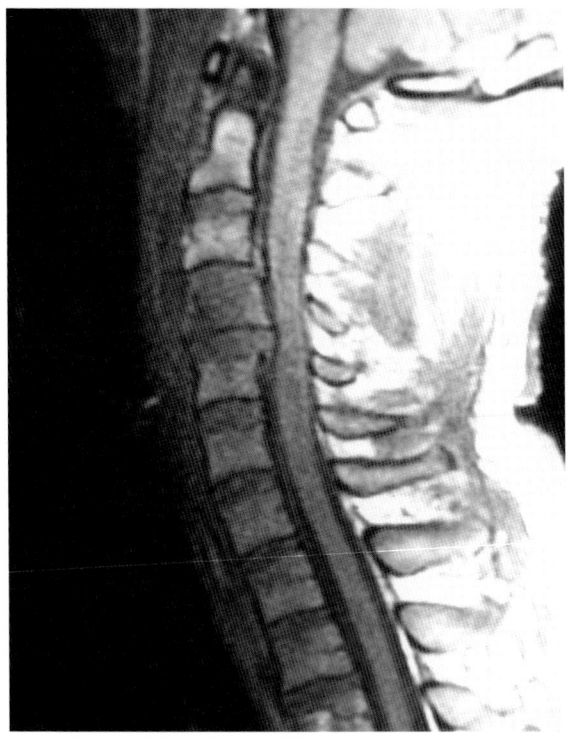

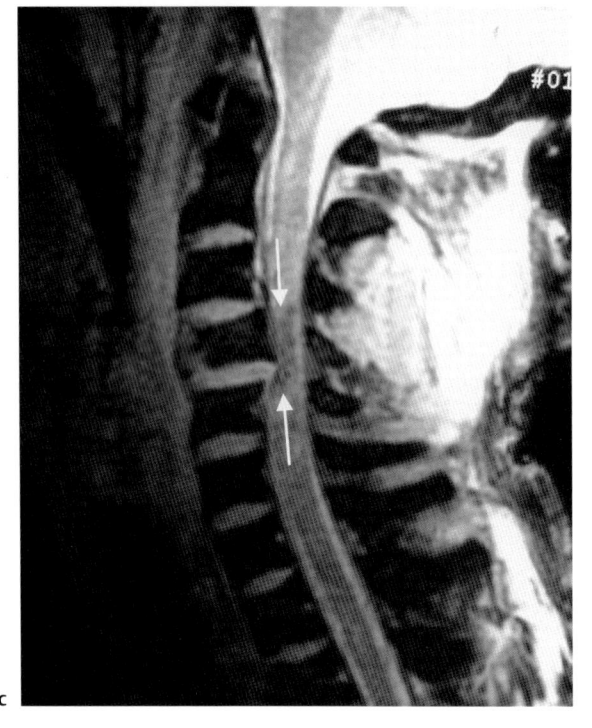

Fig. 7.1 **28-year-old man status trailer falling on neck with resultant C4 vertebral body, facet, and lamina fractures.** This examination was performed at 1.5T. **a** Sagittal T2W image demonstrates the C4 vertebral body fracture with mild retropulsion into the spinal canal. There is an extensive hyperintense signal consistent with edema in the spinal cord (*long white arrows*). An area of hypointense signal is present in the spinal cord presumably from hemorrhage (*short white arrow*). **b** Sagittal T1W image demonstrates at most minimal hypointensity at the area of injury. **c** A sagittal gradient-echo image demonstrates the hemorrhage as hypointense in the spinal cord (*arrows*). Extensive prevertebral soft tissue swelling is present in the mid and upper cervical spine.

In the acute setting hemorrhage in the spinal cord is deoxyhemoglobin and appears as described above. With the passing of time hemorrhage in the spinal cord will progress to methemoglobin. The time frame by which hemorrhage in the spinal cord progresses to methemoglobin based upon the changing signal intensity of the blood has been reported to range from 3 to 10 days.[5,6,24,26,27,30,31] Hematomas in the spinal cord in general will show signal intensity changes progressing from the rim of the hematoma to the center. The signal intensity change consists of the development of a hyperintense rim around the center, which appears isointense on T1W images and hypointense on T2W images.[6,27–30] However, the T1W images will develop the ring of hyperintense signal in the hematoma prior to the T2W images. The earlier T1W change corresponds to the development of intracellular methemoglobin whereas on the T2W images the hematoma will not become hyperintense until enough extracellular methemoglobin is formed (Table 7.1, p. 101).[28,29]

Prognostic Role of MR Imaging in Neurological Outcome

Spinal cord injury as demonstrated by MRI in humans' in-vivo corresponds to abnormalities found in animal models of spinal cord trauma. The commonly occurring hemorrhage and edema in spinal cord trauma has been well documented by MRI, and MRI nicely demonstrates the rarely occurring cord transection (Fig. 7.**2**). Cord swelling is also found at the regions of injury on MRI examinations. Spinal cord compression from bone fragments, disk material, or hemorrhage is well demonstrated on MRI. A normal spinal cord may also be demonstrated on MRI in patients with neurological abnormalities.

The MRI appearance of the spinal cord in the setting of trauma can help predict the neurological outcome. Patients with normal appearing spinal cords uniformly have a good outcome, patients with only spinal cord edema do worse, and patients with hemorrhagic spinal cord injuries have even poorer neurological outcomes compared to patients with only edema. Patients with transected cords, of course, uniformly have the worst neurological outcomes. However, besides patients with transected cords, there is certainly variability seen in the neurological outcome between individual patients.

A classification of spinal cord injuries that has been found to be useful in characterizing injuries includes three patterns.[6,27,30] Pattern type 1 is thought to represent hemorrhage, pattern type 2 is thought to represent edema (Fig. 7.**3**), and pattern type 3 is presumed to contain both edema and blood (Fig. 7.**1**).[6,27,30] The type 1, hemorrhage pattern, correlates with severe neurological deficits and poor outcome.[6,27,30] type 2 had the best outcome and type 3 injury outcomes were variable.[6,27,30]

Expanding the number of patterns of characterization of traumatic spinal cord injury to six has been proposed.[31] The additional types of patterns include a normal pattern, a compression pattern, and a transection pattern. Patients with a normal spinal cord pattern do not have any neurological sequelae on follow-up.[31] The compression pattern and especially the transection pattern indicate poor neurological outcome.[31] However, the cord compression pattern, demonstrating severe obliteration of the spinal cord and significant alteration of cord morphology, did have a somewhat variable neurological outcome.[31] With the cord compression pattern seven of nine patients described had complete spinal cord injuries and no change in clinical outcome, but two of the patients had only incomplete spinal cord injuries and favorable outcomes.[31] Others report cord compression detected on the initial MRI or residual cord compression seen on MRI after reduction is associated with greater neurological compromise.[5,23] Yamashita et al found that if the spinal cord had normal signal on T1W and T2W images, the patients had a good prognosis despite initially having severe cord compression.[23] The presence of abnormal signal on T1W images indicates greater

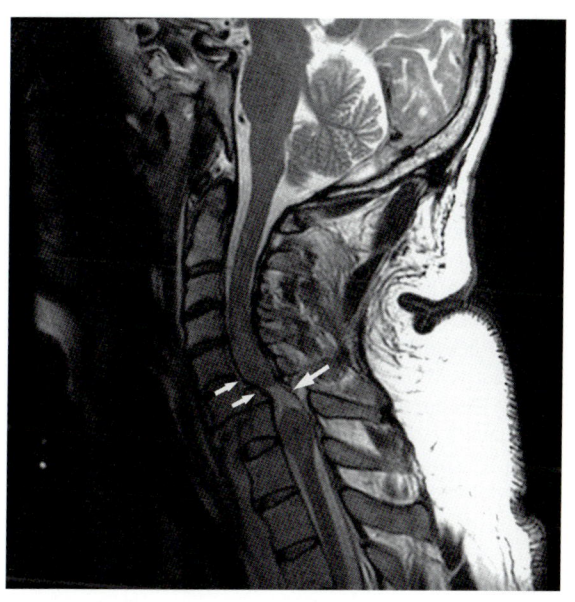

Fig. 7.**2** **46-year-old man status post motor vehicle rollover with bilateral jumped facets**. A sagittal T2W image of the cervical spine demonstrates a 50% spondylolisthesis of C6–C7 with an associated spinal cord transection. Edema and spinal cord swelling surrounds the area of transection (*large arrow*). Behind C5 and C6 vertebral bodies there is a small epidural hematoma present (*small arrows*).

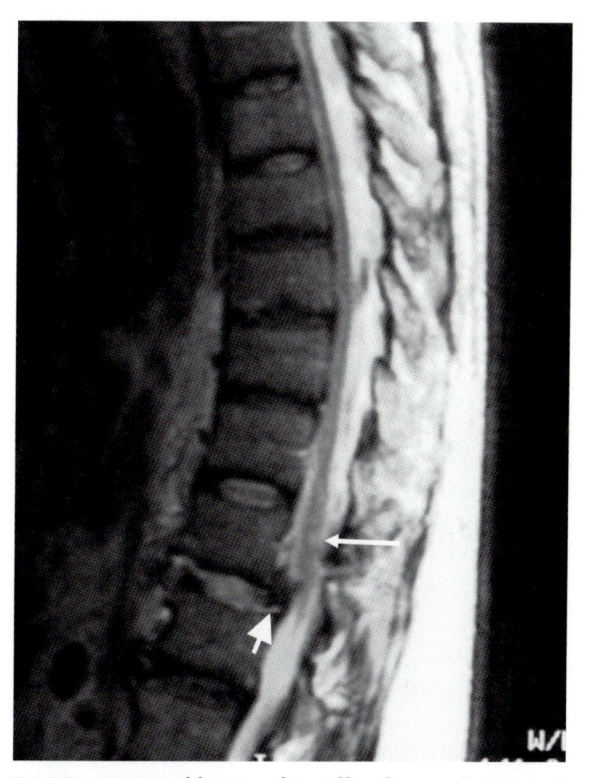

Fig. 7.**3** **48-year-old man who suffered a crush injury at work**. He has a T12 on L1 fracture subluxation and was not moving his lower extremities at presentation. This is a sagittal T2W image that demonstrates a small area of hyperintense signal consistent with edema in the spinal cord at the T12 level (*long arrow*). There are several millimeters of spondylolisthesis of the T12 vertebral body compared to the L1 vertebral body (*short arrow*). There was excellent recovery of motor function and he was walking with a cane at 2 months after the injury.

injury and a poor prognosis, although this study did not differentiate if the T1W changes were from hemorrhage or edema.[23] Others have not found cord compression on the initial examination to be an important indicator of neurological outcome.[22]

The presence of hemorrhage in the spinal cord after spinal cord injury is associated with a significantly greater decrease of motor function than if there was no hemorrhage detected by MRI.[32] Hemorrhage was never detected without edema in this study as has been previously described as a type 1 pattern.[6,30] It is possible that no edema was detected because all the patients underwent MRI with a 1.5T scanner within 72 hours of injury. The edematous portion of an injury on studies that have a greater time delay to imaging may have time to resolve.[32] Smaller hemorrhages may also have been detected due to improved spatial and contrast resolution of the study.[32] Eighty-five percent of subjects with complete motor deficits had hemorrhagic lesions on their initial exams,[32] but hemorrhage was not always associated with a complete motor deficit as has been previously described.[5,33] In fact, 21% of incomplete motor injuries were found to have evidence of spinal cord hemorrhage on initial examination.[32] Schaefer et al described a couple of small spinal cord hemorrhages in patients who exhibited limited improvement of their motor deficits.[34]

Neurological outcome has been associated with the extent of edema in the spinal cord after spinal cord injury.[5,32,34,35] The greater the extent of edema that is present in the spinal cord, the poorer the neurological outcome. A worse neurological outcome was found by Schaefer et al to be associated with edema extending over one segment.[34,35] Each segment consists of a vertebral body and the associated disk below the associated vertebral body. The length of the edema and the severity of the impairment were also found by Flanders et al to correlate, and that patients with complete motor deficits had longer lesions than those with incomplete injuries.[32]

Diffusion-weighted (DW) MRI may help to further differentiate the types of pathophysiological insult to the spinal cord due to trauma. The differentiation of secondary ischemia or apoptosis occurring in the spinal cord as well as the amount of initial spinal cord disruption from trauma may be facilitated with DW MRI.[36] The detected diffusion changes in the spinal cord may help to direct future treatment of spinal cord injuries.

Vascular Injury

When spinal trauma occurs the arteries that supply the spinal cord and the arteries adjacent to the spinal column are at a high risk of injury. The arteries are frequently injured in cervical spinal trauma but these injuries do not usually result in neurological deficits. However, the arterial injuries associated with spinal trauma can result in devastating neurological deficits.[37,38]

Dissection or occlusion of the vertebral arteries places the arteries that arise from them at risk of injury too. If there is vertebral artery injury and lack of collateral flow the vessels that arise from the vertebral arteries that may cause neurological deficits if injured include the posterior inferior cerebellar arteries, the anterior and posterior spinal arteries, and radicular arteries if they have anterior or posterior radiculomedullary branches that supply the spinal cord. With a vertebral artery injury the basilar artery is also at risk for thrombosis and a brain stem infarction can result.[39]

Individual variation complicates the description of the blood supply to the spinal cord. Additional arteries that can potentially supply the spinal cord in the cervical region include the deep cervical arteries, the superior intercostal arteries, and occasionally the ascending cervical artery in the neck.[40,41] Below the cervical region radicular arteries that arise from intercostal arteries can variably supply the spinal cord and can also be damaged. The unpaired great radicular artery of Adamkiewicz in the lower thoracic and lumbar region almost exclusively supplies the spinal cord. In 80% of cases the artery of Adamkiewicz arises on the left side between the T7 and L4 levels.[41] Arterial contributions to the conus medullaris may also include the lateral sacral arteries, iliolumbar arteries, and middle sacral arteries.[40,41]

Due to the variability of the pattern of radicular arteries that supply the spinal arteries in the thoracic region, it is not possible to associate a particular infarct pattern with a specific level of traumatic injury. The variability results not only from which radicular arteries are injured but also depends on which radicular arteries are actually supplying the spinal cord given individual variations. One small radiculomedullary artery may be all that is supplying the upper thoracic cord and because of this the upper thoracic cord is considered a watershed area. The unpaired great radicular artery of Adamkiewicz almost exclusively supplies the spinal cord in the lower thoracic and lumbar region, rendering this area of the spinal cord being particularly vulnerable to ischemia.

Vertebral Artery Injury

Due to the vertebral arteries being closely related to the cervical spine they are at particular risk of injury due to cervical spine trauma. The C6 transverse foramen is usually the first foramen that the vertebral artery enters as it extends cranially from its origin. There is nearly a vertical orientation of the vertebral artery as it runs through the transverse processes of C6 to C1. The vertebral artery at C1 extends posteriorly and horizontally from the transverse foramen along the posterior arch of C1. The artery then pierces the dura matter and enters the intracranial cavity and continues cranially until it forms the basilar artery, usually by joining the vertebral artery from the contralateral side. It is the segment of the vertebral artery that passes through the transverse foramina that is at particular risk of injury with cervical spine trauma.

Vertebral artery trauma may result from varied causes ranging from sports injuries, penetrating

Fig. 7.4 **37-year-old man involved in a single car motor vehicle accident.** a An axial image from a CTA demonstrates a fracture of the left C6 facet and transverse process with associated displacement and obliteration of the transverse foramen and complete left vertebral artery occlusion (*arrow*). b Sagittal CTA reconstruction of the left vertebral artery shows a focal occlusion of the artery (*arrow*) c Coronal CTA reconstruction of the right vertebral artery shows a mild irregularity (*arrow*). d Time-of-flight MRA shows a more pronounced right vertebral artery irregularity (*large arrow*) and occlusion with no distal flow in the left vertebral artery (*small arrows*).

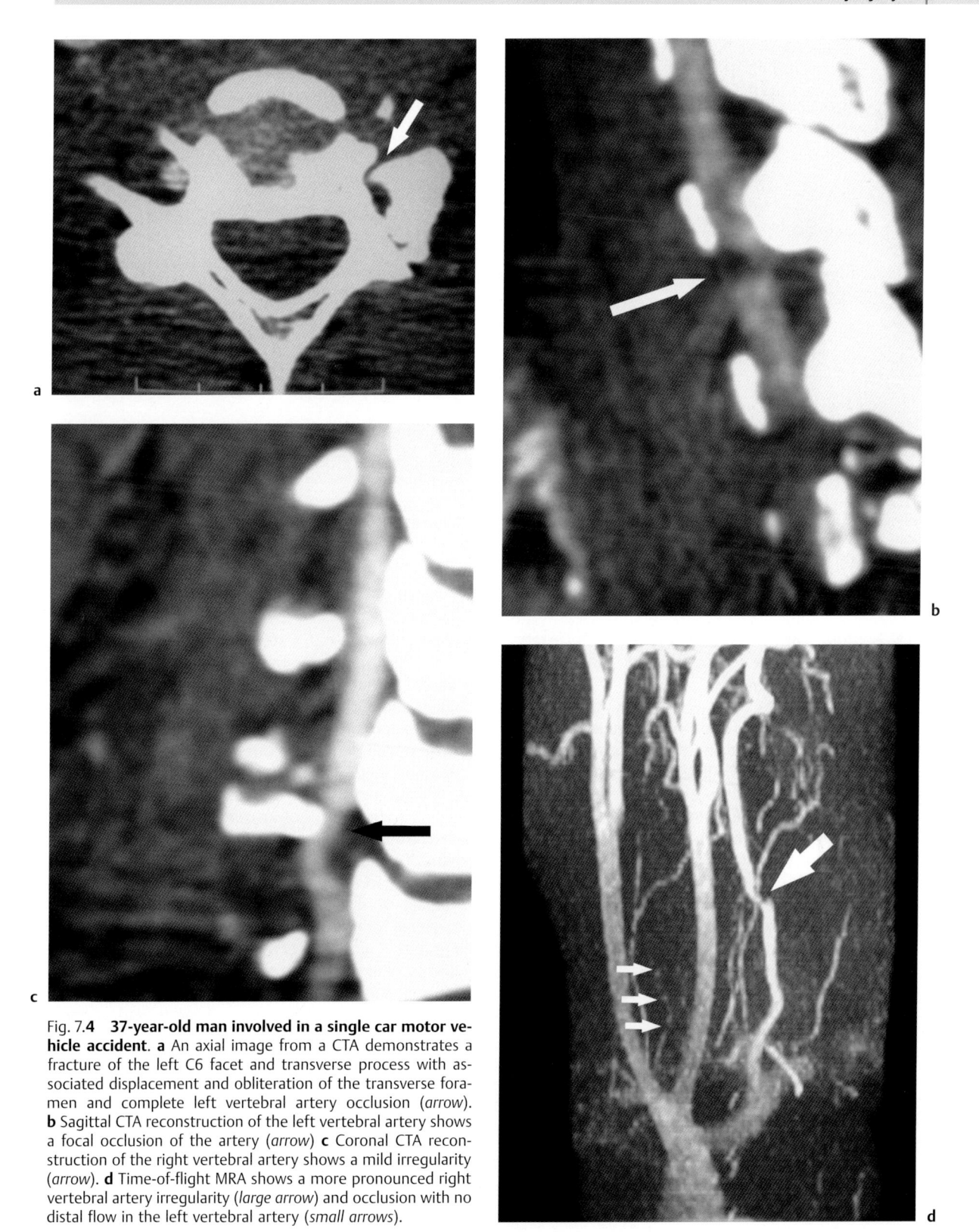

wounds from knife injuries and gunshot wounds, and chiropractic manipulation. Vertebral artery injuries are associated with blunt trauma to the cervical spine and certain fracture patterns increase the likelihood of vertebral artery injury. The risk of vertebral artery injury is particularly prevalent if there is an associated transverse foramen fracture (Fig. 7.4). This, however, is not always the case (Fig. 7.5). Subluxations and dislocations of the facets, burst fractures, and compression fractures also increase the risk of vertebral artery in-

Fig. 7.5 **44-year-old male involved in an all-terrain vehicle rollover with a fracture dislocation at C6–C7. a** Axial image from a CTA demonstrates the left facet is fractured off and displaced laterally and posteriorly with an associated fracture in the transverse foramen (*small arrows*). The artery is patent (*large arrow*). **b** Sagittal reconstructed image demonstrates the left vertebral artery is patent (*arrow*).

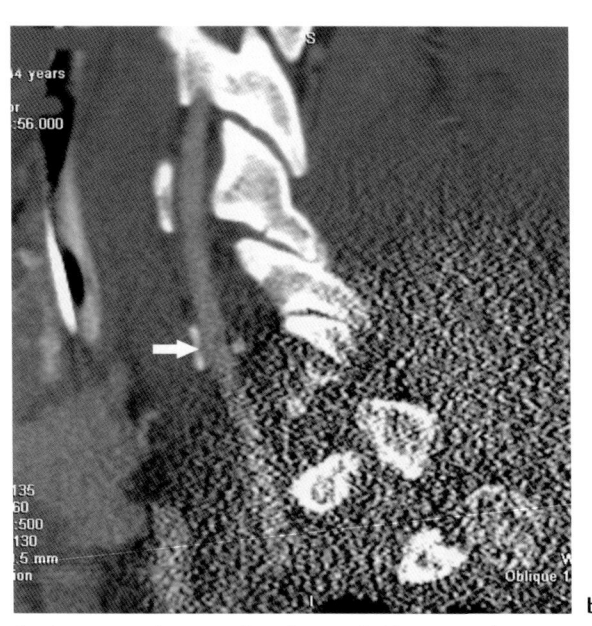

jury. Neurological symptoms associated with vertebral artery injury can be severe but the risk of neurological symptoms is quite low.[37,42,43]

A variety of symptoms are associated with a vertebral artery injury and these may include headache, neck pain and stiffness, pulsatile tinnitus, vomiting, hemiparesis, diplopia, ataxia, dizziness, hemiparesthesia, dysphagia, dysmetria, dysphonia, nystagmus, basilar transient ischemic attacks, Horner's syndrome, hypoesthesia, aphasia, dysnomia, and facial weakness.[7,8,44] Death is the worst outcome resulting from vertebral artery dissections.[39,45] Knowing the associated signs and symptoms of vertebral arterial injury is important so early suspicion can be raised and a work-up can be initiated to detect if an arterial injury is present.

Conventional angiography was utilized to evaluate the vertebral arteries for injury secondary to blunt trauma in a prospective study by Willis et al and the study demonstrated angiographical abnormalities in 16 of 26 patients (62%) (Fig. 7.**6**).[37] However, four of the detected abnormalities did not clearly represent injuries and consisted of arterial stretching and/or mild vasospasm and a vascular blush in and adjacent to a fractured vertebral body. An arterial injury meeting strict definition was observed in 12 of the 26 patients (46%). Occlusion of the vertebral artery (nine), pseudoaneurysm (one), intimal flap (one), and arterial dissection (one) were the strictly defined abnormalities. The vertebral artery occlusions were noted to be at the origins of the vertebral arteries or were located at the level of the injury. No definite neurological symptoms resulted from any of the injuries. Cothren et al found vertebral artery injuries with associated cervical spine fractures from blunt trauma to consist of: (40/89) irregularity of the vessel wall or a dissection/intramural hematoma with < 25% stenosis; (20/89) intraluminal thrombosis or raised intimal flap, or dissection/intramural hematoma with > 25% stenosis; (5/89) pseudoaneurysms; (24/89) vessel occlusions.[59]

Secondary to the criteria utilized by Willis et al to choose which patients in the study would undergo angiography there was a bias of the results towards finding a high percentage of vertebral artery injuries.[37] Patients with injuries of insufficient severity were excluded from angiography. The study required the blunt trauma to the spine to have produced a subluxation from a locked or perched facet, facet destruction with evidence of instability, or a fracture involving the transverse foramen before patients would undergo angiography.[37] Cothren et al found that one third of patients who were at high risk due to their cervical fractures had vertebral artery injuries and 77% of patients with vertebral artery injuries had cervical spine fractures.[59]

Conventional angiography has also been proven by others to demonstrate all types of cerebrovascular traumatic arterial injuries in the neck.[46–50] Types of injuries to the carotid and vertebral arteries identified include intimal irregularity, dissection, intraluminal thrombus, thrombosis/occlusion, transection, and pseudoaneurysms.[46–50] Surprisingly, Miller et al found no strokes in 43 patients with vertebral artery injury but in a prior study they had found a 14% stroke rate in vertebral artery injury.[48] Strokes occurred in 20% of patients with blunt vertebral injuries and 23% with blunt carotid injuries by Biffl et al.[50] Biffl et al in a different study found the only independent predictor of blunt vertebral artery injury to be cervical spine fracture.[46]

Conventional angiography compared to CTA and MRA has been found to be markedly better for detect-

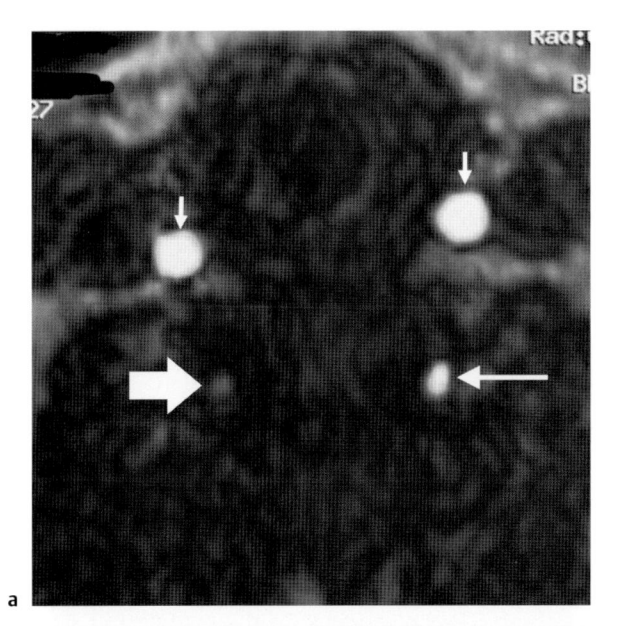

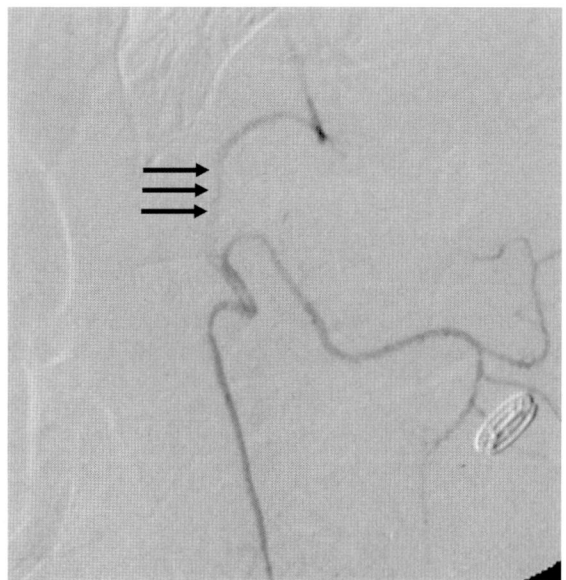

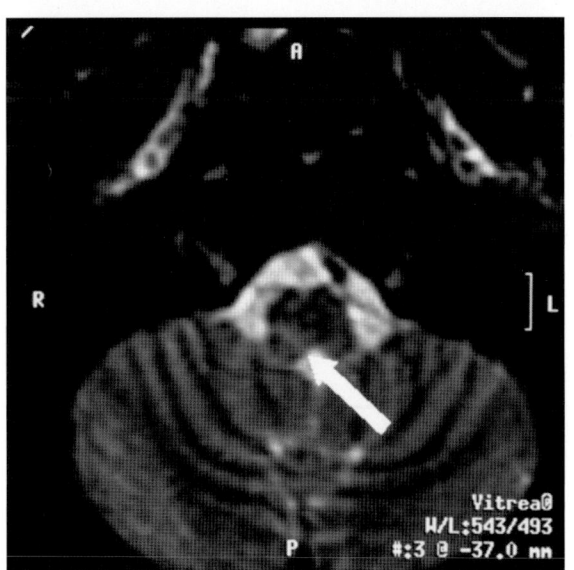

Fig. 7.6 **45-year-old woman who developed neck pain and a headache associated with right face and left leg numbness after having chiropractic neck manipulation. a** Time-of-flight MRA of the neck demonstrates minimal flow in the right vertebral artery (*fat arrow*). The *long arrow* points to the left vertebral artery, and the *small arrows* point to the internal carotid arteries. **b** A right vertebral artery conventional angiogram demonstrates at the C1–C2 vertebral levels luminal irregularity and narrowing of the vertebral artery consistent with a dissection (*arrows*). **c** The dissection resulted in a lateral medullary infarction as demonstrated on a T2W axial image (*arrow*).

ing cerebrovascular injuries.[48,49] Both CTA and MRA have been found to misrepresent vascular abnormalities in certain cases (Fig. 7.7).[48,49] However, the noninvasive techniques are able to detect and classify vascular abnormalities, and both CTA and MRA are far less risky than conventional angiography. Computed tomographic angiography and MRA should definitely be used to screen for vertebral artery injury when conventional angiography is not available.

The demonstration of vertebral artery injuries by magnetic resonance imaging (MRI) and magnetic resonance angiography (MRA) has been evaluated.[7,8,44,51] The actual hematoma in the wall of the artery can be detected by MRA and MRI and this is a great benefit over imaging with conventional angiography in the evaluation of dissection, and MRI and MRA are noninvasive techniques (Fig. 7.8a). For demonstrating vertebral artery dissections, Levy et al found the sensitivity and specificity of MRA and MRI to be 20% and 100%, and 60% and 98%, respectively, when compared to conventional angiography.[51] The presence of an increase in the external diameter of the artery and a narrowing of the lumen of the artery are the criteria that were used to diagnosis dissection on MRI/MRA. The MRI appearance of dissected vertebral arteries has also been found to include visualizing a crescentic, annular, or rounded area of thickening surrounding or replacing the normal arterial flow void.[7,8,44] On MRI throughout the entire dissected vertebral artery there may also be a hyperintense signal and poor or absent visualization of the vessel (Fig. 7.9).[7] Others have found the sensitivity of MRA ranges from 47% to 75% and the specificity ranges from 67% to 97%.[48,49] Presumably, due to the small size of the vertebral arteries and the lower resolution of MRI and MRA compared to conventional angiography, the latter continues to remain useful.[51]

The signal intensity of the hematoma in the wall of a dissected artery on MRI and MRA changes with time.

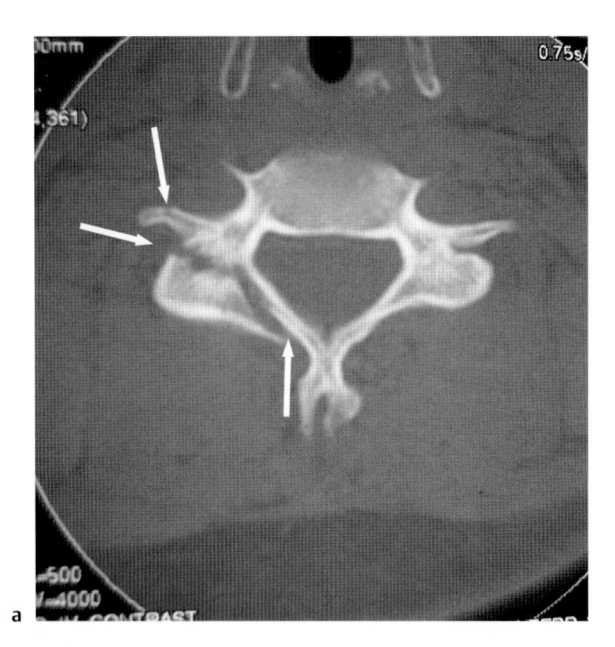

Fig. 7.7 **22-year-old male status post motor vehicle accident**. He suffered right transverse process fractures at C2 and C3 in addition to a right facet, lamina, and transverse process fracture at C6. **a** An axial CT at C6 demonstrates the right facet, transverse process, and lamina fracture (*arrows*). **b** A gadolinium-enhanced MRA shows irregular thickening of the right vertebral artery diffusely worrisome for injury (*arrows*). **c** A conventional angiogram demonstrates a normal right vertebral artery. The etiology of the apparent thickening of the right vertebral artery on the MRA is uncertain and may be related to motion or venous enhancement.

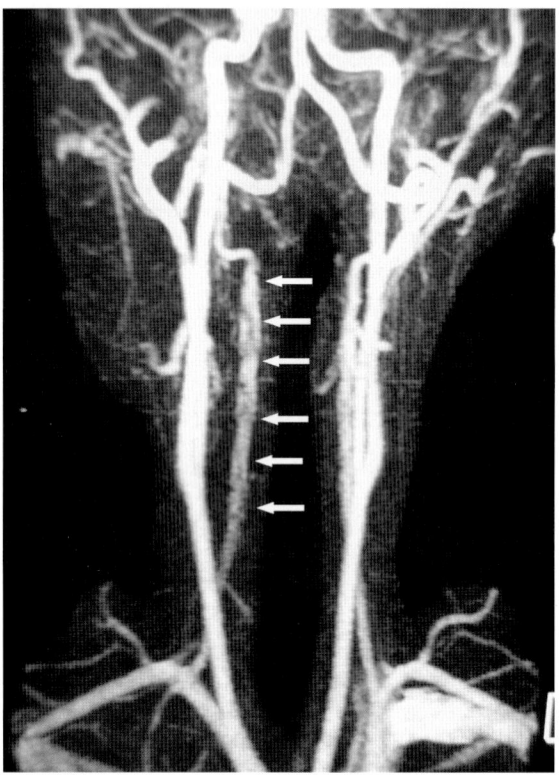

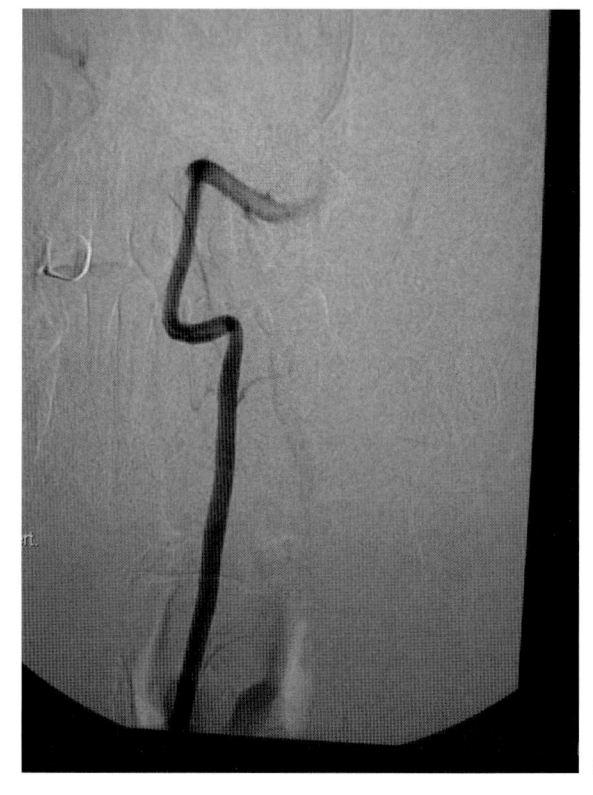

On T1W images the hematoma in the arterial wall has most often been described as having hyperintense signal intensity, and isointense to hyperintense on proton-density and T2W images.[7,8,51,52] An isointense signal on T1W images and hyperintense signal on T2W and proton-density weighted images in the acute stage, up to 36 hours post-trauma, has been seen to be present in the arterial wall hematoma of a dissected vertebral artery.[8] Hypointense signal on T2W images as seen with acute hematomas in the brain or spinal cord at higher field strengths due to the presence of deoxyhemoglobin in an acute hematoma, has not been reported as would be expected in a dissection. It should be kept in mind that arteries on MRI can have increased signal intensity not only due to the presence of hematoma but due to entry phenomenon and from slow blood flow.

The same signal intensity as seen on T1W images will be seen on time-of-flight (TOF) MRA in hemorrhage, including intramural hemorrhage, in a dissection. Intramural hemorrhages have been found to be nicely demonstrated by TOF MRA.[51-53] Magnetic resonance angiography capabilities are limited by the small size of the vertebral artery.[8,51] However, the TOF MRA tech-

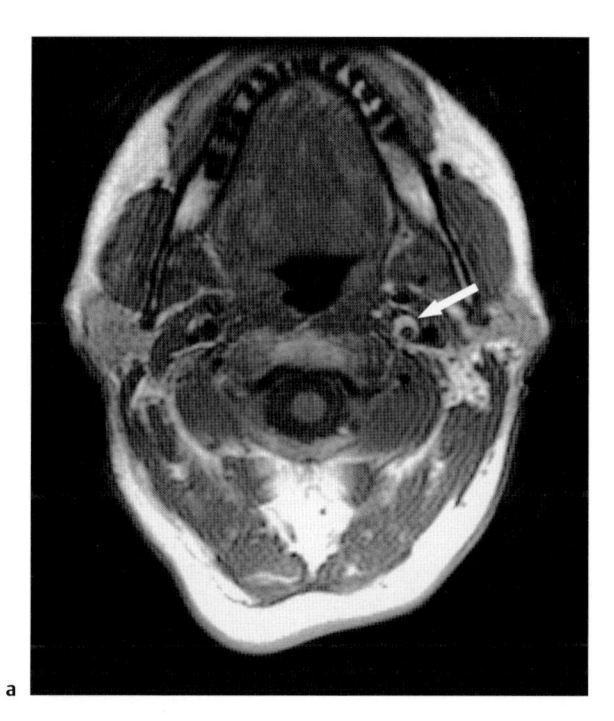

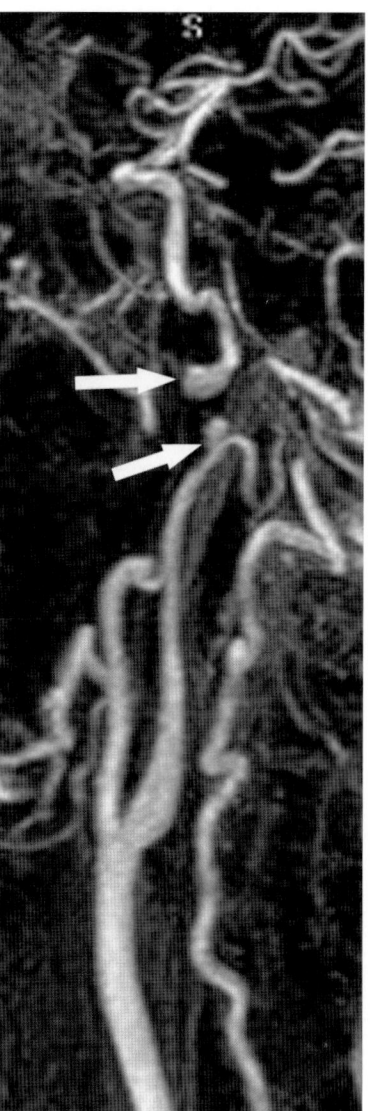

Fig. 7.8 a An axial T1W image demonstrates a dissected left internal carotid artery with a crescent that is hyperintense due to the hematoma in the arterial wall (*arrow*). b A gadolinium-enhanced MRA demonstrates a flow gap surrounded by two areas of dilation consistent with the area of dissection and two pseudoaneurysms that were subsequently proven at conventional angiography (*arrows*).

nique should be used rather than a phase-contrast technique for examining dissections in either the carotid arteries or the vertebral arteries because phase-contrast techniques will not demonstrate the hematoma in the wall of a dissected vessel as they are not sensitive for detecting blood products. Time-of-flight MRA may also be useful to perform in addition to a gadolinium-enhanced MRA, which is insensitive to blood products, to evaluate for an intramural hematoma in cases of suspected arterial dissection.

A number of authors have utilized MRA and MRI to evaluate for vertebral artery injuries associated with blunt cervical spine trauma.[45,54–57] A prospective study was performed by Friedman et al involving 37 patients over a 6-month period.[45] Within 24 hours of injury the patients usually had a MRA and MRI. Vertebral artery injury was found at a rather high rate (24%).[45] One patient with two vertebral artery dissections had a devastating outcome and died in the hospital but otherwise there were few neurological symptoms in these patients. All of these patients had major non-penetrating cervical spine trauma. Vertebral arterial injury in patients with cervical trauma has been found by others to occur at similar rates (19.7–25%) and

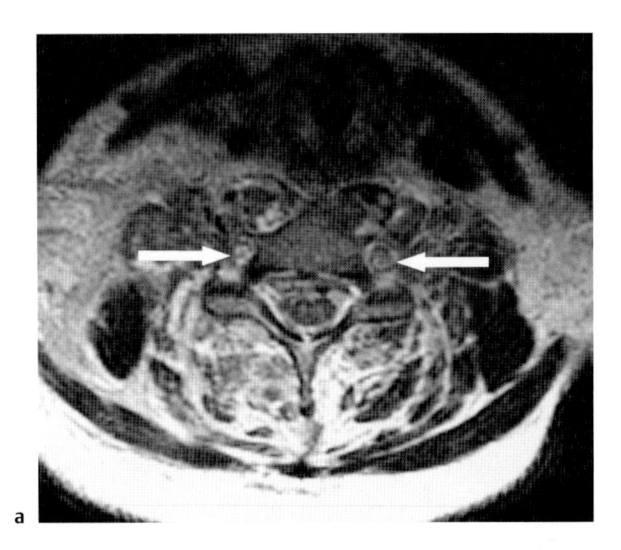

Fig. 7.9 **62-year-old male status post fall with a fracture dislocation at C5–C6 with fractures into the left transverse foramen and distracted facets on the right**. a Axial T2W image demonstrates hyperintense signal in the vertebral arteries instead of flow voids. May also see thickening due to hematoma in the arterial walls. b Left vertebral artery demonstrates occlusion just past the origin on a gadolinium-enhanced MRA. c Right vertebral artery demonstrates a proximal flow gap consistent with occlusion on gadolinium-enhanced MRA. The vertebral artery occlusions are likely due to dissections and were proven on conventional angiography.

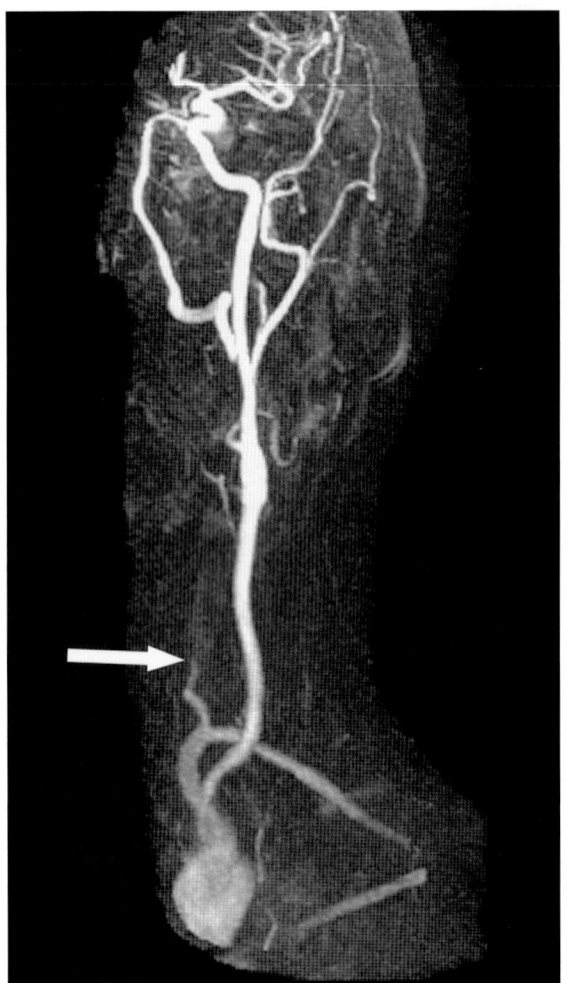

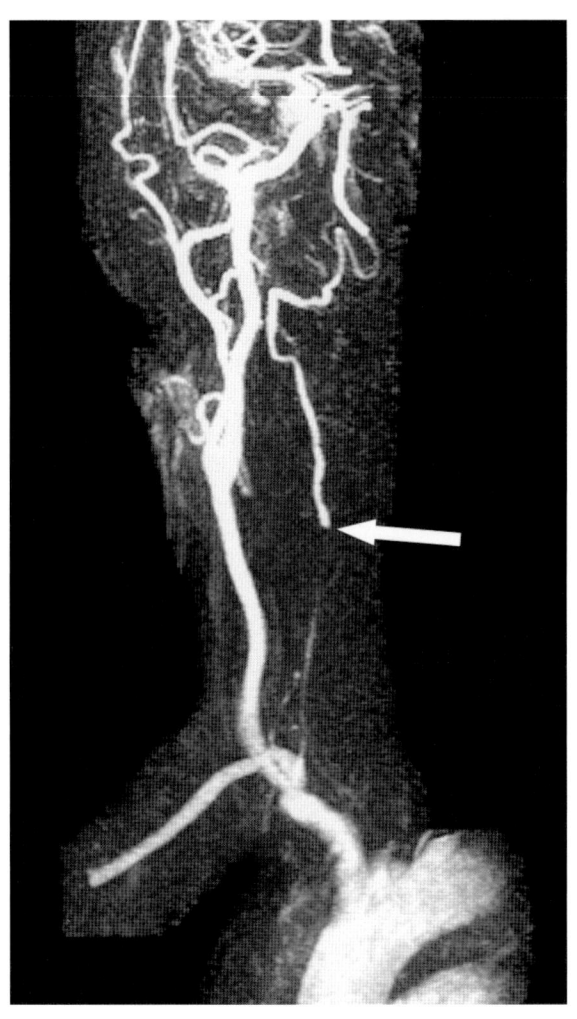

minimal or no neurological symptoms were experienced in these patients.[54,55] Weller et al found only a 10.5% incidence of vertebral artery injury in patients with cervical spine trauma.[57]

The findings seen on MRI and MRA in these studies included dissections, occlusions, focal areas of narrowing, and nonvisualization of the traumatically injured vertebral arteries.[45,54–57] The absence of flow on T1W images was found to indicate occlusion and a high signal on T1W images indicated a clot according to Veras et al.[56] Another technique that is promising for imaging vertebral dissections including the demonstration of pseudoaneurysms is gadolinium-enhanced MR angiography (Figs. 7.**8**, 7.**9**).[44]

Computed tomographic angiography has been found to be useful in studying arterial injuries, including vertebral arterial injuries, secondary to blunt cervical injuries (see Figs. 7.**4**, 7.**5**).[9] Only two of the patients studied had cervical spine fractures.[9] The performance of CTA has not been found to significantly increase the time of the diagnostic work-up.[9]

Studies have reported differences in the type of fractures and cervical spine injuries associated with injuries to the vertebral arteries, but there is certainly a common theme present. The only injury highly predictive of vertebral artery injury found by Willis et al consisted of comminuted fractures of the transverse foramen with bone fragments in the transverse foramen.[37] Weller et al found that all four patients in his study with vertebral artery injuries had fractures through the transverse foramen.[57] Another study found that in patients with transverse process fractures, vertebral angiography demonstrated a high proportion of vertebral arterial injuries.[58] Interestingly, Woodring et al found that transverse process fractures are associated with a brachial plexopathy and cervical radiculopathy in 10% of cases.[58]

Patients with prereduction subluxations greater than 3 mm (38%) versus patients with subluxation < 3 mm (17%), although not statistically significant, were found in a greater proportion of cases to have vertebral arterial injury.[45] Also, patients having complete motor and sensory deficits, indicating more severe trauma, were correlated with the presence of a vertebral arterial injury by Friedman et al.[45] In a study by Parbhoo et al 10 out of 30 patients with unifacet dislocation had a vertebral artery injury and 1 out of 14 patients with bifacet injury had a vertebral artery injury.[55] All patients in a study by Veras et al evaluating vertebral artery occlusion after trauma had facet joint dislocations and/or fractures involving the transverse foramen and the mechanism of injury was usually distractive flexion with a resultant fracture dislocation at C5–C6.[56] Flexion distraction, usually with an associated facet dislocation or a flexion compression injury, was found in a study by Giacobetti et al in 10/12 patients with vertebral artery injury.[54] Fractures that have also been associated with vertebral artery injuries include: burst, compression, odontoid, C1 body and Jefferson, bifacet dislocations, and comminuted fractures.[37,54–57] Cothren et al found that vertebral artery injury is associated with complex cervical spine fractures involving subluxations (55%), extension of fractures into the transverse foramen (26%), or upper C1 to C3 fractures (18%).[59]

Conclusion

Magnetic resonance imaging is unequaled in its in-vivo ability to demonstrate traumatic injuries to the spinal cord. It is the only imaging technique that allows accurate visualization of edema and hemorrhage in the spinal cord and MRI also nicely demonstrates the degree and cause of associated spinal cord compression. The type and extent of traumatic injury to the spinal cord detected by MRI can be used to help predict neurological recovery. Diffusion-weighted magnetic resonance imaging in the future may further enhance the ability of MRI to investigate and categorize traumatic spinal cord injuries. The role of MRI in the chronically injured spinal cord is dealt with in Chapter 13.

Arterial injuries including dissections and pseudoaneurysms due to spinal trauma have been found to be best demonstrated by conventional angiography, but it is an invasive technique. Computed tomographic angiography, MRA, and MRI have been demonstrated to detect a wide variety of traumatic arterial injuries and with improvements in technology they should better approximate the accuracy of conventional angiography. With blunt cervical spinal trauma the vertebral arteries are at a heightened risk of injury when there are significant facet subluxations and dislocations, facet fractures, and fractures through the transverse foramina.

Technological advances continue to improve MRI, MRA, and CTA. These improvements, be it faster computed tomographic scanning, new magnetic resonance sequences, or higher-strength MRI scanners, promise to further advance the imaging of neurovascular spinal injuries. The accurate imaging of neurovascular spinal injuries should only continue to improve and provide even better information to guide patient therapies and prognostic information concerning patient outcomes.

References

1. Silberstein M, Tress BM, Hennessy O. Prediction of neurologic outcome in acute spinal cord injury: the role of CT and MR. *AJNR Am J Neuroradiol.* 1992;13(6):1597–1698.
2. Goldberg AL, Rothfus WE, Deeb ZL et al. The impact of magnetic resonance on the diagnostic evaluation of acute cervicothoracic spinal trauma. *Skeletal Radiol.* 1988;17(2):89–95.
3. Katzberg RW, Benedetti PF, Drake CM et al. Acute cervical spine injuries: prospective MR imaging assessment at a level 1 trauma center. *Radiology.* 1999;213(1):203–12.
4. Wittenberg RH, Boetel U, Beyer HK. Magnetic resonance imaging and computer tomography of acute spinal cord trauma. *Clin Orthop.* 1990;260:176–85.
5. Flanders AE, Schaefer DM, Doan HT, Mishkin MM, Gonzalez CF, Northrup BE. Acute cervical spine trauma: correlation of MR imaging findings with degree of neurologic deficit. *Radiology.* 1990;177(1):25–33.
6. Kulkarni MV, McArdle CB, Kopanicky D et al. Acute spinal cord injury: MR imaging at 1.5T1. *Radiology.* 1987;164(3): 837–43.
7. Sue DE, Brant-Zawadzki MN, Chance J. Dissection of cranial arteries in the neck: correlation of MRI and arteriography. *Neuroradiology.* 1992;34(4):273–278.
8. Mascalchi M, Bianchi MC, Mangiagico S et al. MRI and MR angiography of vertebral artery dissection. *Neuroradiology.* 1997;39(5):329–340.
9. Rogers FB, Baker EF, Osler TM, Shackford SR, Wald SL, Vieco P. Computed tomographic angiography as a screening modality for blunt cervical arterial injuries: Preliminary results. *J Trauma.* 1999;46(3):380–5.
10. Assenmacher DR, Ducker TB. Experimental traumatic paraplegia: the vascular and pathological changes seen in reversible and irreversible spinal-cord lesions. *J Bone Joint Surg Am.* 1971; 53(4):671–80.
11. Yashon D, Bingham WG, Faddoul EM, Hunt WE. Edema of the spinal cord following experimental impact trauma. *J Neurosurg.* 1973;38(6):693–697.
12. Kakulas BA. Pathology of spinal injuries. *Cent Nerv Syst Trauma.* 1984;1(2):117–129.
13. Tator CH, Fehlings MG. Review of the secondary injury theory of acute spinal cord trauma with emphasis on vascular mechanisms. *J Neurosurg.* 1991;75(1):15–26.

14. Hughes JT. *Pathology of the Spinal Cord.* Philadelphia: W.B. Saunders Company; 1978.
15. Reyes O, Sosa I, Kuffler DP. Neuroprotection of spinal neurons against blunt trauma and ischemia. *P R Health Sci J.* 2003; 22(3):277–86.
16. Kim DH, Vaccaro AR, Henderson FC, Benzel EC. Molecular biology of cervical myelopathy and spinal cord injury: role of oligodendrocyte apoptosis. *Spine J.* 2003;3(6):510–9.
17. Duncan EG, Lemaire C, Armstrong RL, Tator CH, Potts DG, Linden RD. High-resolution magnetic resonance imaging of experimental spinal cord injury in the rat. *Neurosurgery.* 1992;31(3):510–519.
18. Schouman-Claeys E, Frija G, Cuenod CA, Begon D, Paraire F, Martin V. MR imaging of acute spinal cord injury: Results of an experimental study in dogs. *AJNR Am J Neuroradiol.* 1990; 11(5):959–65.
19. Chakeres DW, Flickinger F, Bresnahan JC et al. MR imaging of acute spinal cord trauma. *AJNR Am J Neuroradiol.* 1987; 8(1):5–10.
20. Weirich SD, Cotler HB, Narayana PA et al. Histopathologic correlation of magnetic resonance imaging signal patterns in a spinal cord injury model. *Spine.* 1990;15(7):630–638.
21. Hackney DB, Asato R, Joseph PM et al. Hemorrhage and edema in acute spinal cord compression: demonstration by MR imaging. *Radiology.* 1986;161(2):387–390.
22. Mascalchi M, Dal Pozzo G, Dini C et al. Acute spinal trauma: Prognostic value of MRI appearances at 0.5T. *Clin Radiol.* 1993; 48(2):100–108.
23. Yamashita Y, Takahashi M, Matsuno Y et al. Acute spinal cord injury: magnetic resonance imaging correlated with myelopathy. *Br J Radiol.* 1991;64(759):201–209.
24. Beers GJ, Raque GH, Wagner GG et al. MR imaging in acute cervical spine trauma. *J Comput Assist Tomogr.* 1988;12(5):755–61.
25. Silberstein M, McLean K. Fast magnetic resonance imaging in spinal trauma. *Australas Radiol.* 1995;39(2):118–123.
26. Tarr RW, Drolshagen LF, Kerner TC, Allen JH, Partain CL, James AE. MR imaging of recent spinal trauma. *J Comput Assist Tomogr.* 1987;11(3):412–417.
27. Cotler HB, Kulkarni MV, Bondurant FJ. Magnetic resonance imaging of acute spinal cord trauma: preliminary report. *Spine.* 1990;15(3):161–8.
28. Gomori JM, Grossman RI, Goldberg HI, Zimmerman RA, Bilaniuk LT. Intracranial hematoma: Imaging by high-field MR. *Radiology.* 1985;157(1):87–93.
29. Zimmerman RD, Heier LA, Snow RB, Liu DPC, Kelly AB, Deck MDF. Acute intracranial hemorrhage: Intensity changes on sequential MR Scans at 0.5T. *AJR Am J Roentgenol.* 1988(3); 150:651–661.
30. Bondurant FJ, Cotler HB, Kulkarni MV, McArdle CB, Harris JH. Acute spinal cord injury a study using physical examination and magnetic resonance imaging. *Spine.* 1990;15(3): 161–168.
31. Ramon S, Dominguez R, Ramirez L et al. Clinical and magnetic resonance imaging correlation in acute spinal cord injury. *Spinal Cord.* 1997;35(10):664–673.
32. Flanders AE, Spettell CM, Tartaglino LM, Friedman DP, Herbison GJ. Forecasting motor recovery after cervical spinal cord injury: value of MR imaging. *Radiology.* 1996;201(3):649–655.
33. Marciello MA, Flanders AE, Herbison GJ, Schaefer DM, Friedman DP, Lane JI. Magnetic resonance imaging related to neurologic outcome in cervical spine cord injury. *Arch Phys Med Rehabil.* 1993;74(9):940–946.
34. Schaefer DM, Flanders AE, Osterholm JL, Northrup BE. Prognostic significance of magnetic resonance imaging in the acute phase of cervical spine injury. *J Neurosurg.* 1992; 76(2): 218–223.
35. Schaefer DM, Flanders AE, Northrup BE, Doan HT, Osterholm JL. Magnetic resonance imaging of acute cervical spine trauma: correlation with severity of neurologic injury. *Spine.* 1989;14(10):1090–1095.
36. Schwartz ED, Hackney DB. Diffusion-weighted MRI and the evaluation of spinal cord axonal integrity following injury and treatment. *Exp Neurol.* 2003;184(2):570–89.
37. Willis BK, Greiner F, Orrison WW, Benzel EC. The incidence of vertebral artery injury after midcervical spine fracture or subluxation. *Neurosurgery.* 1994;34(3):435–442.
38. Choi JU, Hoffman HJ, Hendrick EB, Humphreys RP, Keith WS. Traumatic infarction of the spinal cord in children. *J Neurosurg.* 1986;65(5):608–610
39. Vishteh AG, Coscarella E, Nguyen B, Sonntag VK, Mcdougall CG. Fatal basilar artery thrombosis after traumatic cervical facet dislocation. *J Neurosurg Sci.* 1999;43(3):195–9.
40. Gillilan L. The arterial supply of the human spinal cord. *J Comp Neurol.* 1958;110(1):75–100.
41. Dommisse GF. The blood supply of the spinal cord. A critical vascular zone in spinal surgery. *J Bone Joint Surg Br.* 1974; 56(2):225–235.
42. Harrop JS, Sharan AD, Vaccaro AR, Przybylski GJ. The cause of neurologic deterioration after acute cervical spinal injury. *Spine.* 2001;15;26(4):340–346.
43. Woodring JH, Lee C, Duncan V. Transverse process fractures of the cervical vertebrae: are they insignificant? *J Trauma.* 1993;34(6):797–802.
44. Leclerc X, Lucas C, Godefroy O et al. Preliminary experience using contrast-enhanced MR angiography to assess vertebral artery structure for the follow-up of suspected dissection. *AJNR Am J Neuroradiol.* 1999;20(8):1482–1490.
45. Friedman D, Flanders A, Thomas C, Millar W. Vertebral artery injury after acute cervical spine trauma: rate of occurrence as detected by MR angiography and assessment of clinical consequences. *AJR Am J Roentgenol.* 1995;164(2): 443–447.
46. Biffl WL, Moore EE, Offner PJ et al. Optimizing screening for blunt cerebrovascular injuries. *Am J Surg.* 1999;178(6):517–522.
47. Kerwin AJ, Bynoe RP, Murray J et al. Liberalized screening for blunt carotid and vertebral artery injuries is justified. *J Trauma.* 2001;51(2):308–314.
48. Miller PR, Fabian TC, Croce MA et al. Prospective screening for blunt cerebrovascular injuries. *Ann Surg.* 2002;236(3): 386–393.
49. Biffl WL, Ray CE, Moore EE, Mestek M, Johnson JL, Burch JM. Noninvasive diagnosis of blunt cerebrovascular injuries: A preliminary report. *J Trauma.* 2002;53(5):850–856
50. Biffl WL, Ray CE, Moore EE et al. Treatment-related outcomes from blunt cerebrovascular injuries: importance of routine follow-up arteriography. *Ann Surg.* 2002 May; 235(5):699–706.
51. Levy C, Laissy JP, Raveau V et al. Carotid and vertebral artery dissections: three-dimensional time-of-flight MR angiography and MR imaging versus conventional angiography. *Radiology.* 1994;190(1):97–103.
52. Oelerich M, Stogbauer F, Kurlemann G, Schul C, Schuierer G. Craniocervical artery dissection: MR imaging and MR angiographic findings. *Eur Radiol.* 1991;9(7):1385–1391.
53. Kirsch E, Kaim A, Engelter S et al. MR angiography in internal carotid artery dissection: improvement of diagnosis by selective demonstration of the intramural haematoma. *Neuroradiology.* 1998;40(11):704–709.
54. Giacobetti FB, Vaccaro AR, Bos-Giacobetti MA et al. Vertebral artery occlusion associated with cervical spine trauma. A prospective analysis. *Spine.* 1997;15;22(2);188–192.
55. Parbhoo AH, Govender S, Corr P. Vertebral artery injury in cervical spine trauma. *Injury.* 2001;32(7):565–568.
56. Veras LM, Pedraza-Gutierrez S, Castellanos J, Capellades J, Casamitjana J, Rovira-Canellas A. Vertebral artery occlusion after acute cervical spine trauma. *Spine.* 2000;1;25(9):1171–1177.
57. Weller SJ, Rossitch Jr E, Malek AM. Detection of vertebral artery injury after cervical spine trauma using magnetic resonance angiography. *J Trauma.* 1999;46(4):660–666.
58. Woodring JH, Lee C, Duncan V. Transverse process fractures of the cervical vertebrae: are they insignificant? *J Trauma.* 1993;34(6):797–802.
59. Cothren CC, Moore EE, Biffl WL et al. Cervical spine fracture patterns predictive of blunt vertebral artery injury. *J Trauma.* 2003;55(5):811–813

8 Trauma to the Pediatric Spine

P. N. M Tyrrell and V. N. Cassar-Pullicino

Introduction

The anatomy and biomechanics of the pediatric spine differ significantly from that of the adult. These differences are related to intrinsic age-related tissue differences and the capacity for growth, remodeling, and regeneration. These differences also vary with growth and development of the spine and give rise to different patterns of injury in the immature spinal skeleton.

The interpretation of the pediatric cervical spine can be difficult for those unfamiliar with the normal pattern of development and ossification of the spine. There is a real risk of both false-negative and false-positive interpretative errors.[1] An understanding of this helps to avoid pitfalls in interpretation. There are a number of predictable epiphyses, apophyses, and synchondroses that may be misinterpreted radiographically as fractures. There is also a wide range of normal variants with specific morphological and radiological characteristics. In addition spinal movement patterns also differ from those expected in the adult.

The appearance of the secondary ossification centers in the growing spine can be associated with radiographically subtle but significant physeal injuries. Although the pediatric spine assumes many of the adult radiographic features by the age of 8 years, as in the peripheral skeleton, potential injuries related to these relatively vulnerable physes should be given due diagnostic consideration.

The incidence of spinal injury in childhood and adolescence is variably reported between 1 % and 9 % of the total reported spinal injuries. This implies that accident and emergency staff and radiologists are unlikely to see this injury on a regular basis in the same hospital. This lack of experience and teaching material increases the risks of missed diagnosis. Cervical spine injuries in particular may be more common than is currently recognized as they are easily overlooked on plain radiographs. Aufdermaur identified injuries through endplates of vertebral bodies in an autopsy study, but only 1 in 12 was suspected to have sustained a spinal injury before autopsy.[2] Road traffic accidents and falls are the most frequent mechanism of injury in the childhood group as a whole. However, in the older child and adolescent, sports-related injuries including diving, surfing, and cycling account for a number of cases.

The pattern of cervical spine injury affecting the child differs from that in the adult. In the younger child (< 8 years), there is a predominance of upper cervical spine injury over the lower cervical region, which is the opposite of that seen in adults. The upper cervical spine is more vulnerable to injury due to a number of anatomical and physiological features. These include the unique pattern of ossification of C1 and C2, the poorly developed neck musculature, the relatively large size of the head compared to the cervical spine in the child, the fulcrum of movement being located in the upper cervical spine in the young child as opposed to the mid to lower cervical region seen in the older child and adult, ligamentous laxity, and underdeveloped skeleton of the spinal motion segments. Adult type of injuries (over 8 years of age) occuring in the pediatric age group will not therefore be the emphasis of this chapter as they are covered in previous chapters.

There are a number of subsets of spinal injury that are predominant or even unique to children. Trauma to the spine occurring at birth is rare, and although uncommon, trauma to the spine in nonaccidental injury has become increasingly recognized, while SCIWORA (*spinal cord injury without radiographic abnormality*) is more commonly seen in children than in adults.

In order to understand the different patterns of injury and avoid errors of interpretation it is important to be familiar with the development of the spine, its radiological appearances and the range of normal variants before embarking on the imaging of the various pathological conditions.

Development of the Vertebral Column

The term *centrum* describes the central part of a developing vertebra. It encloses the notochord and gives rise to most of the vertebral body. A "neural process" extends dorsally on each side of the neural tube and later in the fetal period the right and left processes unite to complete the neural arch, which forms the vertebral arch and a small portion of the vertebral body. In the centrum, endochondral ossification commences at approximately 9 weeks of fetal life. Bipartite centers (anterior and posterior) associated with the arrangement of the blood vessels may be encountered. Coronally cleft vertebrae may occur up to the age of 4 years and are considered to be a normal variation of endochondral ossification[3] that depends on varying patterns of vascular distribution.[4] The junctional area between the centrum and the neural arch is termed the neurocentral synchondrosis.

At birth most vertebrae have three ossific areas—one for the centrum and one for each half of the neural arch. The ossific center of a centrum in the newborn is ovoid on a lateral radiograph. The ossific center of each vertebral centrum is separated from that of the neural arch by the broad radiolucent synchondrosis that contains uncalcified cartilage. Bony union takes place here between 3 and 6 years. Anteriorly and posteriorly there are small indentations or clefts that represent vascular channels running through the ossific center. As normal growth occurs, the vertebral bodies as seen on a lateral radiograph become more rectangular, while the height of the vertebral body compared with the disk space increases.

In early childhood the vertebral endplate has a thick hyaline cartilage component. Growth forces at the diskovertebral interfaces, which are both elliptical in their enlargement contours, have an effect on the distribution of the cartilage components (physes) superiorly and inferiorly. There are no separate epiphyseal ossification centers in the growing human vertebrae, but due to the mechanics in operation the growth cartilage becomes increasingly thin centrally, with a thicker periphery laterally and anteriorly which becomes the ring apophysis. First visible at approximately 5 years they represent an annular recess that surrounds the vertebral body and will form the secondary ossification center of the vertebral endplate. The recess is filled with cartilage. Initially on lateral radiographs the ring apophysis appears set in a superior and inferior groove anteriorly at the borders of the developing vertebra. This is an area of active growth and remodeling carrying significant biomechanical shearing, compressive forces and not just traction stresses. Small calcific foci begin to appear in this cartilaginous rim at 6–8 years in girls and 7–9 years in boys.[5] Ossification of this ring apophysis may not occur simultaneously in the superior and inferior components and must not be mistaken for a fracture. These foci slowly ossify and gradually unite to form a bony vertebral ring—the vertebral ring apophysis. The vertebral ring apophysis/growth plate parallels the superior and inferior vertebral margins and in infants and young children it extends substantially over the superior and inferior aspects of the anterior vertebral margin.[5] The fusion of individual foci to form a unified rim is complete at 12 years. Prior to that, the child's spine assumes adult characteristics by ages 8–10 years.

The neural arches of C1 and C2 show well-developed ossific areas bilaterally at birth, but perichondral ossification of the neural arches here and elsewhere is not complete at birth. The spinous processes do not yet possess their own ossific centers and are formed during the first year by amalgamation of the neural arches. This begins in the lumbar area and spreads to be complete in the cervical spine in the second year. Union may not occur in the atlas until the fourth to sixth year and in the sacrum until the seventh to tenth year. Fusion between the base and apex of the dens usually occurs by 12 years.

Secondary centers of ossification (apophyses) form along the tips of the spinous processes during the years of adolescent growth (11–14 years), formed as small ossific centers that eventually cap the entire tips of the spinous processes. These unite with the spinous processes when vertebral growth is complete. The tips of the transverse processes in the lumbar region show occasional development of secondary ossific centers.

The first two cervical vertebrae are atypical. The central pillar of the axis develops as three segments: (i) the tip of the dens; (ii) the base of the dens; (iii) the centrum. Ossification occurs in the order of the centrum, the base of the dens (appearing at birth) and finally the tip of the dens, the latter occurring before 2 years but not constantly present. The base of the dens has two centers of ossification.

Normal Variants

Visualization of the spine in its developmental stage reveals different stages of ossification. On the radiograph areas of lucency may be representative of cartilaginous development, so knowledge of the expected appearance and approximate age of appearance of different ossification centers will help in interpretation. Synchondroses have smooth well-corticated margins and occur at characteristic sites and awareness of this will avoid misinterpretation of these as fractures. The atlas and the axis have a different developmental and hence morphological appearance to the other vertebrae.

The ossification center for the anterior arch of the atlas is present in 20% at birth but usually appears during the first year. It may, however, be absent resulting in failure of anterior fusion leaving a cleft. The body of C1 joins the neural arches by synchondroses that close by the seventh year, but the ring of C1 reaches its normal adult size by the fourth year (Fig. 8.**1**). The pattern and sequence of ossification of the axis, including the centrum, the odontoid process, and the apex of the odontoid process have been referred to above. The basilar odontoid synchondrosis usually fuses between 3 and 6 years of age but closure may be delayed. This should not be mistaken for a fracture. The vestigial form may still be visible up to the age of 11 years, represented by a fine sclerotic line, but should be clearly differentiated from a fracture line that will appear clearly lucent. This vestigial remnant can remain discernible on CT and MRI images into adult life. Fractures of the peg typically occur above the level of the synchondrosis and may ultimately give rise to an os odontoideum (see later). The ossification center at the apex of the odontoid process appears at approximately 2 years of age and fuses to the larger odontoid process at approximately 12 years. Sometimes the appearance of the apical ossification center may be delayed, or it may even not appear at all.

Disturbances in alignment of the vertebral bodies in the cervical spine may arouse concern about underlying occult injury. Hypermobility, ligamentous laxity, and incomplete ossification may be responsible for these appearances. A number of normal variants occur in a child, which would give rise to alarm if seen in the adult patient. These include:

Pseudo Jefferson fracture (pseudospreading of C1). In young children the ossification of the lateral mass of

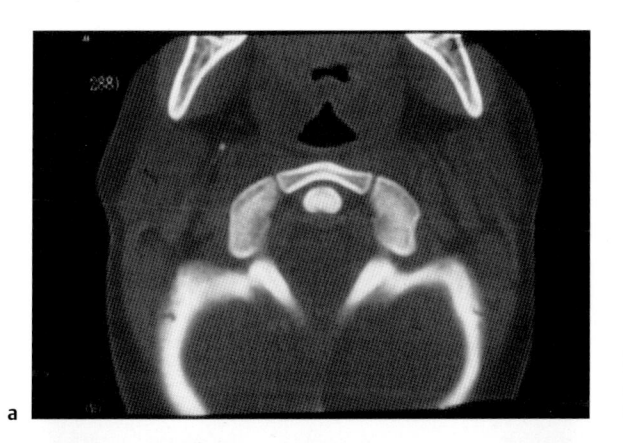

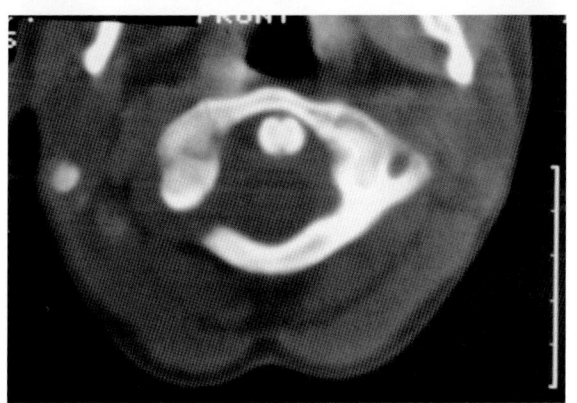

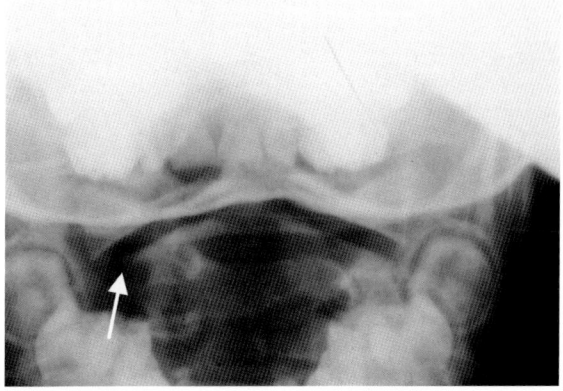

Fig. 8.1 **a** Axial CT of the normal development of the C1 vertebra with the odontoid peg equidistant from the synchondroses of the anterior body of C1. Pseudo Jefferson fracture of C1 with lateral offset on the radiograph on the right (*arrow*) (**b**) due to unequal growth at the synchondroses of C1 producing elongation on the right as judged by the odontoid peg (**c**).

C1 often exceeds that of the ossification of C2 giving rise to what has been called the pseudospread of C1 on C2 (Fig. 8.1).

Pseudosubluxation of the body of C2 on C3 is a well-recognized phenomenon. Forward movement of the second cervical vertebra on the third during flexion and extension of the spine is noted. The phenomenon is a combination of forward shift and flexion of the second cervical vertebra on the third. Pseudosubluxation of up to 4 mm is acceptable in a child. Bailey indicated that attention to both symmetry of the curve and the relative positions of adjacent cervical vertebrae is necessary to identify this phenomenon.[6] Cattel and Filtzer described a method for measuring the degree of anteroposterior movement of C2 on C3.[7] They noted marked to moderate anterior displacement in 39 of 160 children aged 1–16 years and a definite tendency towards anterior displacement in 28 out of 160. Hypermobility with ligamentous laxity were thought to be a contributory factor but also the relative horizontal plane of the articular processes in the upper cervical region as described by Sullivan and colleagues may allow greater forward gliding of C2 on C3.[8] Anterior wedging, a further normal variant (see below) may also contribute to the appearance. Swischuk described a line to help differentiate physiological from pathological C2 anterior displacement.[9] If a line is drawn between the anterior margin of the spinous processes of C1 and C3, in physiological subluxation the anterior aspect of the spinous process of C2 should lie within 2 mm of this line (Fig. 8.2). If it lies more than 2 mm either anterior or posterior to this line then pathological subluxation is present.[10] Cattel and Filtzer also observed posterior displacement in extension at the C2/C3 level.[7] Anterior displacement of C3 on C4 was also observed in 14 % of cases. The radiographic depiction of pseudosubluxation, however, must always be correlated with the clinical status. In instances of persistent cervical symptoms further imaging and follow-up will still be required despite the radiographic demonstration of pseudosubluxation to exclude a hidden injury (Fig. 8.2).[11] The underlying anatomic and physiological factors promoting C2/C3 pseudosubluxation are also in play in a traumatic event, rendering this level susceptible to trauma. Indeed 7 out of 11 patients with presumed pseudosubluxation were shown to have a true injury.[12]

Vertebral pseudowedging. Anterior wedging is merely a radiographic appearance of the vertebrae due to the pattern of vertebral ossification and is not morphological. The apparent wedging of vertebral bodies has been observed by a number of authors on lateral views of the cervical spine. Immature vertebral bodies are oval in shape with smooth rounded corners and gradually become more rectangular in shape with age. A study by Swishuk et al[13] demonstrated that in infants and young children some developed a wedging deformity of the vertebral body ossification center involving the anterosuperior corner of the vertebral body (Fig. 8.4). Swischuk studied the lateral cervical spine radiographs of 481 children ranging in age from birth to 19 years and confirmed that cervical vertebral bodies generally mature from an ovoid shape to a rec-

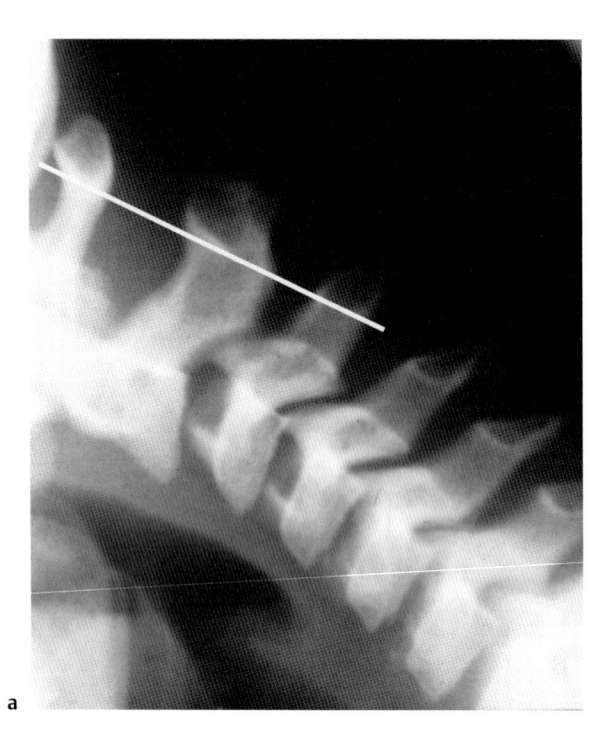

Fig. 8.2 Pseudosubluxation of the body of C2 on C3 confirmed by the continuous spinolaminal line drawn between C1 and C3 (**a**). Despite the radiographic appearance, due to ongoing symptoms appropriate treatment and follow-up was required which revealed a hidden injury of the osteo-ligamentous attachment at C2/C3 highlighted by new bone formation (*arrow*) (**b**).

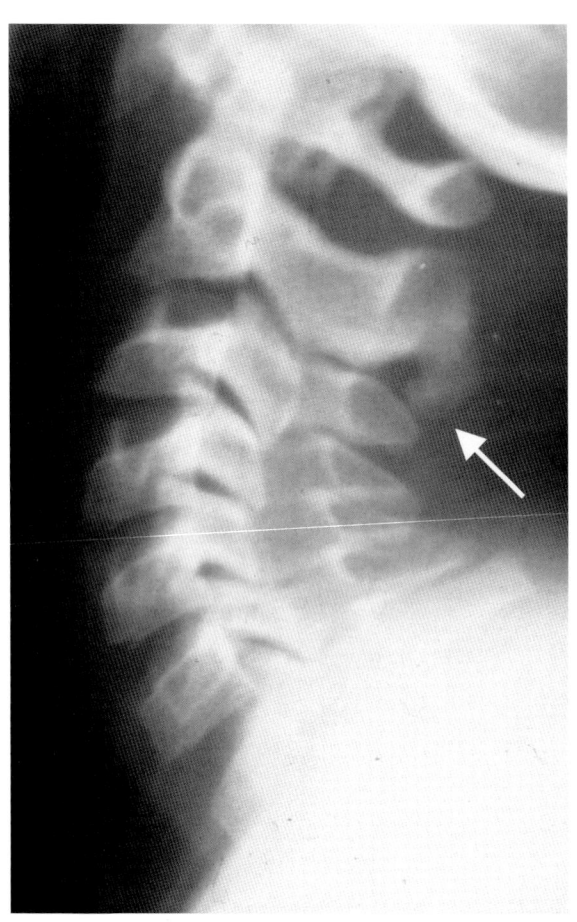

tangular adult shape, but that at the level of C3 some infants and children develop a wedging deformity of the vertebral body ossification center. This appearance was occasionally seen at C4 but was not seen at other levels. The incidence of this anterior wedging decreased with increasing age, being present in 14/481 patients between birth and 3 years, and seen only in 2/481 patients between 13 and 19 years.[13] It was postulated that chronic exaggerated hypermobility caused chronic repetitive impaction of the vertebral body of C3 by C2. Thus hypermobility of the upper cervical spine in infants and children is most pronounced at the C2/C3 level, which is also the fulcrum of movement in this age group, and can be associated with a number of normal variants. These include anterior wedging, actual anterior displacement of the vertebral body, or marked angulation at the C2–C3 level.

Congenital spondylolysis. Farndon and Fielding in 1981 used the term "pedicle defect" to encompass a congenitally absent pedicle, congenital spondylolysis, and persistent synchondrosis.[14] In the cervical region C6 is most commonly involved. The lytic defect may be uni- or bilateral. There may be dysplasia of the posterior elements and a compensatory change in levels above and below the vertebra involved (Fig. 8.**3**).[15,16] Patients may give a history of neck or shoulder pain precipitating the radiographic examination or it may be detected incidentally during imaging following a history of trauma. The abnormality is usually suspected or clearly diagnosed from features on the radiograph. These include the well-corticated margins of the spondylolytic defect, hypoplastic facets, and spina bifida occulta. CT can readily confirm these findings (Fig. 8.**3**). The lesion can be difficult to detect on MRI but absence of the spinous process on sagittal sequences should alert one to the possibility of the diagnosis.[15]

The space between the posterior aspect of the anterior arch of the atlas and the front of the odontoid peg (atlanto-axial or atlanto-odontoid distance) normally measures approximately 4 mm in children (the equivalent adult distance is 2–3 mm). This wider distance in the child is due radiographically to the lucent unossified atlanto-dens cartilage with a degree of ligamentous laxity. The atlanto-odontoid space can widen in flexion up to 5 mm.

There may be overriding of the anterior arch of the atlas on the odontoid process in extension. In Cattel and Filtzer's study[7] overriding was said to be present

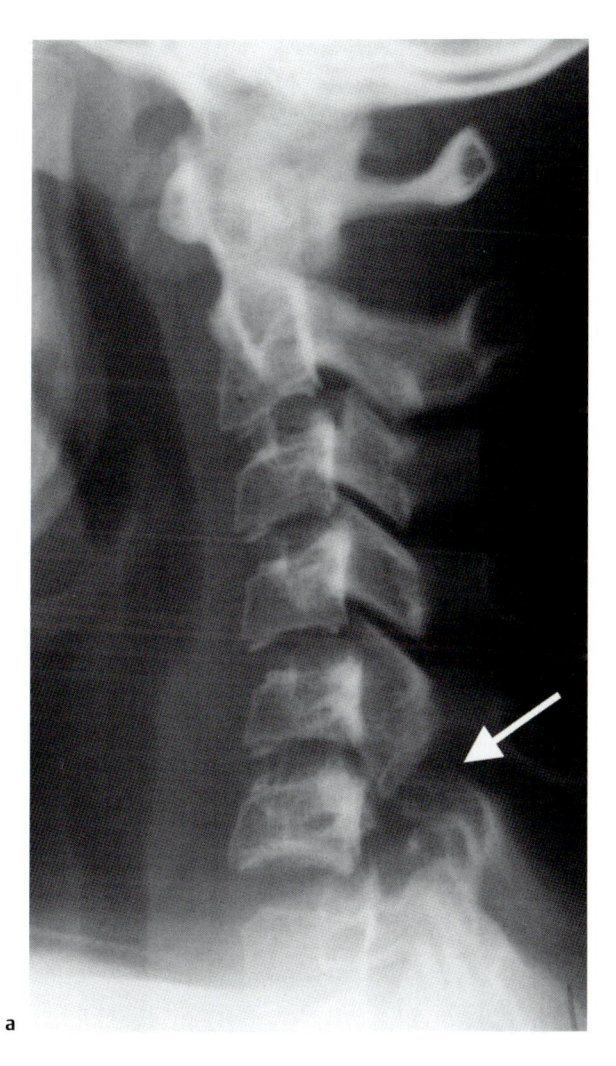

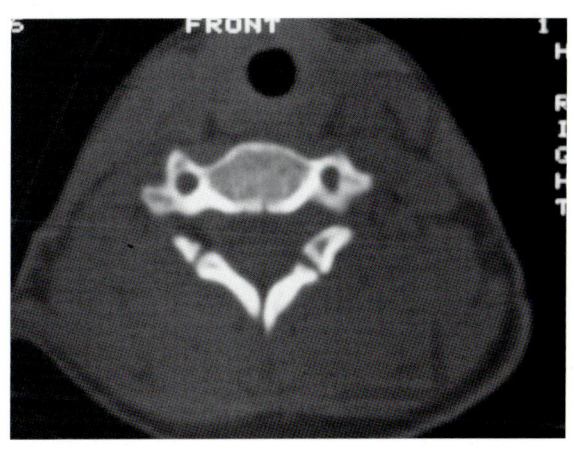

Fig. 8.3 Congenital spondylolysis of C6 seen on the lateral cervical radiograph (*arrow*) (**a**), with evidence of failed fusion at all synchondrotic sites at C6 on the CT (**b**).

when more than two thirds of the visible anterior arch of the atlas lay above the superior margin of the odontoid process.

Absence of the normal lordotic curvature in the neutral position in adults can be considered to represent spasm and be indicative of underlying bone or soft tissue injury. Absent lordosis has, however, been observed by Juhl et al[17] and Fineman et al[18] as occurring in normal subjects and, therefore, not necessarily indicative of injury.

Marked angulation at a single intervertebral level was observed by Cattel and Filtzer[7] and was felt to probably be the result of the relative laxity of the interspinous, interlaminar, and posterior longitudinal ligaments.

In Cattel and Filtzer's study absent flexion curvature of the spine between the second and seventh cervical vertebrae with the neck in flexion was described.[7]

There is a wide range of normal variants occurring in the pediatric spine.[19] Many of these variants relate to hypermobility related to ligamentous laxity and to incomplete ossification, which renders a very different appearance than that seen with the adult spine.

Birth Injury

Injury to the spinal cord is a tragic event that can occasionally occur as a complication of traumatic birth delivery. When it occurs it is usually in association with a breech presentation involving the lower cervical and upper thoracic spine. Although the vertebral column with its intact ligaments is flexible and can stretch, there is a very limited degree of elasticity afforded to the spinal cord and "over stretch" may result in cord injury. When cord injury occurs in association with a breech presentation this is usually at the cervicothoracic junction probably as a result of traction. This contrasts with the high cervical cord injury, which is the usual injury that occurs with a cephalic presentation, and is thought to be due to rotation.[20] There is usually little to find on spinal radiography. The diagnosis is often suspected on the basis of the history of a difficult delivery, neurological signs, and respiratory symptomatology, including pneumonia occurring secondary to weak respiratory muscles. MRI is valuable in demonstrating cord signal abnormality.

Nonaccidental Injury (NAI)

The true incidence of NAI induced spinal injury is unknown. In part this is due to the previous lack of routine acquisition of AP and lateral views of the spine in suspected NAI cases. It is unusual to see obvious vertebral fractures in cases of nonaccidental injury. In this setting the presentation is more likely to be that of neurological disturbance in the presence of normal radiographs. This is because of the elasticity of the spine. Severe shaking or other trauma may induce cord hemorrhage or edema in the absence of actual fracture. In Brown's review of 103 cervical spine injuries in children, the three cases of child abuse were all associated with SCIWORA.[21] Studies,[22] however, have demonstrated that most changes are anteriorly located with subtle compression fractures of vertebrae, some of which may extend into the growth plate. Posterior neural arch fractures are unusual. These have been identified at postmortem. "Typical" fracture patterns have been described as in the paper by Kleinman and Marks.[22] They reported on the postmortem radiological and histopathological findings in 10 cases of vertebral body fractures occurring in infants and young children. Three patterns were noted: (1) Compression only—mild compression deformity (<25%) of the anterior half of the vertebral bodies without disruption of the endplate. (2) Fracture with superior endplate extension. These fractures involved the anterosuperior aspect of the vertebral body with extension into the anterior aspect of the endplate. This tended to undermine a variably sized bone fragment. Histologically the fractures entered the cartilaginous growth plate of the superior endplate. (3) Combined lesions. With increasing compression deformity of the vertebral bodies, extension of the fracture into the proliferative zone of the superior cartilaginous growth plate was more extensive. In cases of nonaccidental injury there is usually evidence of injury elsewhere in the skeleton particularly in relation to long bones and/or rib fractures.

Cervical Spine Injuries

Atlanto-Occipital Dissociation (AOD)

The higher incidence of upper cervical injuries in children compared with adults is also reflected in this injury, which is twice as frequent in the pediatric age group. This rare injury is usually fatal, but in survivors the diagnosis can be clinically difficult to make. In the first instance these victims are usually suffering from severe polytrauma, especially head injuries. In addition the clinical picture is variable with a spectrum of neurological (cranial nerve, quadriplegia, sub-brain stem complete loss), respiratory, and cardiovascular (hypotension, tachycardia, cardiac arrest) dysfunction. The mainstay of diagnosis is based on radiological appearances which are readily appreciated if there is residual atlanto-occipital dissociation at the time of examination. In some instances it is not an easy diagnosis to make when spontaneous anatomical reduction and alignment is restored, but this can become apparent on the lateral radiograph taken immediately after skull traction. The Powers ratio is helpful in identifying the presence of AOD being based on two simple measurements. The distance between the anterior rim of the foramen magnum and the posterior arch of the atlas is divided by the distance between the posterior rim of the foramen magnum and the anterior arch of the atlas. Values greater than 1.0 are abnormal while less than that are definitely normal. This measurement however has been shown to be unreliable when anterior injuries reduce spontaneously, in posterior atlanto-occipital injury, in the presence of an atlas fracture or congenital cranio-vertebral junction osseous abnormalities. To overcome this problem the dens-basion distance can be measured as well as the interspinous C1/C2 and C2/C3 distances. A dens-basion distance over 14 mm was the mainstay of diagnosis in 11 patients with atlanto-occipital dissociation.[23] A C1/C2:C2/C3 ratio greater than 2.5 indicates ligamentous injury. In instances of equivocal radiological measurements, CT and MRI can be employed to identify malalignment and cranio-cervical hemorrhage, respectively. MRI may also be useful if the neurological status deteriorates to exclude hydrocephalus and retropharyngeal pseudomeningocele complications.

Fractures of C1

The Jefferson fracture is a comminuted fracture of the atlas involving both the anterior and the posterior arches of the ring. Most Jefferson fractures occur as a result of a significant impact on the head, such as a fall, or a blow to the vertex. The force is transmitted through the occipital condyles and into the atlas. Although a rare injury in the young child, it needs to be differentiated from both a normal variant appearance and developmental defects. The fracture may also occur through the neuro-central synchondroses, which may remain unfused until the age of 7, and this is best diagnosed by CT.[24, 25] This injury is also rarely unilateral involving one of the anterior synchondroses.

On the lateral view there may be prevertebral soft tissue swelling. This can sometimes be difficult to appreciate in the very young child and also may not always be present. A fracture line may be visible on the lateral projection. On the open-mouth view, however, there is bilateral offset or spreading of the lateral articular masses of C1 in relation to the apposing articular surfaces of C2. The degree of offset may help differentiate between a stable and an unstable injury. A stable Jefferson fracture (in which the transverse ligament is intact) is implied by total offset of the two sides of less than 7 mm. An unstable fracture (in which the transverse ligament has ruptured) is demonstrated by lateral displacement in excess of 7 mm, often together with an increase in the atlanto-axial distance on the lateral view. On occasion the lateral masses of C1 and C2 are aligned on one side but offset on the other. This implies the same as bilateral offset. This situation of bilateral offset of the lateral masses of C1 upon C2 is seen in two other situations—pseudo Jefferson fracture [pseudospreading (see above)] and the presence of developmental defects in C1.[26,27] In this latter situation the bilateral offset amounts to no more than 2 mm on each side whereas offset is usually associated in a Jefferson fracture with a spread of more than 3 mm on each side. The clinical history will be paramount in helping to differentiate between a true fracture and a normal variant or developmental anomaly. Pseudospreading is not uncommonly seen in young children whereas Jefferson fractures are rare.

Injury of C2

Sherk at al noted that lesions of the atlas and axis accounted for 16% of a large series of adult cervical spine injuries whereas they comprise up to 70% of cervical spine injuries in children.[28] The differentiation between a congenital anomaly, a developmental anomaly such as persistent synchondrosis, and a fracture can be difficult. There have been a number of reports in the literature highlighting difficulties in precise diagnosis.[29–32] Classic radiographic features, which are significant findings in the adult and help direct one to a diagnosis, are not always present or are difficult to appreciate in the pediatric cervical spine. Prevertebral soft tissue swelling may not be present in infants, especially in the absence of anterior ligamentous injury. When it is present it may be difficult to assess due to the presence of normal adenoidal tissue or as a result of buckling of the airway in the flexed position.

Some authors have reported spondylolysis of C2 in adults suggesting that it may represent a persistent neurocentral synchondrosis. Schwishuk, however, has stated that the posterior arch synchondroses of C2 are not visible on true lateral views of the cervical spine.[9] If an osseous defect is seen it should be considered to represent a fracture or more remotely a congenital defect. Osseous defects can occur in dysplasias, especially sclerosing dysplasias and pyknodysostosis. Thus, if an unexplained osseous defect is seen, the possibility of a more generalized bone disorder should also be considered in the young person. Mondschein highlighted several radiographic findings that helped to distinguish congenital spondylolysis from a hangman's fracture.[30] The presence of an osseous gap in the region of the pars interarticularis with smooth clearly defined cortical margins on either side is in favor of a spondylolysis. If there is no prevertebral soft tissue swelling and no evidence of instability on flexion/extension views then this would also favor a spondylolytic defect. On a follow-up radiograph, or CT, small foci of ossification may be seen in the defect. It has been highlighted, however, that if there is a positive history of trauma, such an osseous defect should be treated as being traumatic in origin and follow-up with serial plain films and/or CT may lead to the definitive diagnosis.

Odontoid fracture in young children virtually always occurs as a Salter–Harris type I epiphyseal separation of the growth-plate at the base of the dens. As these dens-centrum injuries involve the cartilaginous plates of the axis during the period prior to fusion, they are more accurately termed traumatic disruptions of the synchondroses or synchondrotic slips (Fig. 8.**4**). Two forms exist[33]—one is a disruption of the synchondrosis between the odontoid process/C2 vertebral body unit and the neural arches of C2.[29] This may result in an anterior displacement and angulation of the odontoid process/C2 vertebral body unit. The other form is simply a slippage of the odontoid process with respect to the C2 vertebral body. Anterior displacement or angulation of the odontoid is usually seen on the lateral radiograph. Diagnosis in injuries without displacement can be difficult on radiography. Care with interpretation, however, is required. Vigoroux et al reported angulation of the odontoid process in approximately 4% of normal children.[34] Thin-section CT can be helpful, showing the lack of integrity of the synchondrosis with the parent bone. CT is also helpful in monitoring treatment. An anteriorly displaced odontoid process in younger children can almost always be reduced by gentle manipulation into extension with the position maintained by halo traction and a Minerva jacket. Healing usually occurs without too many problems. Neurological deficit is uncommon unless associated with a head injury especially when associated with 50% or more displacement.[35]

Traumatic subluxation of the axis may be difficult to differentiate from physiological subluxation in children. Traumatic subluxation will be associated with a clinical history of a probable hyperflexion injury, together with neck pain, and tenderness at the C2 spinous process. Sequential radiographs may be required to confirm progression of subluxation and local kyphosis. In time calcified avulsion fragments may be visible adjacent to the bifurcate C2 spinous process. These ossified fragments may be due to an avulsion injury of the supraspinous ligament in acute flexion. Multifidus muscle, cervical semispinalis muscle, and interspinous ligaments are attached to the tip of the spinous process. Secondary cartilaginous ossification centers are present at the tips of the spinous processes. Hence, ossified fragments may result from an avulsion of the apophyses of the spinous process, which are often seen in adolescents. These ossification centers appear at approximately 14 years of age and fuse at approximately 25 years of age. These secondary centers of ossification are located bilaterally, close to the tips of the bifurcate spinous process. It is this bilaterality that suggests that the ossified fragments have resulted from previous avulsion of cartilaginous centers as opposed to a more central avulsed fragment.

Os Odontoideum

Trauma rather than failure of fusion of two ossific centers is the more likely cause of the os odontoideum in otherwise skeletally normal children.[36] It is a separate ossicle separated by a variable gap from the hypoplastic dens.[37] The os odontoideum is an oval or round ossicle

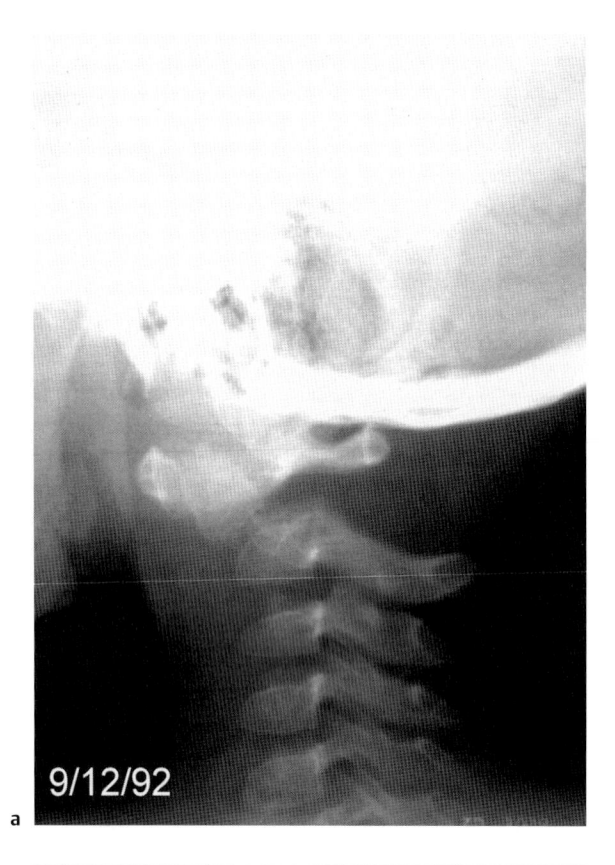

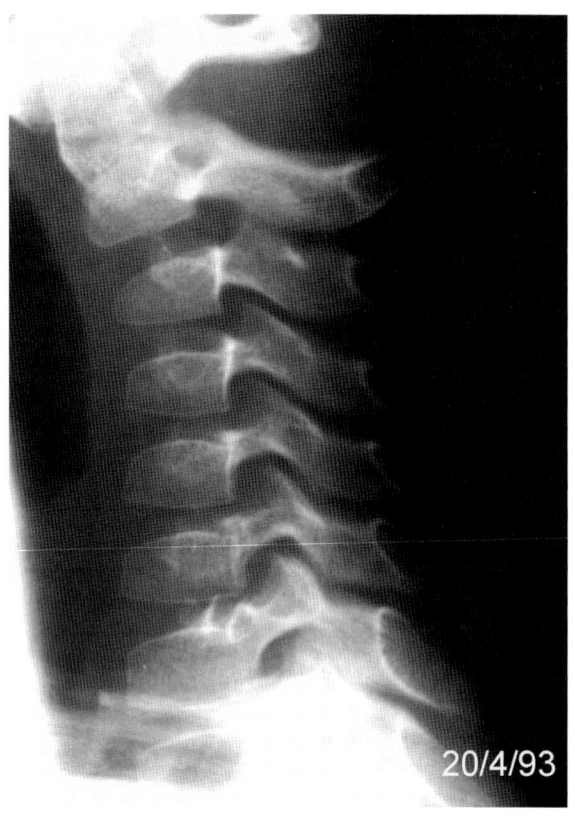

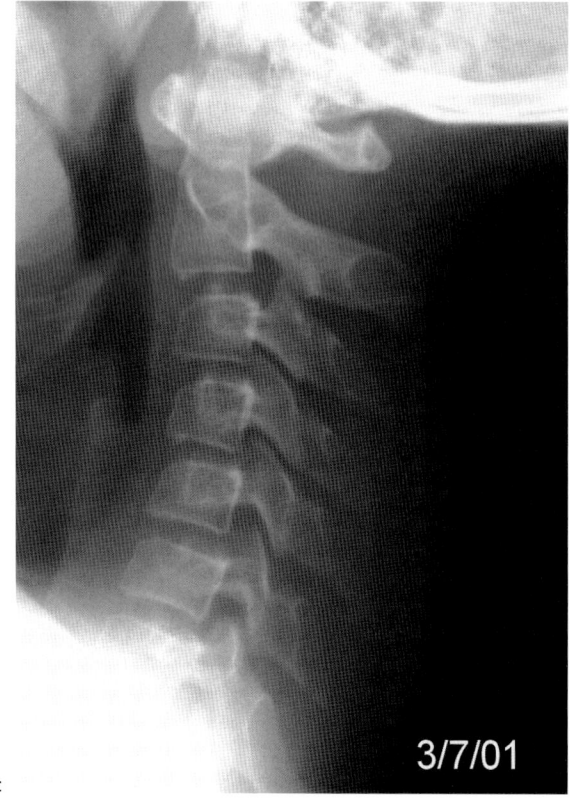

Fig. 8.4 Salter–Harris type I acute synchondrotic separation with forward displacement of the C2 odontoid peg on its body and prevertebral soft tissue swelling (**a**). Lateral follow-up cervical radiograph about 4 months after closed reduction and stabilization showing fusion of the odontoid peg with the body of C2 in a satisfactory position and pseudowedged appearances of the sub-axial vertebrae (**b**). Normal appearing C2 vertebra as well as sub-axial vertebral bodies on a lateral cervical radiograph 9 years after injury (**c**).

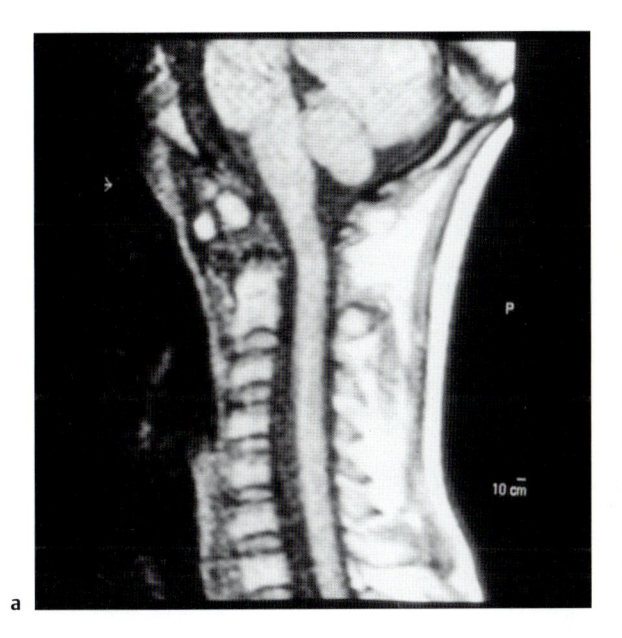

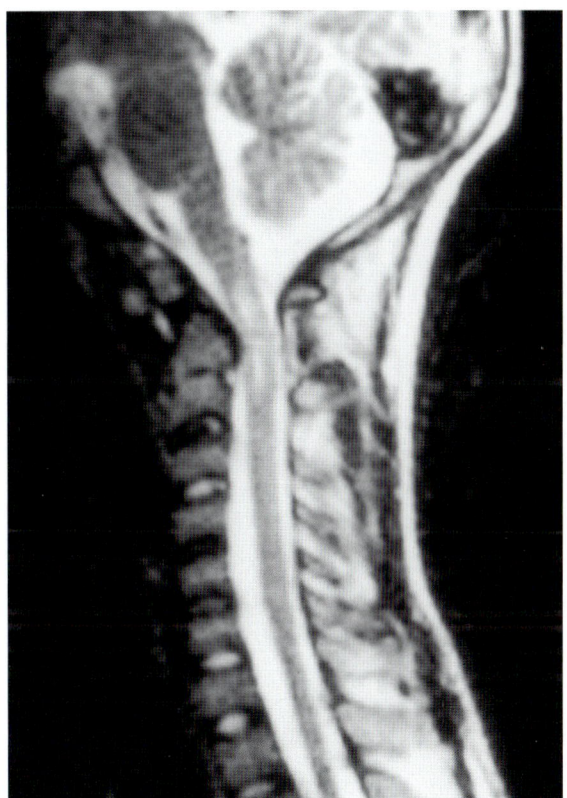

Fig. 8.5 High cervical cord injury in a boy with unsuspected os odontoideum sustained following a dive in a swimming pool seen on sagittal T1 (**a**) and T2 (**b**) MR image.

with a smooth corticated margin located either in the normal position (orthotopic) of the odontoid process or near the base of the occipital bone (dystopic) in the area of the foramen magnum inferior to the clivus. A review of 35 patients with this finding suggested that trauma is the etiology of the lesion.[36] Cervical pain was the most common reason for presentation. Most patients had instability of the affected spinal segment. As movement of the os odontoideum is unpredictable and its effect on the cord in individual cases unknown, each case requires flexion/extension MRI. Acute neurological deficit can occur during play at school, diving, minor trauma etc if the remaining weak ligaments are disrupted (Fig. 8.5) and the cord injured.

Atlanto-Axial Dislocation

Atlanto-axial horizontal separation consists of excessive motion of the atlas on the axis (> 5 mm) due to rupture of the transverse ligament resulting in an unstable injury. Children with acute cervical fractures and dislocations have atlanto-axial dislocation in 10% of cases with minimal neurological signs. Flexion/extension lateral cervical radiographs show excursion greater than 5 mm between the anterior cortex of the dens and the posterior cortex of the anterior ring of C1. It is an uncommon injury in children but there is an increased incidence in Down's syndrome, Klippel–Feil deformity, and skeletal dysplasias. In young children (< 7 years) the synchondrosis at the base of the dens is more likely to fail rather than the transverse ligament of the atlas.

Atlanto-Axial Rotatory Fixation

Atlanto-axial rotatory fixation (AARF) is the preferred term for the condition not infrequently known as atlanto-axial rotatory subluxation or atlanto-axial rotatory dislocation. AARF is preferred since rotatory fixation usually occurs within the normal range of rotation of the joint. There is a wide range of normal movement at the atlanto-axial joint. The normal range of cervical rotation is approximately 90° to either side and half this rotation occurs at the atlanto-axial joint. Studies have measured a range of total rotation (rotation to each of the right and left sides) from 45° to 88.5° (mean 69.25°).[38] Early studies suggest that rotation is initiated at the atlanto-axial joint and C1 rotation is complete before rotation of C2 and the lower cervical vertebrae begins.[39] Pang and Li have studied the dynamic behavior of C1 and C2 during normal voluntary head rotation in children using CT examination.[40] They found that when C1 rotates from 0° to 23° it moves alone, with C2 remaining stationary at approximately 0°. When C1 rotates from 24° to 65°, C1 and C2 move together, but C1 always moves at a faster rate, C2 being pulled by yoking ligaments. From 65° onwards, C1 and C2 move in exact unison with a fixed maximum separation angle of approximately 43°, head rotation being carried out exclusively by the subaxial segments. During rotation the ipsilateral lateral mass of C1 rotates posteriorly into the spinal canal thus narrowing it. However, this rarely produces symptoms. The spinal canal is at its roomiest at this level. Mazarra and Fielding have shown that 64° of right or left atlanto-axial rotation is required to produce

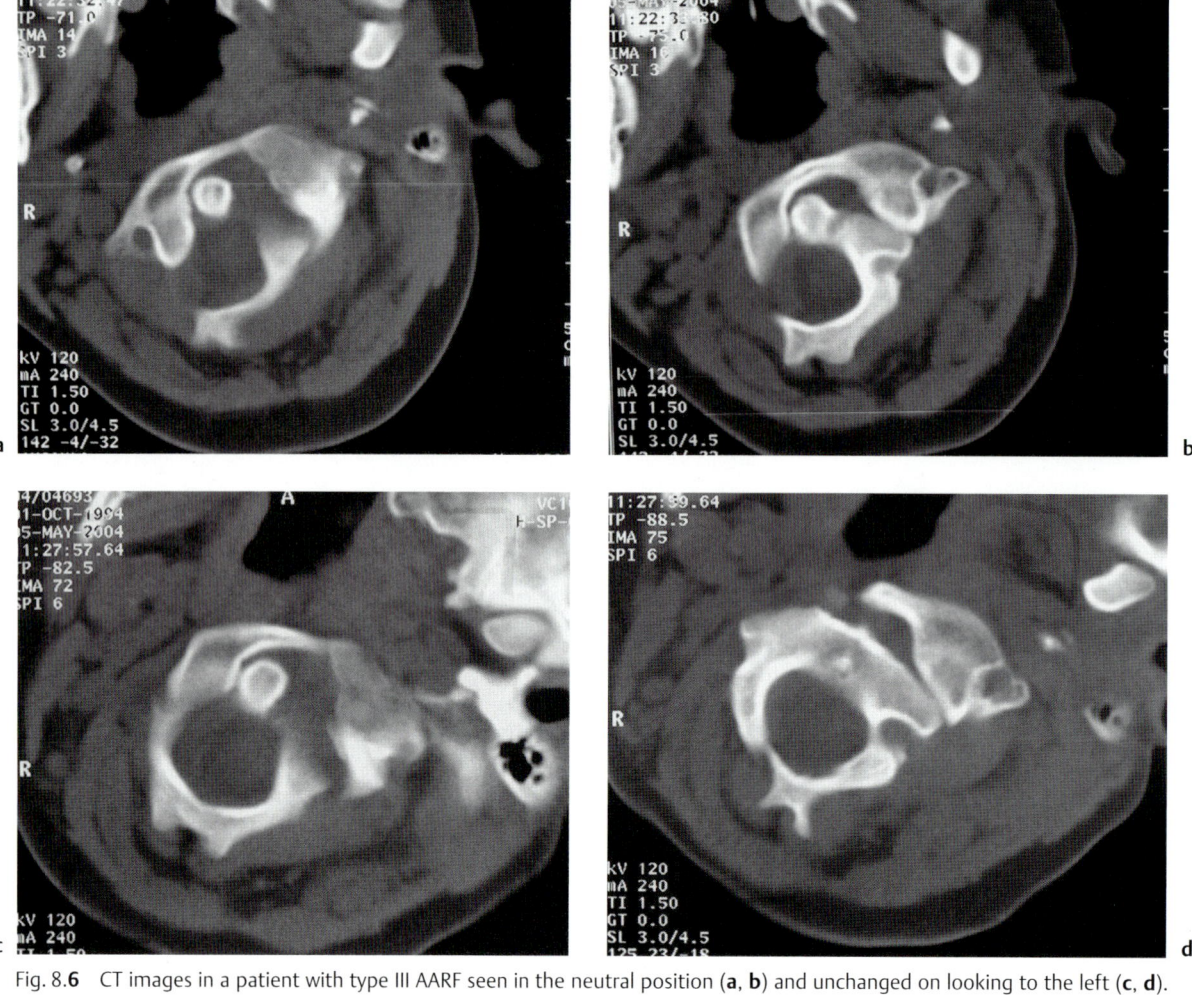

Fig. 8.6 CT images in a patient with type III AARF seen in the neutral position (**a**, **b**) and unchanged on looking to the left (**c**, **d**).

spinal cord compression.[41] A wide range of movement at the atlanto-axial joint is facilitated by the relative transverse lie of the lateral articulations. This wide range of movement, however, may be at the expense of stability. The transverse ligament of the atlas, which passes behind the odontoid peg, helps to control anterior movement of the atlas relative to C2. The paired right and left alar ligaments, which pass from the postero-lateral aspect of the odontoid process to the occipital condyles, limit rotation of the atlas on the axis.

Although AARF can occur as a result of minor or major trauma it is commonly atraumatic. Clinically, atlanto-axial rotatory fixation presents with torticollis and a reduced range of neck rotation. The head is tilted to one side and rotated to the opposite side producing a "cocked robin" position with slight flexion. Neurological compromise is unusual unless there is associated anterior or posterior atlanto-axial displacement. Fielding and Hawkins classified atlanto-axial rotatory fixation into four types.[42]

- Type I rotatory fixation without anterior displacement of the atlas. This is the most common type, oc-
curs within the normal range of rotation of the joint and has the odontoid peg as its pivot point.
- Type II rotatory fixation with anterior displacement of 3–5 mm. This is the second most common type, is associated with deficiency of the transverse ligament and has one of the lateral atlanto-axial joints as its pivot point.
- Type III rotatory fixation with anterior displacement of more than 5 mm. This degree of displacement implies deficiency of both the transverse and the alar ligaments.
- Type IV rotatory fixation with posterior displacement of the atlas. This is the least common type and occurs with a deficient odontoid process.

Types II–IV may be associated with compromise of the spinal canal resulting in neurological signs.

Most cases of childhood torticollis resolve spontaneously. In a few the rotatory deformity becomes fixed and irreducible. The fixation usually occurs within the normal range of rotation of the atlanto-axial joint. The commonest cause for atlanto-axial rotatory

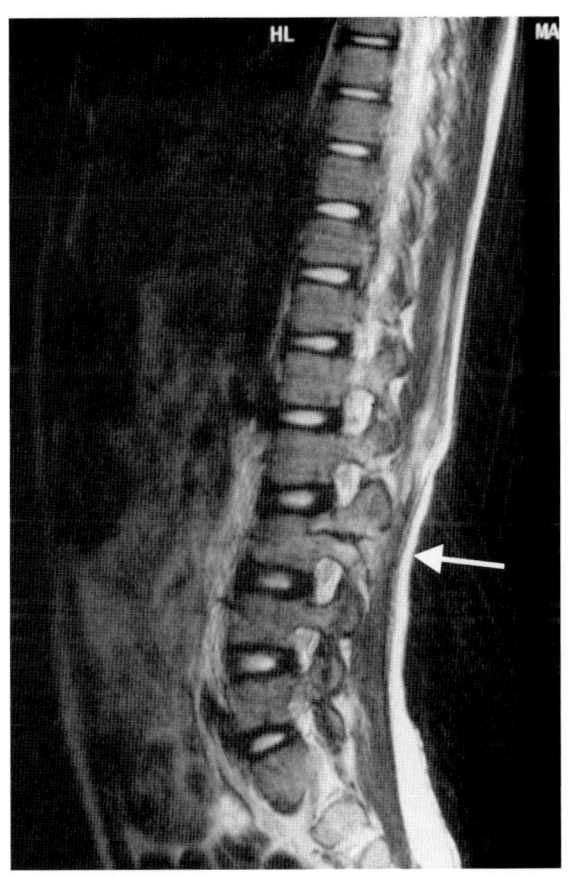

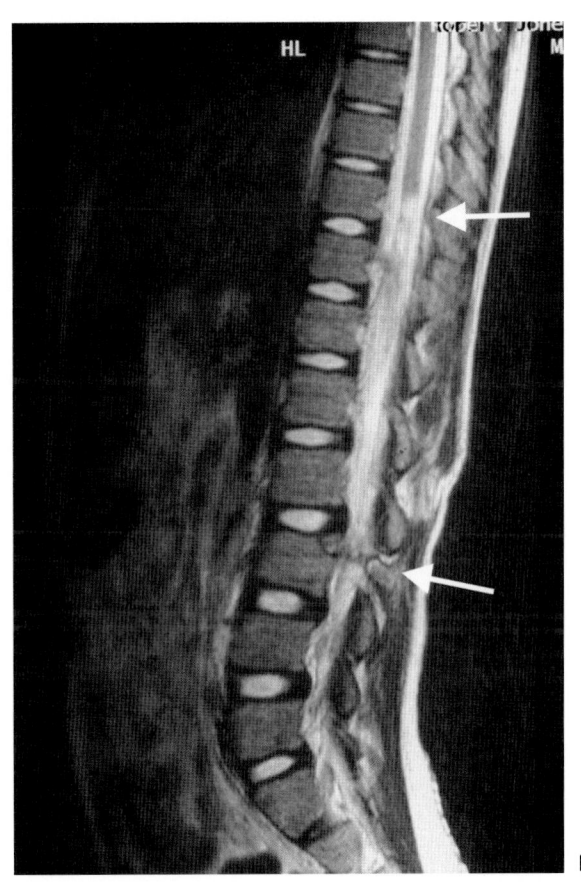

Fig. 8.7 Lap-belt injury in a road traffic accident in an adolescent victim producing a flexion-distraction osteo-ligamentous injury at the L2/L3 level (*arrows*) with a higher cord traumatic lesion at T10 (*arrow*) seen on T2 MR images (**a**, **b**).

fixation is idiopathic. Other etiologies include trauma, infection, or surgery in the head or neck region (Grisel's syndrome), rheumatoid arthritis, and also congenital anomalies of the upper cervical spine. Grisel's syndrome has been described as atlanto-axial rotatory fixation occurring secondary to ligamentous laxity and inflammation following infection or surgery.[43]

The position of the child's neck makes radiographic positioning difficult.[44] The distinction on radiography between abnormal C1/2 due to AARF from a similar appearance of C1/2 in a normal child with the head rotated is difficult. Despite obtaining a good lateral view of either the atlas or the axis, it proves impossible to obtain a normal C1/C2 relationship in the lateral position. This difficulty, together with the clinical presentation should arouse suspicion of the condition. CT beautifully demonstrates the C1/C2 relationship in the axial plane (Fig. 8.**6**). Although MRI may be able to demonstrate this relationship, the osseous detail is not quite as clear, despite the advantages of nonionizing radiation and the excellent depiction of the soft tissues. Utilizing these cross-sectional imaging techniques it is also important to check the alignment between C1 and the occiput to exclude an associated atlanto-occipital rotatory fixation. CT may be diagnostic for types II–IV AARF. However, static CT will not allow differentiation between benign torticollis and type I rotatory fixation and in order to do this, a dynamic study is required. To carry out this dynamic study, an axial CT is initially performed in the neutral position, followed by repeat scans with maximal voluntary ipsilateral and then contra-lateral rotation of the head. In patients with rotatory fixation little or no motion of the atlas on the axis with this maneuver occurs (Fig. 8.**6**). In the CT of patients with transient torticollis a reduction or a reversal of the rotation will be demonstrated. The duration of symptoms and deformity dictate the recommended treatment.

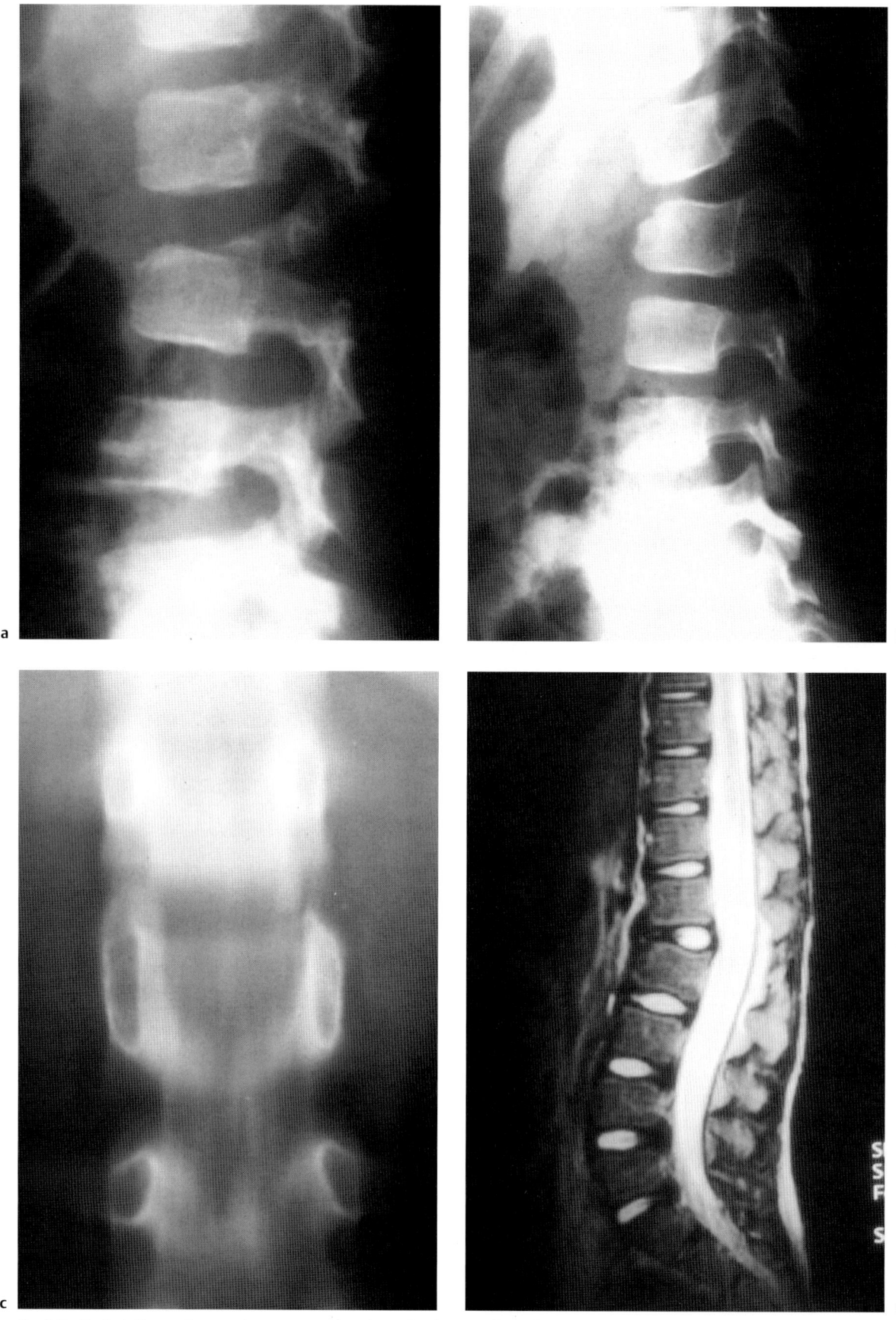

Fig. 8.8 Typical Chance fracture in a young girl at the L2 level seen on the lateral radiograph in the acute stage (**a**), with solid union of the pedicle fractures on lateral (**b**) and frontal tomographic follow-up (**c**). Note the residual instability at the L1/L2 disk level above with reduced disk height anteriorly and widened interfacetal and interspinous distance (**b, d**).

Thoracolumbar Spine Injury

Injury to the cervical spine is more commonly seen in the young child than thoracolumbar spinal injuries. As the child grows, however, the spine assumes more of the characteristics of the adult and the distribution of injuries begins to resemble that seen in the adult with a greater preponderance of injuries in the thoracic and lumbar region. Injuries in the thoracolumbar region in children most frequently occur in association with road traffic accidents (RTAs), sporting injuries, and related to child abuse. Interestingly, while injuries in the cervical spine due to RTAs are not infrequently due to lack of child restraints, injuries due to RTAs in the thoracolumbar spine are frequently related to a lap-belt restraint resulting in a flexion-distraction injury, the so-called lap-belt or Chance fracture (Fig. 8.**7**, see page 123). In this type of injury the fulcrum of movement lies anterior in the vertebral column. There is tension failure of the posterior and middle columns with a variable degree of anterior compression. The distraction commences posteriorly through the supraspinous and interspinous ligaments or the spinous process and may involve a fracture of the laminae or facet joint disruption and extend into the postero-superior apophysis of the vertebra (Fig. 8.**8**). The degree of bony involvement is variable but there is always significant soft tissue disruption. The middle column injury is usually through the bone or the apophysis and not through the posterior disk, which is the more usual in the adult. These injuries are often associated with abdominal wall contusion (ecchymosis) and intraabdominal injuries to both solid and hollow viscera, the diagnosis of which is often delayed.[45–47]

The higher incidence of this type of injury in children as compared to adults is principally because of a higher center of gravity, small anteroposterior dimensions of the abdomen and seat-belt problems. The traditional lap-belt was designed for adults and meant to be worn over the anterosuperior iliac spines of the pelvis. If worn by a child, the lap-belt tends to ride high over the mid-abdomen. In sudden flexion, as might occur with sudden braking, the only anchor is the anterior abdominal wall. Also, a child's center of gravity is higher than that of an adult because of an increased head to body ratio.[48] This leads to an increased force of flexion across a fixed lap-belt and helps to explain the nature of the distraction injury and the associated abdominal wall and visceral injuries.[45,46]

The burst fracture is an axial compression fracture most frequently occurring at the thoracolumbar junction. Typical features of this include a variable degree of anterior wedge compression (usually at least 30%), a break in the posterior vertebral body line with retropulsion of a bone fragment into the spinal canal. This is associated with a fracture through the inferior endplate. There may also be a sagittal fracture of the posterior neural arch. The burst fracture is to be differentiated from a simple anterior wedge compression fracture—the major differentiating feature being the presence of a retropulsed fragment into the spinal canal in the burst type. This injury in its complete form is unstable due to involvement of at least two columns.

The commonest type of injury in the thoracic spine in the child is a vertebral compression fracture. These injuries are frequently associated with sporting activities such as cycling or skiing. The compression is usually 20% or less and multiple-level compression fractures are more common than single-level injury (Fig. 8.**9**). This is likely related to the extreme flexibility and ligamentous laxity seen in the growing skeleton. Although these fractures may heal completely with remodeling to normal alignment, there is a risk of progressive kyphotic deformity especially if the endplates have been disturbed at the time of injury. The superior endplate is involved twice as often as the inferior endplate in compression vertebral fractures (Fig. 8.**10**).

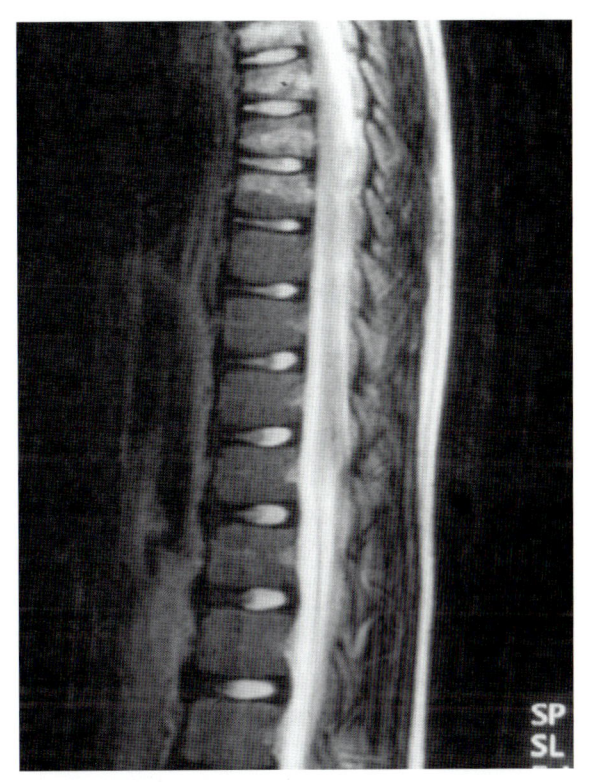

Fig. 8.**9** Multiple contiguous thoracic acute vertebral body compression fractures following a snow-boarding accident seen on a T2 sagittal MR image.

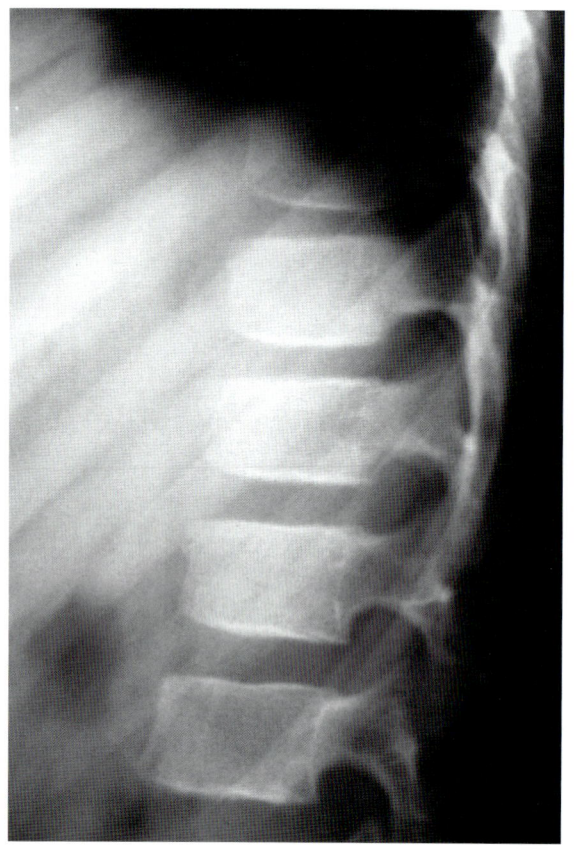

Fig. 8.10 Lateral radiographs of the thoracolumbar junction of a boy taken on the day (**a**) and 4 weeks (**b**) after a fall from a tree showing clear evidence of an acute intraosseous disk herniation at the L1 vertebral level with reduced T12/L1 disk height.

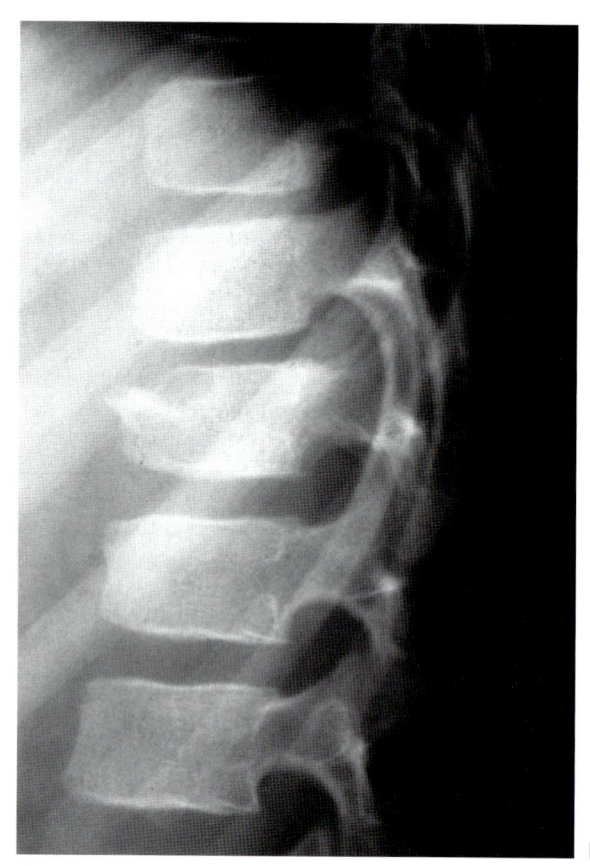

Physeal Injury

The physis is the weakest point in the axial skeleton when subjected to tensile forces. Partial or complete physeal separations can occur at the vertebral endplates, odontoid synchondrosis, apophysis etc (Fig. 8.**11**). By age 8 all the ossification centers have fused with the exception of the apical odontoid epiphysis, ring apophysis, and the secondary ossification centers of the neural arches that appear at puberty. At 7–8 years of age, small linear foci of ossification develop in the endplate cartilages. Abnormalities of the ossified displaced portion seen radiographically are the mainstay of diagnosis. Diagnosis of this injury before the appearance of ossification in the ring apophysis is difficult if not impossible.

Physeal injuries can occur anywhere in the spine but are very important in the sub-axial portion of the cervical spine where they usually involve the inferior growth plate and can be multiple. Although strictly speaking the Salter–Harris classification refers to epiphyseal/physeal interface injuries, one can apply the same classification to injuries in the growth zones of the vertebral body even though they are at the apophyseal/physeal junction. The vertebral endplate injury is often subtle and can separate from the body with perfect relocation following a complete Salter–Harris type I injury, which is more common in infants and young children and may be a factor in SCIWORA. Salter–Harris type III injuries occur in older children and adolescents as the physis begins to close. Due to the difficulties in identifying injuries to the cartilaginous components of the spine on radiographs, the true incidence of these injuries is not known, especially as the injured segments can recoil to virtually normal alignment.

Radiographically the clues include widening of the intervertebral disk space and identification of the displacement of the calcified components of the apophysis from their normal location in relation to the vertebral bodies. The type I injuries are more difficult to detect radiographically than type III injuries. In the cervical spine the type I Salter–Harris injuries usually involve the inferior endplate (Fig. 8.**12**). The absence of well-developed uncinate processes in children less than 8 years of age may predispose to this type of injury and in turn to SCIWORA. After this age the protective effect of the uncinate process makes this type of injury unlikely and only partial in nature (type III). In type I injuries, as the shearing forces pass through a purely cartilaginous plane there is minimal trauma to the adjacent vertebral body. Furthermore as these injuries are also associated with distracting forces, the vertebral bodies even on MR imaging may not show any evidence of injury (Fig. 8.**13**). Radiography is much better at depicting subtle displacement of the fractured apophysis than

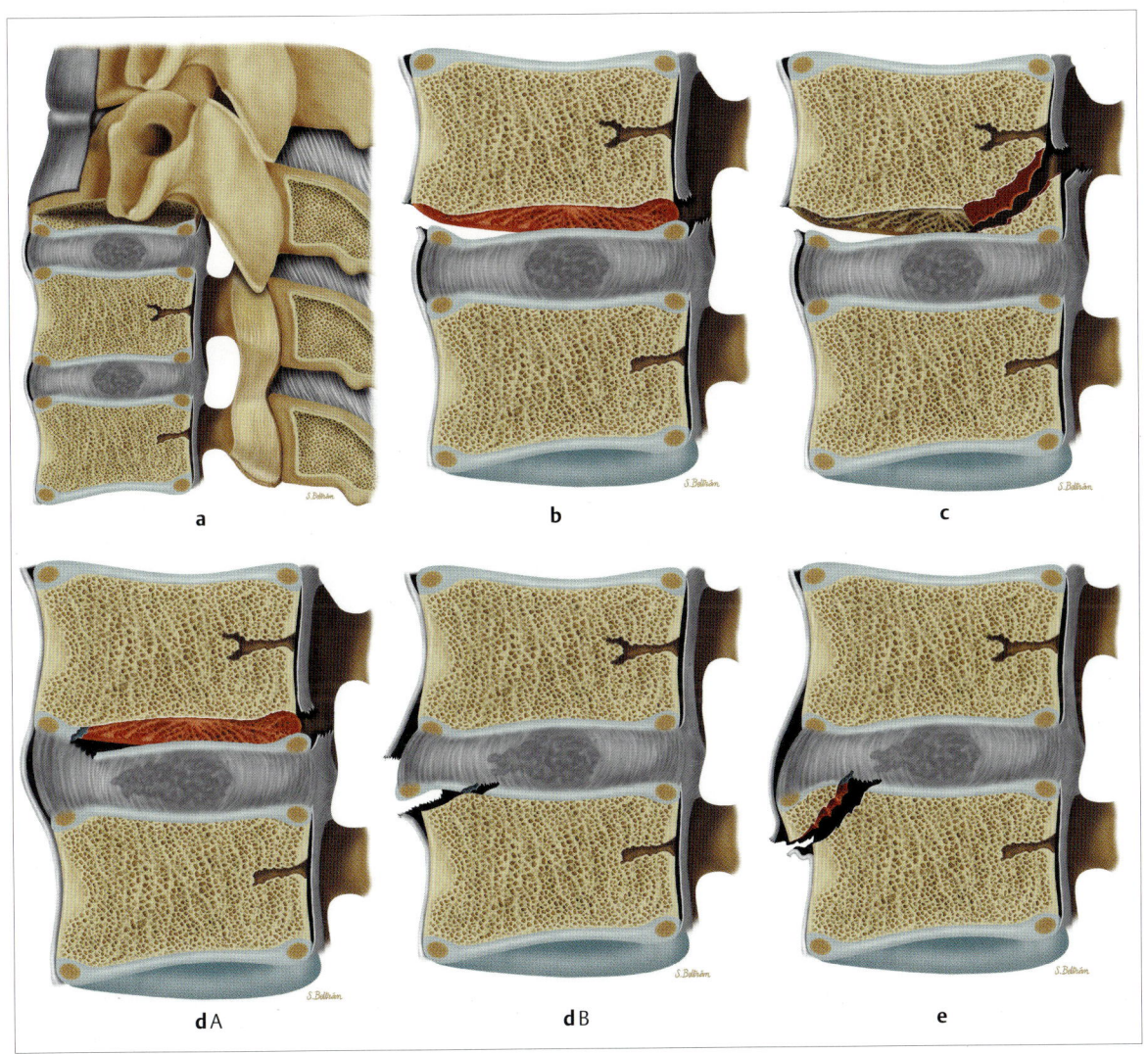

Fig. 8.11 Diagrammatic representation of vertebral growth plate injuries. **a** Normal appearance indicated by intact attachment of the intervertebral disk to the growing vertebral bodies. Note the morphological characteristics of the disk with the vertebral endplates and physis, the ossification centers at the corners of the vertebral bodies, and the intact overlying anterior (ALL) and posterior longitudinal (PLL) ligaments. **b** Type I: There is complete separation of the physeal interface with the inferior aspect of the vertebral body with tears of the ALL and PLL resulting in vertebral displacement. Note that the intervertebral disk is intact as is its annular attachment. **c** Type II: There is incomplete separation at the physeal interface with the inferior aspect of the vertebral body along with a fracture at the postero-inferior corner of the vertebra. Note the torn ALL and PLL, intact intervertebral disk status and its annular attachments. **d** Type III: (A, B) The injuries disrupt the physis and its continuity involving the disk causing intervertebral disk disruption. In type A the PLL is torn but the ALL and annular attachment are preserved anteriorly. In type B the ALL and anterior attachments are disrupted with intact PLL and posterior annular attachments. **e** Type IV: There is a fracture of the vertebral body that traverses the physis to involve the intervertebral disk.

MR imaging, particularly as the normal appearing ossification components of the ring apophysis are not well depicted by MR imaging (see Fig. 8.15). The type I injuries clearly indicate a highly unstable spine status even when they recoil to virtual anatomical alignment (Fig. 8.14). In the odontoid peg the injury's potential for healing without surgery after closed reduction is high but operative treatment is usually required in injuries of the sub-axial position of the spine. As the type III and type IV injuries indicate incomplete separation from the vertebra (Figs. 8.15, 8.17), they heal well by conservative treatment and immobilization (Fig. 8.16). Physeal injuries are also seen in the thoracolumbar spine and the type I Salter–Harris endplate separation is often a component of flexion-distraction seat-belt injuries.

In cervical ring apophyseal avulsion injuries avulsion of the ring apophysis anteriorly occurs at the superior apophysis in hyper-flexion injury, while extension trauma causes avulsion of the inferior ring apophysis.[49] Jonsson et al study commented on the chronic appearance of these injuries.[49] Follow-up of avulsion of the superior apophysis was associated with a bow-shaped superior border, whereas previous avulsion of the inferior ring apophysis demonstrated a large "osteophyte" projecting from the corner of the involved vertebral body (Fig. 8.16).

8 Trauma to the Pediatric Spine

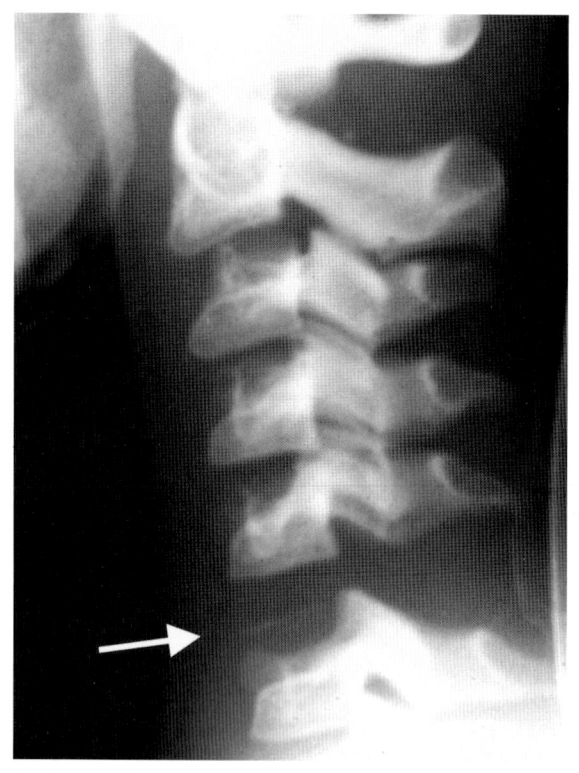

Fig. 8.12 Salter–Harris type I injury through the inferior physis of the C5 vertebra with distraction of the C5/C6 interfacetal and interspinous distance (**a**). Note the inferior apophysis of C5 has an intact relationship with the C5/C6 disk (*arrow*). The unstable nature of this injury is highlighted by the failed conservative treatment with a chronic dislocation on the follow-up radiograph (**b**).

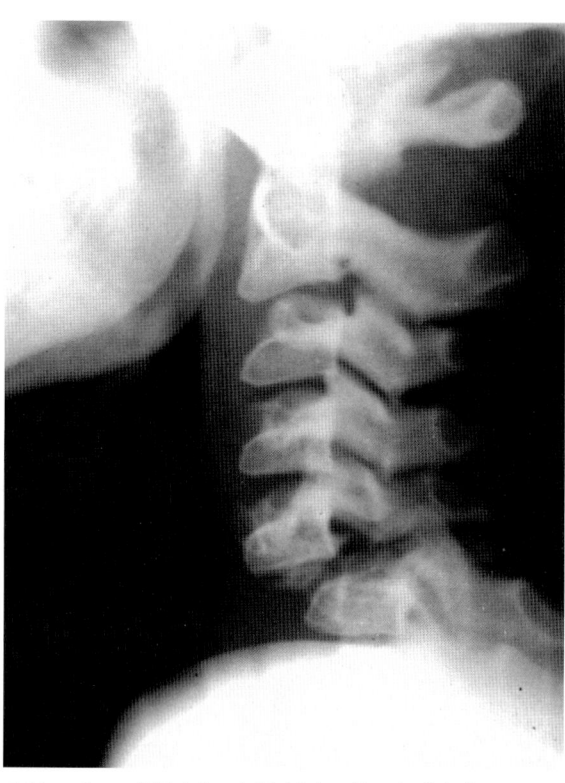

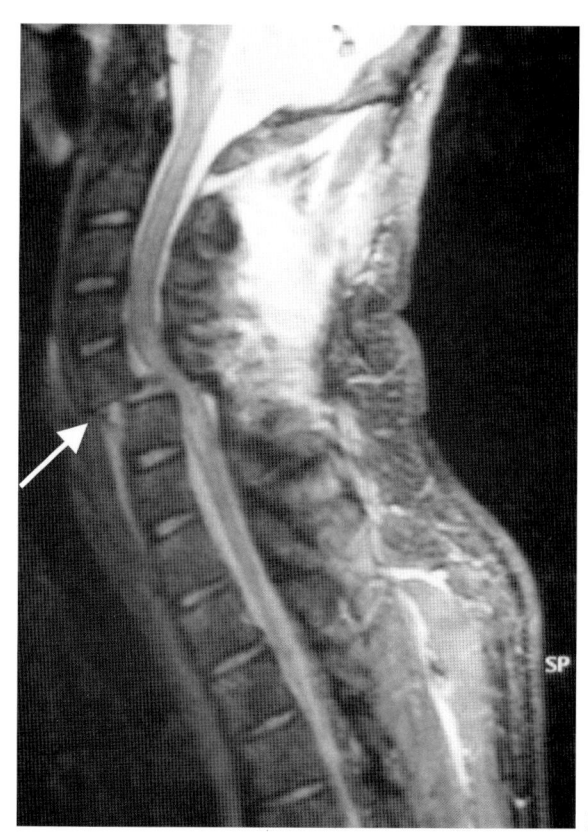

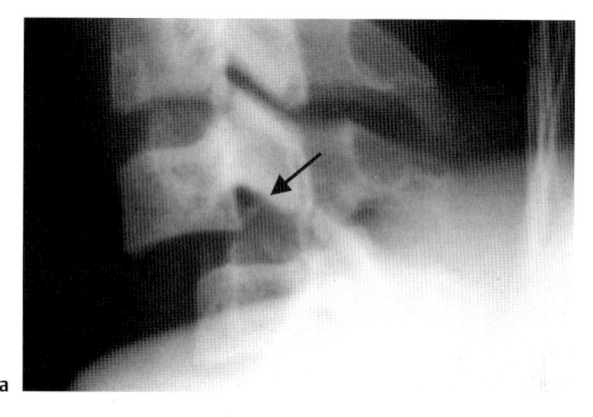

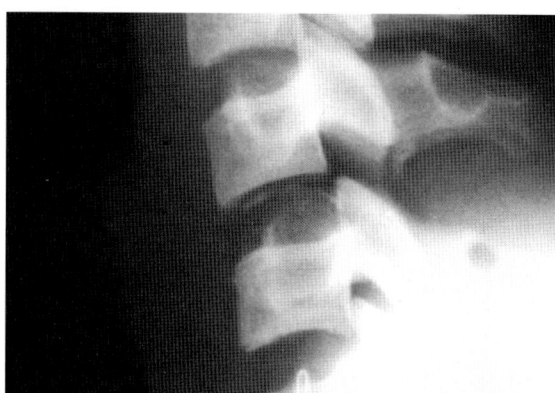

Fig. 8.13 Bilateral C5/C6 facet dislocation with a type I Salter–Harris injury through the inferior physis of C5, which along with the intact C5/C6 disk (*arrows*) prevented relocation of C5 on C6 (**a**, **b**) on skull traction. **c** Eventual relocation showing the separation of C5 from C6 through the inferior physis of C5.

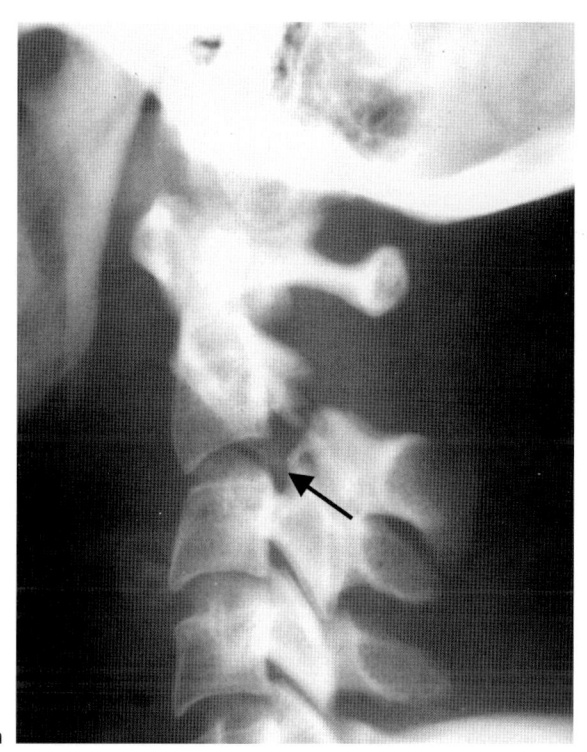

Fig. 8.14 Bilateral posterior neural arch fractures at C2 with markedly widened prevertebral soft tissue space and focal kyphotic deformity at C2/C3 level. Note the trans-physeal separation (Salter–Harris type I) through the inferior endplate of C2 (*arrow*) on the radiograph (**a**) and STIR sagittal image (**b**), along with the C1/C2 soft tissue injury and absence of any bone marrow edema in the C2 vertebra.

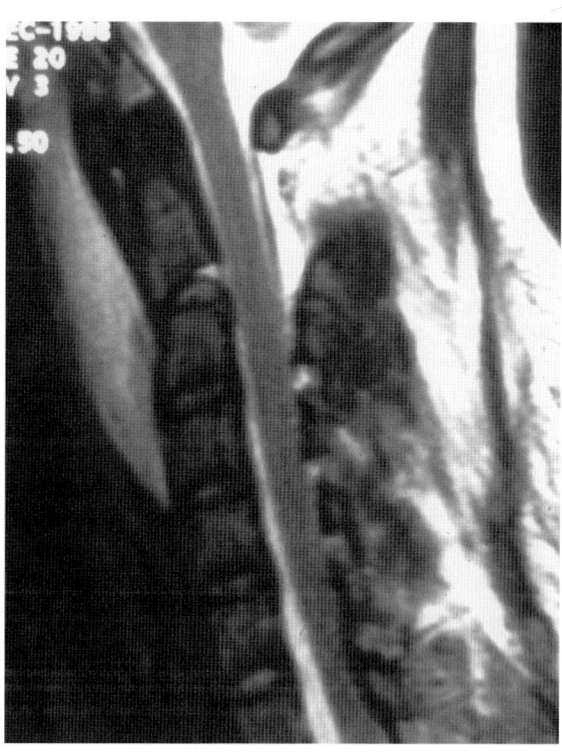

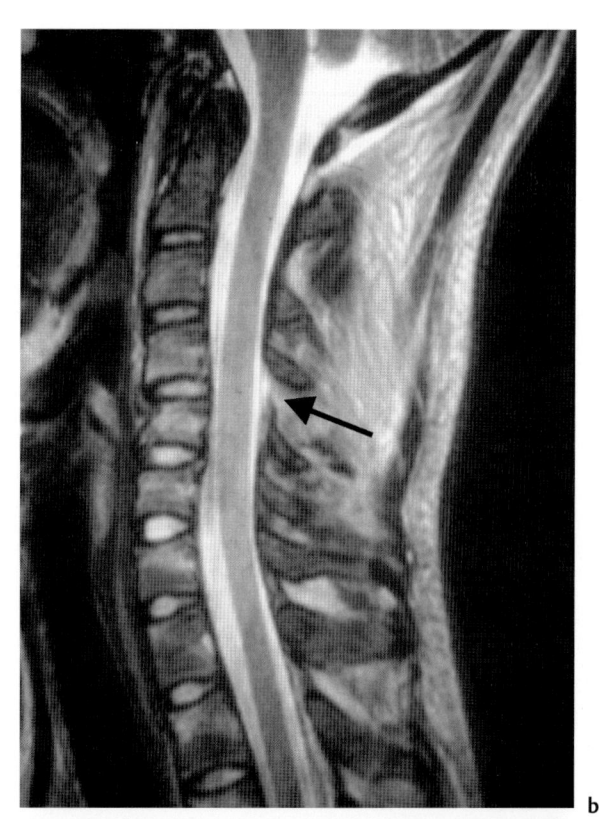

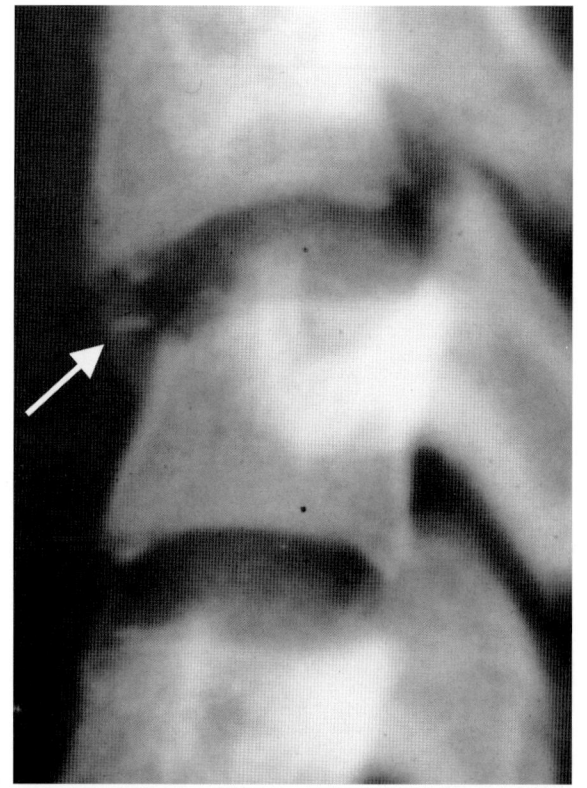

Fig. 8.15 C4/C5 cervical injury of the posterior ligamentous complex (*arrow*) associated with a Salter–Harris type III injury of the physis involving the anterosuperior corner of the C5 vertebra. Note the displacement of the fractured ring apophysis on the radiograph (**a**), the difficulty in appreciating this on the MR T2 sagittal image (**b**), and the multiple injuries in the cervical and upper thoracic vertebral bodies, including damage to the posterior ligaments (arrow).

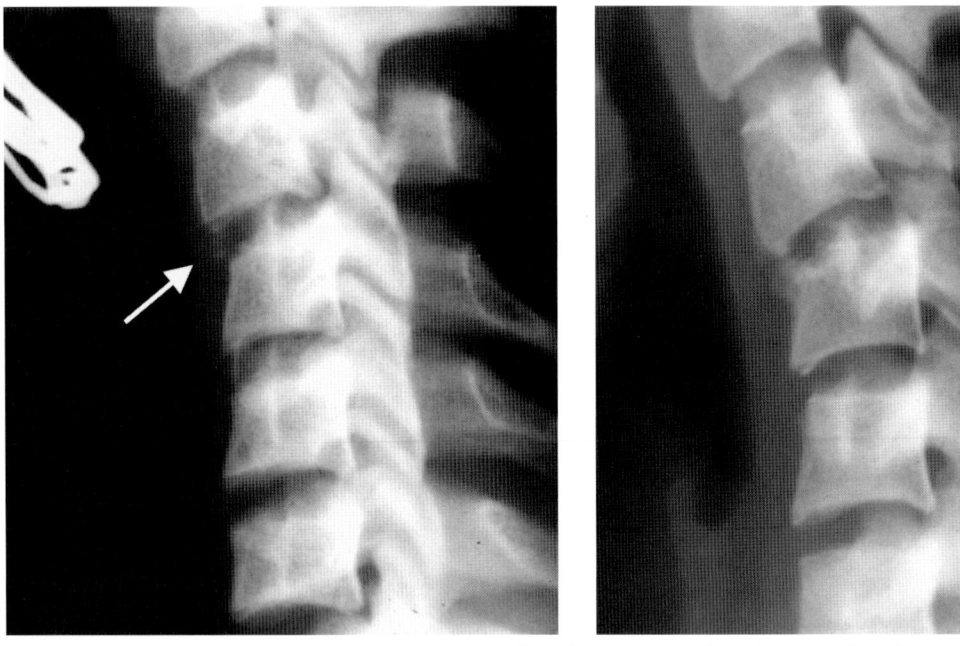

Fig. 8.16 C3/C4 injury (*arrow*) with type III Salter–Harris physeal injury anteriorly in the acute phase (**a**) and 8 weeks later showing posttraumatic new bone formation (**b**).

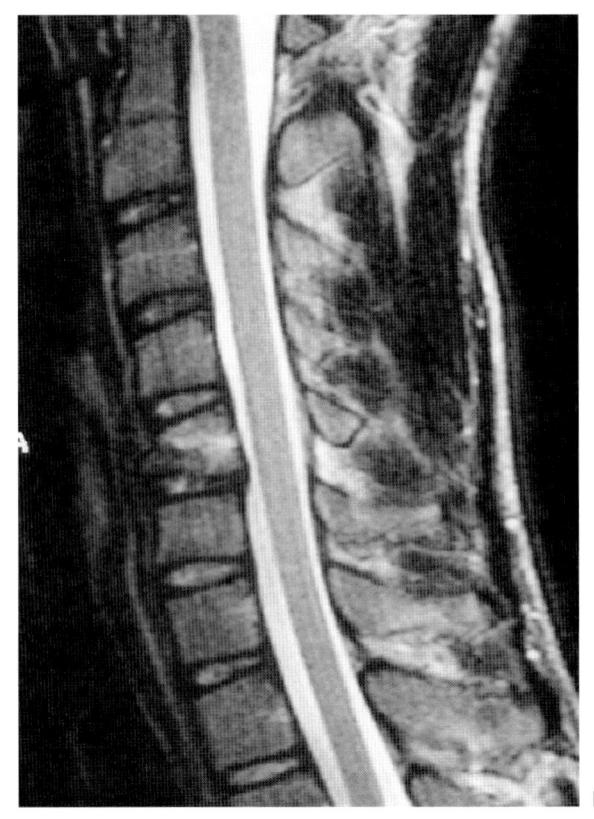

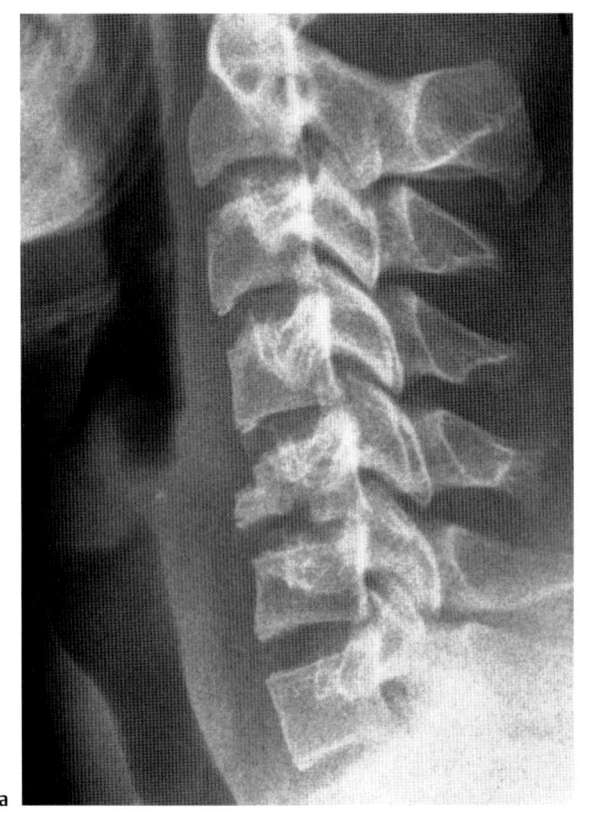

Fig. 8.17 Salter–Harris type IV fracture involving the antero-inferior portion of the C5 vertebral body with damage to the facet joint capsules and the interspinous ligament at the same level (**a**). Note the edema within the vertebral body of C5 and in the interspinous space at C5/C6 on the T2 sagittal MR sequence (**b**).

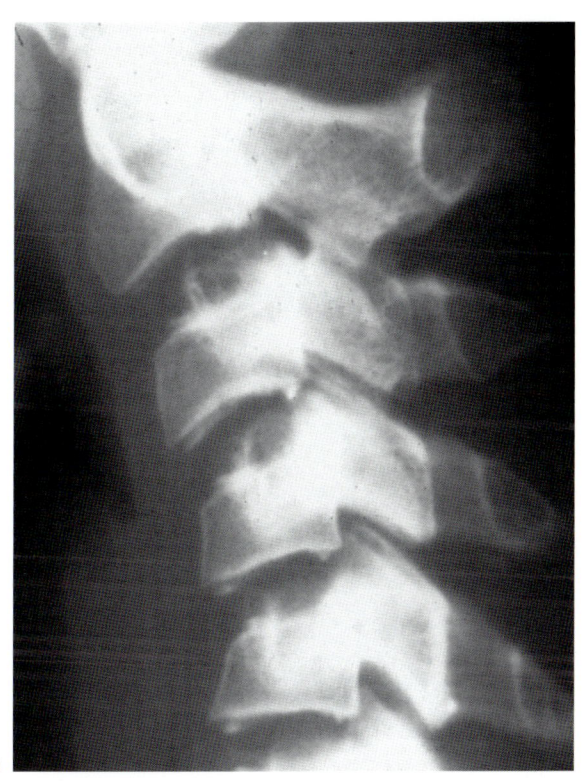

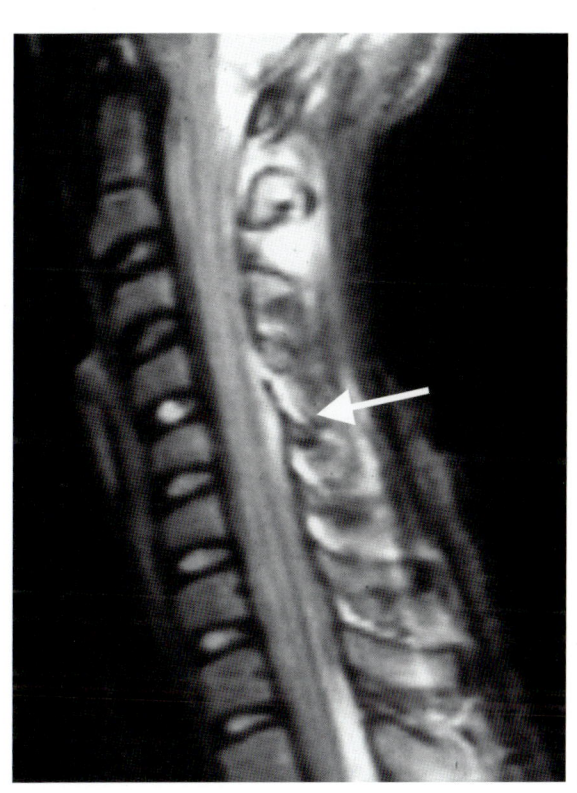

Fig. 8.18 Intact vertebral components, ring apophyses, and physes at all levels (**a**) despite the presence of posterior ligamentous complex disruption at the C4/C5 level (*arrow*) (**b**).

SCIWORA

SCIWORA (*spinal cord injury without radiographic abnormality*) is more commonly identified in children and young adults where ligamentous laxity and flexibility of the developing spine may be associated with tearing or contusion of the cord due to over-stretching before any obvious soft tissue or bone disturbance occurs in the vertebral column. Although more common in children under 10 years of age, it is also well described in adults. SCIWORA occurs in 15–25% of all pediatric cervical spine injuries.[50,51] C2 is the most common level and the most common age is less than 3 years.[52] The term SCIWORA was introduced in the days before MRI was available. In the absence of radiographic and CT abnormality, MRI can clearly detect soft tissue disruption (Fig. 8.18). However, cord signal abnormality can occur in the absence of other evidence of soft tissue injury and perhaps in this instance the term should more correctly be spinal cord injury without imaging abnormality (Fig. 8.19).

Leventhal, in 1960, showed that the spinal column can elongate up to approx. 5 cm without disruption, while the relatively inelastic spinal cord ruptures with just 0.6 cm elongation (Fig. 8.20).[53] Kokoska et al's series showed SCIWORA to be associated with partial cord injury in approximately 80% of cases.[50] Brown et al in their series, however, demonstrated that in adolescents with neck trauma and no evidence of radiographic abnormality but evidence of spinal cord injury, 75% of sporting injuries had this diagnosis.[21] In their series all patients suffering from child abuse had SCIWORA. According to Pang and Pollack in 1989 the sole predictor of outcome in SCIWORA is neurological status at presentation.[54] Patients with incomplete neurological injury tend to have a good outcome. The prognosis for complete neurological injury, however, is similar to that with radiographically evident spinal injury elsewhere.[54-57] Analysis of findings on MRI reveal five classes of post SCIWORA cord findings—complete transection, major hamorrhage, minor hamorrhage, edema only, and normal—which are highly predictive of prognosis and outcome.[58] The possibility of exacerbating a neurological injury in the presence of initial plain radiographs which are normal, needs to be considered. The critical importance of a careful clinical history and examination cannot be over-emphasized. In the younger child in particular help from parents needs to be sought to exclude any subtle sensory neurological symptoms such as pins and needles, tingling, or shock-like sensations after the initial traumatic event. If there is such a history then a MRI scan and careful flexion–extension radiographs seeking evidence of instability need to be carried out. Pang et al noted that over 50% of children with SCIWORA had delayed onset of paralysis up to 4 days after injury.[54] Injury prevention, prompt recognition, use of MRI and electrophysiological verification, and timely bracing of SCIWORA patients remain the chief measures to improve outcome.[58] The prognosis can be improved if the syndrome is diagnosed early.[59]

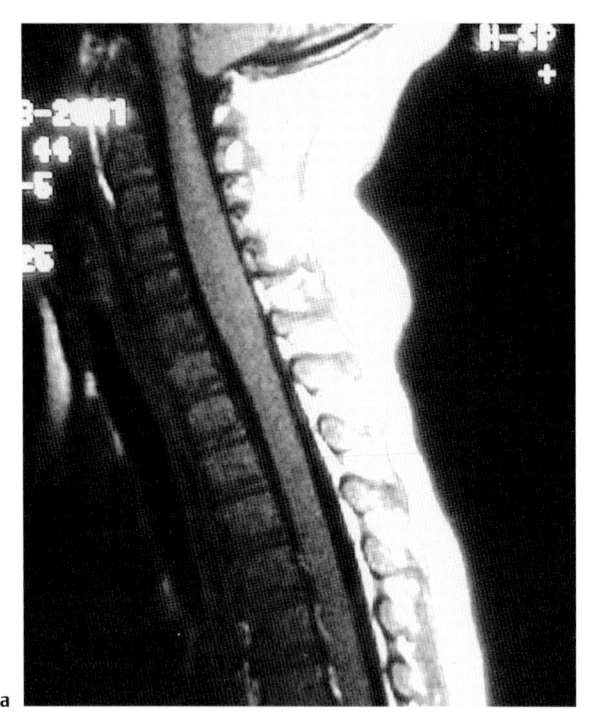

Fig. 8.**19** Acute SCIWORA shown on T1 (**a**) and T2 (**b**) sagittal MR images in a 2-year-old girl with marked edema and hemorrhage within the cervical cord but no evidence of injury to the vertebral column.

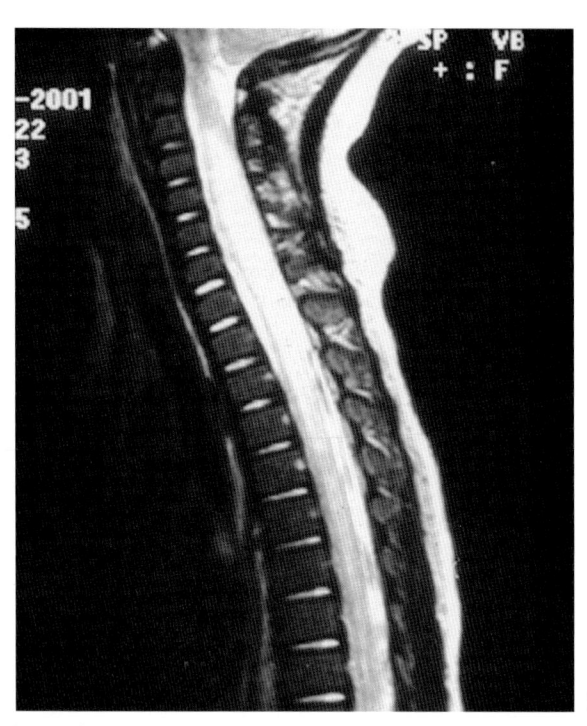

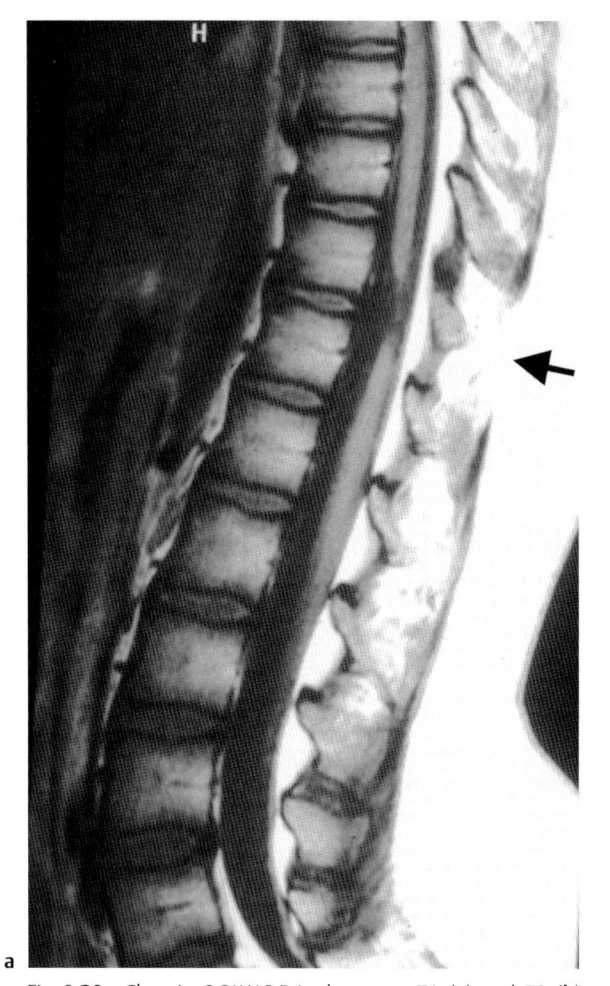

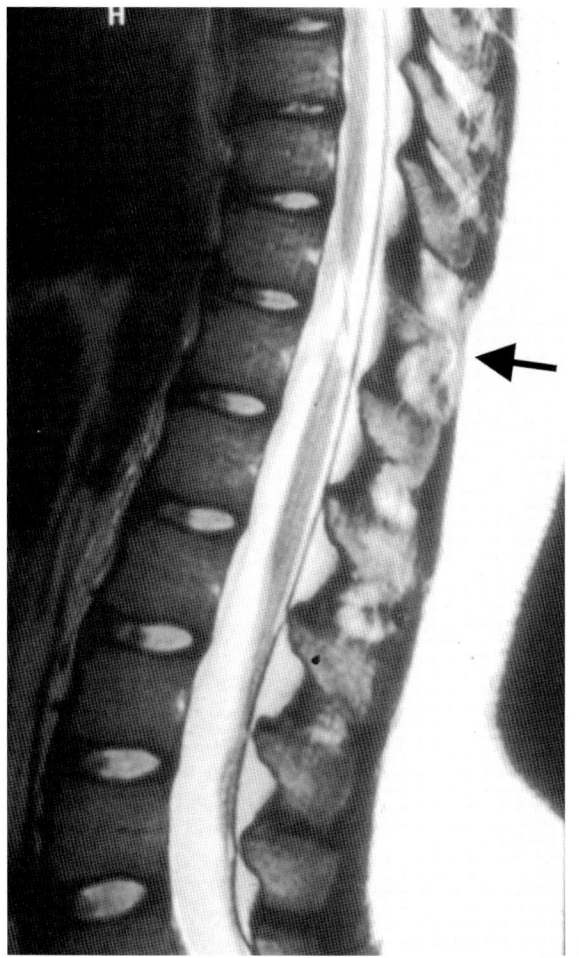

Fig. 8.**20** Chronic SCIWORA shown on T1 (**a**) and T2 (**b**) sagittal MR images in an 18-year-old girl, 8 years after injury to the thoracic cord at the T11/T12 level. Note the atrophy of the cord and deficiency of the posterior ligaments at this level (*arrows*).

Slipped Vertebral Apophysis

The term slipped vertebral apophysis is used to denote partial separation with displacement of a portion of the apophysis. This can occur anywhere along the outline of the ring apophysis but is more commonly seen on a lateral radiograph anteriorly or posteriorly, producing a limbus vertebra. Fractures of the posterior vertebral limbus typically occur in adolescents before the vertebral rim apophysis has fused with the parent bone and are usually associated with disk herniation and its symptoms, but can also become symptomatic in adulthood after fusion. Some authors have suggested that such a fracture in the skeletally mature may imply that the vertebral endplate is defective. These vertebral limbus fractures are typically located in the superior or inferior endplate of the vertebral body, where they involve differing degrees of fragmentation of the peripheral ring apophysis. These fractures can be diagnosed on plain radiographs but a greater incidence is detected on MRI, and is most frequently seen with CT or CT myelography. Takata et al classified these fractures into three types:

- Type I: a simple separation of the entire margin of the limbus.
- Type II: an avulsion fracture of some of the substance of the vertebral body including the margin.
- Type III: a more localized fracture.[60]

Epstein and Epstein introduced a type IV fracture, which spanned the entire length and breadth of the posterior vertebral body (see Chapter 9.2).[61]

Spondylolysis

The spondylolytic defect is never present at birth, but develops during the early growing period (often before the age of 6 years). It is a chronic stress related injury rather than an acute insult. This subject is dealt with in further detail in Chapter 9.1.

Prognosis

Following trauma, the orderly sequential evolution of the mesenchymal, cartilaginous, and osseous stages of vertebral development are disrupted leading to distortion of the structural morphology of one or more of the vertebrae. The posterior elements reach maturity in terms of the potential for longitudinal growth by the end of the first decade, compared with the vertebral bodies, which continue to grow normally until the age of 18 years. The pediatric spine will still have a variable period of growth to complete following the injury and its treatment, dependent on the age at injury.[62] The spine is also adaptable and malleable above and below the injured segments.

Physeal injuries usually heal rapidly (Fig. 8.**4**, 8.**16**) and the objective therapeutically is to assure alignment during the healing period. The wedge compression fractures of the pediatric vertebral bodies in the sagittal plane usually reconstitute the vertebral height especially in children less than 10 years old. The physis can continue to grow even after damage allowing restoration of height if they are not damaged. If the endplates are fractured there is usually no correction. In the absence of spinal cord injury progression of the traumatic spinal deformity is rare. Children's vertebral bodies when injured tend to remodel, subsequent deformity is rare and not progressive. In the review by Horal et al, 53% were normal at follow-up with a high incidence of solid interbody fusion and no significant disability.[63] However, the residual kyphosis especially following cervical vertebral fractures is less well tolerated in the child. In these instances posterior growth continues making the potential for increasing kyphotic deformity a problem. This is particularly the case if the anterior growth potential of one or more vertebrae is destroyed by the anterior fusion as the method of operative fixation in the young child.

In spinal cord injury it is the paraplegia and not the spinal column injury that influences the risk of deformity. Children with spinal cord injury commonly develop spinal deformity at or below the level of injury. The patient's age at the time of injury is the single most important factor in the development of scoliosis.[64] If the injury takes place before the adolescent growth spurt the deformity is severe and invariable. The deformity of the spine is also likely to progress more rapidly with high cord lesions and the degree of spasticity. In this situation there is also a risk of associated pelvic obliquity which increases the risk of ischial pressure sores on the weight-bearing points (Fig. 8.**21**). Correction is needed if the scoliotic curve is more than 40°. If, however, the curve progresses rapidly, an MRI of the spine is required before any corrective surgery to exclude posttraumatic syringomyelia as an associated etiological factor to the scoliotic deformity.

Chronic instability is also a potential problem at the site of vertebral column injury in the child, especially if a laminectomy is done for decompression at the thoracolumbar junction. The unstable spinal segment can also have a slowly deleterious effect on the spinal cord and its function due to chronic trauma resulting in further loss of neurological function. This particular complication is best seen at the C1/C2 level in instances of os odontoideum (Fig. 8.**22**). The potential for neurological recovery following severe incomplete spinal cord injury in children and adolescents is good.[65,66]

References

1. Avellino AM, Mann FA, Grady MS, Chapman JR, Ellenbogen RG, Alden TD, Mirza SK. The misdiagnosis of acute cervical spine injuries and fractures in infants and children: the 12-year experience of a level I pediatric and adult trauma center. *Childs Nerv Syst.* 2005;21(2):122–127. Epub 2004 Dec 18.
2. Aufdermaur M. Spinal injuries in juveniles. Necropsy findings in 12 cases. *J Bone Jt Surg.* 1974;56B:513–519.
3. Reichmann S, Lewin T. Coronal cleft vertebrae in growing individuals. *Acta Orthop Scand.* 1969;40:3–22.

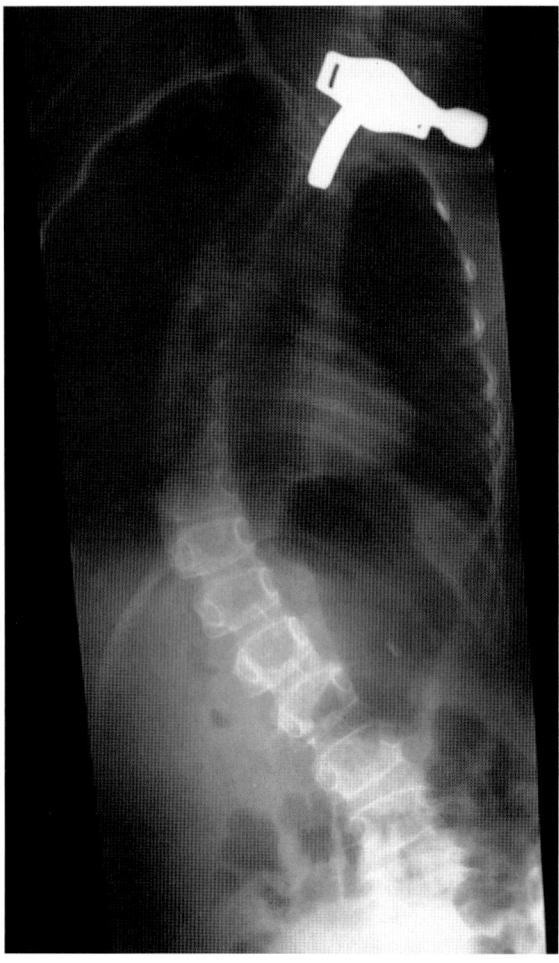

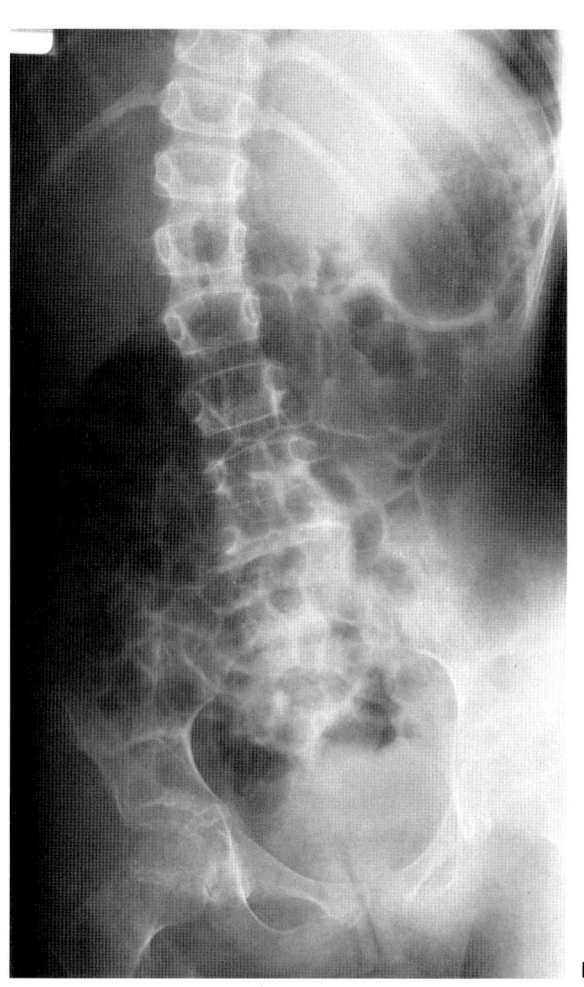

Fig. 8.21 Spinal deformity with a paralytic scoliosis (a) in a boy who had sustained a high quadriparesis aged 2 due to C1/C2 traumatic dislocation, associated with pelvic obliquity (b).

4. Tanaka T, Uhthoff HK. Coronal cleft of vertebrae, a variant of normal endochondral ossification. *Acta Orthop Scand.* 1983; 54:389–395.
5. Bick EM, Copel JW. The ring apophysis of the human vertebra. *J Bone Jt Surg.* 1951;33A:783–787.
6. Bailey DK. The normal cervical spine in infants and children. *Radiology.* 1952;59:712–719.
7. Cattel HS, Filtzer DL. Pseudosubluxation and other normal variations in the cervical spine in children. *J Bone Jt Surg.* 1965; 47A:1295–1309.
8. Sullivan CR, Bruwer AJ, Harris LE. Hypermobility of the cervical spine in children: A pitfall in the diagnosis of cervical dislocation. *Am J Surg.* 1958;95:636–640.
9. Schwischuk LE. Anterior displacement of C2 in children: physiologic or pathologic? A helpful differentiating line. *Radiology.* 1977;122:759–763.
10. Matsumoto M, Toyama Y, Chiba K, Fujimura Y, Fukui Y, Kobayashi K. Traumatic subluxation of the axis after hyperflexion injury of the cervical spine in children. *J Spinal Disord.* 2001; 14(2):172–179.
11. Wakeley CJ, Cassar-Pullicino VN, McCall IW. Case of the month: Not so pseudo. *Br J Radiol.* 1991;64:375–376.
12. Pennecot GF, Leonard P, Peyrot Des Gachons S, Hardy JR, Pouliqen JC. Traumatic ligamentous instability of the cervical spine in children. *J Pediatr Orthop.* 1984;4(3):339–345.
13. Swischuk LE, Swischuk PA, John SD. Wedging of C3 in infants and children: usually a normal finding and not a fracture. *Radiology.* 1993;188:523–526.
14. Farndon DF, Fielding JW. Defects of the pedicle and spondylolisthesis of the second cervical vertebra. *J Bone Jt Surg.* 1981; 63B:526–528.
15. Redla S, Sikdar T, Saifuddin A, Taylor BA. Imaging features of cervical spondylolysis—with emphasis on MR appearances. *Clin Radiol.* 1999;54:815–820.
16. Schwartz JM. Case 36: Bilateral cervical spondylolysis of C6. *Radiology.* 2001;220:191–194.
17. Juhl JH, Miller SM, Roberts GW. Roentgenographic variations in the normal cervical spine. *Radiology.* 1962;78:591–597.
18. Fineman SOL, Borrelli FJ, Rubinstein BM, Epstein H, Jacobson HG. The cervical spine: transformation of the normal lordotic pattern into a linear pattern in the neutral posture. A roentgenographic demonstration. *J Bone Jt Surg.* 1963;45A:1179–1183.
19. Lustrin ES, Karakas SP, Ortiz AO et al. Pediatric cervical spine: normal anatomy, variants and trauma. *RadioGraphics.* 2003; 23:539–560.
20. Franken EA. Spinal cord injury in the newborn infant. *Pediatr Radiol.* 1975;3:101–104.
21. Brown R, Brunn MA, Garcia VF. Cervical spine injuries in children: A review of 103 patients treated consecutively at a Level I pediatric trauma centre. *J Pediatr Surg.* 2001;36(8): 1107–1114.
22. Kleinman PK, Marks SC. Vertebral body fractures in child abuse. Radiologic-histopathologic correlates. *Invest Radiol.* 1992;27:715–722.
23. Bulas DI, Fitz CR, Johnson DL. Traumatic atlanto-occipital dislocation in children. *Radiology* 1993;188:155–158.

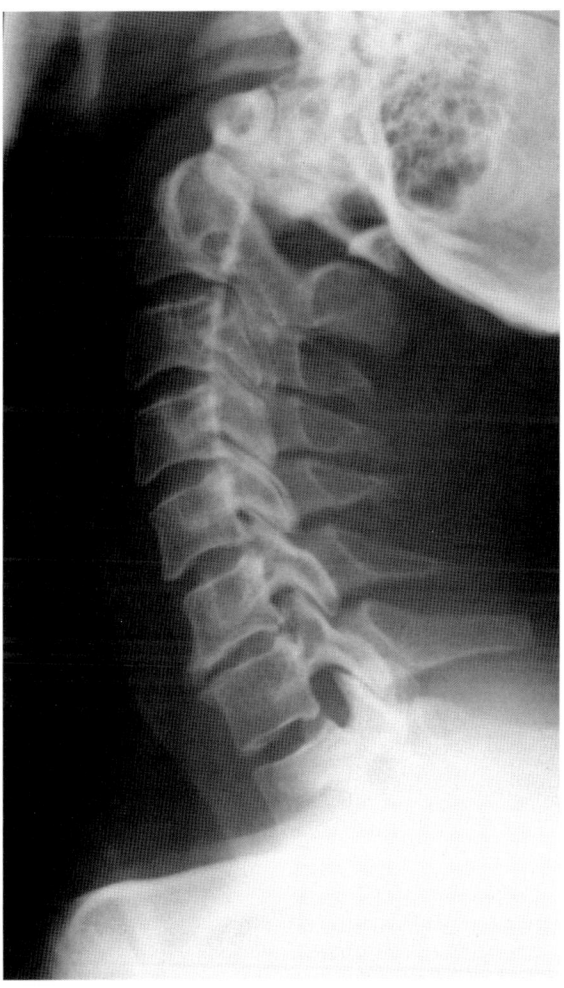

Fig. 8.22 Chronic C1/C2 instability related to os odontoideum with posterior subluxation on the radiograph in extension (**a**), associated with marked atrophy of the upper cervical cord (**b**) on the T1 MR image.

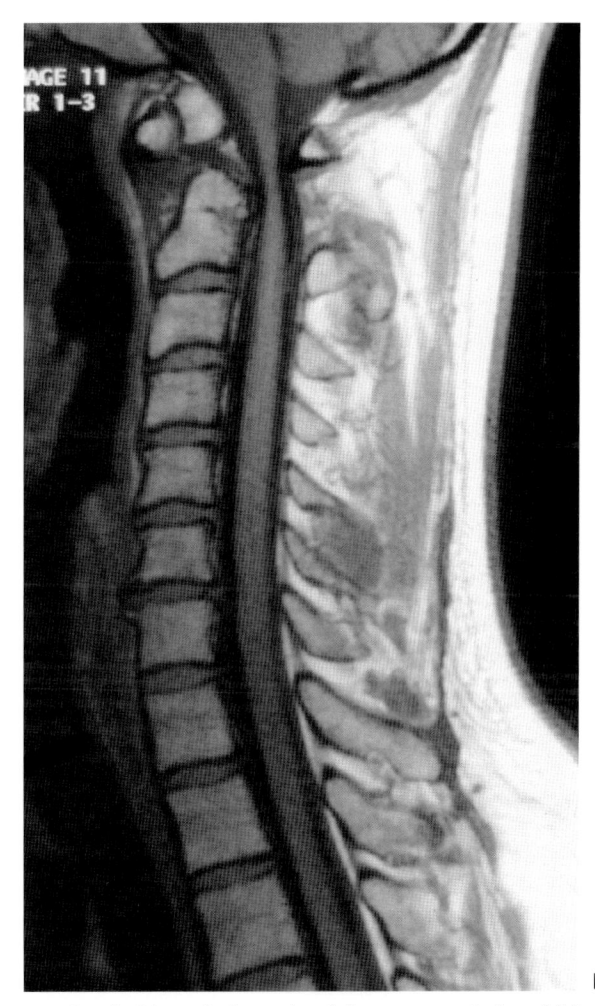

24. Galindo MJ, Francis WR. Atlantal fracture in a child through anterior and posterior congenital arch defects: A case report. *Clin Orthop Relat Res.* 1983;178:220–222.
25. Thakar C, Harish S, Saifuddin A, Allibone J. Displaced fracture through the anterior atlantal synchondrosis. *Skeletal Radiol.* 2005;34:547–549.
26. Gehweiler Jr JA, Daffner RH, Roberts Jr L. Malformations of the atlas vertebra simulating the Jefferson fracture. *AJR.* 1983; 140(6):1083–1086.
27. Saifuddin A, Renwick IGH. Case of the Month: A pain in the neck. *Br J Radiol.* 1993;66:379–380.
28. Sherk HH, Schut L, Lane JM. Fractures and dislocations of the cervical spine in children. *Orthop Clin North Am.* 1976;7(3): 593–604.
29. Williams III JP, Baker DH, Miller WA. CT appearance of congenital defect resembling the Hangman's fracture. *Pediatr. Radiol.* 1999;29:549–550.
30. Mondschein J, Karasick D. Spondylolysis of the axis vertebra: A rare anomaly simulating hangman's fracture. *AJR Am J Roentgenol.* 1999; 172:556–557.
31. Parisi M, Lieberson R, Shatsky S. Hangman's fracture or primary spondylolysis: a patient and a brief review. *Pediatr Radiol.* 1991;21:367–368.
32. Hasue M, Kikuchi S, Matsui T, Machida H, Kirokawa T, Kataoka O. Spondylolysis of the axis. Report of four cases. *Spine.* 1983; 8:901–906.
33. Vining D, Benzel EC, Orrison W. Childhood odontoid fractures evaluated with computerised tomography. A Case Report. *J Neurosurg.* 1992;77:795–798.
34. Vigouroux RP, Baurand C, Choux M et al. Les traumatismes du rachiscervical chez l'enfant. *Neurochirurgie.* 1968;14:689–702.
35. Sherk HH, Nicholson JT, Chung SMK. Fractures of the odontoid process in young children. *J Bone Joint Surg (Am).* 1978;60: 921–924.
36. Fielding JW, Hensinger RN, Hawkins RJ. Os odontoideum. *J Bone Jt Surg.* 1980;62A:376–383.
37. Choit RL, Jamieson DH, Reilly CW. Os odontoideum: a significant radiographic finding. *Pediatr Radiol.* 2005;35(8): 803–807. Epub 2005 Apr 28.
38. Roche CJ, King SJ, Dangerfield PH, Carty HM. The atlanto-axial joint: physiological range of rotation on MRI and CT. *Clin Radiol.* 2002;57:103–108.
39. White AA, Panjabi MM. Kinematics of the spine. In: White AA, Panjabi MM, eds. *Clinical Biomechanics of the Spine.* Philadelphia, PA: JB Lippincott; 1978:87–125.
40. Pang D, Li V. Atlantoaxial rotatory fixation: Part 1–Biomechanics of normal rotation at the atlantoaxial joint in children. *Neurosurgery.* 2004;55(3):614–25; discussion 625–6.
41. Mazarra JT, Fielding JW. Effect of C1–C2 rotation on canal size. *Clin Orthop Rel Res.* 1988;237:115–119.
42. Fielding JW, Hawkins RJ. Atlanto-axial rotatory fixation (fixed rotatory subluxation of the atlanto-axial joint). *J Bone Jt Surg.* 1977; 59A:37–44.
43. Mathern G, Batzdorf U. Grisel's Syndrome. *Clin Orthop Rel Res.* 1989;244:131–146.
44. Roche CJ, O'Malley M, Dorgan JC, Carty HM. A pictorial review of atlanto-axial rotatory fixation: key points for the radiologist. *Clin Radiol.* 2001;56:947–958.

45. Rumball K, Jarvis J. Seat belt injuries of the spine in young children. *J Bone Jt Surg.* 1992;74B:571–574.
46. Sivit CJ, Taylor GA, Newman KD, Bulas DI, Gotschall CS, Wright CJ, Eichelberger MR. Safety-belt injuries in children with lap-belt ecchymosis: CT findings in 61 pateints. *AJR Am J Roentgenol.* 1991;157: 111–114.
47. Santschi M, Echave V, Laflamme S, McFadden N, Cyr C. Seat-belt injuries in children involved in motor vehicle crashes. *Can J Surg.* 2005;48(5):373–376.
48. Agran PF, Dunkle DE, Winn DG. Injuries to a sample of seat-belted children evaluated and treated in a hospital emergency room. *J Trauma.* 1987;27:58–64.
49. Jonsson K, Niklasson J, Josefsson PO. Avulsion of the cervical spinal ring apophysis: acute and chronic appearance. *Skeletal Radiol.* 1991;20:207–210.
50. Kokoska ER, Keller MS, Rallo MC, Weber TR. Characteristics of paediatric cervical spine injuries. *J Pediatr Surg.* 2001;36(1): 100–105.
51. Birney TJ, Hanley EN. Traumatic cervical spine injuries in childhood and adolescence. *Spine.* 1989;14(12):1277–1282.
52. Osenbach RK, Menezes AH. SCIWORA in children. *Paediatr Neurosci.* 1989;15:168–175.
53. Leventhal HR. Birth injuries of the spinal cord. *J Paediatr.* 1960;56:447–453.
54. Pang D, Pollack IF. Spinal cord injury without radiographic abnormality in children—the SCIWORA syndrome. *J Trauma.* 1989;29:654–664.
55. Pang D, Wilberger J. Spinal cord injury without radiographic abnormalities in children. *J Neurosurg.* 1982;57:114–129.
56. Dickman CA, Zabramski JM, Hadley MN, et al. Paediatric spinal cord injury without radiographic abnormalities. Report of 26 cases and review of the literature. *J Spinal Disord.* 1991;4: 296–305.
57. Kriss VM, Kriss TC. SCIWORA (spinal cord injury without radiographic abnormality) in infants and children. *Clin Pediatr.* 1996;35:119–124.
58. Pang D. Spinal cord injury without radiographic abnormality in children, 2 decades later. *Neurosurgery.* 2004;55(6): 1325–1342; discussion.
59. Launay F, Leet AI, Sponseller PD. Pediatric spinal cord injury without radiographic abnormality: a meta-analysis. *Clin Orthop Relat Res.* 2005;433:166–170.
60. Takata K, Inque S, Takahashi K, Ohtsuka Y. Fracture of the posterior margin of a lumbar veretebral body. *J Bone Jt Surg.* 1988;70A (4):589–594.
61. Epstein NE, Epstein JA. Limbus lumbar vertebral fractures in 27 adolescents and adults. *Spine.* 1991;16(8):962–966.
62. Vogel LC, Hickey KJ, Klaas SJ, Anderson CJ. Unique issues in pediatric spinal cord injury. *Orthop Nurs.* 2004;23(5): 300–8; quiz 309–310.
63. Horal J, Nachemson A, Scheller S. Clinical and radiological long term follow up of vertebral fractures in children. *Acta Orthop Scand.* 1972;43:491–503.
64. Lancourt JE, Dickson JH, Carter RE. Paralytic spinal deformity following traumatic spinal cord injury in children and adolescents. *J Bone Jt Surg.* 1981;63A:47–53.
65. Wang MY, Hoh DH, Leary SP, Griffith P, McComb JG. High rates of neurological improvement following severe traumatic pediatric spinal cord injury. *Spine.* 2004;29(13):1493–7; discussion E266.
66. Carreon LY, Glassman SD, Campbell MJ. Pediatric spine fractures: a review of 137 hospital admissions. *J Spinal Disord Tech.* 2004;17(6): 477–482.

9.1 Sports Injuries: Spondylolysis

F. Kainberger

Introduction

Spondylolysis is an interruption of the pars interarticularis of the vertebral pedicles due to abnormal stress. This is usually a chronic recurrent form of stress, and acute episodes of trauma causing pars fractures are rare. Clinically, it manifests mainly during the second decade of life and it is in most cases located in the fifth lumbar segment. Spondylolysis is most commonly observed in males and has a male to female occurrence ratio of 2–3:1, as well as a higher probability of occurrence with inherited traits.[1,2]

Although some patients are asymptomatic, spondylolysis seems to be the most significant cause of lower back pain in athletes and in this group it is observed to occur more frequently than in the general population.[3,4] Certain movement patterns associated with various types of sports (Table 9.1.**1**) may be causal in the development of spondylolysis in athletes as well as in other physically active individuals.[5] Most notably younger, skeletally immature, athletes are at higher risk of spondylolysis during times of rapid skeletal growth.[6] There is also a racial preponderance with a prevalence of 5–7% in Europeans, 9% in Bantus, 7–10% in Japanese, and up to 50% in Eskimos.[7]

The development of spondylolysis is thought to derive from differential stress applied to the pars interarticularis of the vertebral arch. Therefore, spondylolysis is classified as a stress fracture of the vertebral arch and the numerous theories concerning its etiology may in principle relate to this concept.[8,9] Brocher hypothesized in 1950 that spondylolysis develops from a congenital cleft.[10] Such a defect, however, does not occur in this part of the vertebral arch, in which the perichondral ossification centers are located.[11] So far spondylolysis has not been observed in neonates.[7] Spondylolysis seems to develop in childhood around 6 years of age without clinical symptoms.[1,8] Niethard et al attributed the frontal orientation of the facet joints of the lower spine to a reduction of stability in this area and an increase in mobility, thus resulting in increased mechanical stress.[12] In the early Medieval period, the prevalence of spondylolysis in an area of south-western Germany has been shown to have been the same as its prevalence in the same area today.[13]

Low stress-resistance is mainly due to an elongation and thinning of the pars and is exaggerated by a prominent lordosis of the lumbar spine. Such lordosis especially develops between 6 and 8 years of age and is associated with a physiological flexion of the hip joints. Radiological evidence of a lumbosacral transitional vertebra (Fig. 9.1.**1**), a congenital cleft of the posterior arch of the S1 segment (spina bifida occulta), or of a zygapophyseal joint anomaly is strongly associated with spondylolysis of L5.[9] Spina bifida occulta has been described to occur in between 13% and 58% of cases concomitant with spondylolysis.[12] Spondylolysis also occurs in patients with Marfan's syndrome and Ehlers–Danlos syndrome; in the latter disease it may be severe. Osteogenesis imperfecta and osteopetrosis are other forms of systemic diseases related to spondylolysis.

Repeated microfractures are mainly related to hyperextension movements, thus amplifying the lordotic state. Muscle strength and tension may influence the development of spondylolysis through shortening or tightness of the hamstring muscles of the thigh with increased tension on the posterior vertebral arches of the lower lumbar spine. Weakening of the spinal and the anterior abdominal wall muscles is a precursor in the development of spondylolysis, too, whereas strengthening parts of these muscles should have a preventive effect.

In the later course of spondylolysis, fibrous or bony callus formation at the pars defect site may develop. Bony outgrowths, facet joint arthrosis, or instability may lead to nerve root impingement with leg pain, numbness, or weakness.

With longer exposure to applied forces the isthmic form of spondylolisthesis may develop. It is a forward movement of the body of one of the lumbar vertebrae on the vertebra below it, whereas the posterior joints and the neural arches are aligned with the posterior elements of the inferior vertebral body. A fully dislocated vertebral body is named "spondyloptosis."

Table 9.1.1 "Fingerprints" of vertebral injury

Applied force	Type of activity
Repetitive hyperextension maneuvers	Gymnastics, wrestling, diving, throwing sports, basketball, volleyball, pole vaulting, certain swimming styles (butterfly), high diving
Strong muscle forces	Body building, wrestling, hockey
Repeated monotonous exercises	Rowing
Rotational motion creating unilateral defects	Throwing sports, golf
High and various degrees of movement	Football, track and field athletics, dancing, figure skating

9.1 Sports Injuries: Spondylolysis

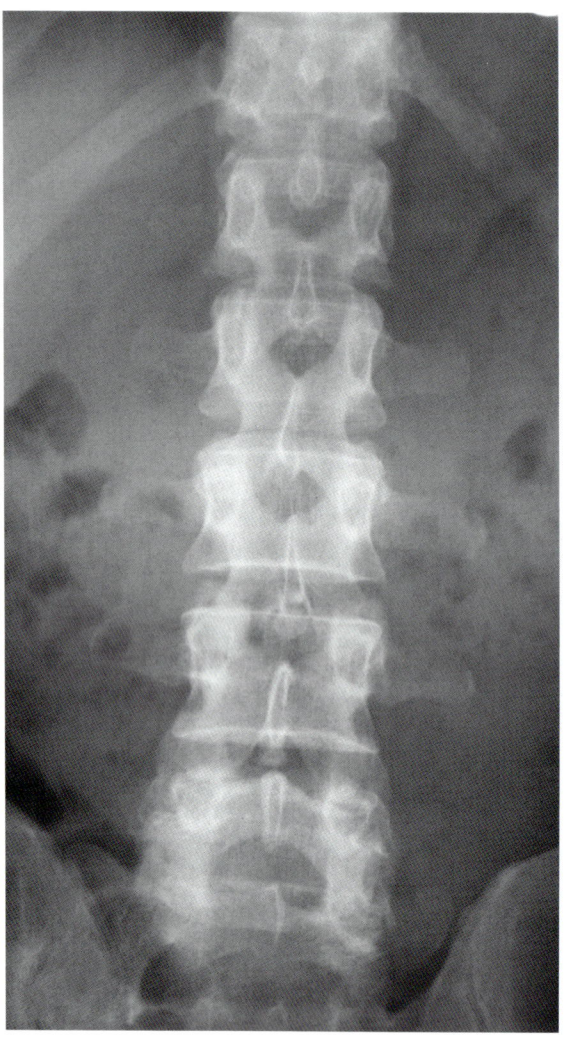

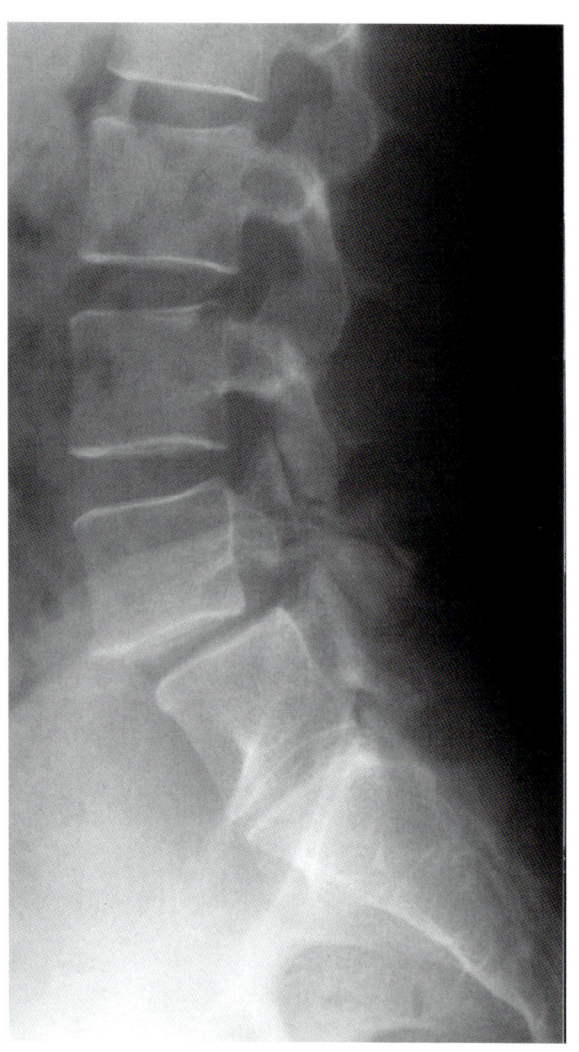

Fig. 9.1.1 Spondylolysis and spondylolisthesis with a concomitant transitional vertebra.

Spondylolisthesis occurs in the preadolescent and is found in up to 50% of athletes with persistent back pain. Symptoms may not occur until later in life. In a longitudinal study by Fredrickson et al three-quarters of all individuals with spondylolysis had an identifiable pars defect on plain films by age 6, and approximately 75% of these patients had evidence of a slip at that time.[1] Further progression of the slip in adulthood is rare.[14]

Indications for Imaging

Imaging investigations should be performed if back pain more persistent than simple myalgia is observed. The typical pain associated with spondylolysis is dull and occasionally unilateral, sometimes radiating into the buttocks or even the groin.[15] The pain increases during exercise with hyperextension and rotational movements. Hyperlordosis, stiffness of the hip joints, and pain or cramps in the hamstring muscles or in the erector spinae may be associated findings. Signs of neural impingement with L5 root compression or in some rare cases with cauda equina syndrome may indicate severe spondylolisthesis. A history of trauma is not observed, but subclinical backache for a longer period of time is typical. Today, the extreme form of slipped vertebra with heart-shaped buttocks, high iliac crests, and a relatively short torso is rarely observed.

Predisposing factors include history of a first-degree relative with a slipped vertebra, rare callus formation, and a young age of onset.[16]

The primary imaging investigation is done with conventional radiographs. More specialized investigation includes magnetic resonance imaging (MRI), computed tomography (CT), and scintigraphy. Following European referral criteria these modalities are classified with an evidence level of "C" on a scale A–C.[17] Many cases of spondylolysis identified by some of the newer imaging techniques are not noted concurrently on conventional radiograms. MRI is performed to detect associated disk prolapse and to delineate the extent of neural impingement. CT is the modality of choice to confirm or rule out spondylolysis by displaying the morphology of the vertebral arch in great detail. Nuclear medicine studies should be applied if the results of other imaging modalities are negative, however, generally they are of lesser importance considering the modern multi-planar capabilities of CT and MRI.

Follow-up imaging studies may be indicated for the athlete if there is an urgent requirement for a return to competition. In general, nonoperative treatment of spondylolysis is reported to result in successful pain relief in approximately 80% of athletes, independent of radiographic evidence of healing of the defect.[5] As it is difficult in children and preadolescents to predict the risk and the extent of vertebral slipping, radiological monitoring may be indicated in patients involved in sporting activities that are associated with a higher risk of spondylolysis, especially in throwing sports, gymnastics, and rowing (Table 9.1.**1**).[4,7,18]

Investigation Techniques

Radiography

Conventional radiographs should be exposed in the lateral and antero-posterior direction and in many cases an interruption of the pars interarticularis can be detected on the lateral views. As there is an overlap of the right and left pars, oblique views with 45° angulation may be helpful. Amato et al found that lateral oblique views and a lumbosacral lateral spot view (Fig. 9.1.**2a**) are superior to anteroposterior and lateral views of the lumbar spine.[19] Flexion and extension views of the lumbar spine are helpful to measure the extent of hypermobility or instability in the spondylolytic and in the neighboring segments (Figs. 9.1.**2**, 9.1.**3**). Correct display of the vertebral arches is, however, not always easy because of the nontomographical character of plain films and especially in patients with associated scoliosis where an interruption of the isthmus may be obscured (Fig. 9.1.**4**). Saifuddin et al analyzed 69 spondylolytic defects with CT and found a wide variation between individuals with only 32% of the lesions aligned within 15° of the 45° lateral oblique plane.[20] Unfortunately, no internationally accepted labeling of the angulated views with respect to the left and right side exists; labels may refer to the side of the patient's body as well as to the beam direction.

Fluoroscopy may be of help in selected cases to observe atypical movement patterns; however, considering radiation protection issues there is no justification in routine diagnosis.

Computed Tomography

CT with its multi-planar capabilities is the modality of choice to document spondylolysis (Fig. 9.1.**5**). Images reconstructed in a sagittally angulated plain parallel to the course of the pars interarticularis are the most useful for displaying not only an interruption of the pars but also its length and shape. Moreover, repair mechanisms and associated abnormalities of the facet joints or intervertebral foramina can be detected with CT. Furthermore, CT allows us to define the exact angles of spondylolysis as well as of the slipping of a vertebra. Investigations should be performed with a multi-row multidetector unit to obtain images with a high resolution in all planes. Where single-row machines are only available, the technique of reverse angle gantry tilt may be applied with images oriented perpendicular to the vertebral arch.

Magnetic Resonance Imaging

MRI is useful for detecting osseous clefts, bone marrow edema, or fat marrow conversion due to mechanical overload. It is of specific importance for assessing the spinal capacity and causes of neural impingement. With a standardized technique of investigation including sagittal T1W and T2W or STIR sequences a gap of the pars interarticularis is more easily detected than with axial slices (Fig. 9.1.**6**). Angulation parallel to the orientation of the disk space means that axial sequences are also oriented parallel to the fracture line. Stoller et al recommended peripheral parasagittal images, particularly T2W images or T1W images acquired without an interslice gap.[21] MRI myelography with T2W sequence parameters may be of help for documenting the narrowing of the thecal sac.

Nuclear Medicine Studies

In several studies bone scans were shown to be superior to plain film radiography.[9] It could be demonstrated that this technique is suitable for documenting the repair of low-degree pars defects. Further studies have shown that single-photon emission computed tomography (SPECT) is even more sensitive.[22] In contrast to other imaging modalities, nuclear medicine studies are suitable for determining whether a lesion is metabolically active or not.

Ultrasound

Tallroth et al described sonography as being useful for measuring the degree of spondylolisthesis.[23] This technique has not been routinely used so far.

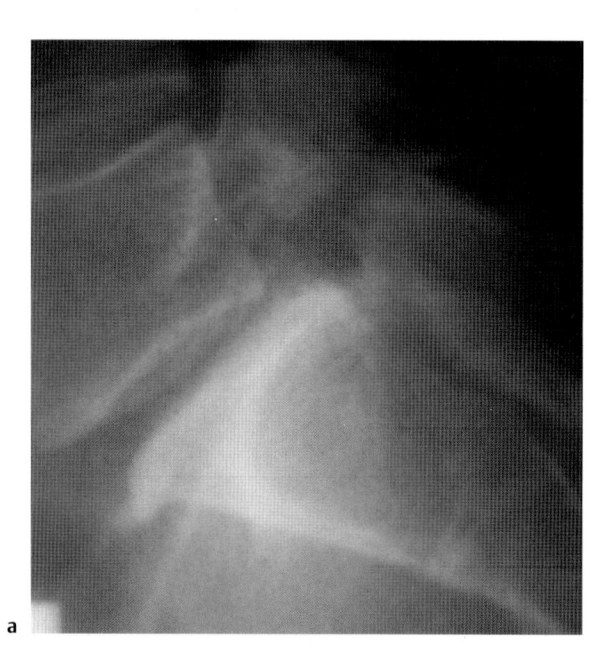

Fig. 9.1.2 Spondylolysis with a typical cleft is best seen on the lateral spot view (**a**) and the hyperlordotic state of the lumbar spine on flexion and extension views (**b**, **c**).

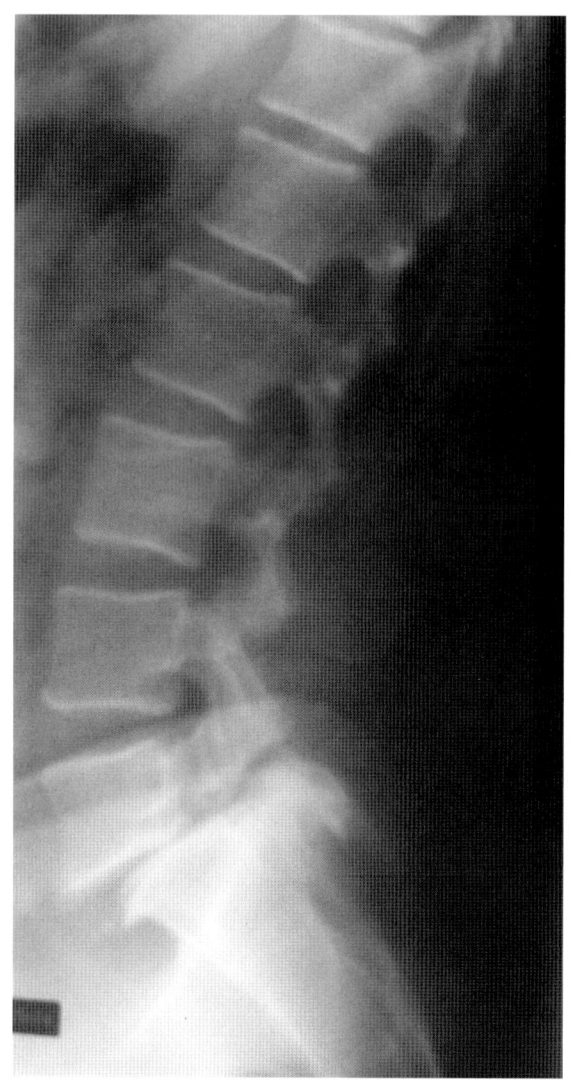

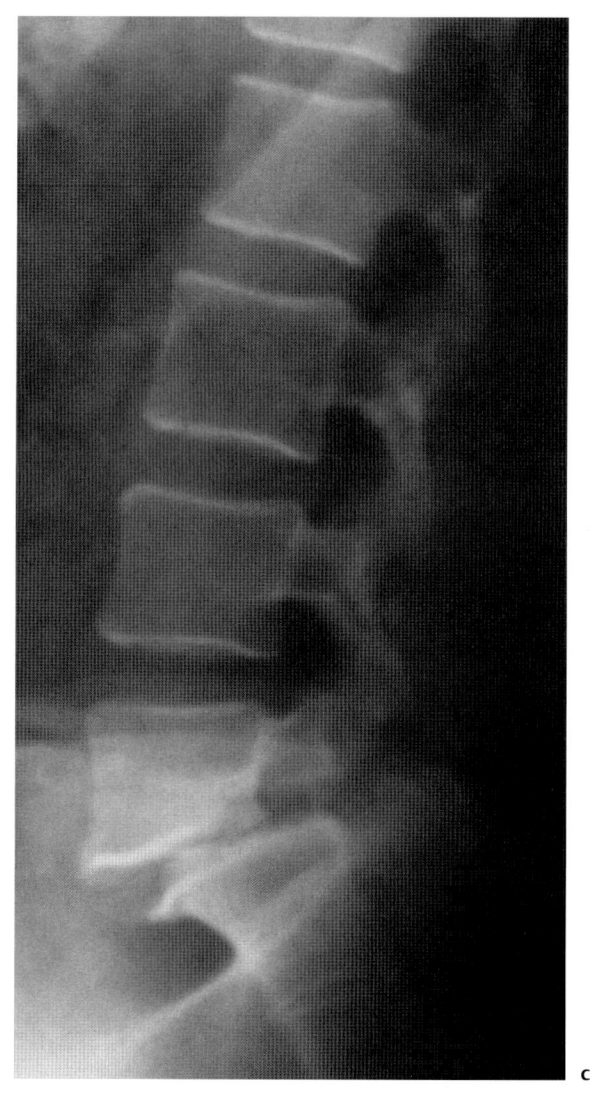

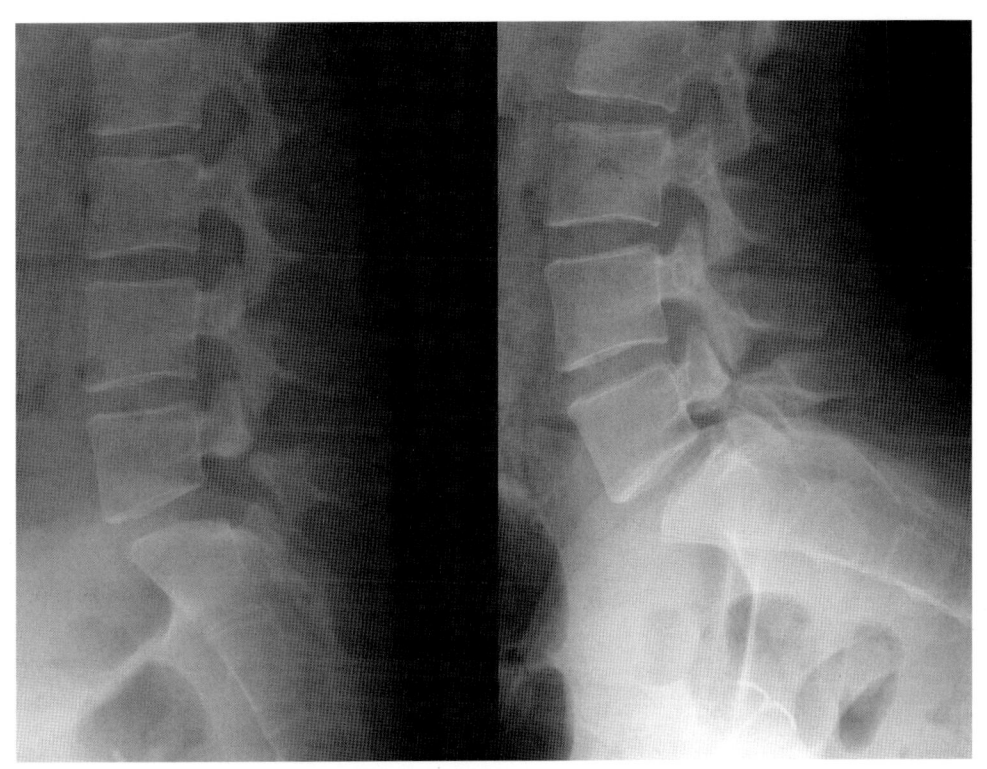

Fig. 9.1.3 A flexion and extension view with segmental instability associated with spondylolysis in L5 and hypermobility in the L3–L4 segment.

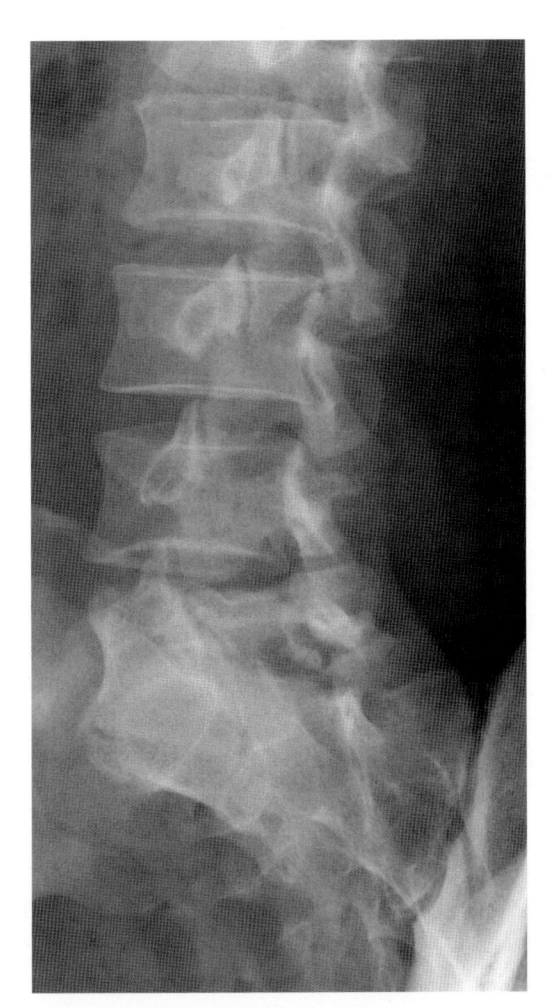

Fig. 9.1.4 A spondylolytic defect in L5 only partially visible due to the overlaying structures of the spine and the pelvis.

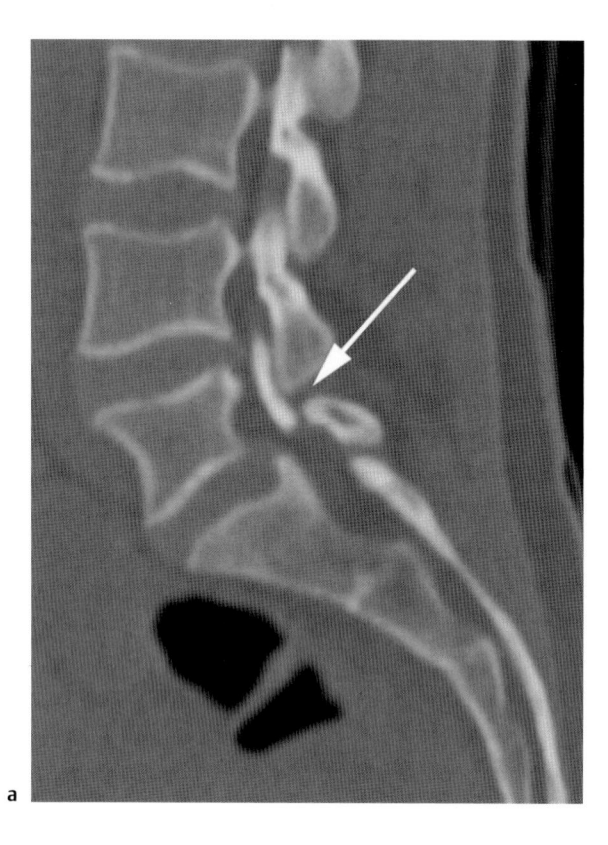

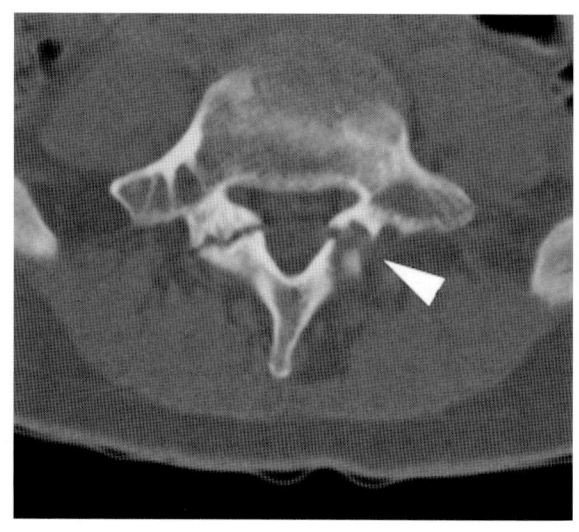

Fig. 9.1.5 **a** A reformatted sagittal image with a spondylolytic defect in L5 (*arrow*) that is only in part visible on the axial image **b** (*arrowhead*) due to the partial volume effect.

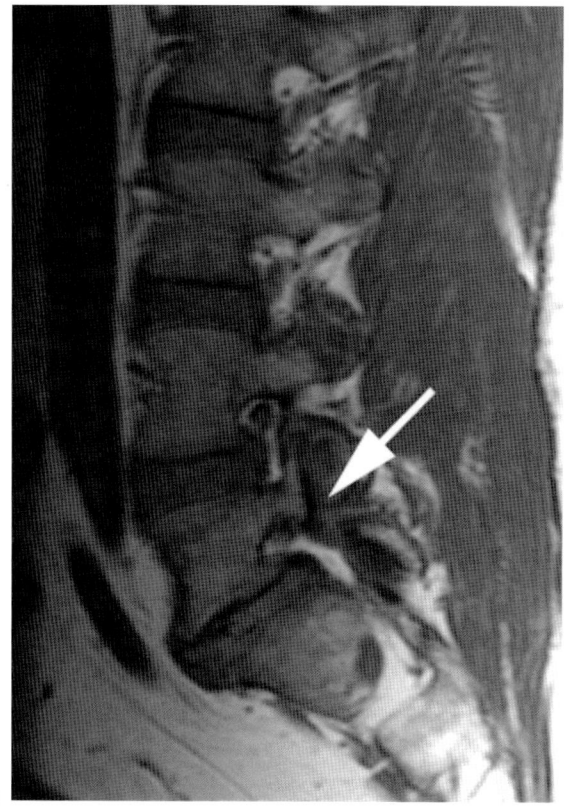

Fig. 9.1.6 **a** Sagittal T1W hypointense sclerotic pars defect (*arrow*) with a slight compression of the spinal nerve in the adjacent intervertebral foramen. **b** The corresponding conventional radiogram with cleft (*arrowhead*).

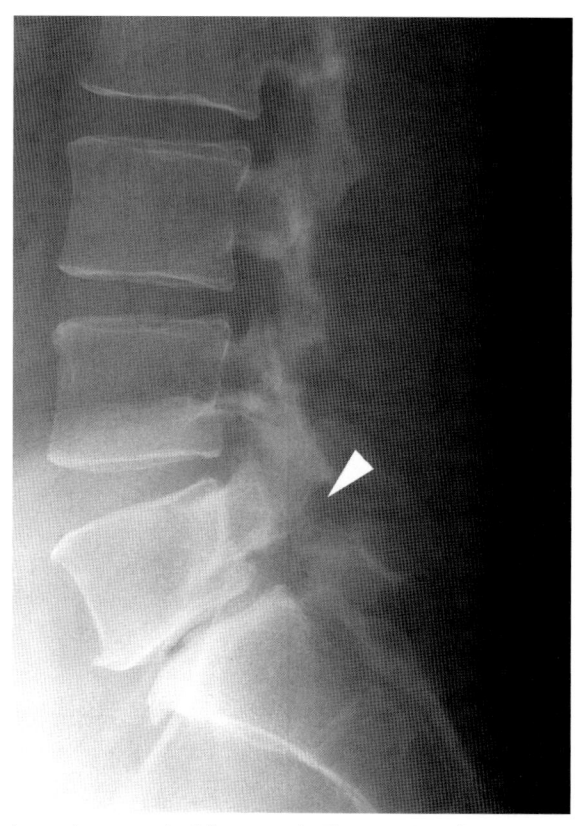

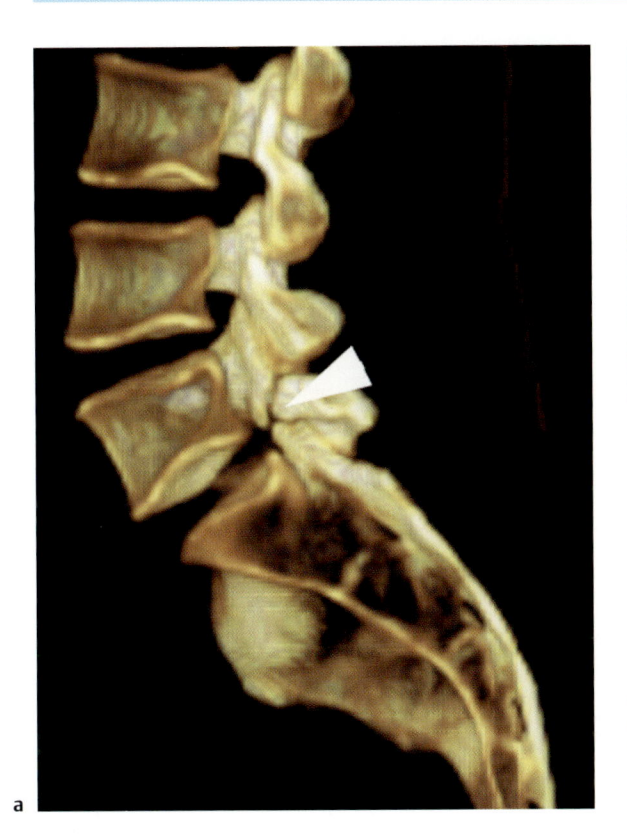

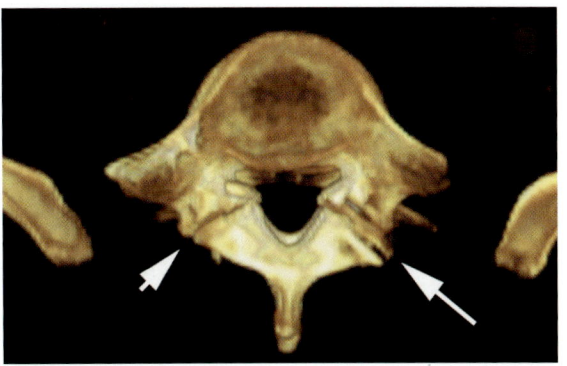

Fig. 9.1.7 **a** CT volume reconstruction with typical pars defect (*arrowhead*) in the fifth lumbar segment. **b** On the axial image a lytic pars defect is visible on the left side (*long arrow*) behind the facet joint (double facet joint sign). Erosive osteoarthritis of the contralateral facet joint (*small arrow*).

Image Interpretation

Imaging Anatomy

The pars interarticularis, i.e., "interarticular portion" or isthmus vertebrae, is a clinical description for the part of the vertebral arch running between the superior and the inferior articular processes.[24] It consists mainly of cortical bone and contains almost no bony trabeculae. It forms an obtuse angle with the plane of the horizontal vertebral body axis and is specifically prone to mechanical stress applied from backward and forward levers (Fig. 9.1.7). The greatest forces occur at the L5–S1 segment, where the cross-sectional area of the pars is only 0.75 cm^2.[15,25] Therefore, the vast majority of spondylolytic defects occur at the L5 level in 85–95% of cases, whereas at L4 only 5–15% of lesions are observed (Fig. 9.1.8) and other vertebral segments are only rarely involved.[9] Multi-segmental involvement may be observed.[26] After post-operative spinal fusion monosegmental instability in the adjacent vertebra may occur (Fig. 9.1.9). The orientation of the lumbar facet joints, in contrast to degenerative spondylolisthesis, does not play a direct role in the development of isthmic spondylolysis.[27] Superimposition of the transverse processes has been termed "pseudospondylolysis." It may be visible especially in the mid third of the lumbar spine on lateral radiograms and should not be mistaken for a real pars defect.[28]

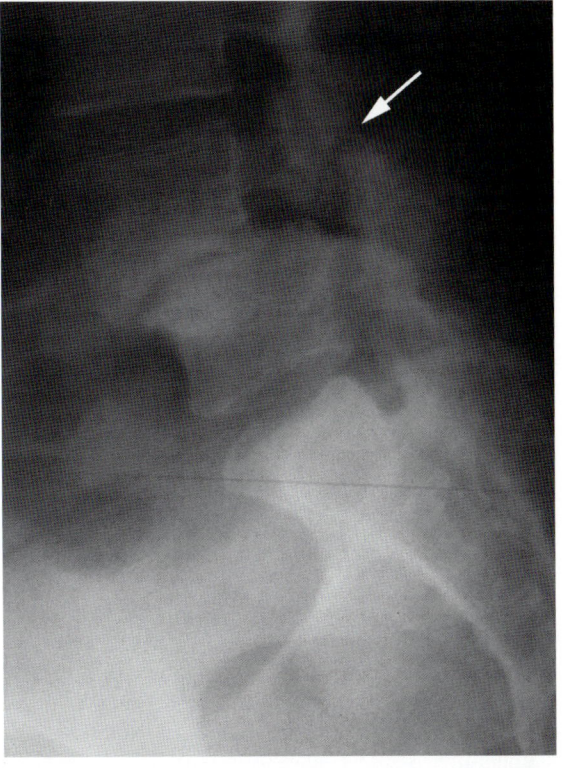

Fig. 9.1.8 Spondylolysis in the fourth lumbar segment (*arrow*) with spondylolisthesis and secondary degeneration of disk space.

9.1 Sports Injuries: Spondylolysis

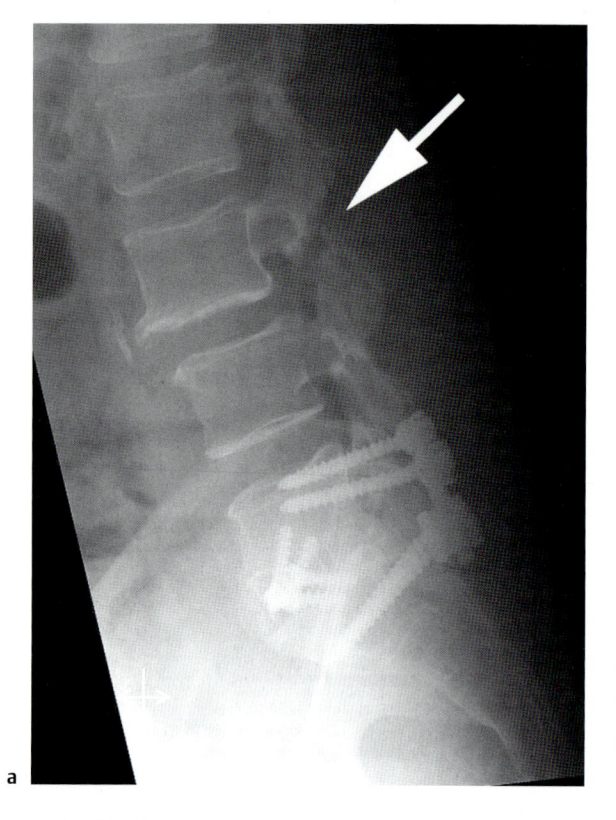

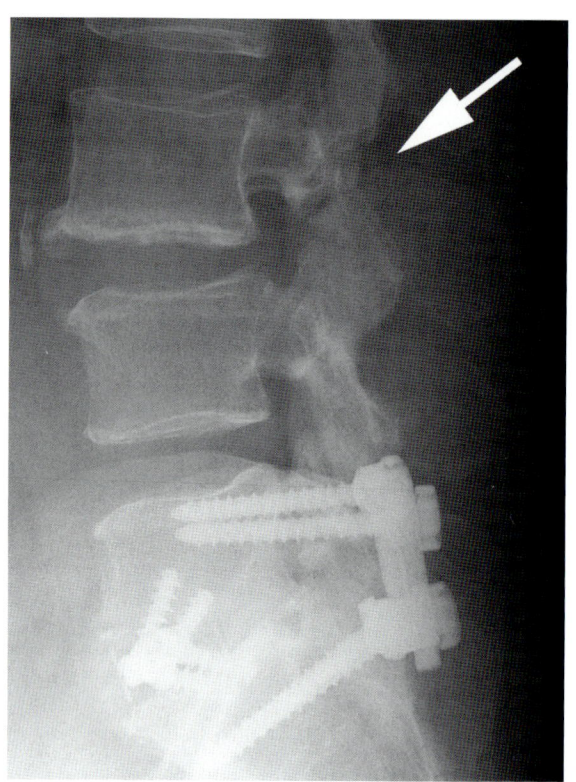

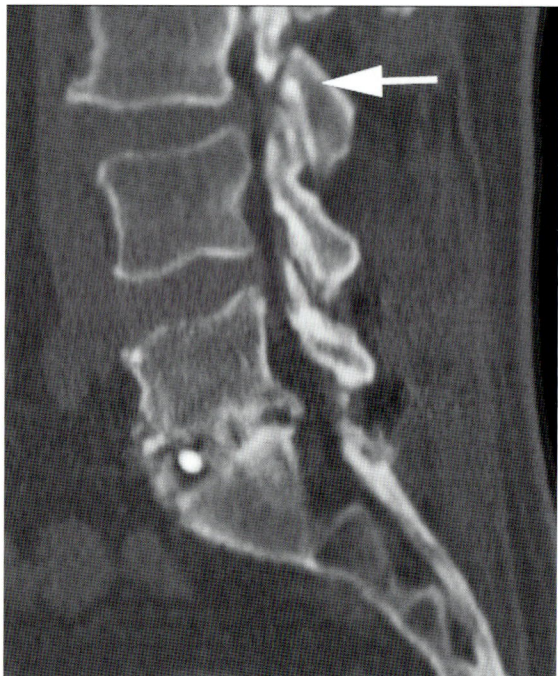

Fig. 9.1.**9** Post-operative spondylolysis (*arrows*) in the L3 segment with (**a**, **b**) hypermobility on flexion and extension views and (**c**) protrusion of the "disk at risk" on reformatted CT.

Signs

On the basis of therapeutic and prognostic aspects the direct findings of spondylolysis, including its predisposing conditions and the post-traumatic or degenerative sequels, may be grouped into an early phase with a good prognosis of healing and a late phase with a higher rate of recurrence after conservative treatment.[7,18,29]

In the early phase there is a small fracture line visible in the pars interarticularis. On oblique views its appearance between the superior and inferior articular facets has been attributed to a collar of "LaChapele's dog" or "Scotty dog" (Fig. 9.1.**10**). Three alignment patterns have been regarded as predisposing for the development of spondylolysis: hyperlordosis, scoliosis, and spina bifida occulta. Hyperlordosis and the position of the sacrum influence the degree of shear

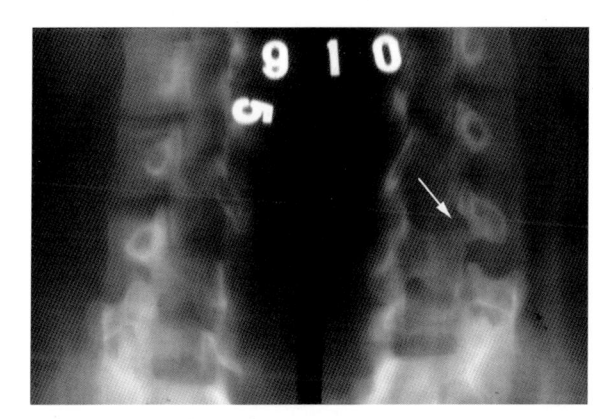

Fig. 9.1.**10** Conventional ("oblique") tomogram with unilateral spondylolysis visible as a collar (*arrow*) of the "Scotty dog".

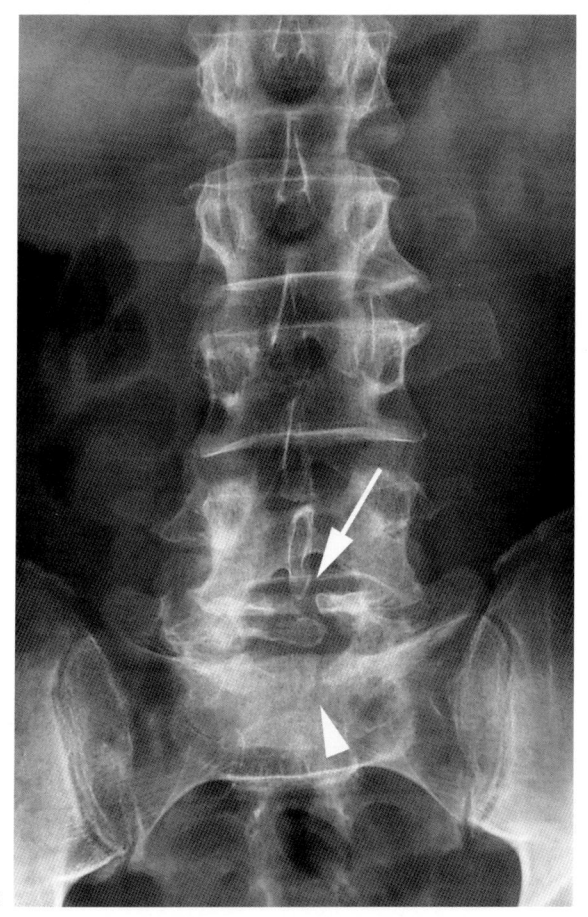

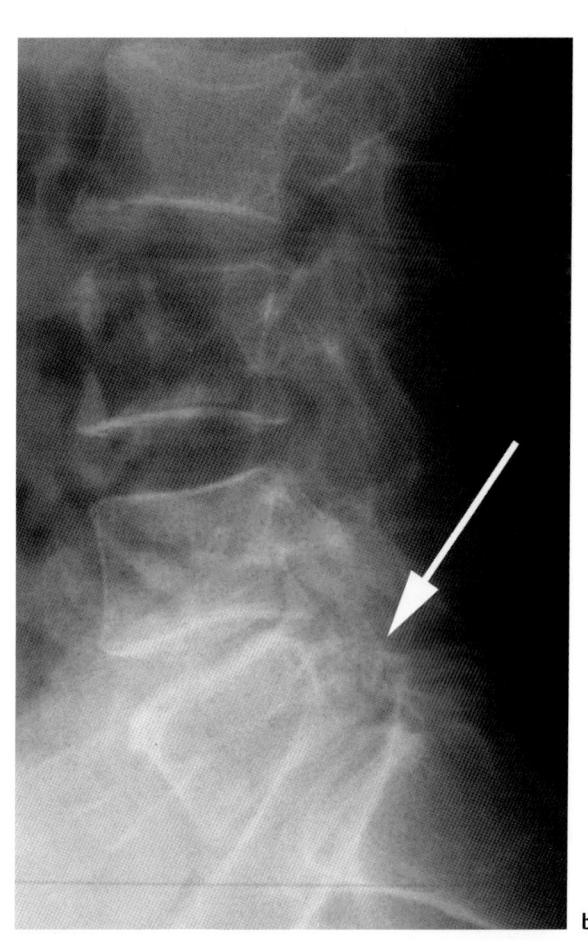

Fig. 9.1.**11**   **a** Spina bifida occulta type I (*arrowhead*) and type II (*arrow*) associated with (**b**) a fragmented type of spondylolysis (*long arrow*).

forces on the neural arch.[30] Three types of spina bifida occulta have been described: type I with a wide cleft, type II with slightly attaching ends of the vertebral arch, and type III with the ends overlapping each other.[12] Types II and III are those which are associated with spondylolysis and indicate a developmental retardation of the lower spine (Fig. 9.1.**11**). The perivertebral tissues, the disk space, the facet joints, and the bony structures of the involved vertebra are not involved in the early phase of lysis.

In the late phase the fracture within the pars interarticularis line has widened to more than 3 mm. A segmental hypermobility may be observed on flexion and extension views. There is a complex mechanism of abnormal gliding with the involved vertebra being partially fixed by the facet joints, thus "jumping" in a temporary retrolisthesis during anteflexion. Such abnormalities may become visible with fluoroscopy and are indicative of the enormous stress applied on the vertebral junctions. This may lead to entrapment of the spinal nerves and degeneration of the facet joints and the intervertebral disk. With CT, an incomplete ring sign on axial imaging may simulate "extra" facet joints. In unilateral spondylolysis, reactive sclerosis on the con-

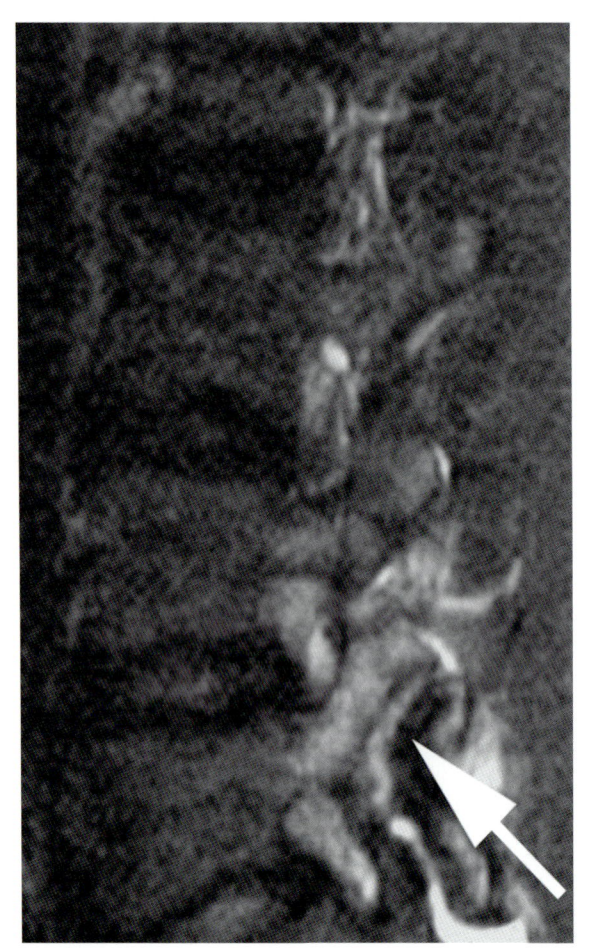

Fig. 9.1.**12** A type I stress reaction with edema on a fat-suppressed T2W image in the pars interarticularis (*arrow*).

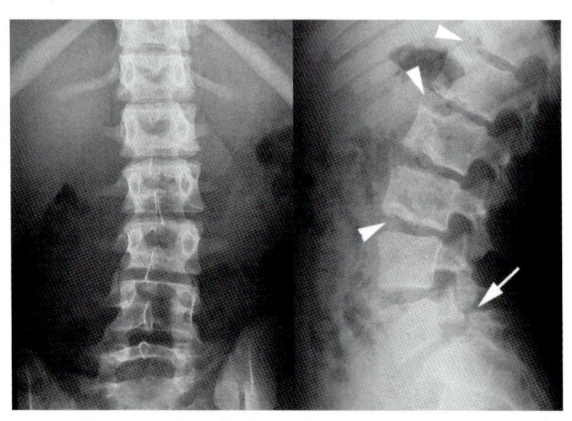

Fig. 9.1.**13** Typical triad of spinal overuse in a young wrestler with spondylolysis (*arrow*), scoliosis, and endplate reactions (*arrowheads*).

tralateral side of the vertebral arch may occur. Lytic defects and foraminal narrowing are visible on reformatted images. Signs with MRI include a focally decreased signal or fragmentation in the pars on sagittal and axial T1W and T2W sequences, an elongation of the spinal canal at the level of the pars defect and a more horizontal configuration of the affected neural foramina on sagittal imaging with or without loss of fat surrounding the exiting nerve roots. Reactive marrow changes which are similar to those described for endplate changes and degenerative disk disease may be seen in the adjacent pedicles in 40% of patients with spondylolysis.[31] A type 2 pedicle change with hyperintensity on T1W images and isointensity or hyperintensity on T2W images is the most frequent pattern of pedicle signal intensity observed. Stäbler et al stress the high importance of type 1 reactions (Fig. 9.1.**12**) for the early diagnosis of spondylolysis.[32] Sherif and Mahfouz described epidural fat interposition between the dura mater and spinous process of L5 as an indirect sign of spondylolysis on midsagittal MR imaging of the lumbar spine.[33]

Degeneration of the vertebral junctions and osseous abnormalities may be associated with disk bulging, spur formation, or ligament thickening with reduction of the diameters of the spinal canal, thus lowering the spinal capacity and leading to acquired vertebral stenosis (see Fig. 9.1.**8**).

Differential Diagnosis

Other Forms of Overuse of the Spine

Lower back pain or pain in the buttocks is not uncommon in athletes and several other forms of overuse may be associated with spondylolysis:

- This is especially true for the triad of hyperlordosis, scoliosis, and endplate deformities (Fig. 9.1.**13**). The latter are often classified with the term *atypical Scheuermann's disease*.
- Degeneration of the vertebral junctions, i.e., disk herniation, facet joint syndrome, or interspinous bursitis are in many cases late sequels of repetitive movements.
- Sacroiliac joint disease less commonly accounts for lower back pain in athletes.
- Other types of stress fractures are rare. They may occur as sacral stress fractures or as facet joint stress fractures.[34,35]
- Spinal process apophysitis has been reported to mimic spondylolysis on scintigrams.[36]

Congenital Clefts

Besides isthmic type spondylolysis other clefts that are of congenital origin may be observed in the posterior part of the vertebral arch.[11,24] Median posterior clefts are most commonly observed, other forms are the paraspinal, retroisthmic, and the retrosomatic cleft.

Spondylolisthesis

Overall, the risk of progression of spondylolysis to spondylolisthesis is about 4%.[37] The only predictive variable was an initial slip of more than 20%.[38] Muschik et al found a progression to spondylolisthesis during the early growth spurt of puberty.[39]

The degree of spondylolisthesis has been quantified by Meyerding who divided the sagittal diameter of the subjacent vertebra into four segments and classified

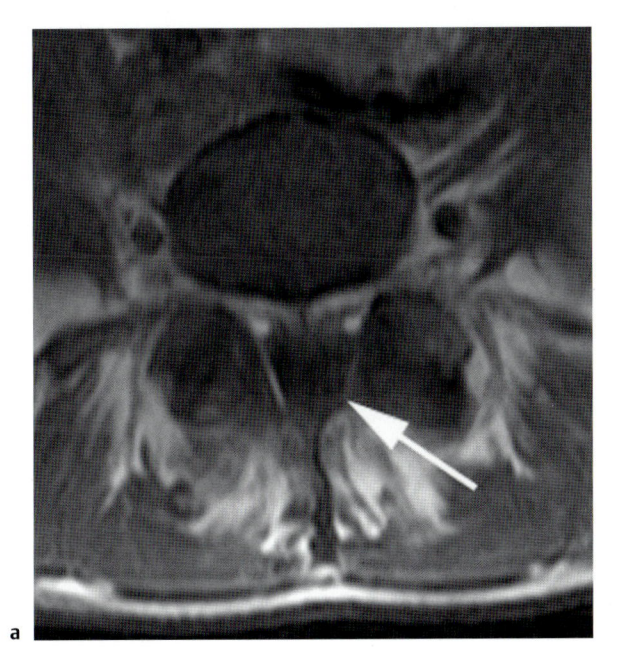

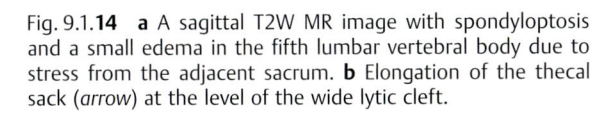

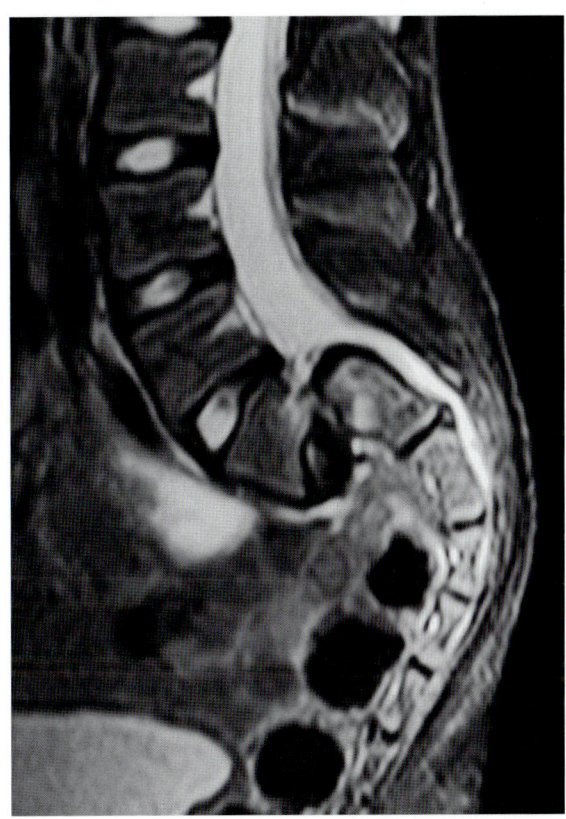

Fig. 9.1.**14 a** A sagittal T2W MR image with spondyloptosis and a small edema in the fifth lumbar vertebral body due to stress from the adjacent sacrum. **b** Elongation of the thecal sack (*arrow*) at the level of the wide lytic cleft.

the extent of the slip from I to IV.[40] Sim measured the distance between the posterior aspects of the slipped vertebra and the vertebra below it and thus calculated the percentage of slip.[41] The measurements of vertebral translation and angulation are associated with a good intra- and interobserver variation.[42] Owing to its etiology spondylolisthesis may be classified into five types (Table 9.1.**2**).

In isthmic or spondylolytic spondylolisthesis, the anteroposterior diameter of the spinal canal is increased at the level of the pars defect (Fig. 9.1.**14**). Sclerotic reactions of the pars that mimic spondylolysis especially in a healed pars may cause a partial volume artifact from a spur arising from the superior facet slightly lateral to the pars. Hypertrophic bone and fibrocartilaginous overgrowth at the pars defect often produce lateral recess or central canal stenosis and neural foraminal stenosis may occur without central canal stenosis. The posterior aspects of the two involved vertebrae may be seen in the same axial image.

Degenerative spondylolisthesis, also referred to as pseudospondylolisthesis, occurs in older patients and is associated with disk degeneration. It is more often seen in the L4–L5 segment with forward displacement of the superior vertebral body secondary to medial superior erosion of the inferior facet and is often associated with vertically oriented facet joints. In the absence of a pars defect, which would decompress the central canal, narrowing of the anteroposterior diameter of the spinal canal occurs, causing severe central spinal stenosis in addition to lateral recess stenosis, neural foraminal stenosis, or both. The contours of the thecal sac may have an hourglass or constricted outline.

Neoplasms

In some rare cases, neoplasms may simulate sclerotic reactions of the vertebral arch. Osteoid osteoma most commonly accounts for such an appearance. On CT images, a typical nidus is seen in most of these cases. Other osseous neoplasms with sclerotic reactions are osteoblastoma and malignant osseous tumors as well as metastases, but they are rarely observed.

Table 9.1.**2** Classification of spondylolisthesis[8]

Type I:	Dysplastic or congenital, caused by insufficiency or agenesis of the superior articular facet
Type II:	Isthmic, with a defect in the pars interarticularis that may be (1) a fatigue fracture, (2) an elongated but intact pars, or (3) an acute fracture
Type III:	Degenerative, resulting from long-standing intersegmental instability
Type IV:	Traumatic, caused by fractures in areas of the posterior elements other than the pars interarticularis
Type V:	Pathologic, due to generalized or localized bone disease

Conclusion

Diagnostic imaging plays a key role in the primary diagnosis of spondylolysis and an increasing role in the follow-up. Spondylolysis is regarded as a form of overuse with a strong relationship to sport and is in fact the most common type of bony overuse injury of the spine. As in other types of overuse, critical anatomical zones and a certain vulnerable phase during life can be identified, in this case the pars interarticularis in the second decade of life. The clinical problem with spondylolysis is the associated back pain, but even more important is the potential of degenerative facet joint disease and of developing isthmic spondylolisthesis.

Taking into account athletic scholarships or professional contracts a definite diagnosis based on dedicated sports-related algorithms should be established more urgently than for the normal nonathletic patient. Screening with MR imaging needs a dedicated protocol.[44] In conclusion, the clinical and imaging characteristics of the athlete's spine reflect the intimate relationships among congenital dispositions, adaptation of the shape to specific sports-related requirements, and definite functional and morphological pathology.

References

1. Fredrickson BE, Baker D, McHolick WJ, Yuan HA, Lubicky JP. The natural history of spondylolysis and spondylolisthesis. *J Bone Joint Surg Am.* 1984;66(5):699–707.
2. Roche M, Rowe G. The incidence of separate neural arch and coincident bone variations: a survey of 4,200 skeletons. *Anat Rec.* 1951;109((7)):233–252.
3. Rossi F, Dragoni S. Lumbar spondylolysis: occurrence in competitive athletes. Updated achievements in a series of 390 cases. *J Sports Med Phys Fitness.* 1990;30(4):450–452.
4. Soler T, Calderon C. The prevalence of spondylolysis in the Spanish elite athlete. *Am J Sports Med.* 2000;28(1):57–62.
5. Bono CM. Low-back pain in athletes. *J Bone Joint Surg Am.* 2004;86A(2):382–96.
6. Stinson JT. Spondylolysis and spondylolisthesis in the athlete. *Clin Sports Med.* 1993;12(3):517–28.
7. Engelhardt M, Reuter I, Freiwald J, Böhme T, Halbsguth A. Spondylolysis and spondylolisthesis and sports. *Orthopäde.* 1997;26(9):755–759.
8. Wiltse LL, Newman PH, Macnab I. Classification of spondylolisis and spondylolisthesis. *Clin Orthop.* 1976;117(1):23–29.
9. Standaert CJ, Herring SA. Spondylolysis: a critical review. *Br J Sports Med.* 2000;34(6):415–422.
10. Brocher J. Die Dysplasie des Wirbelbogens. Eine pathologische Studie zum Spondylolisthesisproblem. *Rofo.* 1950; 73((11)): 719–725.
11. Töndury G, Theiler K. *Entwicklungsgeschichte und Fehlbildungen der Wirbelsäule.* Stuttgart: Hippokrates-Verlag; 1990.
12. Niethard FU, Pfeil J, Weber M. Ätiologie und Pathogenese der spondyloltischen Spondylolisthese. *Orthopäde.* 1997;26(9):750–754.
13. Weber J, Czarnetzki A. Paleopathology of the lumbar spine in the early medieval period. *Z Orthop Ihre Grenzgeb.* 2002;140(6):637–643.
14. Floman Y. Progression of lumbosacral isthmic spondylolisthesis in adults. *Spine.* 2000;25(3):342–347.
15. Harvey J, Tanner S. Low back pain in young athletes. A practical approach. *Sports Med.* 1991;12(6):394–406.
16. Wimberly RL, Lauerman WC. Spondylolisthesis in the athlete. *Clin Sports Med.* 2002;21(1):133–145.
17. Armstrong P, Ringertz H, Bischof Delaloye A. *Referral guidelines for imaging.* Luxembourg: European Commission Directorate-General for the Environment; 2001.
18. Miller SF, Congeni J, Swanson K. Long-term functional and anatomical follow-up of early detected spondylolysis in young athletes. *Am J Sports Med.* 2004;32(4):928–933.
19. Amato M, Totty WG, Gilula LA. Spondylolysis of the lumbar spine: demonstration of defects and laminal fragmentation. *Radiology.* 1984;153(3):627–629.
20. Saifuddin A, White J, Tucker S, Taylor BA. Orientation of lumbar pars defects: implications for radiological detection and surgical management. *J Bone Joint Surg Br.* 1998;80(2):208–211.
21. Stoller D, Hu S, Kaiser J. Spine. In: D Stoller, ed. *Magnetic Resonance Imaging in Orthopaedics and Sports Medicine.* Philadelphia: Lippincott-Raven Publishers; 1996.
22. Lusins JO, Elting JJ, Cicoria AD, Goldsmith SJ. SPECT evaluation of lumbar spondylolysis and spondylolisthesis. *Spine.* 1994;19(5):608–612.
23. Tallroth K, Ylikoski M, Taavitsainen M. Sonographic measurement of vertebral dislocation in spondylolisthesis. *J Pediatr Orthop.* 1987;7(5):538–540.
24. Platzer W. *Musculoskeletal System.* Stuttgart: Thieme; 1999.
25. Dietrich M, Kurowski P. The importance of mechanical factors in the etiology of spondylolysis. A model analysis of loads and stresses in the human lumbar spine. *Spine.* 1985; 10(6):532–542.
26. Al-Sebai MW, Al-Khawashki H. Spondyloptosis and multiple-level spondylolysis. *Eur Spine J.* 1999;8(1):75–77.
27. Grobler LJ, Robertson PA, Novotny JE, Pope MH. Etiology of spondylolisthesis. Assessment of the role played by lumbar facet joint morphology. *Spine.* 1993;18(1):80–91.
28. El-Khoury GY, Yousefzadeh DK, Kathol MH, Mulligan GM. Normal roentgen variant: pseudospondylolysis. *Radiology.* 1981;39(1):72.
29. Morita T, Ikata T, Katoh S, Miyake R. Lumbar spondylolysis in children and adolescents. *J Bone Joint Surg Br.* 1995;77(4):620–625.
30. Sward L. The thoracolumbar spine in young elite athletes. Current concepts on the effects of physical training. *Sports Med.* 1992;13(5):357–364.
31. Ulmer JL, Mathews VP, Elster AD, Mark LP, Daniels DL, Mueller W. MR imaging of lumbar spondylolysis: the importance of ancillary observations. *AJR Am J Roentgenol.* 1997;169(1):233–239.
32. Stäbler A, Paulus R, Steinborn M, Bosch R, Matzko M, Reiser M. Spondylolysis in the developmental stage: diagnostic contribution of MRI. *Rofo.* 2000;172(1):33–37.
33. Sherif H, Mahfouz AE. Epidural fat interposition between dura mater and spinous process: a new sign for the diagnosis of spondylolysis on MR imaging of the lumbar spine. *Eur Radiol.* 2004;14(6):970–973.
34. White JH, Hague C, Nicolaou S, Gee R, Marchinkow LO, Munk PL. Imaging of sacral fractures. *Clin Radiol.* 2003; 8(12):914–921.
35. Fehlandt Jr AF, Micheli LJ. Lumbar facet stress fracture in a ballet dancer. *Spine.* 1993;18(16):2537–2539.
36. Mannor DA, Lindenfeld TN. Spinal process apophysitis mimics spondylolysis. *Am J Sports Med.* 2000;28(2):257–260.
37. Danielson BI, Frennered AK, Irstam LK. Radiologic progression of isthmic lumbar spondylolisthesis in young patients. *Spine.* 1991;16(4):422–425.
38. Seitsalo S, Osterman K, Hyvarinen H, Tallroth K, Schlenzka D, Poussa M. Progression of spondylolisthesis in children and adolescents. A long-term follow-up of 272 patients. *Spine.* 1991;16(4):417–421.
39. Muschik M, Hahnel H, Robinson PN, Perka C, Muschik C. Competitive sports and the progression of spondylolisthesis. *J Pediatr Orthop.* 1996;16(3):364–369.
40. Meyerding H. Spondylolisthesis. *Surg Gynecol Obstet.* 1932; 4(4): 371–377.
41. Sim G. Vertebral contour in spondylolisthesis. *Br J Radiol.* 1973; 46(5):250–254.
42. Tallroth K, Ylikoski M, Landtman M, Santavirta S. Reliability of radiographical measurements of spondylolisthesis and extension-flexion radiographs of the lumbar spine. *Eur J Radiol.* 1994;18(3):227–231.
43. Junghanns H. *Die Wirbelsäule unter den Einflüssen des täglichen Lebens, der Freizeit, des Sports.* Stuttgart: Thieme; 1986.
44. Campbell RS, Grainger AJ, Hide IG, Papastefanou S, Greenough CG. Juvenile spondylolysis: a comparative analysis of CT, SPECT and MRI. *Skeletal Radiol.* 2005;34:63–73.

9.2 Sports Injuries: Diskovertebral Overuse Injuries

J. J. Rankine

Introduction

Chronic overuse injury of the immature spine can damage not only the posterior elements, but the anterior structures of the spine as well. The role of chronic overuse in damaging the vertebral body endplates is less clear-cut than stress fractures of the posterior elements. This is because Scheuermann's disease, characterized by endplate abnormalities and kyphosis, can occur in relatively sedentary individuals. There is clear evidence for a genetic predisposition to developing Scheuermann's disease, but with increasing participation of adolescents in high-level sports it has become clear that mechanical factors are important. This chapter examines the evidence for the importance of mechanical factors in causing endplate abnormalities and discusses imaging strategies for the athlete with back pain. The controversial area of the role of chronic overuse injury in the etiology of disk degeneration and herniation is discussed.

Anatomy

The vertebral endplate consists of a layer of cartilage that covers the surface of the disk, separating the disk from the adjacent vertebral body. It is debatable whether the endplates are strictly components of the disk or whether they actually belong to the vertebral body, but they are often described as being part of the intervertebral disk.[1] The intervertebral disk is composed of a central nucleus pulposus with a surrounding annulus fibrosus. The nucleus pulposus is a semi-fluid mass of mucoid material, rather like toothpaste. The annulus fibrosus consists of collagen fibers that surround the nucleus pulposus in concentric rings. The endplate lies on the superior and inferior surfaces of the intervertebral disk, so the nucleus pulposus is in direct contact with the endplate (Fig. 9.2.1). The endplates are attached to the subchondral bone of the vertebral body. In small pockets over the surface of the subchondral bone, the bone is deficient allowing the marrow cavity to abut the surface of the endplate. The intervertebral disk has no direct blood supply, and indeed is the largest avascular structure in the body. The pockets of deficient subchondral bone facilitate the diffusion of nutrients from blood vessels in the marrow space and are important for the nutrition of the endplate and intervertebral disk. They do, however, represent relative areas of weakness, which can allow the nucleus pulposus to herniate directly into the vertebral body, forming a Schmorl's node.

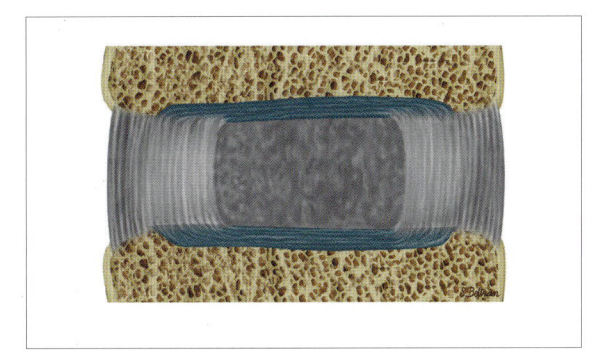

Fig. 9.2.1 **Diagrammatic representation of a sagittal slice through the intervertebral disk.** The nucleus pulposus is in direct contact with the cartilage of the vertebral endplate.

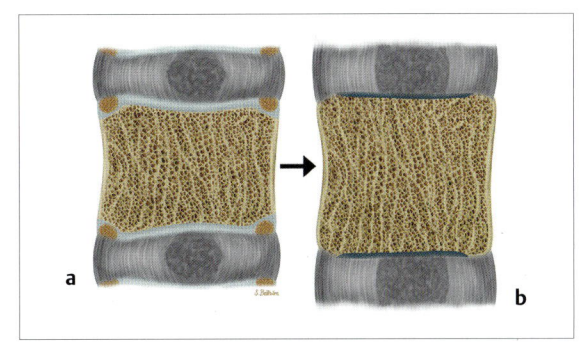

Fig. 9.2.2 **a** Sagittal slice through the vertebral body and disk in adolescence. The ring apophysis is separated from the vertebral body by a thin layer of hyaline cartilage and is an area of relative weakness. **b** The ring apophysis fuses with the vertebral body. The peripheral fibres of the adult annulus have a bony attachment, while the more central fibres insert into the vertebral endplate.

In the immature spine, a cartilaginous growth plate on the superior and inferior surfaces of the vertebral body achieves growth in vertical height. At maturity the subchondral bone plate develops on the vertebral body side of the growth plate, with the cartilaginous endplate on the other. Until the endplate ossifies, the cartilaginous growth plate of the immature spine is relatively weak and prone to injury, resulting in endplate abnormalities.

The ring apophysis develops between the ages of 7 and 9 years. It consists of a ring of ossification at the edge of the cartilaginous plate. It fuses with the vertebral body at some time, usually between the ages of 14 and 18 years (Fig. 9.2.2). Before fusion, the ossification

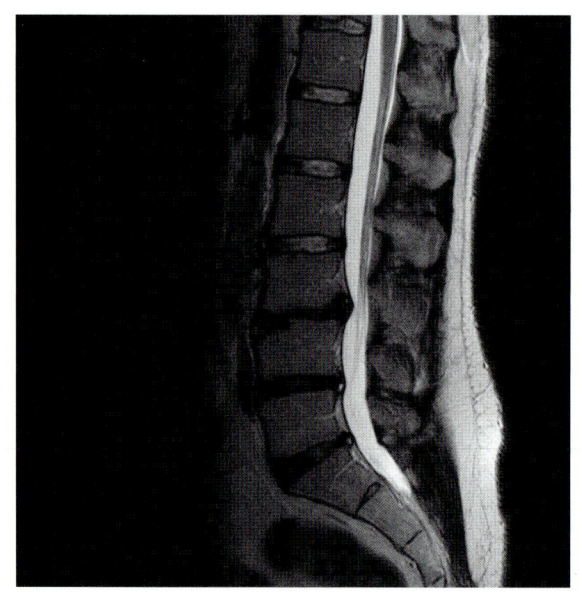

Fig. 9.2.3 **Sagittal T2W MRI through the lumbar spine.** L3/L4 limbus vertebrae. The intervertebral disk has prolapsed between the ring apophysis and vertebral body at the superior endplate of L4, permanently separating the apophysis from the body.

is separated from the rest of the vertebral body by a thin layer of hyaline cartilage and this area represents a relative region of weakness. Herniation of the nucleus pulposus can occur through this region, permanently separating the ring from the vertebral body forming a limbus vertebra (Fig. 9.2.3).

Scheuermann's Disease

In 1921 Scheuermann described a condition characterized by vertebral body wedging resulting in a kyphosis of the lower thoracic spine.[2] Hereditary factors have long been thought to be important in the pathogenesis of the disease.[3,4] In 1977 Alexander proposed a theory that there were two types of Scheuermann's disease.[5] The classical form, as described by Scheuermann, occurs around the T7 to T10 levels, while the traumatic form occurs lower down at the thoracolumbar junction. This type, found in young athletes undergoing a variety of sports, has been termed "atypical Scheuermann's."[6,7] It should be of no surprise that mechanical factors have their greatest affect on the spine at this level, since this is the region of greatest mobility in the thoracic and lumbar spine. The thoracolumbar junction includes the T11 and T12 vertebrae, as the floating ribs at these levels provide no structural support, unlike the bony ring of spine, ribs, and sternum higher up the thoracic spine. The mechanical forces induced by chronic sporting activities particularly affect the anterior portion of the vertebral body, and this is an important distinction to make from the classical Schmorl's nodes.

Schmorl described a herniation of the intervertebral disk through the endplate in 1927.[8] Schmorl's nodes are very common and occur in 19% of asymptomatic individuals,[9] and occur equally frequently in athletic and nonathletic individuals.[10,11] An acute herniation of the disk into the vertebral body is usually not visible on a plain radiograph until bone repair forms a sclerotic edge around the herniation. Unlike chronic Schmorl's nodes, the acute Schmorl's node is a painful condition and is best demonstrated by magnetic resonance imaging, which shows bone edema within the vertebral body (Fig. 9.2.**4**).[12] Little is known of the natural history of the acute Schmorl's node in terms of the MRI appearances, but since it represents an acute fracture, reactive bone edema can be expected for at least 6 months. After this the edema subsides, but the Schmorl's node remains as a chronic lifelong feature. Whilst Schmorl's nodes are undoubtedly a feature of the endplate abnormalities of Scheuermann's disease, the demonstration of Schmorl's nodes in themselves does not constitute a diagnosis of Scheuermann's disease, since this requires anterior endplate abnormalities with wedging. In the athlete with back pain, Schmorl's nodes can largely be discounted as being of any significance, except in the acute stages when they are responsible for an acute onset of back pain.

Atypical Scheuermann's disease, with anterior endplate lesions occurring at the thoracolumbar junction has been demonstrated in relation to athletic activity.[11,13–15] The most commonly investigated groups have been gymnasts and elite skiers. The competitive nature of sports is leading more children into strenuous activity at an earlier age in order to gain an advantage over rival competitors, but this subjects the spine to mechanical forces during a vulnerable period of growth. Most studies have concentrated on the plain radiographic appearances in young athletes. It is generally accepted that there is a poor correlation between plain radiographic findings and patient's symptoms, with many plain radiographic abnormalities being found in asymptomatic individuals.[16,17] The demonstration of endplate abnormalities in the thoracolumbar region on plain radiographs therefore does not necessarily explain a patient's symptoms.

Whilst most studies have simply documented the incidence of endplate abnormalities in athletes, a study by Ogon et al correlated these abnormalities with lower back pain.[18] They performed radiographs on 120 adolescent elite skiers and followed them up for the development of back pain over a 2-year period. The incidence of lower back pain was 12.5%, and severe anterior lesions were significantly associated with the development of lower back pain. Moderate endplate lesions, posterior endplate lesions, and Schmorl's nodes were not associated with back pain. Forty-five percent of the skiers had anterior lesions, and these anterior lesions appear to be the most clinically significant (Fig. 9.2.**5**).

Once the endplate lesions develop, they become a lifelong feature, but most people with Scheuermann's disease do not have symptoms, attributable to their Scheuermann's changes in adult life. Little is known

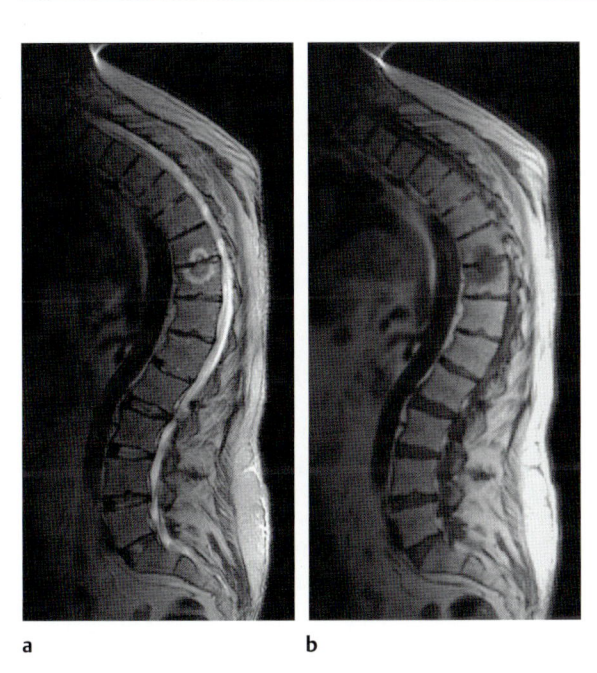

Fig. 9.2.4 **a** Sagittal T2W and **b** sagittal T1W MRI. Acute Schmorl's node formation of the superior and inferior endplates of the T10/T11 intervertebral disk. The semi-circular pattern of bone edema is the result of the shape and position of the disk herniation into the vertebral body. L1 anterior corner injury and T11 and T12 inferior endplate Schmorl's nodes are an old feature, since there is no adjacent bone edema.

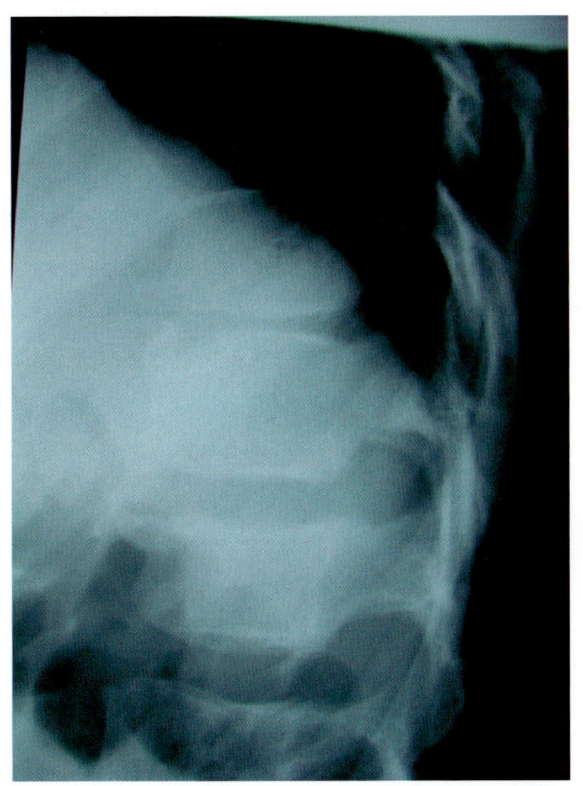

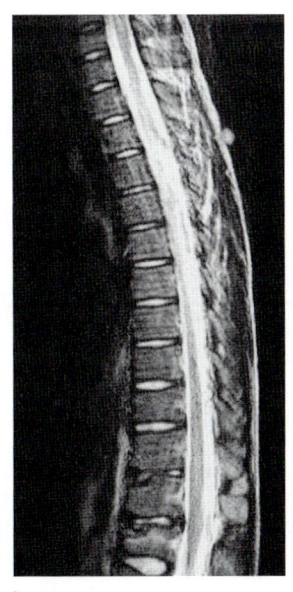

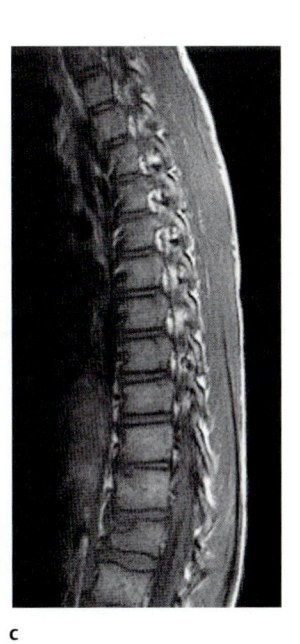

Fig. 9.2.5 **a** Plain radiograph, **b** sagittal T2W, and **c** sagittal T1W MRI in an 11-year-old gymnast. Thoracolumbar anterior endplate lesions. Adjacent bone edema indicates that these are of recent origin.

about the long-term effect of endplate abnormalities in the athlete, but Harreby et al investigated 640 school children over a 25-year period.[19] Using plain radiographs they found abnormalities in 13% of cases, which were mainly changes of Scheuermann's disease. There was no correlation between these abnormalities and lower back pain in adult life. It seems most likely that the symptomatic phase is during the development of the endplate abnormality in adolescent life. The plain radiograph gives no indication of the stage of development of an endplate lesion, unless serial radiographs are performed over time. MRI has the capacity to demonstrate edema associated with the early development of a lesion, and is the investigation of choice in the examination of lower back pain in the athlete (Fig. 9.2.5). The demonstration of a recently formed endplate lesion increases the diagnostic confidence in attributing the lesion as the cause of pain, and advising a reduction in, or complete cessation of training, to which it is always difficult for the high-level athlete to agree. The natural history of the MRI appearances of the early stages of anterior endplate lesion formation is an area that requires further research.

Disk Degeneration

Whilst it appears that endplate lesions are unlikely to result in back pain in the long term, considerable interest has been taken in the role of athletic activity in the development of disk degeneration, which clearly does have implications for the athlete in their later life. Individuals participating in sports that put high demands on the spine, such as wrestling and gymnastics, seem to have a higher incidence of degeneration than age-matched controls.[13] These are also the individuals who appear to have an increased incidence of endplate lesions, suggesting that the degeneration may occur as a secondary feature to the endplate injury.

The cardinal features of disk degeneration on MRI are disk space narrowing and dehydration of the nucleus pulposus. When the nucleus pulposus herniates through an endplate defect, be it an anterior lesion or a simple Schmorl's node, there is an inevitable reduction in the disk height. Furthermore, as the nucleus pulposus herniates from the intervetebral space there is an inevitable reduction in the hydration of the disk (Fig. 9.2.**6**). Whether or not this truly represents disk degeneration is highly debatable, as it would seem likely that these are secondary changes resulting from the herniation of the disk into the vertebral body, rather than a primary disease of the disk itself.

Whilst the etiology of disk degeneration is not fully understood, it is well recognized that the single most important factor influencing the presence, distribution, and severity of disk degeneration is familial influence.[20–22] The occurrence of adolescent disk disease in relatively sedentary individuals, and the striking similarities in the degree and distribution of degenerate changes in identical twins points to a strong genetic influence. Attempting then, to prove the role of environmental factors is fraught with difficulties, without controlling for genetic factors. The role of cigarette smoking in the etiology of degeneration, has been shown in identical twins, where one smoked and the other didn't.[23] There was an 18% greater degree of disk degeneration among the smokers. Perhaps not surprisingly there is a lack of such rigorously genetically controlled studies of the role of athletic activity in the etiology of degeneration.

Whilst it seems clear that disk degeneration, as diagnosed by disk space narrowing and dehydration, is more common in athletes, the role of athletic activity in damaging the annulus is less certain. It is certainly a general public misconception that trauma can lead to disk herniation, or a "slipped disk," a view also expressed in the medical literature.[24,25] It is, however, the experience of spinal surgeons that no more than 14% of patients with disk herniation coming to surgery give a history of physical activity or trauma.[26] An athlete, training for high-level sporting activity inevitably spends a great deal of time devoted to their activity, and it is understandable that they should link the development of symptoms with their activity. Disk herniation is a common finding in asymptomatic individuals,[9,27] so not only may a disk herniation not be caused by the athletic activity, it may well not be responsible for the athlete's symptoms.

The concept that repetitive trauma to the disk could lead to disk degeneration and disk herniation is based on the empirical notion that the disk acts as a "shock absorber," so that the disk absorbs repeated energy applied to the spine rendering it prone to injury and herniation. Biomechanical evidence suggests that disks are not shock absorbers and do not take up any significant energy applied to the body other than the sort of loads that might equate with the normal activity of daily living such as walking.[28] Other than these small quantities and frequencies, it is the spine's natural shock absorbers, the posterior spinal muscles and ligaments that absorb energy. Further biomechanical evidence suggests that when degenerate disks are loaded they do not respond by herniating.[29] In vitro, under grossly unphysiological circumstances, a few normal disks protruded under load, but degenerative disks did not behave in this manner. This was explained by the fact that degenerate disks are dehydrated and have increased fibrous tissue, making them too stiff to respond to loading by herniation.

It has been suggested that mechanical stresses to the disk can result in annular tears,[25] and in turn this weakens the annulus resulting in disk herniation. Annular tears can be seen on MR images as an area of high signal within the annulus on T2W images (Fig. 9.2.**7**). In common with many other degenerative findings on MRI they are frequently encountered in asymptomatic individuals. Jensen et al found annular tears in 14% of asymptomatic individuals.[9] Considerable interest in the annular tear has been addressed to whether or not it indicates a disk, which is painful on stress diskography, and therefore a marker for "diskogenic" back pain. Results of studies have been mixed, with some reports suggesting that the annular tear is

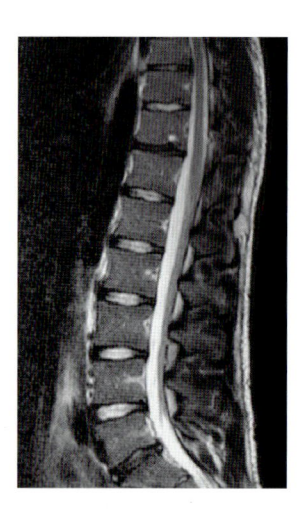

Fig. 9.2.**6** **Sagittal T2W MRI in a professional rugby player.** There is dehydration of the T11/T12 intervertebral disk as a result of herniation of the nucleus pulposus into the T11 vertebral body. The nucleus pulposus is seen as a high signal area within the vertebral body. A more classical degenerative process is affecting the L5/S1 disk.

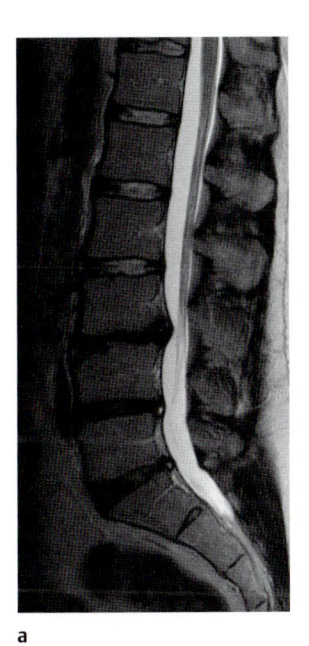

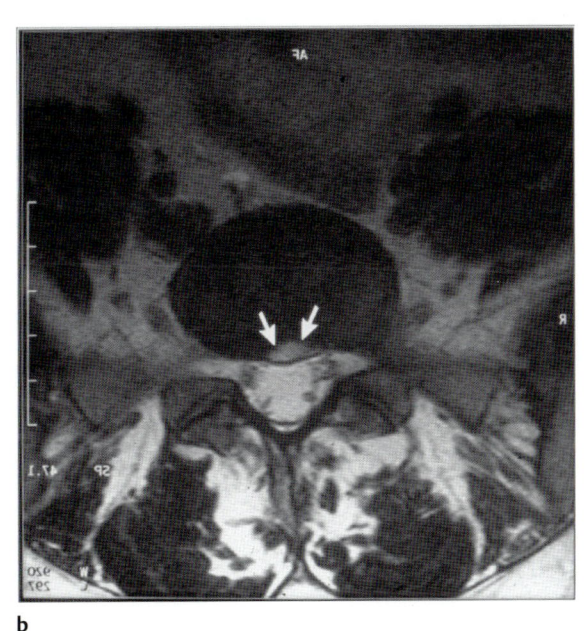

Fig. 9.2.7 Annular tear shown on a sagittal T2W MRI **a** and **b** an axial T2W MRI. There is a high signal focus within the posterior annulus (*arrows*).

associated with a positive stress test,[30-32] whilst other studies have failed to correlate the annular tear, or other signs on MRI with a stress diskogram.[33-35] Further confusion arises with different terms being applied to the same MRI abnormality, with the terms "high intensity zone," "annular fissure," and "annular tear" all being used. The term "annular tears" is a misnomer, since it implies a traumatic etiology. Patients with lower back pain and annular tears do not present with a particular set of symptoms, and they do not report an acute onset of symptoms, as one would expect with a traumatic etiology.[36] The annular tear is part of the degenerative process of the intervertebral disk so the term annular fissure is preferable, since the term fissure implies a degenerative etiology. Caution must therefore be applied in interpreting the significance of an annular tear in an athlete, and it must not be assumed that this is in anyway related to the athletic activity. As with other features of degeneration on MRI, close correlation with the patient's symptoms is essential.

Plain radiographs of the spine are often used as a first-line investigation of spinal problems, but they are not an appropriate form of investigation for the anterior spinal injuries in the athlete. The plain radiograph cannot demonstrate bone edema, and can make no assessment of how long an endplate lesion has been present. Disk space narrowing is only a crude indicator of degenerative disease. As radiographs of both the thoracic and lumbar spine would be required, this constitutes a considerable radiation dose, and serial films to document progression of the lesions and developing kyphosis worsens this burden. MRI, then, is the investigation of choice, both for the initial assessment and in the follow-up of progression. Sequences should include sagittal T1W and sagittal T2W fat saturation, or STIR, sequences of the whole thoracic and lumbar spine. The T1W sequence gives good anatomical detail of the endplate lesion, and the fat-saturated T2W sequence is sensitive to bone edema. In many ways MRI is an overly sensitive investigation and the demonstration of degenerative diseases should be assessed with caution, and closely correlated with the patient's symptoms. The assessment of spinal pain in the adolescent athlete is simplified, as young people usually have a constitutional cause for spinal pain, other than mechanical/degenerative causes. The demonstration of anterior endplate lesions, particularly in the presence of bone edema, is a strong indicator that the athlete should modify their activity, or risk the development of a lifelong kyphotic deformity.

References

1. Bogduk N. *Clinical Anatomy of the Lumbar Spine and Sacrum.* Churchill Livingstone; 1997.
2. Scheuermann HW. The classic: kyphosis dorsalis juvenilis. *Clin Orthop.* 1977;128:5–7.
3. Halal F, Gledhill RB, Fraser C. Dominant inheritance of Scheuermann's juvenile kyphosis. *Am J Dis Child.* 1978;132(11):1105–1107.
4. McKenzie L, Sillence D. Familial Scheuermann's disease: a genetic and linkage study. *J Med Genet.* 1992;29(1):41–45.
5. Alexander CJ. Scheuermann's disease; a traumatic spondylodystrophy? *Skeletal Radiol.* 1977;1:209–221.
6. Greene TL, Hensinger RN, Hunter LY. Back pain and vertebral changes simulating Scheuermann's disease. *J Pediatr Orthop.* 1985;5(1):1–7.
7. Hafner RHV. Localised osteochondritis (Scheuermann's Disease). *J Bone Joint Surg.* 1952;34B:38–40.
8. Schmorl G. Die pathologische Anatomie der Wirbelsaule. *Verh Dtsch Orthop Ges.* 1927;21:3.
9. Jensen MC, Brant-Zawadzki MN, Obuchowski N, Modic MT, Malkasian D, Ross JS. Magnetic resonance imaging of the lumbar spine in people without back pain. *N Engl J Med.* 1994;331(2):69–73.
10. Hellstrom M, Jacobsson B, Sward L, Peterson L. Radiologic abnormalities of the thoraco-lumbar spine in athletes. *Acta Radiol.* 1990;31(2):127–132.
11. Sward L, Hellstrom M, Jacobsson B, Nyman R, Peterson L. Disc degeneration and associated abnormalities of the spine in elite gymnasts. A magnetic resonance imaging study. *Spine.* 1991;16(4):437–443.

12. McCall IW, Park WM, O'Brien JP, Seal V. Acute traumatic intraosseous disc herniation. *Spine*. 1985;10(2):134–137.
13. Sward L. The thoracolumbar spine in young elite athletes. Current concepts on the effects of physical training. *Sports Med*. 1992;13(5):357–364.
14. Sward L, Hellstrom M, Jacobsson B, Karlsson L. Vertebral ring apophysis injury in athletes. Is the etiology different in the thoracic and lumbar spine? *Am J Sports Med*. 1993;21(6):841–845.
15. Sward L, Hellstrom M, Jacobsson B, Peterson L. Back pain and radiologic changes in the thoraco-lumbar spine of athletes. *Spine*. 1990;15(2):124–129.
16. Witt I, Vestergaard A, Rosenklint A. A comparative analysis of X-ray findings of the lumbar spine in patients with and without lumbar pain. *Spine*. 1984;9(3):298–300.
17. La Rocca H, Macnab I. Value of pre-employment radiographic assessment of the lumbar spine. *Can Med Assoc J*. 1969;101(7):49–54.
18. Ogon M, Riedl-Huter C, Sterzinger W, Krismer M, Spratt KF, Wimmer C. Radiologic abnormalities and low back pain in elite skiers. *Clin Orthop*. 2001(390):151–162.
19. Harreby M, Neergaard K, Hesselsoe G, Kjer J. Are radiologic changes in the thoracic and lumbar spine of adolescents risk factors for low back pain in adults? A 25-year prospective cohort study of 640 school children. *Spine*. 1995;20(21):2298–2302.
20. Videman T, Battie MC. The influence of occupation on lumbar degeneration. *Spine*. 1999;24(11):1164–1168.
21. Battie MC, Videman T, Gibbons LE, Fisher LD, Manninen H, Gill K. 1995 Volvo Award in clinical sciences. Determinants of lumbar disc degeneration. A study relating lifetime exposures and magnetic resonance imaging findings in identical twins. *Spine*. 1995;20(24):2601–2612.
22. Battie MC, Haynor DR, Fisher LD, Gill K, Gibbons LE, Videman T. Similarities in degenerative findings on magnetic resonance images of the lumbar spines of identical twins. *J Bone Joint Surg Am*. 1995;77(11):1662–1670.
23. Battie MC, Videman T, Gill K, Moneta GB, Nyman R, Kaprio J, et al. 1991 Volvo Award in clinical sciences. Smoking and lumbar intervertebral disc degeneration: an MRI study of identical twins. *Spine*. 1991;16(9):1015–1021.
24. Commandre FA, Argenson C, Fornaris E, Aboulker C, De Peretti F, Zakarian H. Lumbar spine, sport and actual treatment. *J Sports Med Phys Fitness*. 1991;31(2):129–134.
25. Hadjipavlou AG, Simmons JW, Pope MH, Necessary JT, Goel VK. Pathomechanics and clinical relevance of disc degeneration and annular tear: a point-of-view review. *Am J Orthop*. 1999;28(10):561–571.
26. Naylor A. Late results of laminectomy for lumbar disc prolapse. A review after ten to twenty-five years. *J Bone Joint Surg (Br)*. 1974;56(1):17–29.
27. Boden SD, Davis DO, Dina TS, Patronas NJ, Wiesel SW. Abnormal magnetic-resonance scans of the lumbar spine in asymptomatic subjects. A prospective investigation. *J Bone Joint Surg (Am)*. 1990;72(3):403–408.
28. Smeathers JE. Shocking news about discs. *Curr Orthop*. 1994;8:45–48.
29. Adams MA, Dolan P. Recent advances in lumbar spinal mechanics and their clinical significance. *Clin Biomech*. 1995;10(1):3–19.
30. Aprill C, Bogduk N. High-intensity zone: a diagnostic sign of painful lumbar disc on magnetic resonance imaging. *Br J Radiol*. 1992;65(773):361–369.
31. Schellhas KP, Pollei SR, Gundry CR, Heithoff KB. Lumbar disc high-intensity zone. Correlation of magnetic resonance imaging and discography. *Spine*. 1996;21(1):79–86.
32. Saifuddin A, Braithwaite I, White J, Taylor BA, Renton P. The value of lumbar spine magnetic resonance imaging in the demonstration of anular tears. *Spine*. 1998;23(4):453–457.
33. Ricketson R, Simmons JW, Hauser BO. The prolapsed intervertebral disc. The high-intensity zone with discography correlation. *Spine*. 1996;21(23):2758–2762.
34. Buirski G, Silberstein M. The symptomatic lumbar disc in patients with low-back pain. Magnetic resonance imaging appearances in both a symptomatic and control population. *Spine*. 1993;18(13):1808–1811.
35. Horton WC, Daftari TK. Which disc as visualized by magnetic resonance imaging is actually a source of pain? A correlation between magnetic resonance imaging and discography. *Spine*. 1992;17(6 Suppl):164–171.
36. Rankine JJ, Gill KP, Hutchinson CE, Ross ER, Williamson JB. The clinical significance of the high-intensity zone on lumbar spine magnetic resonance imaging. *Spine*. 1999;24(18):1913–1919.

10 The Rigid Spine

P. H. Lander

Introduction

The spinal motion segment consists of the diskovertebral joint and the zygapophyseal joints of two adjacent vertebrae and their connecting ligamentous tissues. Each motion segment has six degrees of freedom of movement and rotation,[1] and restriction of this motion will alter the biomechanical transmission of compressive, tensile, and rotational forces across the spine. Disorders with progressive ankylosis of the motion segments restrict normal compliance and predispose the rigid spine to fractures with a higher incidence of neurological complications than in the normal population.[2,3] Ankylosing spondylitis (AS) and disseminated idiopathic skeletal hyperostosis (DISH) are the most common acquired etiologies of the rigid spine.[4,5] Congenital failures of segmentation in the spine and operative spinal fusion also contribute to an increased susceptibility to fracture.[2,6]

Ankylosing Spondylitis

Ankylosing spondylitis begins with sacroiliitis, enthesopathic inflammation, and formation of syndesmophytes or thin vertical ossifications within the outer annulus fibrosis at the diskovertebral junction. There is progressive calcification and ossification of the posterior ligaments and the capsule of the facet joints, predominately involving the interspinous and supraspinous ligaments within multiple motion segments of the spine. The thoracic and lumbar spine are typically affected earlier than the cervical spine,[4] however, cervical ankylosis is reported to develop in 75% of patients whose disease duration is 16 years or greater.[7] The prevalence of AS is estimated to be approximately 1–2% of the population.[4]

Disseminated Idiopathic Skeletal Hyperostosis

The prevalence of DISH has been estimated to be 25% in men over 50 years of age, 35% in men over the age of 70, and 15% in women over 50 years of age.[8] Fractures in patients with DISH are consequently more commonly seen than in patients with AS.

The radiological diagnosis of DISH includes flowing ossification or calcification across the anterolateral aspect of four or more contiguous vertebral bodies in the absence of extensive degenerative diskopathy (such as vacuum gas, significant loss of disk height or marginal body sclerosis), the absence of apophyseal joint ankylosis and erosion, or intraarticular osseous fusion of the sacroiliac joints. Involvement of the mid and lower thoracic spine is most frequent, followed by the upper lumbar spine and the mid and lower cervical spine.[5] Although the diagnostic criteria requires ankylosis across three consecutive disk spaces, enthesopathic ossification may involve less than four contiguous vertebral bodies and in some patients, the features of both AS and DISH in the spine may coexist.

While extensive ossification within adjacent motion segments may be present throughout the spine in both AS and DISH there are differences in the anatomical site of ligament ossification as well the extent of extraosseous enthesopathic ossification. As the syndesmophytes of AS become more extensive, a thin continuous undulating contour or bamboo spine is formed. There is progressive ossification of the posterior ligaments including the ligamentum flavum and the capsule of the apophyseal joints with ankylosis of the facet joints in more advanced AS.[4]

The apophyseal joints are uninvolved with DISH, and ankylosis of the ligamentum flavum and supraspinous ligaments is less commonly seen. Anterior longitudinal ligament and anterolateral paravertebral calcifications or ossifications are generally thicker and may be up to 20 mm thick in the thoracic and lumbar spine and 12 mm in the cervical spine in DISH. Ossification of the posterior longitudinal ligament (OPLL) of the cervical spine may present in patients with DISH, and is less frequently seen in the thoracic spine.[5] OPLL is uncommon in AS, although quadriplegia has been described as a complication of cervical trauma with this combination.[9]

Mechanisms and Imaging Techniques

In the presence of multi-segmental ankylosis, the action of compressive, tensile, and shear forces on the spine resembles an extended lever arm of a long bone of the appendicular skeleton.[10] These injuries cause shearing, axial, or oblique transverse fractures with failure in tension of the ossified ligaments and disk, or across the vertebral body with an associated fracture of the posterior column. Fractures are distracted ante-

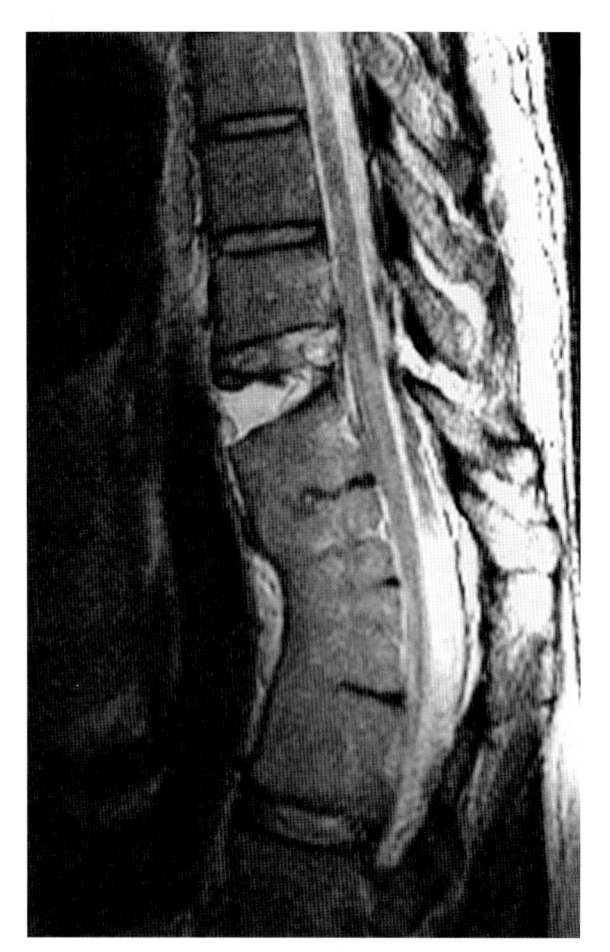

Fig. 10.1 **Transverse fracture within a congenital thoracic anterior nonsegmented bar in a 26-year-old man involved in a nonconstrained motor vehicle accident.** The image shows a sagittal T2W MRI of the thoracic spine. There is increased signal in a transverse fracture of the body of T9 subjacent to the T8–T9 disk within a congenital nonsegmented bar involving T9–T12. The disruption of the posterior ligaments at T8–T9 and anterior widening of the fracture indicate an extension tensile injury.

riorly with an extension injury, or posteriorly with a flexion injury. Since the nucleus pulposus is frequently preserved, a herniation of the nucleus pulposus with fractures traversing the disk may cause nonosseous cord compression. Long segments of ankylosis with AS or DISH renders the spine more prone to fracture, especially in the presence osteoporosis. While a high-velocity traumatic impact frequently results in significant injury, there is commonly a history of relatively low-velocity impact or minor trauma, such as a fall from an upright or seated position at ground level or a history of a glancing blow to the head. New onset of neck, thoracic, or lower back pain even in the absence of any trauma should prompt an imaging investigation for an insufficiency fracture.[10,11]

Conventional radiographs are the first imaging modality performed on patients sustaining minor trauma or complaining of neck pain. However, the lower cervical and cervicothoracic spine are frequently obscured due to the overlying shoulders, and the lack of mobility and often exaggerated cervicothoracic kyphosis limits the usefulness of the swimmers lateral projection. Oblique projections, however, may demonstrate a fracture across the posterior arch. Severe osteoporosis, ossification of the ligaments, and annulus fibrosus distorting the landmarks may delay the diagnosis of bone injury in AS. The enthesopathy in DISH also leads to extensive ossification and calcification that obscures the normal vertebral anatomy. The suspicion of any discontinuity of the anterior vertebral cortex or ossified anterior longitudinal ligament or hyperostosis, particularly in the presence of widening of a portion, or all of the adjacent disk space, should prompt a search for a fracture in the posterior cortex of the vertebral body and the corresponding posterior arch and ossified ligamentous structures.

Cross-sectional imaging is increasingly utilized to corroborate and define the extent of the injury. Since as many as 40% of patients sustaining a cervical spine fracture have been reported to have multiple fractures within the cervical spine or the thoracic spine, additional imaging of the entire spine at presentation is essential.[11] Patients with a severe kyphosis and a transverse fracture are at risk of further neurological injury when placed supine on a spinal board or a radiographic table by causing hyperextension of the fracture, and should be supported in a flexed position.[12]

The development of multi-channel/multi-detector spiral or helical CT scans has markedly improved the visualization of subtle fractures, and these scans have become routine in the assessment of the cervical thoracic junction when overlapping shoulder and other soft tissue densities preclude adequate visualization. Multi-planar high-resolution sagittal and coronal reformatted imaging is especially useful in demonstrating fractures that may be poorly seen in the axial transverse plane and has largely supplanted tomography.[13–15]

Multi-detector spiral CT scans with thin axial collimation and overlapping reconstruction increments of half a slice thickness allow post-processing of high-resolution sagittal and coronal reformatted images that provide excellent bone detail in all planes of the cervical spine from the occiput through the upper thoracic spine. Evaluation of the thoracic and lumbar spine with high-resolution sagittal and coronal reformatted images may also obviate the need for conventional radiographs and CT scans have the advantage of scanning patients with a prominent thoracic kyphosis in the lateral decubitus position.[14,15]

MRI will demonstrate fractures, bone marrow hemorrhage, and contusion and is especially useful in detecting occult unsuspected fractures remote to the primary injury (Fig. 10.1). MRI is most sensitive in the detection of spinal cord contusion, intramedullary hematoma, and compression of the cord from an epidural hematoma, or displaced disk or bone fragments and is the preferred exam if neurological deficit is suspected.[16,17]

A mid-line sagittal STIR imaging series with a large field of view encompassing the cervical and upper thoracic spine in one sequence and the lower thoracic and lumbar spine on a second sequence has been advocated as a minimum screening MRI exam to detect the presence of intraosseous or intraspinal hemorrhage consequent to a fracture and to search for a second occult fracture.[17,18] MRI examination sequences vary with institutional preference and also may include sagittal T1W spin-echo, sagittal T2W fast spin-echo, sagittal inversion recovery (STIR), and sagittal gradient-echo with axial T1W spin-echo, T2W fast spin-echo, and gradient sequence images as well as sagittal and axial T1W fat-suppressed imaging following intravenous gadolinium.

Cervical Spine Injuries

Congenital failure of segmentation of one or more segments such as in the Klippel–Feil syndrome, or the presence of a previous surgical fusion, particularly in the cervical spine, transfers forces to an adjacent mobile spinal motion segment and predisposes these segments to clinical injury (Fig. 10.2).[2,6]

Patients with Klippel–Feil syndrome have been categorized into three main types:
- Type 1 anomaly: the nonsegmentation or congenital fusion is present in three or more levels of the cervical or upper thoracic spine.
- Type 2 anomaly: the nonsegmentation fusion anomaly is isolated to one or two levels in the cervical spine.
- Type 3 anomaly: the cervical fusion is associated with nonsegmentation in the lower thoracic or lumber spine.

The junctional mobile segments in this disorder have been shown to be hypermobile. This excess motion and segmental overload accelerate degenerative disk disease causing disk bulge and spinal stenosis predisposing to injury of the spinal cord (Fig. 10.3).[2,6,19]

Fractures of the odontoid process were associated with a fusion of the upper cervical spine, while single-level lower cervical spine fusion was associated with unilateral facet fracture-dislocation in 20 patients with congenital or post-surgical spinal fusion in a series of 368 patients with cervical spine injury.[2]

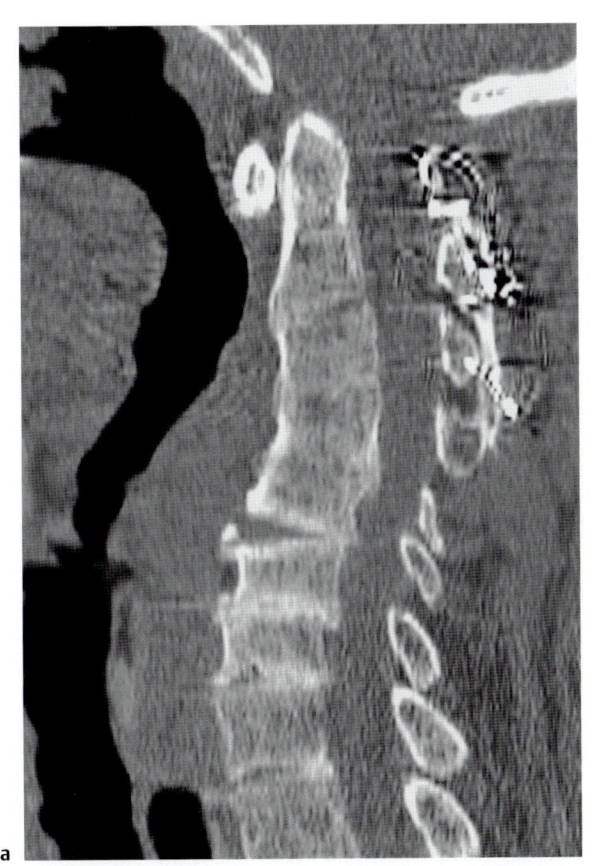

Fig. 10.2 **Disk disruption below a cervical fusion in a 73-year-old man involved in a motor vehicle accident**. A central cord syndrome was diagnosed at presentation. **a** Sagittal CT scan of the cervical spine. A mature posterior interspinous fusion with cerclage wires and secondary anterior kyphotic ankylosis is seen at C2–C5, there is also anterior widening of the C5–C6 disk. The subjacent disks are severely narrowed. **b** Sagittal STIR MR image of the cervical spine. Extensive prevertebral edema is associated with disruption of the C5–C6 annulus and anterior longitudinal ligament. Increased signal in the posterior column reflects the extension injury. Significant cord compression at C5–C6 is due to buckling of the ligamentum flavum and mild retropulsion of C5 on C6. Fluid signal within the central spinal cord reflects cord contusion. No signal abnormality was seen in the cord on T1W images. The apparent narrowing of the cord at C1 is related to a metal susceptibility artifact.

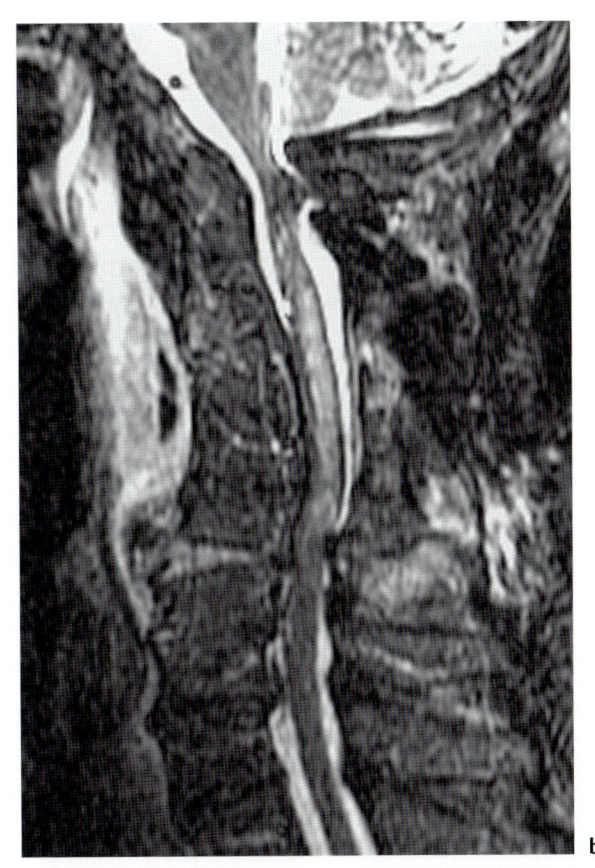

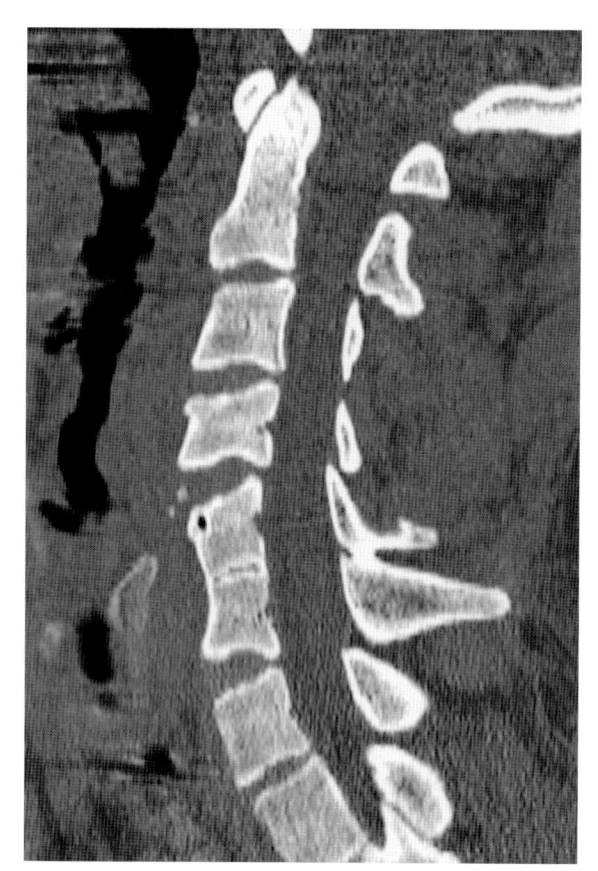

Fig. 10.3 **Congenital Klippel–Feil with a tensile anterior disk disruption of C4–C5 in a 32-year-old man following a motor vehicle accident.** Sagittal CT reformatted image of the cervical spine. Failure of segmentation of the anterior and posterior columns at C5–C6 is typical of a type 2 Klippel–Feil anomaly. Note anterior widening of the disk space at C4–C5 with tiny anterior ossified fragments, minimal posterior translation of C4 on C5, and prevertebral soft tissue swelling. A small subchondral cyst with intraosseous gas at the anterior superior border of the body of C5 is related to degenerative spondylosis at this level. Mild anterior deformity is seen in the superoanterior border of C4 due to prior trauma.

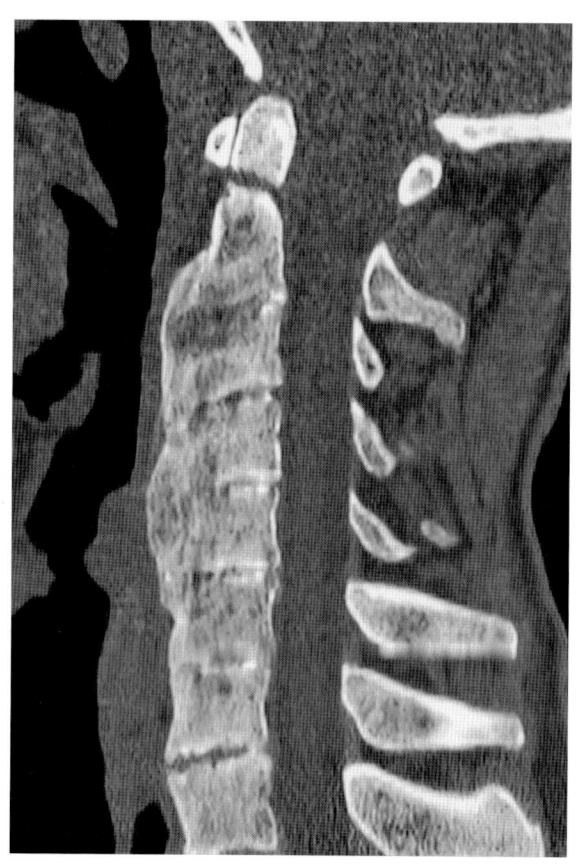

Fig. 10.4 **Type II odontoid fracture in a 59-year-old man with AS who suffered a ground level fall.** Sagittal reformatted CT of the cervical spine. A high transverse fracture of the odontoid process is seen with anterior ankylosis and disk narrowing of C2 through C7. Enthesopathic anterior vertebral ossification indicates a component of DISH. Bilateral ankylosis of the facet joints was demonstrated on other CT images.

Fractures of the cervical spine occurring in preexisting ankylosing spondylitis comprised 2% of a series of 1028 patients with cervical spine injuries.[20] The lower cervical spine and cervicothoracic junction are most commonly injured,[7,10,20] and up to 70% of cervical fractures involve segments C5–T1.[3,10,21] Fractures of the axis and the odontoid in AS have been thought to be rare.[7,22] However, a study of 31 patients with AS and spinal fractures noted 61% of the fractures involved the cervical spine, and 21% of cervical spine fractures involved the C1–C2 segments (Fig. 10.**4**).[10]

Cervical fractures are often extremely unstable because the fracture plane traverses the anterior and posterior columns with distraction and/or displacement of the fragments (Fig. 10.**5**).[7,10] An increased risk of neurological deficit is related to coexistent hemorrhage, edema, contusion or transection of the cord, cord compression due to a displaced disk or bone fragment, or spinal epidural hematoma.[3,10,11,20,21,23,24] Spinal cord injury with AS has constituted from 2% to 3.5% of patients with cervical cord injuries admitted for spinal cord injury.[3,20]

Spinal epidural hematoma and spinal cord compression complicating cervical fractures in patients with AS have a higher incidence than in patients without AS presumably related to tears of the epidural veins leading to an increased incidence of acute spinal epidural hematoma.[3,20,21] Spinal epidural hematomas are characteristically posterior to the cord and are recognized as a biconvex extradural mass with tapering well-defined borders compressing the dura and spinal cord.[25,26] Immediately following a fracture the hematoma may have increased signal on both T1W and T2W images compared to the cord.[26] They may be recognized on a CT scan as an increased density within the spinal canal compared to the spinal cord density.[25,27] Fractures traversing the disk are less likely to be associated with profound neurological deficit than

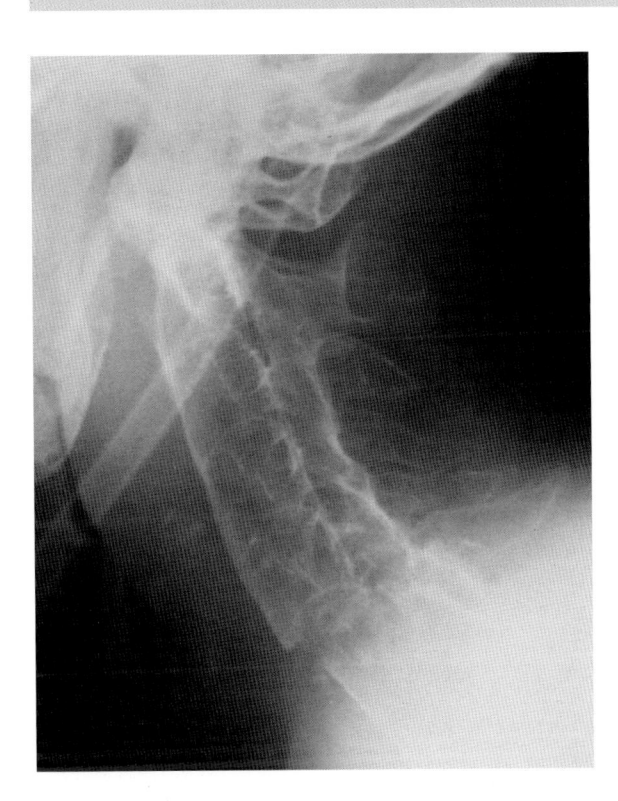

Fig. 10.**5** **Hyperextension fracture of the cervical spine in a 56-year-old man with longstanding AS who suffered quadriplegia at the time of injury.** Lateral cervical spine. Tensile disruption and diastasis of the C5–C6 disk and facet joints with fracture of the ossified ligaments and the spinous processes of C5. Note the anterior column ankylosis with syndesmophytes typical of a bamboo spine.

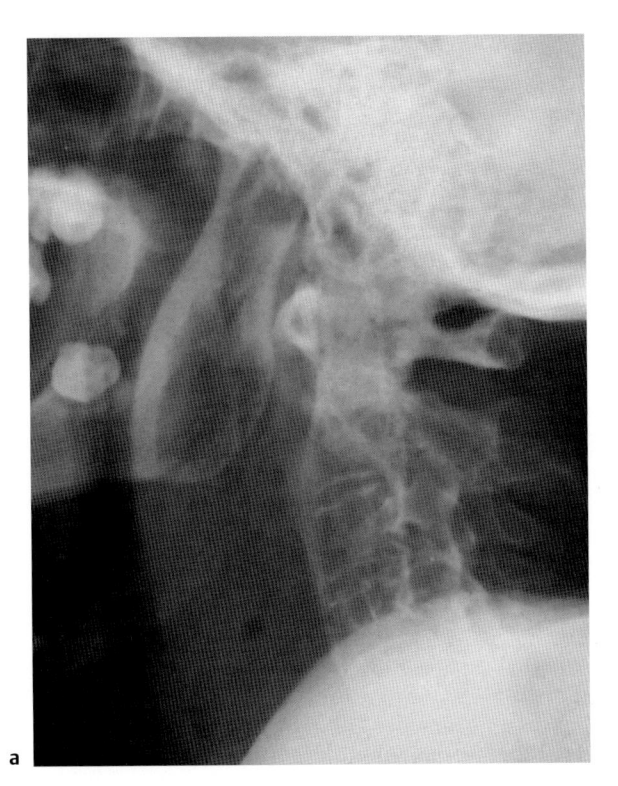

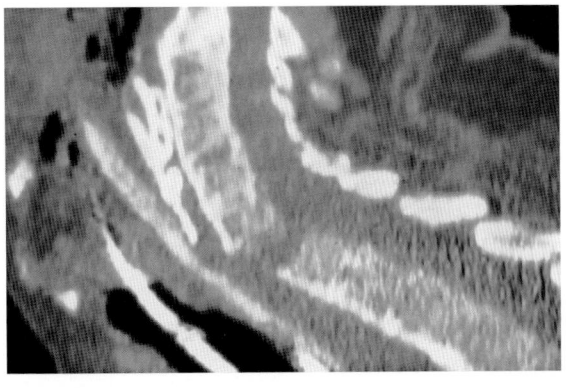

Fig. 10.**6** **Retropharyngeal abscess secondary to a fracture in the cervical spine with AS occurring in a 67-year-old man who fell and complained of dysphagia 1 week after the minor trauma. a** Lateral radiograph of the neck. A large soft tissue mass containing gas displaces the airway and pharynx anteriorly. Note the typical anterior syndesmophytes in this limited assessment of the cervical spine. **b** CT sagittal reformatted image of the cervical spine. A transverse fracture is seen at C6 with ankylosis of the spine. Retained surgical drains are in place following operative drainage of a retropharyngeal and epidural abscess. A small esophageal tear secondary to the fracture was postulated as the etiology for the abscess.

patients with AS whose fracture involves only the vertebral body of the cervical spine.[28] Injury to anterior structures such as the esophagus or trachea may occur with distraction of the anterior fracture fragments and the presence of a retropharyngeal abscess can herald an associated injury to the spine (Fig. 10.**6**).

Injuries of the cervical spine in patients with DISH, although reported less frequently than with AS, are also a consequence of ground level low-velocity injury as well as high-velocity trauma.[29,30,31] Involvement of all segments is reported, including the axis, however the lower cervical spine segments from C4 to T1 are

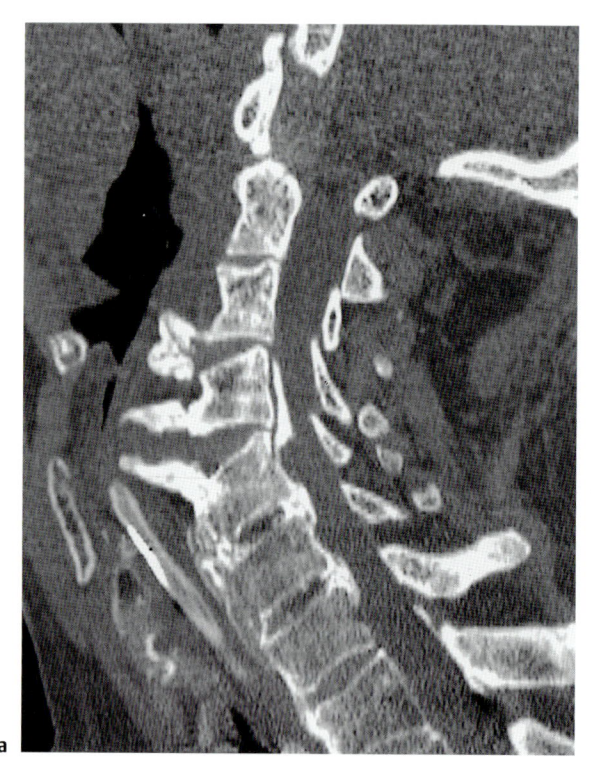

Fig. 10.7 **Hyperextension disk injury in a 77-year-old man with DISH and OPLL who fell approximately 1 m from a ladder and became quadriplegic. a** Sagittal reformatted CT scan of the cervical spine. Widening of the anterior osteophytes and disk space of C3–C4 and C4–C5 reflects an extension injury. Note the ankylosis across the anterior bodies of C5–T1 typical for DISH. Severe central stenosis is due to the thick ossification of the posterior longitudinal ligament (OPLL) minimally displaced from the adjacent posterior cortex of C4. **b** Axial CT C4–C5. Note the separation and displacement of the ossified posterior longitudinal ligament from the posterior cortex of the vertebral body.

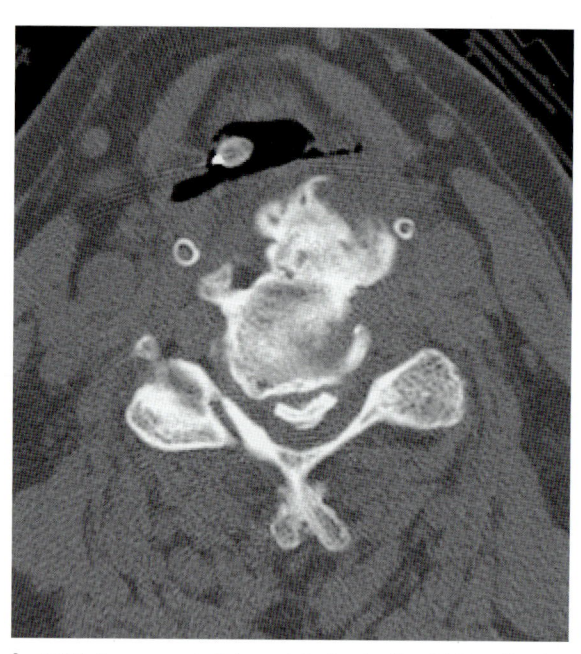

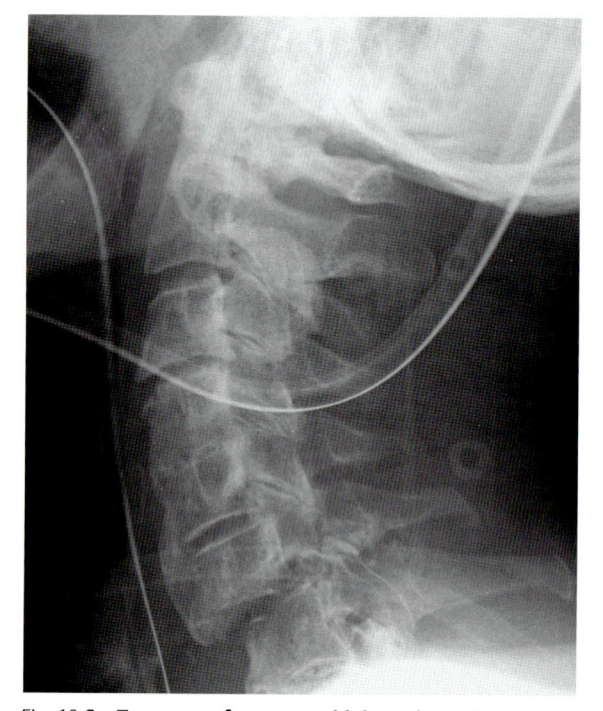

more likely to be injured.[29,30] Extension injuries occur more frequently with DISH than a flexion or shearing mechanism and usually traverse the vertebral body or the hyperostotic ossification of the anterior longitudinal ligament at the level of a disk with disruption of the disk (Fig. 10.7).[29,31] The fractures may traverse the body adjacent to the endplates, a combination of both disk and endplate, or less commonly at the mid vertebral body.[29,30] A fracture of the posterior column or disruption of the capsule and posterior ligaments can be associated with facet joint dislocation (Fig. 10.8). The fractures have been described either within the ankylosed segments or at the junction of an ankylosed segment and a motion segment.[30] Delayed diagnosis is frequent and high mortality rates have been reported ranging from 25% to 40%.[29,30]

A high incidence of neurological injury including quadriplegia and central cord syndrome whether due to trivial or high-impact trauma is reported with these injuries and spinal epidural hematoma has also been reported in a patient with DISH.[23,26,29,30]

Fig. 10.8 **Transverse fracture and bilateral interfacetal dislocation in the cervical spine of a 72-year-old man with DISH.** Image is a lateral radiograph of the cervical spine. A fracture transverses the endplate and adjacent disk at C6–C7 with bilateral facet dislocation and perched facet joints. Typical flowing anterior hyperostosis of DISH is seen anterior at C3–C7.

Thoracolumbar Spine Injuries

Thoracolumbar spine fractures complicating both ankylosing spondylitis and DISH occur frequently with ground level falls or minor trauma as well as major

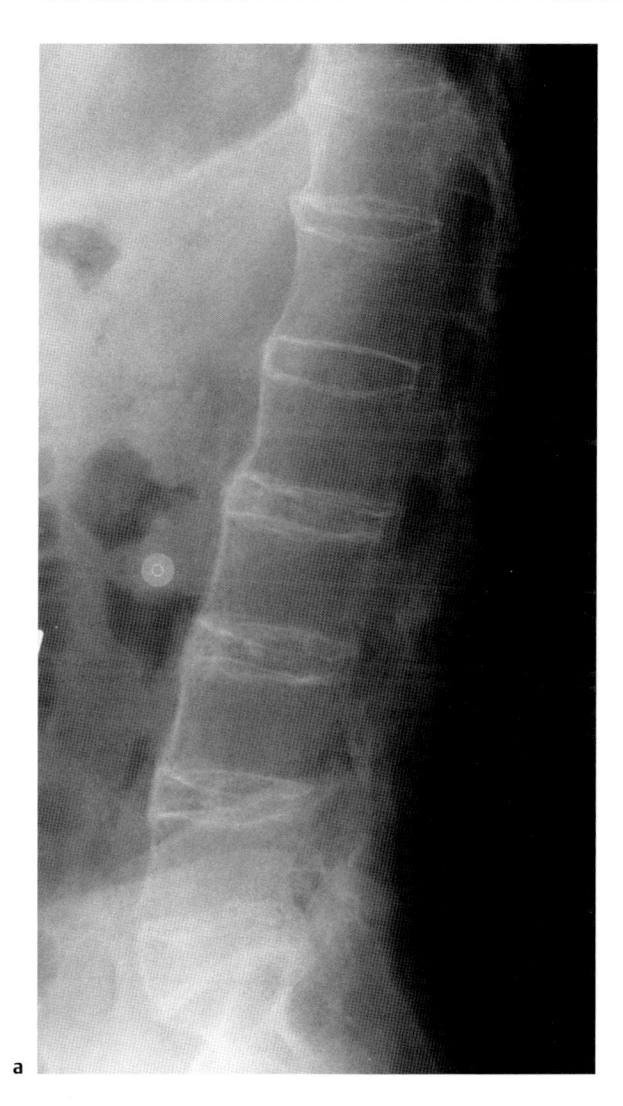

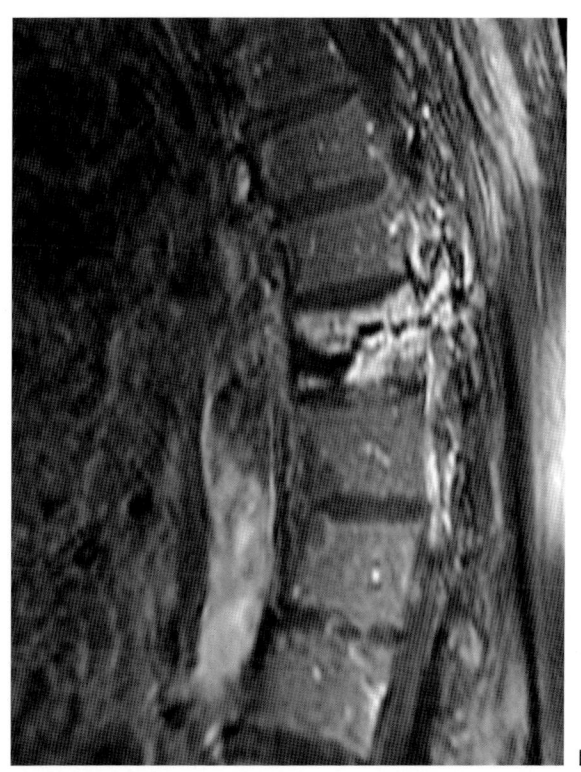

Fig. 10.**9** Transcorporal thoracic fracture in a 65-year-old man with ankylosing spondylitis involved in a minor automobile accident without neurological deficit. **a** Lateral projection of the lumbar spine. Syndesmophytes are present at multiple levels typical of ankylosing spondylitis. **b** Sagittal T1W fat-saturated MR image of the thoracic spine following intravenous gadolinium. Diffuse enhancement of the marrow of the vertebral body and pedicle of T10 demonstrates a low signal within a widened globular transverse fracture. The low signal of the fracture extends into the pedicles indicative of a tensile extensor mechanism.

trauma[32,33] (Fig. 10.**8**). The absence of compensatory motion in patients with multi-level ankylosis of the thoracic and lumbar spine increases the susceptibility of the anterior column to fracture under tension. Smaller magnitude forces are postulated to fracture the ankylosed spine due to the higher tensile stresses generated with relatively small forces in the absence of the preload absorption by normal disks and spinal ligaments.[34] Fractures in AS tend to cluster in the lower thoracic spine and the thoracolumbar junction.[33]

These injuries are typically an axial transverse disruption across the disk space, or fracture of the mid vertebral body or subjacent to an endplate due to an extension tensile force. Anterior widening of the disk and/or slight anterior malalignment designates an extension injury, and is associated with fractures of the posterior column or facet joint subluxation at the same level, or at a level above or below the anterior column fracture (Fig. 10.**9**).[35,36] An oblique fracture of the vertebra indicates a shearing force across the anterior column. A flexion compression injury in the ankylosed spine with tensile distraction of the posterior column is less commonly seen. These injuries present as an anterior wedge compression fracture with a posterior column distraction injury such as facet dislocation. The displacement of the disk or fracture fragments is in the anteroposterior plane usually with avulsion fractures of the adjacent bridging bone of the ossified anterior longitudinal ligament and interspinous ligaments. Neurological deficits are frequent and have been recorded in greater than 50% of patients sustaining an injury.[32,33] Traumatic rupture of the aorta is a rare complication of a tensile distraction fracture with the aorta adherent to the ossified anterior longitudinal ligament.[37] Flexion fracture deformities of the vertebra in the thoracic and lumbar spine are more frequent in patients with AS prior to extensive ankylosis and have been associated with disease-induced osteoporosis.[38]

Fractures of the thoracic and lumbar spine in patients with ankylosing spondylitis are more frequently transdiskal than transvertebral with a greater incidence of neurological complications noted in transvertebral fractures.[35,39]

Transdiskal and transcorporeal fractures have also been recorded in patients with DISH. Transcorporeal fractures have been associated with increased, decreased or unchanged anterior vertebral body height and osteolysis of the medullary trabeculae on

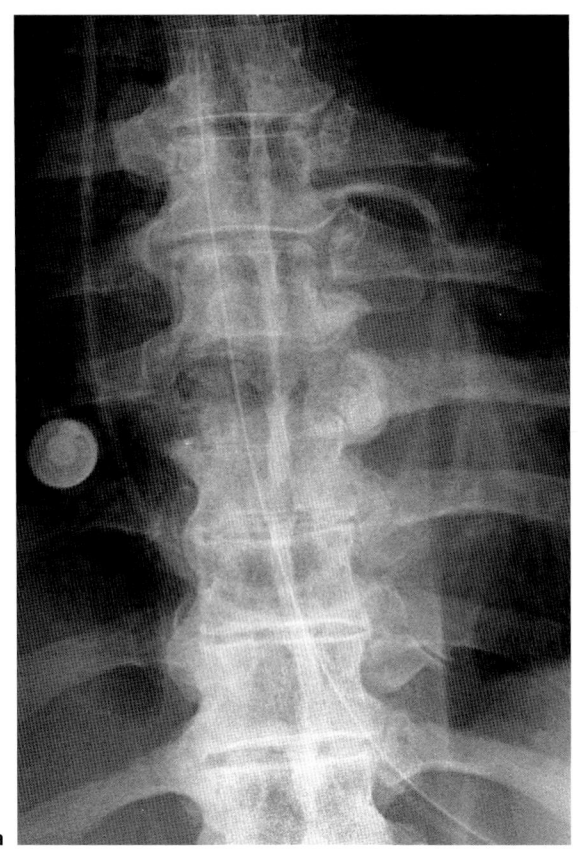

Fig. 10.**10 Transverse fracture of the thoracic spine with DISH in a 52-year-old man involved in a MVA with paraplegia. a** AP radiograph of the thoracic spine. Diffuse flowing hyperostosis across multiple disk spaces is typical of DISH. A wide transverse radiolucency is projected over the body and the pedicles of T7 (*arrow*). **b** CT reformatted parasagittal image. An extension injury through the anterior column has resulted in anterior disk widening and tensile fractures across the anterior hyperostosis of T6–T7. Note the gas within the disk from the adjacent lung herniation into the fracture and widening of the apophyseal joint.

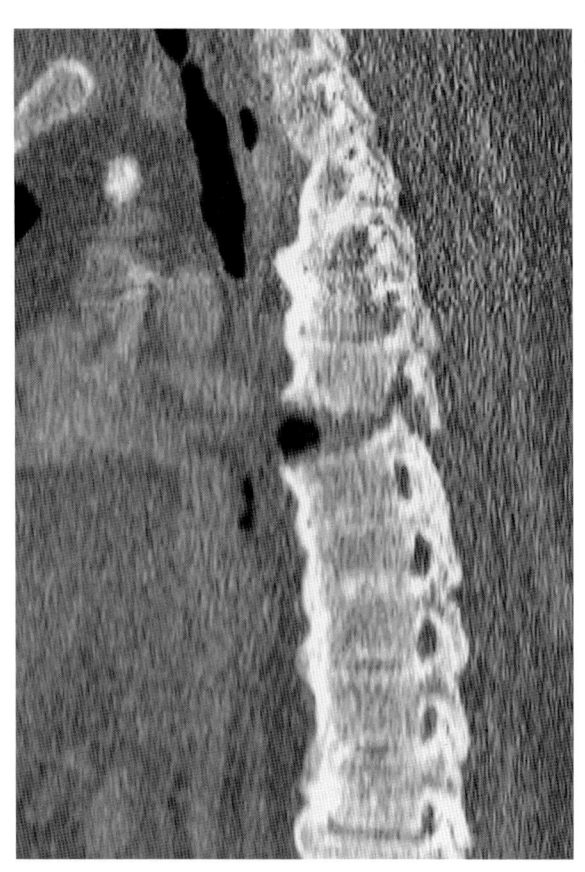

radiographs and CT scans. Anterior or lateral translation at the fracture or disk as well as widening of the anterior disk or anterior vertebral body typical of an extension mechanism is observed associated with posterior column fractures, posterior ligament complex disruption, and facet dislocation (Fig. 10.**10**).[32]

New onset of thoracic and low back pain, regardless of the absence of a history of trauma or the severity of trauma, requires imaging with conventional radiographs. The absence of a demonstrable fracture, however, should prompt further cross-sectional imaging with multi-detector CT scans since conventional radiographs alone may be insufficient to visualize an undisplaced fracture, particularly in the presence of severe osteoporosis. MRI demonstration of bone marrow contusion or hemorrhage on water-sensitive sequences such as STIR or T2W fat saturation are usually diagnostic for bone injury and may demonstrate ligamentous disruption as well as occult fractures at levels remote from the primary injury.[17,18] MRI is essential for the demonstration of spinal cord compression or contusion. Radionuclide bone scans are a useful screening imaging modality to direct cross-section imaging.[41]

MRI findings of fractures in the thoracolumbar spine in patients with AS demonstrate a low signal on T1W images in fractures of the body and levels of transdiskal disruption and the adjacent medulla and a variably high or low signal on T2W images of both anterior and posterior column fractures. Disruption of the calcified anterior longitudinal ligament is frequent and is seen as a step-like disruption of the anterior vertebral body low signal with or without abnormal translation. Variable enhancement of both the anterior and posterior column fractures is seen following intravenous gadolinium (Fig. 10.**9**).[24,39,42]

Fractures of the thoracolumbar spine in patients with DISH demonstrate a low to intermediate signal on T1W images and a high signal on T2W images within the vertebral body. This intravertebral fluid-like signal has been described as a sharp-edged defined triangular shape with the base at the anterior body, which does not enhance following intravenous gadolinium administration. It is postulated that the unusual configuration of this fluid signal is due to a hematoma accumulating within the tensile distracted fragments, or to the presence of post-traumatic osteolysis and early pseudoarthrosis with bone necrosis and repair. Differ-

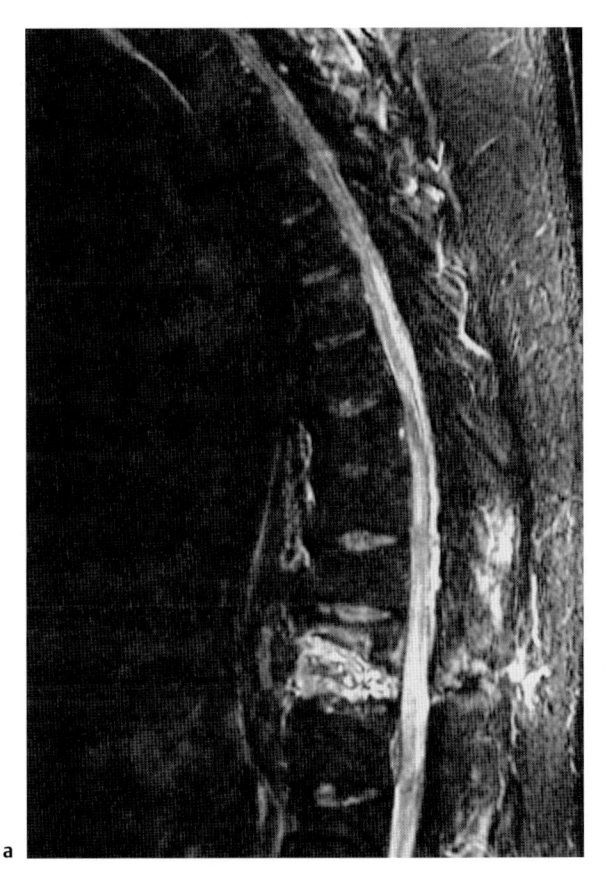

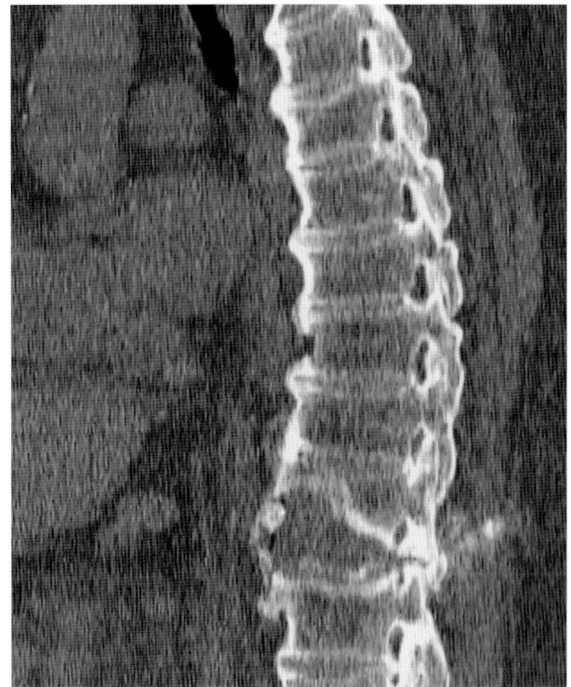

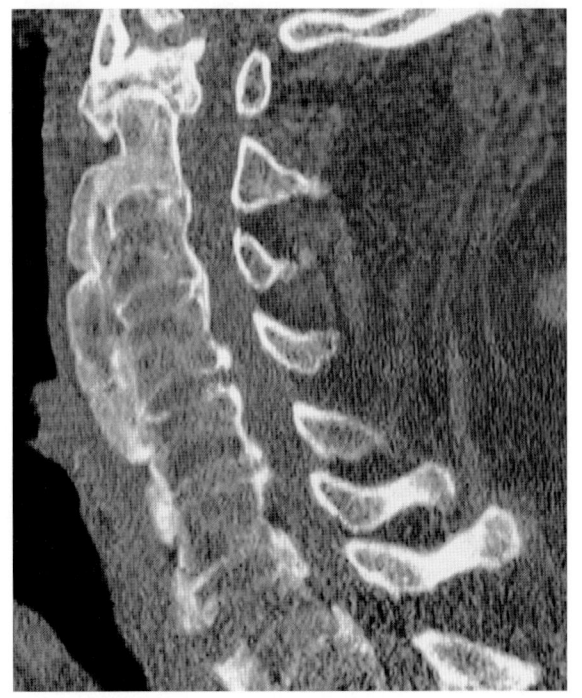

Fig. 10.11 Pseudoarthrosis of the thoracic spine with a transverse fracture of the cervical spine in a 49-year-old man with DISH subsequent to a ground level fall. a Sagittal STIR sequence of the cervicothoracic spine. The increased heterogeneous signal within a wedge-shaped pseudoarthrosis at T11 is associated with an acute transverse fracture of the body of C7 with a prevertebral hematoma. No enhancement of the pseudoarthrosis was seen following intravenous gadolinium. Note the increased signal within the posterior arch of T11. **b** Sagittal reformatted CT of the thoracic spine. A wedge-shaped pseudoarthrosis with sclerotic margins is seen within the body of T11. A fracture was seen in the posterior arch at T11. **c** Sagittal reformatted CT of the cervical spine. Extensive anterior hyperostosis typical of DISH is seen with a transverse fracture of the body of C7.

entiation from tumor necrosis or osteomyelitis is aided by abnormal signal intensities in or adjacent to the posterior column structures due to the presence of fractures in the posterior column or facet dislocation (Fig. 10.11).[32]

Pseudoarthrosis can be seen in AS and DISH and is thought to be a complication of a stress (insufficiency or fatigue type) or minor traumatic transverse fracture across the ankylosed disk or within the vertebral body and the posterior column structures. The rigidity of the adjacent ankylosed segments concentrates flexion and extension forces at the fracture. Persistent motion across the fracture causes a failure of healing and nonunion.[2,32] Another postulated mechanism is a failure of ankylosis across a disk between adjacent ankylosed segments or at the junction between mobile and nonmobile segments that leads to increased stresses and motion at the disk with the development of intradiskal tears and an accelerated disk spondylosis associated with persistent motion and hypertrophy of the facet

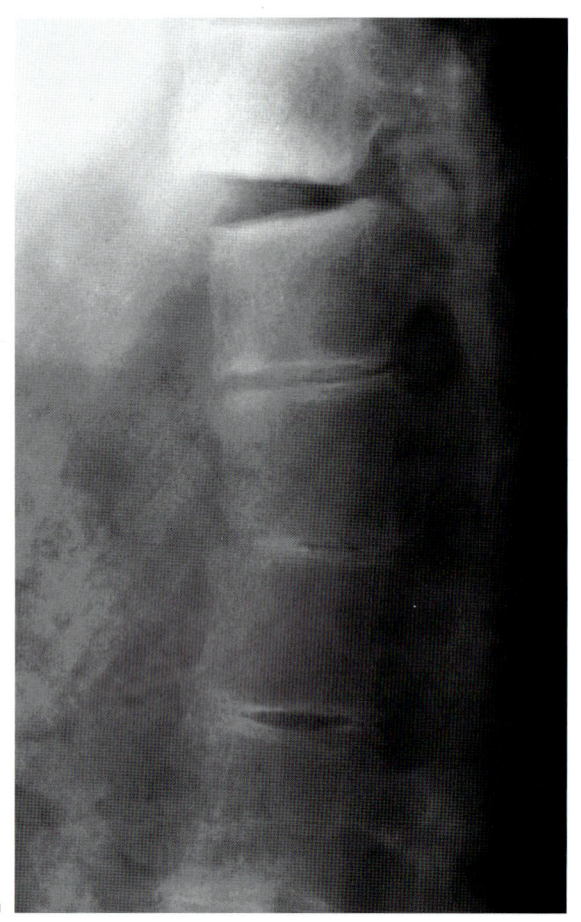

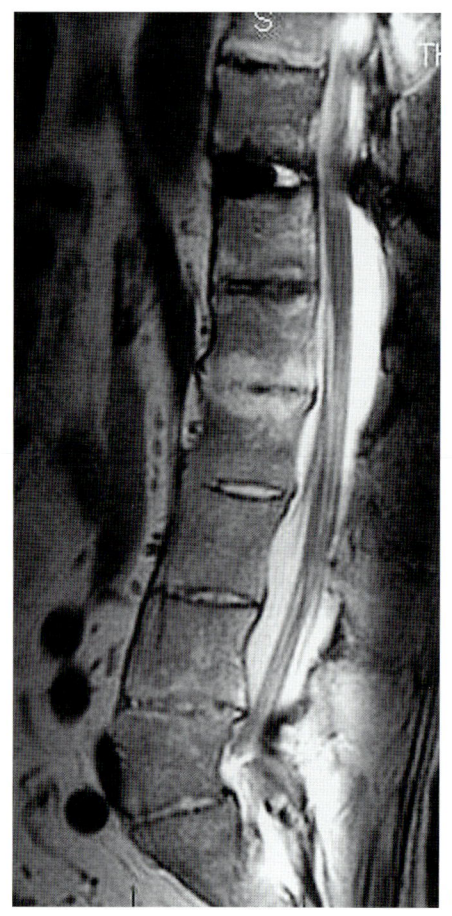

Fig. 10.**12** **Pseudoarthrosis within the thoracolumbar junction in longstanding AS in a 62-year-old man with increasing back pain.** **a** Lateral radiograph of the lumbar spine. A nonankylosed T11–T12 segment with sclerotic margins and intradiskal gas is seen within the lumbar spine. Note the anterior translation of T11. Typical syndesmophytes are present in the distal segments. **b** Sagittal T2W MRI of the lumbar spine. Intradiskal T11–T12 decreased signal anteriorly noted due to susceptibility artifact from intradiskal gas. There is an increased fluid signal posteriorly in this disk pseudoarthrosis. Diffuse disk narrowing and bridging syndesmophytes are present in the other segments. Thecal sac stenosis at T11–T12 and L4–L5 is also present.

joints.[32,43] Other theories include an inflammatory reaction with disk necrosis and proliferation of granulation tissue at the diskovertebral junction.[44]

Pseudoarthrosis occurs almost exclusively in patients with advanced ankylosis. Conventional radiographs and CT scans demonstrate a well-defined radiolucent defect traversing the ankylosed spinal vertebral body or disk within adjacent granulation tissue and typically the development of reactive sclerotic borders at the site of the nonunion or disk degeneration (Fig. 10.**12**).[35,43,45] The CT scan is more sensitive in demonstrating a transverse fracture of the posterior elements or nonankylosed facet joints at the level of the pseudoarthrosis.[45] The MRI appearance of pseudoarthrosis is widening or cavity-like spaces of the fracture lines with a low or intermediate T1W signal and a high or low T2W signal anteriorly.[39] The reparative process leads to fibrovascular tissue proliferation from the adjacent bone marrow and replacement of the fracture or disk with fibrous tissue or cartilage. Fractures of the posterior elements are less frequently seen on MR imaging,[42] but may be associated with replacement of the normal marrow signal with a low T1W and high T2W signal intensity.[32,39]

Early in the development of the pseudoarthrosis differentiation from an acute fracture may be difficult based only on conventional radiographs or the CT scan. Acute injuries typically present with a low signal on T1W sequences and a high signal on T2W images within the fracture line and adjacent bone marrow. However, in a recent study of fractures in AS the fracture site was noted to be low signal on T1W and high signal on T2W images in 70% of patients,[39] while a low T1W signal and low T2W signal was seen in 30% of the patients. The appearance of posttraumatic osteolysis and pseudoarthrosis may mimic or be mistaken for a tumor, infective spondylodiskitis, or neuropathy particularly in association with a widening of the disk or fracture.[32,46,47]

Acknowledgement

Joel Cure, M.D., for the contribution of case material.

References

1. White AA, Panjabi MM. Kinematics of the Spine. In: White AA, Panjabi MM, eds. *Clinical Biomechanics of the Spine*, 2nd ed. Philadelphia, PA: JB Lippincott Co; 1990:86–125.
2. MacMillillan M, Stauffer ES. Traumatic instability in the previously fused cervical spine. *J Spinal Disord*. 1991;4(4):449–454.
3. Tico N, Ramon S, Garcia-Ortun F, Ramirez L, Castello T, Garcia-Fernandez L, Lience E. Traumatic spinal cord injury complicating ankylosing spondylitis. *Spinal Cord*. 1998;36(5):349–352.
4. Resnick D. Ankylosing Spondylitis. In: Resnick D, ed. *Diagnosis of Bone and Joint Disorders*, 4th ed. Philadelphia, PA: W. B. Saunders Co; 2002:1023–1081.
5. Resnick D. Diffuse Idiopathic Skeletal Hyperostosis. In: Resnick D, ed. *Diagnosis of Bone and Joint Disorders*, 4th ed. Philadelphia, PA: W. B. Saunders Co; 2002:1476–1503.
6. Karasick D, Schweitzer ME, Vaccaro AR. The traumatized cervical spine in Klippel-Feil syndrome: imaging features. *Am J Roentgenol*. 1998;170(1):85–88.
7. Murray GC, Persellin RH. Cervical fracture complicating ankylosing spondylitis: a report of eight cases and review of the literature. *Am J Med*. 1981;70(5):1033–1041.
8. Weinfeld RM, Olson PN, Maki DD, Griffiths HJ. The prevalence of diffuse idiopathic skeletal hyperostosis (DISH) in two large American Midwest metropolitan hospital populations. *Skeletal Radiol*. 1997;26:222–225.
9. Ho EK, Leong JC. Traumatic tetraparesis: a rare neurologic complication in ankylosing spondylitis with ossification of the posterior longitudinal ligament of the cervical spine. A case report. *Spine*. 1987;12(4):403–405.
10. Olerud C, Frost A, Bring J. Spinal fractures in patients with ankylosing spondylitis. *Eur Spine J*. 1996;5(1):51–55.
11. Fox MW, Onofrio BM, Kilgore JE. Neurological complications of ankylosing spondylitis. *J Neurosurg*. 1993;78(6):871–878.
12. Moreau AP, Willcox N, Brown MF. Immobilisation of spinal fractures in patients with ankylosing spondylitis. Two case reports. *Injury*. 2003;34(5):372–373.
13. Blackmore CC, Mann Fa, Wilson AJ. Helical CT in the primary trauma evaluation of the cervical spine: an evidence-based approach. *Skeletal Radiol*. 2000;29:632–639.
14. Mann FA, Cohen WA, Linnau Kf, Hallam DK, Blackmore CC. Evidence-based approach to using CT in spinal trauma. *Eur J Radiol*. 2003;48:39–48.
15. Wintermark M, Mouhsine E, Theumann N, Mordasini P, Van Melle G, Leyvraz PF, Schnyder P. Thoracolumbar spine fractures in patients who have sustained severe trauma: depiction with multi-detector row CT. *Radiology*. 2003;227(3):681–689.
16. Cohen WA, Giauque AP, Hallam DK, Linnau KF, Mann FA. Evidence-based approach to use of MR imaging in acute spinal trauma. *Eur J Radiol*. 2003;48:49–60.
17. Finkelstein JA, Chapman JR, Mirza S. Occult vertebral fractures in ankylosing spondylitis. *Spinal Cord*. 1999;37(6):444–447.
18. Green RA, Saifuddin A. Whole spine MRI in the assessment of acute vertebral body trauma. *Skeletal Radiol*. 2004;33:129–135.
19. Hall JE, Simmons ED, Danylchuk K, Barnes PD. Instability of the cervical spine and neurological involvement in Klippel-Feil syndrome. A case report. *J Bone Joint Surg Am*. 1990;72:460–462.
20. Rowed DW. Management of cervical spinal cord injury in ankylosing spondylitis: the intervertebral disc as a cause of cord compression. *J Neurosurg*. 1992;77(2):241–246.
21. Hunter T, Dubo HI. Spinal fractures complicating ankylosing spondylitis. A long-term follow-up study. *Arthritis Rheum*. 1983;26(6):751–759.
22. Miller FH, Rogers LF. Fractures of the dens complicating ankylosing spondylitis with atlantooccipital fusion. *J Rheumatol*. 1991;18:771–774.
23. Mody GM, Charles RW, Ranchod HA, Rubin DL. Cervical spine fracture in diffuse idiopathic skeletal hyperostosis. *J Rheumatol*. 1988;15(1):129–131.
24. Karasick D, Schweitzer ME, Abidi NA, Cotler JM. Fractures of the vertebrae with spinal cord injuries in patients with ankylosing spondylitis: imaging findings. *AJR Am J Roentgenol*. 1995;165(5):1205–1208.
25. Wu CT, Lee ST. Spinal epidural hematoma and ankylosing spondylitis: case report and review of the literature. *J Trauma*. 1998;44:558–561.
26. Ng WH, Lim CC, Ng PY, Tan KK. Spinal epidural hematoma: MRI – aided diagnosis. *J Clin Neurosci*. 2003;95:92–94.
27. Van de Straete S, Demaerel P, Stockx L, Nutin B. Spinal epidural hematoma and ankylosing spondylitis. *J Belge Radiol*. 1997;80:109–110.
28. Harding JR, McCall IW, Park WM, Jones BF. Fracture of the cervical spine in ankylosing spondylitis. *Br J Radiol*. 1985;58:3–7.
29. Hendrix RW, Melany M, Miller F, Rogers LF. Fracture of the spine in patients with ankylosis due to diffuse skeletal hyperostosis: clinical and imaging findings. *AJR Am J Roentgenol*. 1994;162:899–904.
30. Paley D, Schwartz M, Cooper P, Harris WR, Levine AM. Fractures of the spine in diffuse idiopathic skeletal hyperostosis. *Clin Orthop*. 1991;267:22–32.
31. Meyer PR Jr. Diffuse idiopathic skeletal hyperostosis in the cervical spine. *Clin Orthop*. 1999;(359):49–57.
32. LeHir PX, Sautet A, Le Gars L, Zeitoun F, Tubiana JM, Arrive L, Laredo JD. Hyperextension vertebral body fractures in diffuse idiopathic skeletal hyperostosis: a cause of intravertebral fluidlike collections on MR imaging. *Am J Roentgenol*. 1999;173(6):1679–1683.
33. Hitchon PW, From AM, Brenton MD, Glaser JA, Torner JC. Fractures of the thoracolumbar spine complicating ankylosing spondylitis. *J Neurosurg*. 2002;97(2 Suppl):218–222.
34. Wade W, Saltzstein R, Maiman D. Spinal fractures complicating ankylosing spondylitis. *Arch Phys Med Rehabil*. 1989;70(5):398–401.
35. Thorngren KG, Liedberg E, Aspelin P. Fractures of the thoracic and lumbar spine in ankylosing spondylitis. *Arch Orthop Trauma Surg*. 1981;98:101–107.
36. Trent G, Armstrong GW, O'Neil J. Thoracolumbar fractures in ankylosing spondylitis. High-risk injuries. *Clin Orthop*. 1988;227:61–66.
37. Savolaine ER, Ebraheim NA, Stitgen S, Jackson WT. Aortic rupture complicating a fracture of an ankylosed thoracic spine. A case report. *Clin Orthop*. 1991;(272):136–140.
38. Mitra D, Elvins DM, Speden DJ, Collins AJ. The prevalence of vertebral fractures in mild ankylosing spondylitis and their relationship to bone mineral density. *Rheumatology (Oxford)*. 2000;39(1):85–89.
39. Shih TT, Chen PQ, Li YW, Hsu CY. Spinal fractures and pseudoarthrosis complicating ankylosing spondylitis: MRI manifestation and clinical significance. *J Comput Assist Tomogr*. 2001;25(2):164–170.
40. Burkus JK, Denis F. Hyperextension injuries of the thoracic spine in diffuse idiopathic skeletal hyperostosis. Report of four cases. *J Bone Joint Surg Am*. 1994;76(2):237–243.
41. Resnick D, Williamson S, Alazraki N. Focal spinal abnormalities on bone scans in ankylosing spondylitis: a clue to the presence of fracture of pseudarthrosis. *Clin Nucl Med*. 1981;6(5):213–217.
42. Goldberg AL, Keaton NL, Rothfus WE, Daffner RH. Ankylosing spondylitis complicated by trauma: MR findings correlated with plain radiographs and CT. *Skeletal Radiol*. 1993;22(5):333–336.
43. Quagliano PV, Hayes CW, Palmer WE. Vertebral pseudoarthrosis associated with diffuse idiopathic skeletal hyperostosis. *Skeletal Radiol*. 1994;23(5):353–355.
44. Wu PC, Fang D, Ho EK, Leong JC. The pathogenisis of extensive discovertebral destruction in ankylosing spondylitis. *Clin Orthop*. 1988;(230):154–161.
45. Chan FL, Ho EK, Chau EM. Spinal pseudarthrosis complicating ankylosing spondylitis: comparison of CT and conventional tomography. *AJR Am J Roentgenol*. 1988;150(3):611–614.
46. Albertsen AM, Jurik AG. Posttraumatic spinal osteolysis in ankylosing spondylitis as part of pseudoarthrosis. A case report. *Acta Radiol*. 1996;37(1):98–100.
47. Eschelman DJ, Beers GJ, Naimark A, Yablon I. Pseudoarthrosis in ankylosing spondylitis mimicking infectious diskitis: MR appearance. *AJNR Am J Neuroradiol*. 1991;12(6):1113–1114.

11 Spinal Trauma in the Elderly

S. Ehara

Background

The aged population is increasing in most industrialized countries. In Japan, low birth and death rates have contributed to a significant increase in the aged population. Between 2005 and 2010, those aged 65 years or older will comprise 20% of the population, and in 2015 that figure will reach 25%.[1] Such an increase in the aged population will also be observed in North America and Europe.[2] The increased physically active aged population also has a higher chance of major trauma including traffic accidents, and falling at home also contributes to the increased chance of injury to the spine.

Injury to the spine due to major trauma is considered to be common among the young and physically active population, but another peak is present in the older age group of the late 50s and 60s.[3] In our institution, approximately 2/3 of spinal injury patients are older than 50 years, and the mean age is the mid 50s. Although fractures of the spine and dislocations due to major trauma are common in the young age groups, elderly people are more likely to sustain significant injury through minor trauma.

In general, the clinical manifestations of spinal injury in the elderly are more complicated and the diagnosis is more difficult and may be delayed due to variation in associated mental, social, and morphological states. In elderly patients, injury in the cervical spine is less common, and the injuries tend to be less severe; however, mortality rates are relatively high.[4] In addition, the imaging evaluation is more difficult due to associated age-related processes, including spondylosis deformans and paravertebral ligamentous ossification, accentuated kyphosis, compression fractures, and degenerative scoliosis. Detecting traumatic change in the associated degenerative process is important for diagnosing spinal injury in the aged population.

Cervical Spine

Biomechanical Characteristics

Flexion, extension, and axial loading are all causes of injury to the spine, and susceptibility to trauma depends on age, gender, and loading rate. Decreased bone mineral content makes the spine vulnerable to axial loading, but it is more significant in the thoracolumbar vertebrae. Hyperflexion and hyperextension are common mechanisms of cervical spine injury. Cervical spine injury in young patients is usually caused by a high loading rate, but in the elderly, injury also occurs with low loading rates.[5]

The range of motion of the cervical spine decreases with age, due to development of spondylosis deformans, including ligamentous degeneration and ossification.[6] Cervical spine injury with rigid segments most often occurs through or adjacent to such a segment. Increased rigidity may be the reason for the high frequency of upper cervical spine injury in the elderly.[7] Hyperextension injury is often seen in the upper cervical spine in the younger population; however, such injury commonly occurs in the mid and lower cervical levels in the elderly,[8] probably because of decreased tensile strength of the ligaments.

Clinical Features

Clinical evaluation of injured elderly patients is often difficult due to altered physiological and mental states. Cervical spine injury occurs often under the influence of alcohol, or physical or mental disorders, and this may make clinical assessment difficult. Neck pain is still the most significant initial symptom, but other symptoms often conceal neck complaints.

Although traffic accidents are by far the most common cause of injury in the general population, falling is the most common cause of cervical spine injury in most studies of spine injury in the elderly. In the elderly, falling causes 2/3 to 3/4 of cervical spine injury: 78% in Lieberman and Webb's study of patients older than 65 years.[9] Falling down the stairs is the most common injury at home, and it is often associated with loss of consciousness. The cause of the loss of consciousness may be a sign of more serious disorders.

The injury pattern in the elderly may be more complicated than in the younger population. In previous reports on cervical spine injury in the elderly, upper cervical spine injury, particularly dens fractures, is frequent, whereas lower cervical spine injury is more frequent in the younger population.[7,10,11]

On the other hand, the spondylotic spine tends to be injured in the lower cervical spine, which is particularly associated with degenerative changes.[8] This is due to the high frequency of hyperextension injury of the spondylotic lower cervical spine caused by falling. Hyperextension injury is typically common in older people, whereas hyperflexion and compression injury are relatively common in younger people.[12] There are two mechanisms of hyperextension injury: direct anterior craniofacial trauma, where people typically fall and hit their foreheads, and forced hyperextension in rear-end motor vehicle collisions, which is more common in younger and active people.

In hyperextension injury, central cord syndrome is the most common spinal cord injury, in which the pinching of the spinal cord may be caused by the bulged ligamentum flavum during hyperextension.[13] The central cord syndrome tends to occur at more than one level, based on MR imaging.[14] The prognosis of spinal cord injury is generally worse than in younger people.[10,15]

Hyperflexion injury, a common type of injury, is also seen in elderly patients. No specific type of injury is reported to be common in the elderly, but interfacetal fracture-dislocation is a typical injury in the mid and lower cervical spine.

Imaging Techniques

Imaging techniques are essentially the same as in the younger age group.[16] Plain radiography, particularly a high-quality lateral view, is of prime importance as in the younger age group, but associated degenerative or other disorders make the assessment of traumatic change more difficult. Adequately including the lower cervical spine is particularly important in elderly patients.

Although routine use of helical CT for vertebral trauma is controversial, multi-detector row CT (MDCT) makes evaluation of the wide zones of the spinal column easy. When fracture or dislocation is suspected by clinical data, a volume scan with multi-planar reconstruction by MDCT needs to be performed without delay.[17] In multi-trauma patients, evaluation of the whole spine by MDCT is particularly useful to assess multiple levels of traumatic lesions.

MR imaging is indicated whenever there is discrepancy between imaging features and neurological findings.[16] We routinely obtain sagittal T1W spin-echo, sagittal T2W (fast) spin-echo, and axial T2W (fast) spin-echo (or gradient-echo) images after a localizing scan with no contrast medium. Among them, the mid-sagittal T2W images are the most important screening method for the presence or absence of edema or hematoma in the paravertebral soft tissue and spinal cord.[18] Sagittal T1W images are sensitive to the detection of bone marrow trabecular bone fractures and high-signal cord hematoma. Axial T2W images are used to confirm and determine the localization of spinal cord injury, since artifacts often overlie the cord on sagittal images.

Radiological Features

There are no specific types of injury in elderly people, but a dens fracture and hyperextension injury due to falling is relatively common. Associated degenerative changes often modify traumatic change.[19]

SCIWORA (Spinal Cord Injury Without Radiographic Abnormalities)

The lack of findings of trauma is one of the characteristic imaging features of cervical spine injury in old people. Different from SCIWORA in children, trauma findings are hidden by degenerative changes. Senescent and pathological changes overlap, particularly in degenerative changes in the endplate and osteophyte formation, and the differentiation is often difficult. In Bryson et al's study of 174 patients older than 40 years, only 8 patients had findings of acute injury.[20] In Regenbogen et al's study of 88 patients older than 40 years, no bone abnormalities were seen in 28%, and minimal abnormalities were seen in 20%.[8] Another cause of this low sensitivity of plain radiography is probably related to the high frequency of hyperextension injury.

Hyperextension Injury

Hyperextension injury is usually a stable injury, and bone changes on plain radiography are frequently absent (Fig. 11.**1**).[21] Widening of the disk space is often the only finding. Prevertebral hematoma is frequently associated with this injury. In the study of Edeiken-Monroe et al, the combination of diffuse prevertebral soft tissue swelling and normal alignment of the cervical spine were the only findings in 30% of their cases.[22] MR imaging is particularly useful for evaluation of hyperextension injury in demonstrating injuries in the anterior longitudinal ligament and the anterior annulus, and occult endplate fractures.[14] In addition, hemorrhagic necrosis in the spinal cord caused by impaction is only seen on MR imaging.[23] The cord edema tends to extend to multiple levels,[14] but the degree of signal abnormalities varies.

Dens Fracture

The dens fracture has been reported to be the most common spinal injury in the elderly. It can be detected on plain radiography without MR imaging, but the diagnosis is often delayed, as seen in the younger age group (Fig. 11.**2**).[24] The pattern of dens fracture in elderly patients is controversial. An impaction fracture at the base of the dens (type III) may be characteristic in elderly patients with osteoporosis.[25] Posterior displacement of the dens may occur due to hyperextension. Anderson–D'Alonzo type III fractures were commonly seen in one study,[26] but in another study, the type II injury was more common.[27]

Fractures and Dislocations Associated with Rigid Segments

Spondylosis Deformans

Spondylosis deformans is an aging process characterized by degeneration of the intervertebral disks and a degenerative process of the diskovertebral and zygapophyseal joints. The degenerative process is evi-

11 Spinal Trauma in the Elderly

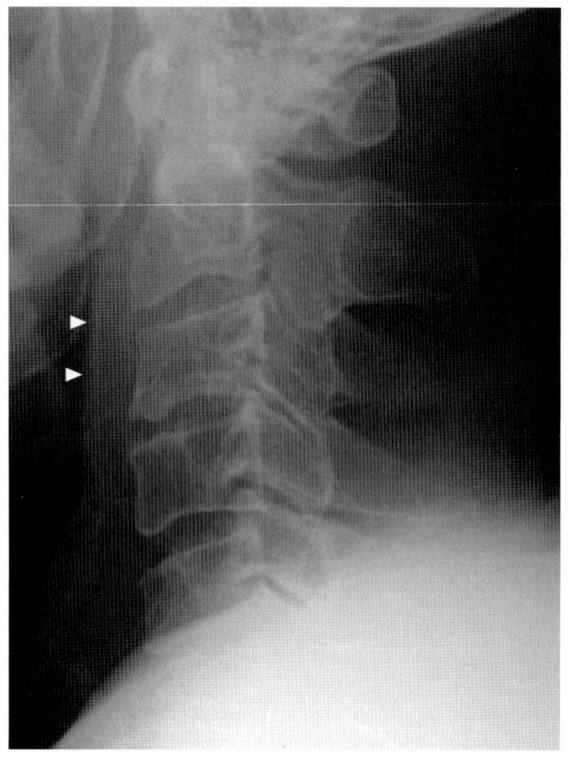

Fig. 11.**1 Hyperextension injury (60-year-old man who fell in the bathroom). a** Lateral radiography. Prevertebral soft tissue is prominent at the C3–C4 level (*arrowheads*). Disk space narrowing and mild osteophyte formation are also seen at C3–C4. The spinal canal is narrow below the C3 level. **b** Sagittal T2W MR image. Signal intensity in the spinal cord is increased at the C3–C4 level with posterior disk protrusion. Increased signal intensity and swelling of the prevertebral soft tissue at the C1–C5 levels represents hematoma (*arrowheads*).

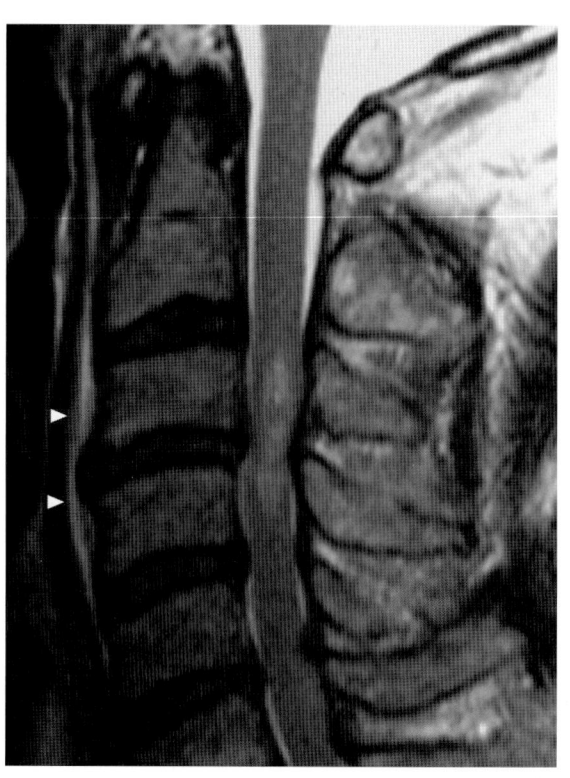

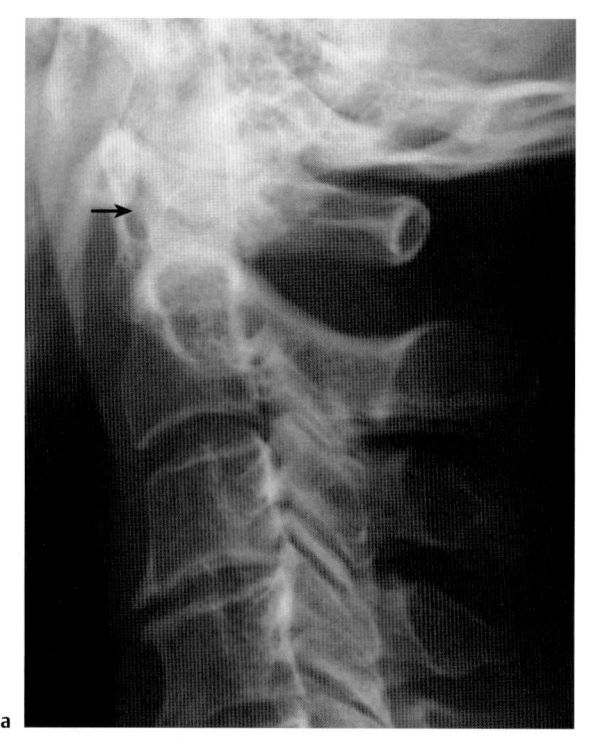

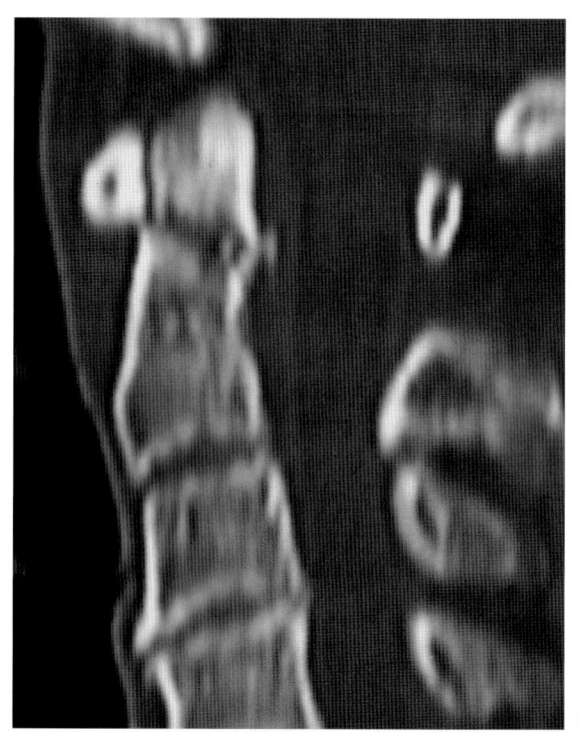

Fig. 11.**2 Dens fracture (67-year-old man involved in a motor vehicle accident). a** Lateral radiography. Prevertebral soft tissue is prominent at the C1–C2 levels. The fracture line is visible (*arrow*), but is difficult to confirm due to the overlying mastoid. **b** CT scan with sagittal reconstruction. The fracture is evident at the base of the dens (Anderson–D'Alonzo type II). The orientation of the fracture line is suggestive of a hyperextension injury.

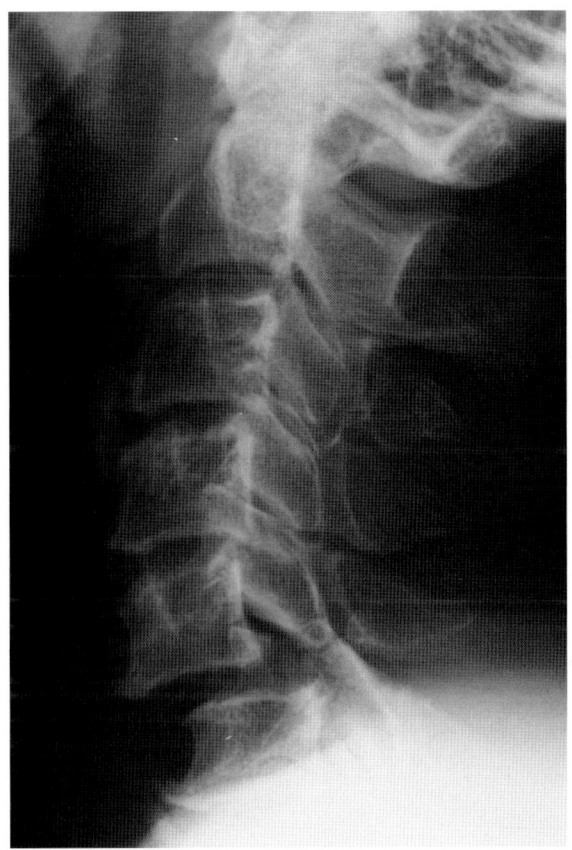

Fig. 11.**3 Bilateral interfacetal fracture-dislocation (62-year-old man involved in a motor vehicle accident). a** Lateral radiography. Bilateral articular processes of C5 are dislocated anteriorly on C6 articular processes. Disk spaces are narrowed and osteophyte formation is noted below the C3 level. **b** Sagittal T2W MR image. C5 body is displaced anteriorly on C6. Disk space narrowing and osteophytes are noted at C3 and below. The signal intensity of the spinal cord is slightly increased (*arrow*).

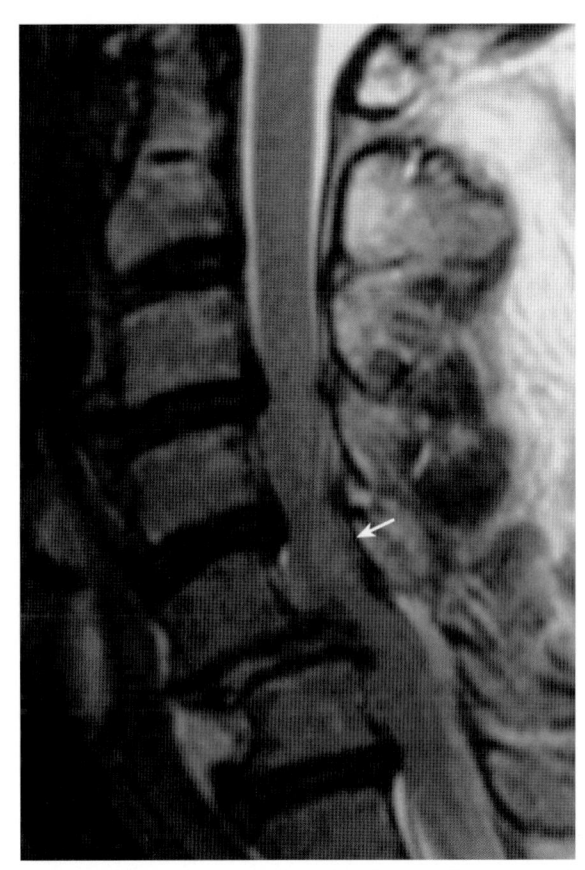

dent in the majority of spine injury cases.[8,20] The loss of flexibility contributes to the increased risk of trauma. The injury tends to occur at or adjacent to the rigid segment, where the stress due to trauma concentrates (Fig. 11.**3**). In addition, the association of spinal canal stenosis may further increase the risk of spinal cord injury. However, the diagnosis is often difficult because of an overlap of the radiological findings of spondylosis and trauma, including mild spondylolisthesis, osteophytes without continuation from the corner of the vertebral bodies, segmental ossification at the annulus fibrosus or anterior longitudinal ligament, and osteophytes of the zygapophyseal joint. Although plain radiography may be adequate for differentiation in many cases, MR imaging also provides clues for differentiating traumatic from degenerative changes, such as spinal cord edema or hematoma, prevertebral hematoma, "fluid" (or blood) collection in the intervertebral disk, disruption of ligaments, and bone marrow edema. The limitation of MR imaging still exists in the difficulty of differentiation between acute traumatic cord edema and chronic cord compression, although the cord lesion tends to be more extensive in the trauma cases.

Paravertebral Ligamentous Ossification (DISH, OPLL)

Paravertebral ligamentous ossification (diffuse idiopathic skeletal hyperostosis [DISH], ossification of the posterior longitudinal ligament [OPLL], ossification of the ligamentum flavum [OLF]) is essentially a disorder of the elderly. It alters biomechanical characteristics due to ankylosis or restricted motion and a narrow spinal canal. Mechanical stress concentrated on a relatively weak segment damages the spinal cord in the narrow spinal canal at the occurrence of a minor trauma. In such patients, the minor trauma often aggravates their preexisting symptoms. The injury is often due to minor trauma, as seen in 11 out of 15 patients in Hendrix at al's series.[28] The fracture pattern is a shear type transverse fracture, similar to that of ankylosing spondylitis, but the spinal canal is narrow in such patients. Fractures typically occur in the lower cervical spine, C5–C7, particularly through the ankylosed segment, involving a weak intervertebral disk or a poorly mineralized body. Fractures also occur at the edge of the ankylosed segment, particularly at the dens in patients with extensive paravertebral ossification.[29] Fracture lines traversing the vertebral column including the anterior and posterior elements are similar to those of ankylosing spondylitis.[28] In patients with OPLL, the posterior longi-

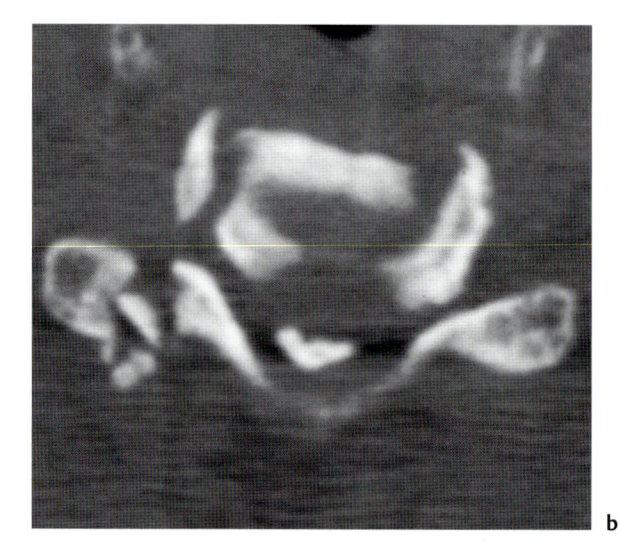

Fig. 11.4 **Fracture of the articular process and lamina with a unilateral interfacetal fracture, associated with OPLL (69-year-old man involved in a traffic accident). a** Lateral radiography. OPLL of the contiguous type is seen at the C1–C5 levels. C5 is slightly displaced posteriorly on C6, and ossified PLL is also displaced into the spinal canal (*arrow*). **b** A CT scan at the C5–C6 disk level. Fractures of the right articular process and lamina are noted at C5. OPLL is displaced into the center of the spinal canal.

tudinal ligament may be disrupted in the spinal canal and the displaced ossified ligament may directly damage the spinal cord (Fig. 11.4).[30] Although MR imaging is not sensitive to the detection of ligamentous ossification, it often helps in detecting spinal cord injury, and ligamentous disruption. Spinal cord damage due to chronic compression is a common finding in patients with a narrow spinal canal. Differentiating such patients from those with traumatic cord edema is difficult, and needs to be based on clinical findings.

Ankylosing Spondylitis

Fractures through the ankylosed spinal column due to ankylosing spondylitis often occur in the older population. The injury often occurs due to minor trauma, typically falling at home. The injury is common in the lower cervical spine and thoracolumbar junction. The fracture through the ankylosed vertebrae is typically a shear-type transverse fracture through the bodies, disks, and posterior elements, and is unstable. Prognosis is reported to be worse in patients with ankylosing spondylitis and cervical spine injury.[31] This is covered separately in Chapter 10.

Thoracolumbar Spine

Biomechanical Characteristics

Biomechanical characteristics of the spinal column change with the aging process. Such changes have been well investigated in the lumbar spine, and biochemical alteration in the ligaments results in diminished tensile, torsional, and shear strength. Loss of mineralization and increased rigidity contribute to an increase in the fracture risk due to minor trauma. Flexion is the major cause of thoracolumbar spine fractures, and rotation and shear are frequently associated factors. An extension injury may occur, but only in the rigid spine.

The preferential loss of horizontal trabeculae in vertebral bodies is the major cause of osteoporotic compression fractures. The vertebral bodies of the thoracolumbar junction are the most common site due to a lack of supporting structures, including the ribs and the sternum. Ankylosis due to spondylosis deformans, inflammatory spondyloarthropathy, and DISH also contribute to an increased fracture risk of adjacent vertebral bodies.

Clinical Features

A simple wedge compression fracture with intact posterior elements is by far the most common injury. The thoracolumbar junction, including the isolated rib-bearing thoracic spine (T11 and T12) and the upper two lumbar vertebrae, is the most common site. In most cases, the history of trauma is not significant. The incidence of the specific trauma episode is not well known, and it may be only seen in less than one-third of the compression fracture cases. Differentiation of the benign osteoporotic fracture and the pathological fracture (e.g., metastasis) is important particularly in patients with a history of malignancy.

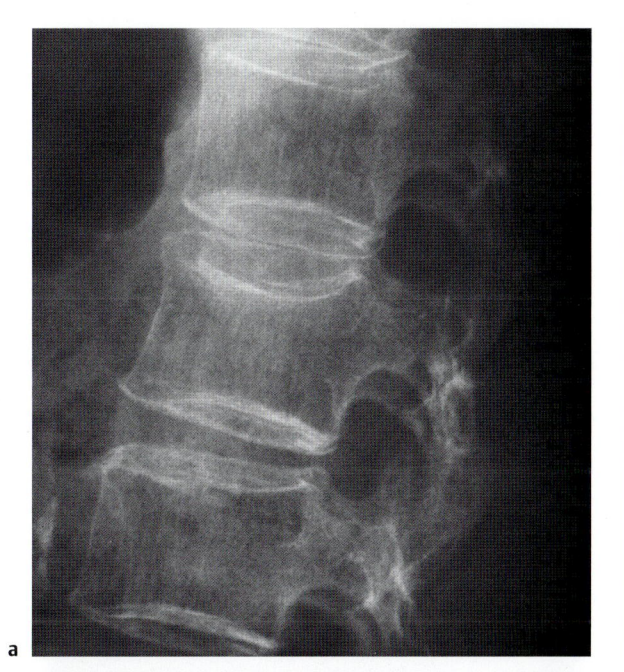

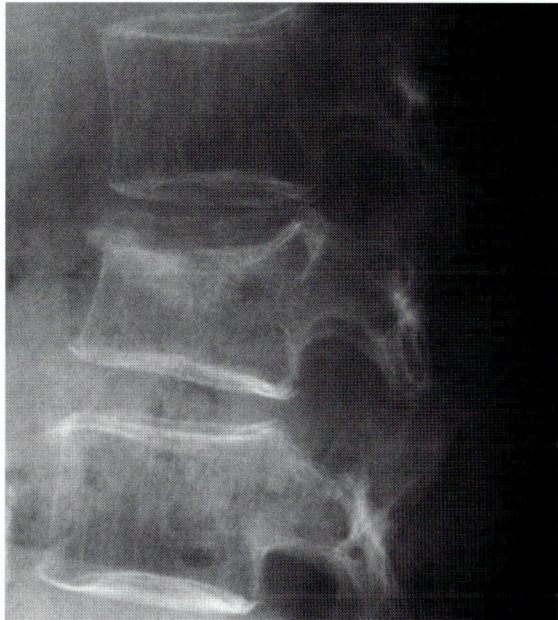

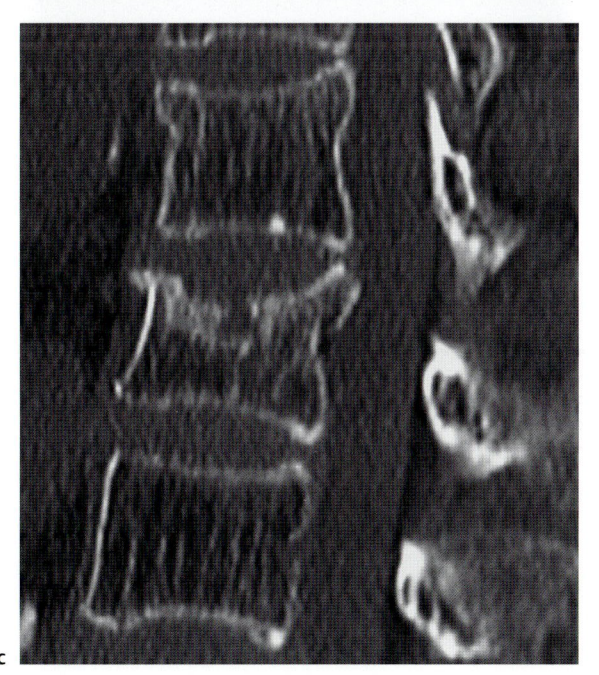

Fig. 11.**5 Osteoporotic compression fracture with progression of collapse (70-year-old woman who fell)**. **a** Lateral radiography obtained soon after the injury. Osteoporosis is evident. The superior endplate of the L2 body is minimally depressed. **b** Lateral radiograph obtained 4 months later. Further collapse and sclerosis of the superior endplate are noted. **c** A CT scan with sagittal reconstruction. In addition to the collapse and sclerosis, a Schmorl's node is noted in the collapsed L2 endplate.

Spine injury due to major trauma is more commonly seen in the cervical spine, rather than the thoracolumbar spine. Mid-thoracic spine fractures and fracture-dislocations are commonly due to major trauma, and is rarely seen in the elderly. Fractures of the sternum and ribs are characteristically associated with thoracic spine fractures. When kyphosis is significant, stress fractures of the sternum may be associated.

Imaging Techniques

Plain radiography is still of prime importance in the case of thoracolumbar spine injury. CT is indicated when a burst fracture or a fracture of the posterior element is suspected. MDCT is particularly useful to cover a wide range of the thoracolumbar spine in multi-trauma patients or patients in whom there is difficulty in localizing injury levels. MR imaging is not usually indicated in the acute phase, but it may be useful when neurological deficit is not explained by the other imaging modalities, and when a pathological fracture is suspected. CT and MR imaging techniques do not differ from their usage for the young population. Quantitative assessment, i. e., dual energy X-ray absorptiometry (DXA), is valuable for osteoporotic fractures.

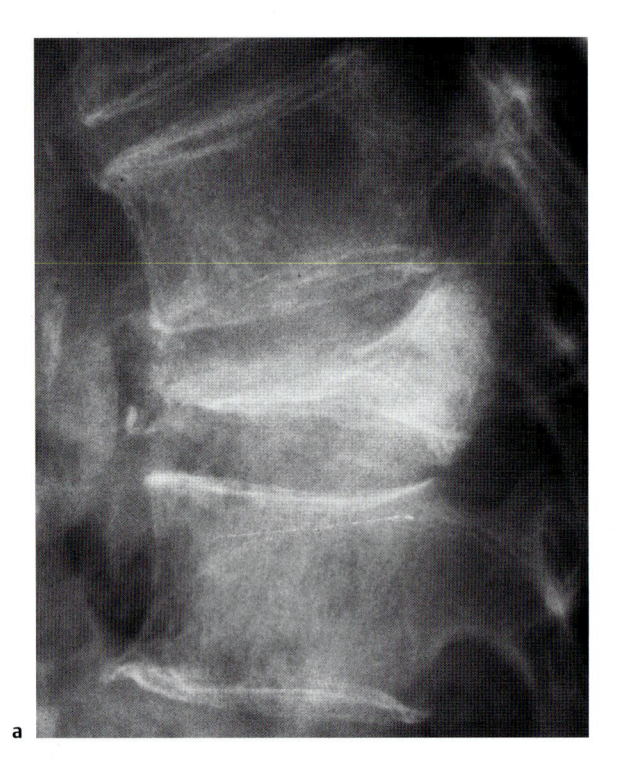

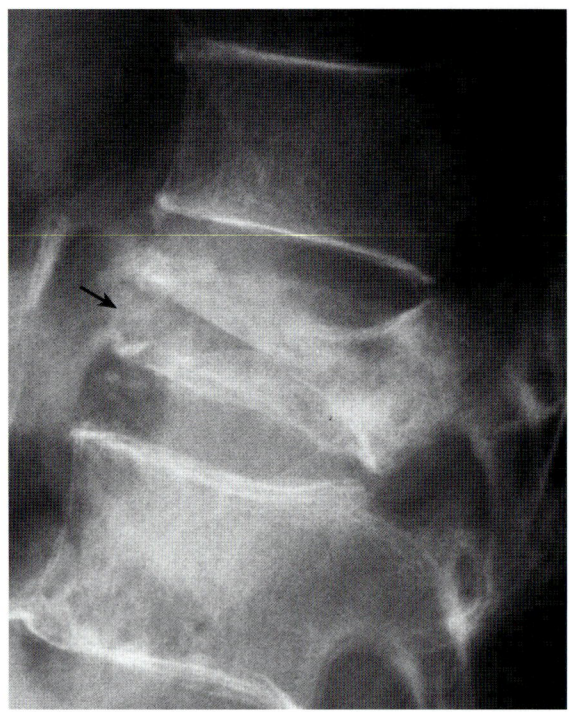

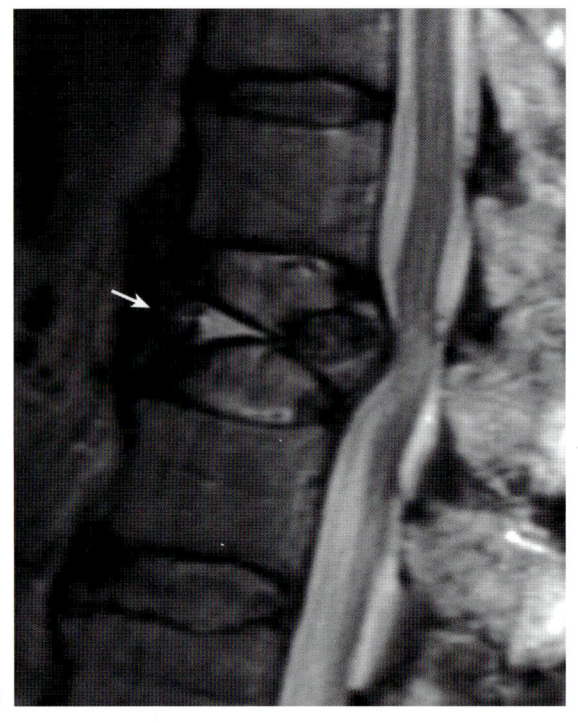

Fig. 11.6 **Kümmell-type vertebral collapse (61-year-old man with persistent pain after falling).** a Upright lateral radiography on flexion. The T12 body is severely collapsed. b Upright lateral radiography on extension. Anterior aspect of the collapsed T12 body is slightly widened, and the density of the widened portion is low, representing a vacuum cleft (*arrow*). c A sagittal T2W MR image. The T12 body is severely collapsed with retropulsion of the posterior aspect of the vertebral body. The high signal in the anterior aspect of the body represents fluid collection (*arrow*) with a gas-fluid level.

Imaging Features

Osteoporotic Compression Fracture

The osteoporotic compression fracture is common, but its prevalence increases with increased age and decreased bone mineral, and is as high as 42%.[32] Osteoporotic fractures of other sites, e. g., the distal forearm, hip, and other levels of the spine, tend to be associated synchronously or metachronously. Flexion typically causes failure of the anterior aspect of the vertebral body. Falling is obviously one definite cause of compression fractures in the elderly who have an osteoporotic spine, but specific traumatic events are not often elicited. Many older patients have painless multiple wedge fractures, and compression fractures are detected often due to unrelated causes.

The findings of an osteoporotic compression fracture may be subtle or underestimated initially (see Fig. 11.5). The endplate depression is subtle on radio-

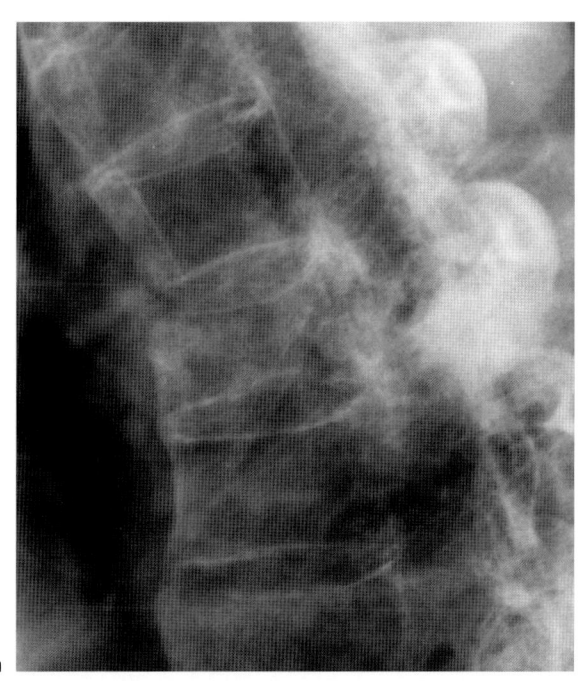

Fig. 11.7 **Shear fracture through the vertebral body of T7 associated with DISH (70-year-old woman with persistent back pain after falling). a** Lateral radiography. Paravertebral ossification and ankylosis are noted. The superior endplate of the T7 body is collapsed with kyphosis. **b** A sagittal T1W MR image. A band of low signal in the body and the posterior element corresponds to the transverse fracture.

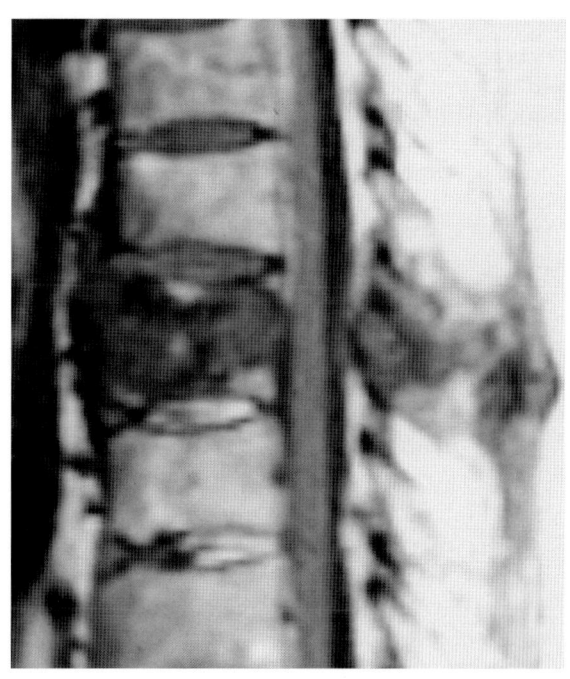

graphy, and it may be reduced in the supine position during the acute phase. A compression fracture is defined as the collapse of only the anterior column with no disruption of the posterior margin of the vertebral body, but typical deformities in the chronic phase include anterior wedging, the central endplate depression resulting in "fish vertebra," and diffusely decreased height. The fracture usually heals uneventfully, but the deformity of the vertebral body may be more significant in the delayed phase even without complications, either due to the initial underestimation or delayed progression of the collapse (see Fig. 11.5). Such a delayed collapse usually occurs within 8 weeks after trauma. Fracture healing is often associated with condensation of the collapsed endplate, and it tends to be significant in a steroid-induced osteoporotic fracture. Such a sclerotic reaction tends to regress gradually over the years. Further progression of collapse may occur, as discussed in the next section (see Chapter 14).

Kümmell-Type Delayed Vertebral Collapse

Osteoporotic compression fractures occasionally result in progressive collapse of the vertebral body, causing severely decreased vertebral body height with retropulsion of the posterior aspect of the vertebral body. It is usually seen in elderly patients, and the thoracolumbar junction is the most common site. In such cases, fracture lines are persistent, and radiographically a vacuum cleft is noted when a distraction force is applied (Fig. 11.6). Such a vacuum cleft has been called Kümmell's disease, or osteonecrosis of the vertebral body. On MR imaging, such unhealed fractures are filled with gas or fluid, depending on the internal pressure. Their true nature is still controversial, but poor blood supply to the collapsed endplate due to aging is considered to result in delayed fracture healing, or pseudoarthrosis.[33] Percutaneous vertebroplasty is currently one of the treatment options.

Fractures Related to Rigid Vertebral Segments

Fractures through or at the end of rigid segments, as seen in the cervical spine, also occur in the thoracolumbar spine, particularly at the thoracolumbar junction. Typical underlying disorders include DISH and ankylosing spondylitis. Transverse fractures through the ankylosed segments are typical such injuries (Fig. 11.7).[34,35] Such fractures are usually unstable and are often associated with neurological deficits. In patients with ankylosing spondylitis, a destructive change in the endplate, called spondylodiskitis or an Andersson lesion, is either due to inflammation or trauma, and it may be difficult to differentiate from an acute traumatic injury.[36] Such a traumatic lesion is often an occult fracture, and can be seen only on MR imaging. In DISH, similar changes due to trauma occur, and the differentiation from pathological fractures may be challenging (see Chapter 10).

Pathological Fracture Secondary to Neoplasm

Metastasis and multiple myeloma are common causes of localized or generalized bone resorption in the elderly patient's spine. Such disorders involve any level of the spinal column, but they are common in the thoracolumbar spine. They are typically associated with a compression fracture due to failure to axial loading or hyperflexion. When localized osteolysis or tumor mass is evident on plain radiography or CT, differentiating such a lesion from an osteoporotic compression fracture is not difficult. However, intertrabecular metastases, which may be seen in one-third of the cases, may not be detected.[37] A benign compression fracture typically presents with a band of signal abnormality subjacent to the collapsed endplate on MR imaging;[38] but the differentiation may still be difficult, and a biopsy or follow-up evaluation is indicated because the sub-endplate region is theoretically a common site of hematogenous metastasis (see Chapter 14).

Conclusion

Injury to the spine in the elderly population may also increase in the future. Diagnosis without delay is important to improve the prognosis. Dens fractures and hyperextension injuries are commonly seen cervical spine injuries due to trauma. Osteoporotic compression fractures are common in the thoracolumbar junction. A degenerative process may be associated with trauma cases and make differentiation difficult. Shear fractures through the ankylosed segment and fractures and/or dislocations at the end of the segment are typical in rigid spines.

References

1. National Institute of Social Security and Demography. *Current status and future of the population in Japan and the world* [in Japanese]. Tokyo: Kosei-Tokei Kyokai; 1999:31.
2. US Census Bureau. Global Population Profile: 2002.
3. Kraus JF, Franti CE, Riggins RS, Richards D, Borhani NO. Incidence of traumatic spinal cord lesions. *J Chronic Dis.* 1975;28:471–492.
4. Irwin ZN, Arthur M, Mullins RJ, Hart RA. Variations in injury patterns, treatment, and outcome for spinal fractures and paralysis in adult versus geriatric patients. *Spine.* 2004;29:796–802.
5. Pintar FA, Yoganandan N, Voo L. Effect of age and loading rate on human cervical spine injury threshold. *Spine.* 1998;23:1957–1962.
6. Kuhlman KA. Cervical range of motion in the elderly. *Arch Phys Med Rehabil.* 1993;74:1071–1079.
7. Ryan MD, Henderson JJ. The epidemiology of fractures and fracture-dislocations of the cervical spine. *Injury.* 1992;23:38–40.
8. Regenbogen VS, Rogers LF, Atlas SW, Kim KS. Cervical spinal cord injuries in patients with cervical spondylosis. *Am J Roentgenol.* 1986;146:277–284.
9. Lieberman IH, Webb JK. Cervical spine injuries in the elderly. *J Bone Joint Surg.* 1994;76B:877–881.
10. Spivak JM, Weiss MA, Cotler JM, Call M. Cervical spine injuries in patients 65 and older. *Spine.* 1994;19:2302–2306.
11. Daffner RH, Goldberg AL, Evans TC, Hanlon DP, Levy DB. Cervical vertebral injuries in the elderly: A 10-year study. *Emerg Radiol.* 1998;5:38–42.
12. Kiwerski J. The influence of the mechanism of cervical spine injury on the degree of the spinal cord lesion. *Paraplegia.* 1991;29:531–536.
13. Weingarden SI, Graham PM. Falls resulting in spinal cord injury: Patterns and outcomes in an older population. *Paraplegia.* 1989;27:423–427.
14. Davis S, Teresi LM, Gradley WG Jr, Ziemba MA, Bloze AE. Cervical spine hyperextension injuries: MR imaging. *Radiology.* 1991;180:245–251.
15. Alander DH, Parker J, Stauffer ES. Intermediate-term outcome of cervical spinal cord-injured patients older than 50 years of age. *Spine.* 1997;22:1189–1192.
16. American College of Radiology. *ACR Appropriateness criteria: Cervical spine trauma.* Reston, VA: ACR; 1995.
17. Nunez DB, Quencer RM. The role of helical CT in the assessment of cervical spine injuries. *Am J Roentgenol.* 1998;171:951–957.
18. Fehlings MG, Rao SC, Tator CH, Skaf G, Arnold P, Benzel E, et al. The optimal radiologic method for assessing spinal canal compromise and cord compression in patients with spinal cord injury. Part II: Results of a multicenter study. *Spine.* 1999;24:605–613.
19. Ehara S, Shimamura T. Cervical spine injury in the elderly: imaging features. *Skeletal Radiol.* 2001;30:1–7.
20. Bryson BL, Warren K, Schwedheim M, Mumford B, Lanaghan PA. Trauma to the aging cervical spine. *J Emerg Nurs.* 1987;13:334–341.
21. Cintron E, Gilula LA, Murphy WA, Gehweiler JA. The widened disk space: a sign of cervical hyperextension injury. *Radiology.* 1981;141:639–644.
22. Edeiken-Monroe B, Wagner LK, Harris JH Jr. Hyperextension dislocation of the cervical spine. *Am J Roentgenol.* 1986;146:803–808.
23. Chakeres DW, Flickinger F, Bresnahan JC, Beattie MS, Weiss KL, Miller C, Stokes BT. MR imaging of acute spinal cord trauma. *Am J Neuroradiol.* 1987;8:5–10.
24. Clark CR, Igram CM, El-Khoury GY, Ehara S. Radiographic evaluation of cervical spine injuries. *Spine.* 1988;13:742–747.
25. Gerhart TN, White AA III. An impacted dens fracture in an elderly woman. *Clin Orthop.* 1982;167:173–175.
26. Pepin JE, Bourne RB, Howkins RJ. Odontoid fractures, with special emphasis to the elderly patients. *Clin Orthop.* 1985;193:178–183.
27. Hanigan WC, Powell FC, Elwood PW, Henderson JP. Odontoid fractures in elderly patients. *J Neurosurg.* 1993;78:32–35.
28. Hendrix RW, Melany M, Miller F, Rogers LF. Fracture of the spine in patients with ankylosis due to diffuse skeletal hyperostosis: Clinical and imaging findings. *Am J Roentgenol.* 1994;162:899–904.
29. Paley D, Schwartz M, Cooper P, Harris WR. Levine AM. Fracture of the spine in diffuse idiopathic skeletal hyperostosis. *Clinical Orthop.* 1991;267:22–32.
30. Ehara S, Shimamura T, Nakamura R, Yamazaki K. Paravertebral ligamentous ossification: DISH, OPLL and OLF. *Eur J Radiol.* 1998;27:196–205.
31. Olerud C, Andersson S, Svensson B, Bring J. Cervical spine injury in the elderly: factors influencing survival in 65 patients. *Acta Orthop Scand.* 1999;70:509–513.
32. Melton LJ III, Kan SH, Frye MA, Wahner HW, O'Fallon WM, Riggs BL. Epidemiology of vertebral fractures in women. *Am J Epidemiol.* 1989;129:1000–1011.
33. Yuh WTC, Mayr NA, Petropoulou K, Beall DP. MR fluid sign in osteoporotic vertebral fracture. *Radiology.* 2003;227:905.
34. Graham B, van Peteghem PK. Fractures of the spine in ankylosing spondylitis: Diagnosis, treatment and complications. *Spine.* 1989;14:803–807.
35. Gelineck J, De Carvalho A. Fractures of the spine in ankylosing spondylitis. *Fortschr Roentgenstr.* 1990;152:307–310.
36. Dihlmann W, Delling G. Disco-vertebral destructive lesions (so-called Andersson lesions) associated with ankylosing spondylitis. *Skeletal Radiol.* 1978;3:10–16.
37. Yamaguchi T. Intertrabecular vertebral metastases: metastases only detectable on MR imaging. *Semin Musculoskeletal Radiol.* 2001;5:171–175.
38. Uetani M, Hashmi R, Hayashi K. Malignant and benign compression fractures: differentiation and diagnostic pitfalls on MRI. *Clin Radiol.* 2004;59:124–131.

12 Therapy—Options and Outcomes

J. M. Trivedi

Introduction

A neurological injury in spine trauma is a devastating event. It results in significant functional disability, high economic costs, and sometimes decreased life expectancy. There have been advances in both nonoperative as well as operative modalities of treatment of patients with spinal injuries. These advances have led to renewed interest in the management of a spinally injured patient. However, despite these advances, controversies exist, regarding the classification of spinal fractures, the use of pharmacological intervention, the timing of surgery, and indeed the use of surgical intervention itself in the management of these fractures. Most of these controversies surround the treatment of thoracic and lumbar fractures. The optimal treatment of patients with thoracolumbar fractures with incomplete neurological deficit is still controversial. The purpose of this chapter is to provide an overview of spinal fractures and discuss therapy options available in the treatment of these fractures. Newer surgical treatments for certain types of fractures are described.

Epidemiology of Spinal Trauma

The incidence of spinal injury in the United States is between 4 and 5.3 per 100 000 of population.[1] This amounts to 12 000 new spinal cord injuries every year. Some degree of neurological deficit may occur in 10–25% of patients with spinal trauma.[2,3] The common causes of spinal trauma include road traffic accidents (45%), falls (20%), and sports (15%).[4] The male to female ratio is 4:1. The overall survival rate for patients with spinal injuries is 86% at 10 years.[4] This tends to decrease as the patient gets older. The annual mortality in the first year following spinal cord injury is reported to be 3.6%.[5]

The establishment of centers for the treatment of patients with spinal injuries has improved the outcome in these patients. Historically, the concept of a spinal injuries center was popularized by Sir Ludwig Guttman at the Stoke Manderville Hospital in England as early as 1943.[6] Many such specialized centers now exist in the developed world. This has resulted in shorter hospitalization, reduced complications, and thus a reduced overall cost in the care of these patients.

Pathophysiology of Spinal Cord Injury

Trauma from the vertebral column is transferred to the spinal cord by one of two mechanisms: either a direct injury, by means of excessive flexion, extension, or rotation of the spinal cord or an indirect injury resulting from impaction of displaced bone, disk fragments, or hematoma. Spinal cord injury may be either compressive or secondary to traction. The latter has a poor prognosis. The consequences of compressive injury depend upon not only the degree of compression but also the duration of compression. Animal studies by Rivlin, Tator, Dolan, and Delamarter have shown that the clinical consequences of cord compression are inversely related to the duration of cord compression.[7,8,9,10] Delamarter and colleagues created spinal cord injuries in dogs using constriction bands.[8,9] They showed that a 50% compression of the cauda equina led to significant electrodiagnostic and neurophysiological changes. At 75% compression there was permanent paraplegia. Recovery following the release of these bands was time dependent. Those animals that underwent decompression either immediately or at 1 hour were electrophysiologically normal at 6 weeks. Those animals that were decompressed after 6 hours did not make significant recovery.

Ducker et al found that experimentally injured primates made significantly more neurological recovery following immediate immobilization.[11]

All these studies, as well as advances in understanding the pathophysiology of spinal injury, form the basis of current principles of treatment of the spinally injured patient. These include the use of pharmacological agents, fracture reduction and stabilization either operatively or nonoperatively, and neurological decompression in these patients.

Anatomical Classification of Spinal Fractures

Holdsworth proposed a "two-column" concept to assess spinal stability.[12] In Holdsworth's model the spine was comprised of anterior and posterior columns. The anterior column comprising of the vertebral body, the intervertebral disk, the anterior longitudinal ligament (ALL), and the posterior longitudinal ligament (PLL) transmits compressive loads. The posterior column responsible for tensile stresses consists of the facet joints, the neural arch, and the interspinous liga-

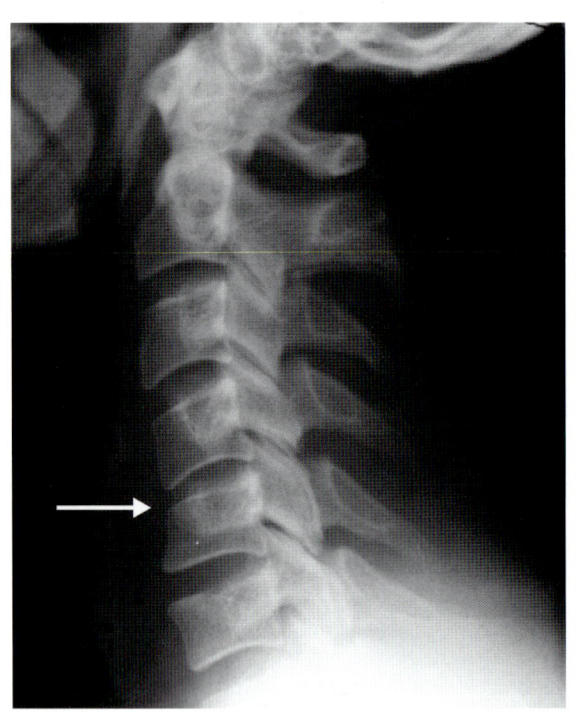

Fig. 12.1 Lateral radiograph of a flexion injury in the cervical spine. Loss of anterior disk height (*arrow*) at C4/C5 level.

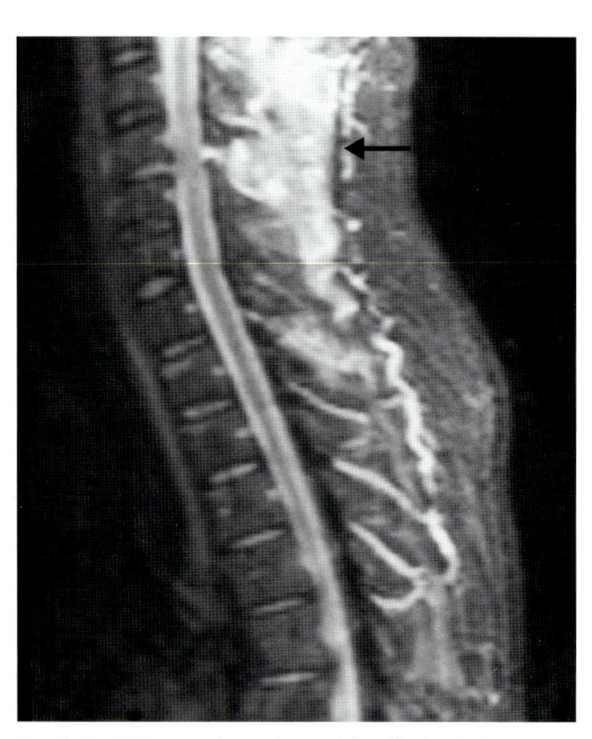

Fig. 12.2 MRI scan of a patient with a flexion injury. Injury to the interspinous ligaments, ligamentum flavum and supraspinous ligaments (*arrow*).

ments. In Holdsworth's model, the posterior ligaments play an important role functioning as a tension band to balance the loads passing through the anterior column.

Denis elaborated on Holdsworth's concept by developing the three-column concept of spinal stability.[13] The anterior column consists of the ALL and the anterior two-thirds of the vertebral body and disk. The middle column comprises of the posterior third of the vertebral body and disk with the PLL. The posterior column includes everything posterior to the PLL. In Denis' model disruption of two columns indicates spinal instability. For vertebral burst fractures the presence of intact posterior ligaments represents a more stable configuration than when these ligaments are disrupted. A detailed appraisal of the relevance of classifications is found in Chapter 4.

Patterns of Injury

The spine exhibits six degrees of freedom of motion about three axes. This results in six possible patterns of injury: compression, extension, distraction, rotation, flexion, and shear. The direction of the force vector and the position of the spine at the moment of impact determine the nature of injury to the spinal column.

Flexion Injury

A compression force in a flexed spine may result in a compression fracture. The anterior column fails in compression. The middle column remains intact. The posterior column may disrupt or remain intact depending upon the severity of the injury. If the posterior column is disrupted, it results in a potentially unstable situation (Figs. 12.**1**–12.**3**).

Burst Fractures

Axial loading force results in a compression failure of anterior and middle columns resulting in a "burst fracture." The vast majority of burst fractures are associated with a retropulsion of bony fragments into the spinal canal. Radiologically, there is a loss of vertebral height with varying degrees of kyphosis, widening of the interpedicular distance and on a CT scan a demonstrable encroachment of the spinal canal from retropulsed bony fragments.

Flexion Distraction Injury

The flexion distraction injury was first described by Chance in 1948.[14] The axis of flexion is anterior and the vertebral column fails in tension. The tensile forces disrupt the posterior ligaments. The forces can produce a pure osseous injury or a mixed osseous-ligamentous injury (Fig. 12.**4**). The former has an excellent potential for healing whereas the latter usually requires operative stabilization to substitute for the failed ligament complex posteriorly (Fig. 12.**5**). The location of force vectors results in a significant association of injury to the abdominal viscera and rates as high as 45 % have been reported.[15]

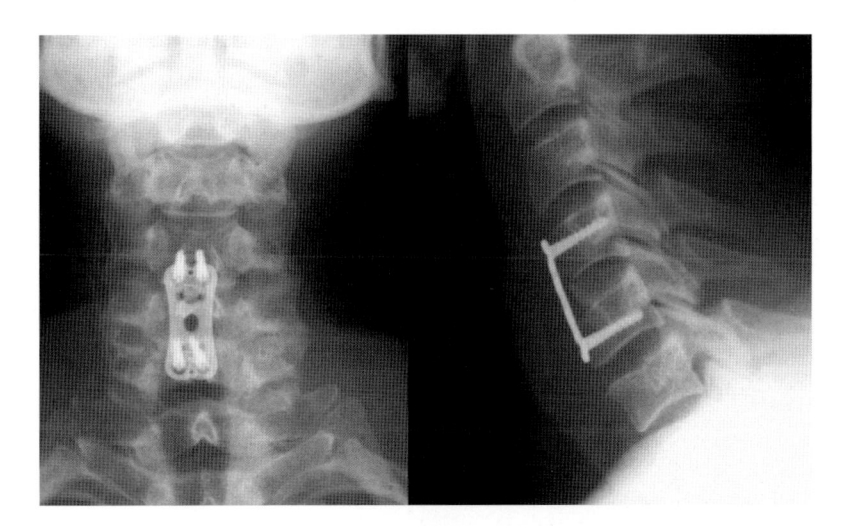

Fig. 12.3 Surgical stabilization for flexion injury of the cervical spine.

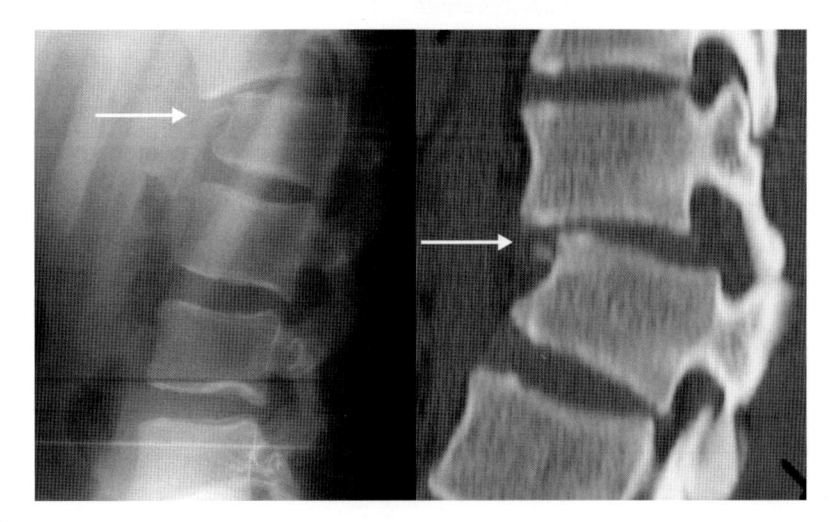

Fig. 12.4 Flexion distraction injury at the thoracolumbar junction (*arrows*) associated with dislocation.

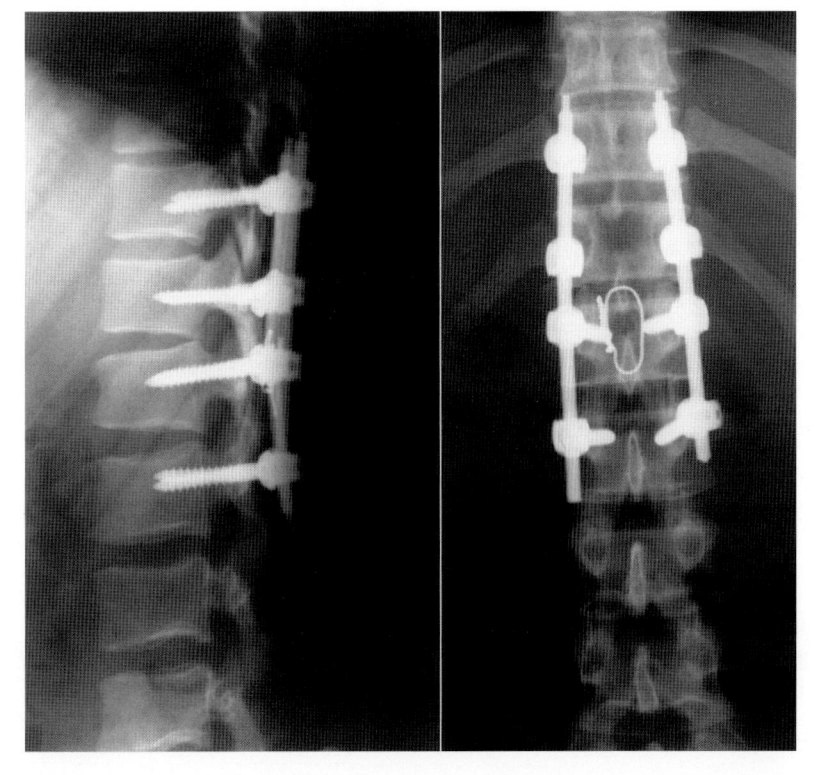

Fig. 12.5 Surgical stabilization of the flexion-distraction injury with posterior instrumentation using pedicle screws.

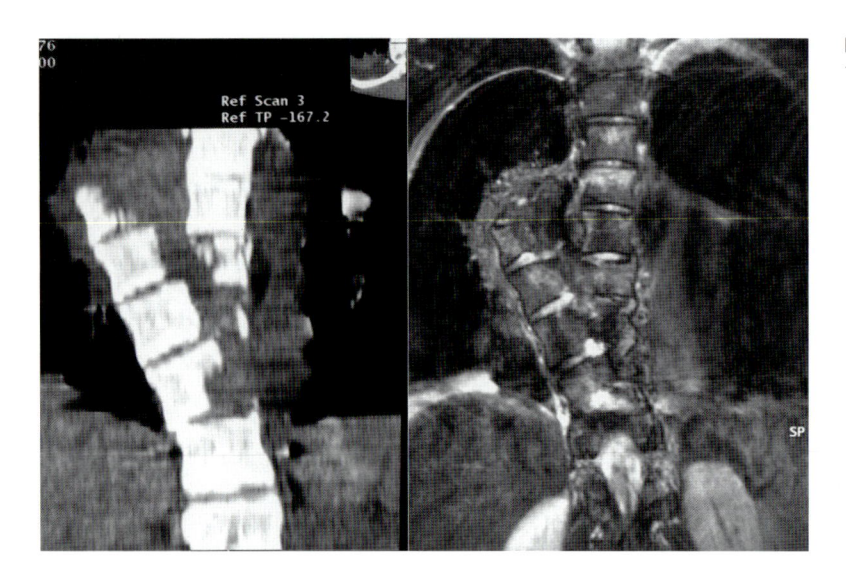

Fig. 12.6 Flexion rotation injury in the thoracic spine.

Flexion Rotation

This injury is caused by a combination of flexion and rotation forces. The posterior ligaments and joint capsules are disrupted and the vertebral body may be disrupted obliquely. In the cervical spine this results in facet dislocations and in the thoracic and lumbar spine it may cause fracture dislocation (Fig. 12.6).

Management

Initial Management

At the scene of the accident, the management of a patient with a spinal injury should follow the protocols laid down by the ATLS system. This involves emphasis on maintenance of the airway, breathing, and circulation. Those suspected of having a spinal injury should be immobilized on a spinal backboard with adequate immobilization of the cervical spine. The most effective method of initial cervical immobilization is the use of bilateral sand bags and taping of the patient across the forehead to a spinal board along with the use of a Philadelphia collar. Immobilization gear should be removed only after radiographs have been interpreted as normal.

Multiple injuries are not uncommon in patients sustaining a spinal injury. As a result, a spinally injured patient may be hypotensive on initial assessment. The treating physician should also be aware of neurogenic shock, which is defined as vascular hypotension with associated brachycardia as a result of spinal injury. This usually results from traumatic disruption of the sympathetic outflow between T1 to L2 and the subsequent unopposed vagal tone, which results in bradycardia and hypotension. Evaluation of the bulbocavernous reflex may provide a clue towards the presence of spinal shock. An absent bulbocavernous reflex associated with a loss of sensory-motor function signifies spinal shock. The degree of hypotension, bradycardia, and the incidence of cardiac arrest are related to the severity of neurological injury. Piepmeier et al in a review of 45 patients with a cervical spinal cord injury found that 87% of Frankel A patients had a pulse rate lower than 55 beats per minute, with a 21% incidence of cardiac arrest.[16] Only 62% of patients with Frankel B neurological status had a pulse rate of less than 55 beats per minute and none had cardiac arrest. Efforts must be made to regulate the blood pressure as the injured spinal cord loses its ability to auto-regulate blood pressure. Thus prolonged hypotension may increase the ischemia of the injured spinal cord.

The initial examination must include inspection of the spine and a neurological assessment. Inspection of the back may reveal laceration, bruising, and swelling. Palpation of the spine will reveal tenderness and a possible step off, gap or malalignment of the spinous processes. The neurological examination should include assessment of spinal cord and nerve root integrity. The spinal cord usually extends up to the lower border of L1 in adults and injuries cephalad to this level may involve the cord. Injuries at the lower lumbar level by contrast involve the cauda equina. The presence of sacral sparing suggested by the presence of anal tone and perianal sensation is an important prognostic finding as it signifies an incomplete spinal cord injury.

Attempts should be made to realign the spinal column if possible. In the cervical spine this may be done through the use of skeletal traction applied through the medium of tongs. Gardner-Wells tongs are most commonly used and are fast and easy to apply, requiring no assistance. In the thoracolumbar spine traction is less successful and emergency surgical reduction may be required to restore anatomical alignment.

Several authors have reported neurological deterioration in patients with cervical dislocations undergoing traction and reduction.[17–19] This has been attributed to the high incidences of disk herniations in patients with facet dislocations (Figs. 12.7, 12.8).

Fig. 12.7 Dislocation of C4 on C5.

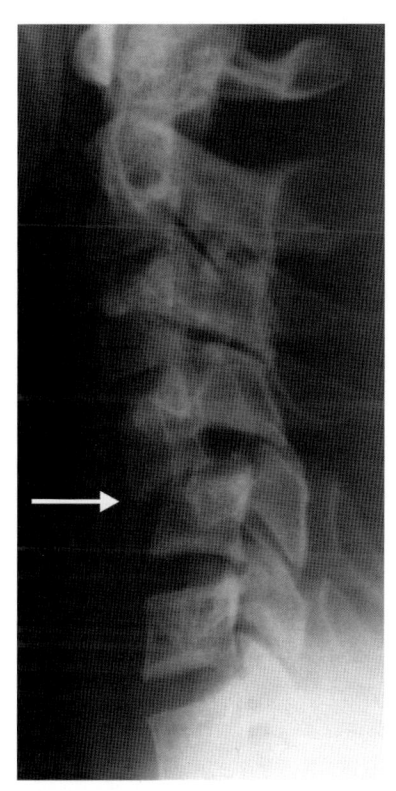

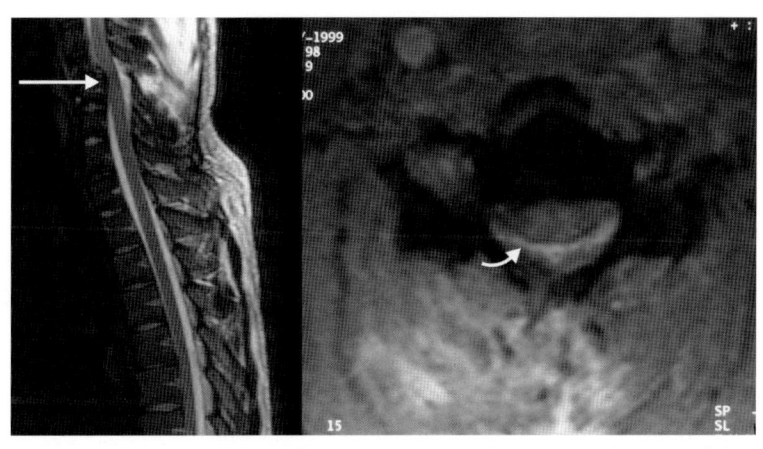

Fig. 12.8 Sagittal (**a**) and axial (**b**) MR images scan of a patient with a cervical dislocation. *Arrows* indicate disk herniation within the spinal canal at the C4/C5 level.

Theoretically, during reduction, the herniated intervertebral disk can remain posterior to the vertebral body and even in the spinal canal causing neurological injury as reduction of the dislocation is undertaken. This has prompted the use of MRI scanning prior to closed reduction of the cervical spine using traction. Other large studies have refuted this showing no neurological deterioration in reduction attempted in awake and cooperative patients.[20,21] If an MRI scan can be obtained expeditiously then it should be done. An MRI should always be obtained if the patient is uncooperative or will require reduction under anesthesia. If the scan demonstrates a disk herniation then a three-stage operative procedure may be required. The first stage is an anterior approach to the cervical spine through which the herniated disk is removed. The anterior wound is then closed temporarily and the patient is carefully turned over to allow for a posterior procedure in which the dislocation is reduced. This may involve a partial facetectomy of the superior articular facet if simple levering of the facets does not result in reduction. Thereafter, the injured level may be stabilized with an interspinous wire fixation before turning the patient over again to complete the anterior procedure through an anterior interbody fusion and plating (Fig. 12.9).

Nursing of the spinally injured patient should be aimed at minimizing complications of decubitus ulceration. This can be done through the use of a special selection of beds such as the turning frames of Stryker/Foster or the Rotorest bed. Some of these beds such as the Rotorest bed can allow application of traction in various planes.

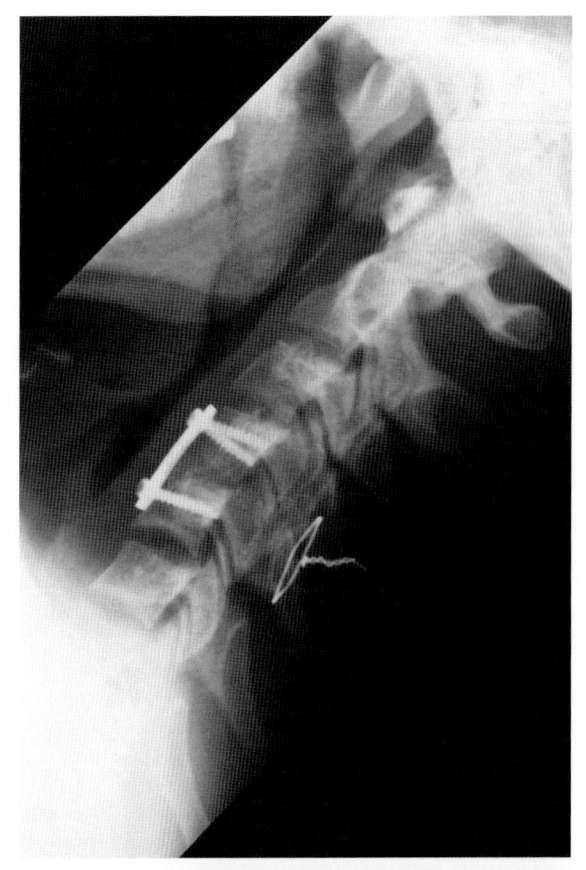

Fig. 12.9 **Three-stage surgery for a patient with a cervical dislocation.** Stage 1: anterior approach with removal of the disk. Stage 2: Posterior reduction and stabilization with interspinous wiring. Stage 3: Anterior stabilization.

Pharmacological Intervention

The secondary phase of spinal cord injury following trauma involves enzymatic lipid peroxidation and ischemia.[22–24] In animal studies high doses of methylprednisolone were found to reduce the effects of secondary injury to the spinal cord. Bracken et al have conducted three studies on the use of methylprednisolone in spinally injured patients (NASCIS I, II, and III).[22–24] In NASCIS II, methylprednisolone was given in a dose of 30 mg/kg body weight as a bolus followed by 23-hour infusion at 5.4 mg/kg. Naloxone was administered in a dose of 5.4 mg/kg of bolus followed by a 24-hour infusion at 4 mg/kg. These two drugs were compared with a placebo in patients randomized within 12 hours of injury. Patients treated with methylprednisolone within 8 hours of injury experienced significantly improved neurological function over placebo-treated patients 6 weeks, 6 months, and 1 year post-injury. Naloxone treatment was no better than control. However, a predictable trend towards increased complications were seen in the steroid group including a two-fold increased incidence of wound infection.

In the third trial (NASCIS III), 48-hour administration of methylprednisolone was compared with a 24-hour maintenance therapy. The basis of this study was that posttraumatic lipid peroxidation in the spinal cord is known to last beyond 24 hours. In the third trial a 48-hour maintenance treatment with tirilazad mesylate, which is a potent lipid peroxidation inhibitor, was also studied 6 weeks and 6 months following injury. Patients treated within 3 hours of injury recovered equally in all three treatment groups. This recovery was maintained at 1-year follow-up. The rate of recovery, however, was slower between 6 months and 1 year and in those patients where treatment was initiated more than 3 hours after injury. Those receiving a 48-hour schedule of methylprednisolone showed greater recovery in motor function, overall functional independence, and self-care than the 24-hour methylprednisolone group. The relative improvements at 1 year, however, were modest. There was a significant increase in severe pneumonia seen at 6 weeks after the 48-hour methylprednisolone treatment.

The above studies would suggest that high doses of steroid shortly after spinal injury might be of benefit. However, this is still controversial. Short et al in a scientific review on the use of high dose methylprednisolone found that many large studies did not satisfy validity criteria.[25] Of the three clinical trials and six cohort study publications that did satisfy validity criteria there was inconclusive evidence on the use of steroids. Coleman et al have likewise challenged the statistical design of the NASCIS II and III studies.[26] Hurlbert concluded that the efficacy of methylprednisolone was weak and 24-hour administration of methylprednisolone must be considered to be experimental.[27]

Recent studies have concentrated on the use of gangliosides particularly GM1 ganglioside in these patients.[28] Vitamin E has an antioxidant effect and may be useful in these patients. However, the need to give the drug before the injury limits its application.[29] Other drugs that have been experimented with include calcium channel blockers as well as osmotic diuretics.[30] Both these failed to provide evidence of clinical effectiveness with regard to spinal cord injury.

Nonsurgical Management of Spinal Fractures

Modalities for nonsurgical treatment of patients include:
- Recumbency
- Use of specific orthoses
- Observation alone

Treatment by Recumbency

Historically, this has been popularized by several authors including Sir Guttman, Bedbrook, and Nicoll.[6,31,32]

Outcomes

Frankel et al reporting the results of patients treated with postural reduction and prolonged recumbency found that of 394 patients with thoracolumbar injuries only 2 patients developed late instability that required further surgery.[33] Ten percent of patients with complete paraplegia made significant motor recovery. Sixty-eight percent of patients with incomplete injuries likewise made recovery of at least one Frankel grade. The limitation of this study was that 70 patients who died within 3 months of injury were excluded from analysis.

Rechtine reviewed the results of long-term bed rest in 150 patients with thoracic and lumbar fractures.[34] These were compared with 120 patients who were treated surgically within the same period (10 years). He found that complications totaled 32% in the surgical group and 22% in the nonsurgical group. Mortality was 3.3% in the surgical group and only 2% in the nonsurgical group.

Weinstein et al published the long-term results of nonoperative treatment for fractures of the thoracolumbar spine.[35] The average length of follow-up was 20.2 years and the average length of hospitalization averaged 34 days. They reported no complications related to treatment. Seventy-eight percent of patients had no neurological deficit at the time of their original injury and no patient demonstrated worsening of their Frankel grading. Seventeen percent improved their neurological status. Eighty-eight percent of the patients contacted were able to work sometime after their injury in their pre-injury occupation or capacity.

Orthotic Management

The rationale behind the use of orthosis is to limit motion of the injured segment and if possible decrease the loads in the spinal column. Bracing is more widely

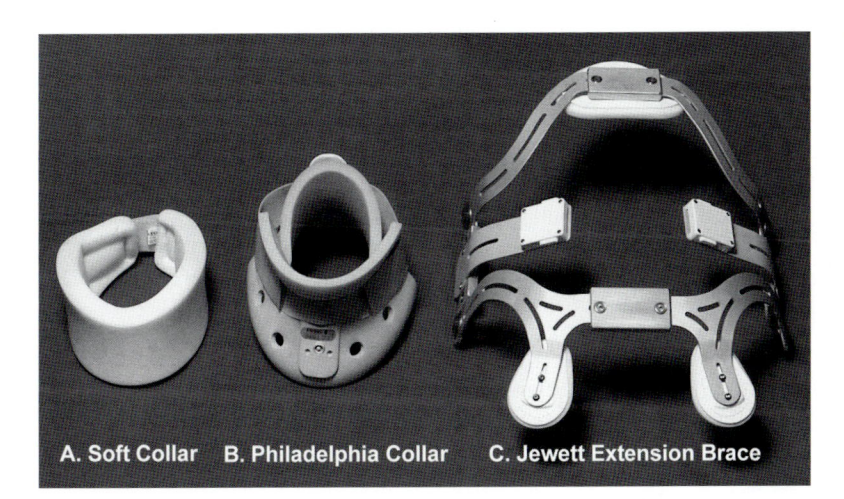

Fig. 12.**10** Cervical and thoracic orthoses in spinal trauma.

used for thoracolumbar injuries. The principle of treatment here is to provide a three-point pressure. Norton and Brown observed that braces that did not fix adequately to the pelvis tended to produce a concentration of force in the upper lumbar and thoracolumbar regions.[36] Fidler and Plasmans found that canvas corsets reduced the motion of the lumbar segments to approximately two-thirds of normal.[37] The spica was the only method of immobilization that significantly decreased motion below the third lumbar vertebra. A commonly used brace for thoracolumbar injuries is the Jewett hyperextension brace. Nagel and associates found that the Jewett brace reduced flexion by 40% but had no affect on lateral bending and rotation.[38] To control motion in multiple planes a total contact orthosis is more effective (Fig. 12.**10**).

Observation Alone

Certain fractures may be deemed to be "stable" on initial presentation. White and Punjabi define instability as a "loss of ability of the spine under physiologic loads to maintain relationships in such a way that there is neither damage nor subsequent irritation to the spinal cord or nerve roots and in addition there is no development of incapacitating deformity or pain."[39] Stable fractures such as a wedge compression fracture, with less than 40% loss of anterior vertebral height in the thoracic spine may be treated with pain relief and early mobilization. Serial radiographs may be required to make sure there is no increase in deformity.

Surgical Treatment of Spinal Fractures

Principles

The goals of surgery are (1) to reduce fractures and dislocation; (2) stabilize injured segments; and (3) prevention and limitation of neurological injury. Secondary goals include (4) deformity correction and (5) rapid rehabilitation.

Controversies concerning surgical treatment include the timing of surgery and the choice of surgical approach (anterior or posterior).

Indications for surgery include:
- Dislocations and major ligament disruptions. Ligament injuries in the spine behave similarly to ligament injuries involving other joints. These are potentially unstable and are therefore best treated surgically.
- Patient with neurological deficit secondary to a spinal injury who also has a concomitant upper thoracic injury. Here surgical stabilization is indicated so that the patient may be mobilized early in order to avoid pulmonary complications.
- Patients with progressive neurological deficit with radiologic evidence of neural compression. Surgery is required here to effect decompression of the neural structures in order to prevent further deterioration.
- Open spine fractures: treatment of these injuries follows the principles of compound fracture management in the long bones.

Choice of Approach; Anterior or Posterior Surgery

Anterior, posterior, and combined anterior-posterior approaches have been described in the treatment of thoracic and lumbar fractures. Surgery involving the anterior approach alone works well in a setting of injured anterior and middle columns, when the posterior column has remained intact. A posterior-only technique is suitable for flexion-distraction injuries and in those patients where spinal stabilization is the goal and decompression is not required (see Fig. 12.**5**). The latter situation arises in the treatment of a complete neurological injury where spinal fixation may offer immediate stabilization facilitating early rehabilitation and obviating the need for a cumbersome orthosis.

In a setting of significant three-column disruption with neurological compromise, a combined anterior and posterior approach offers the advantages of thorough decompression and the greatest degree of iatrogenic spinal stability.

The advantages of posterior surgery include less morbidity and less potential for disturbance of the vascular supply to an already injured cord. The advan-

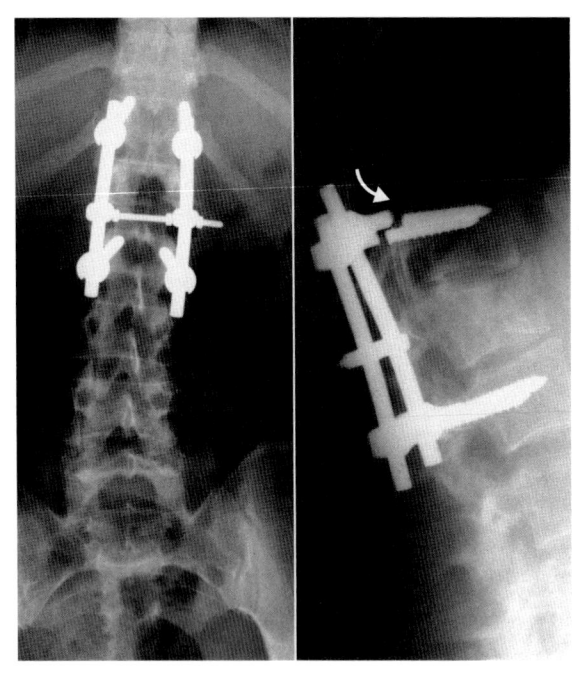

Fig. 12.11 Short segment posterior stabilization for a burst fracture. Note the broken pedicle screw (curved arrow).

Several posterior instrumentations exist. These vary from the simple rod hook system popularized by Harrington to the more recent multi-segmental systems as well as pedicular screws. In-direct spinal canal decompression may be achieved by ligamentotaxis. This depends on the integrity of Sharpey fibers and the annular ligament attachments to the displaced bony fragments. When a distraction force is applied posteriorly, ligamentotaxis results in an anteriorly directed force on the displaced bony fragments thus effecting reduction of the fracture. This technique is effective only in the first 2 or 3 days after injury.

When a simple rod hook system is used, longer segments of the spinal column may need to be fused to maintain fracture reduction. Short segment fixation using the CD instrumentation has been shown to have a poor outcome. McLain et al in their review of 19 patients found hardware failure and a loss of reduction in 10 patients (Fig. 12.11).[57] To overcome the disadvantage of fusing a longer area of the spinal column the concept of rod long and fuse short has been introduced. The method involves fusing only the two levels adjacent to the injured vertebra while spanning additional levels cephalad and caudad to the injured vertebra. The instrumentation is subsequently removed at a year from the injury. The disadvantage of this is the requirement for two surgical procedures with the subsequent procedure required to remove the rods. There is also an increased incidence of accelerated arthritis in the immobilized segments and a tendency for kyphosis following removal of instrumentation. The evolution of the modern pedicle screw-based posterior spinal stabilization systems have allowed for more reliable fixation while fusing fewer motion segments. Using these systems it is now possible to incorporate only two levels cephalad and caudad to the injured vertebra and obtain a satisfactory long-term outcome through the posterior alone fixation technique. A short segment posterior fixation is the treatment of choice for a flexion-distraction injury with an intact anterior osteo-ligamentous hinge.

tage of anterior surgery includes the possibility of obtaining a more thorough canal clearance in patients with significant canal compromise.

A review of the literature does not reveal a distinct advantage of one approach over the other. Gertzbein found that anterior surgery was likely to be more beneficial in improving complete bladder impairment compared to posterior surgery.[43] Dall and Stauffer in their series found that neurological recovery did not correlate with the treatment method (posterior instrumentation alone versus posterior stabilization followed by anterior decompression).[50] Edwards et al in their review of 122 patients found excellent maintenance of alignment in terms of kyphosis and vertebral height in patients treated posteriorly with rods that were centered over the pedicle of the fractured vertebra.[51] Kaneda et al reviewing 27 patients with thoracolumbar burst fractures treated by anterior decompression and fusion found that 73% of their patients had neurological improvement of at least 1 Frankel grade.[52] Anderson et al have shown that anterior decompression increases axoplasma flow, decreases ischemia, and leads to improvement of neurological function.[53,54] McAfee et al reviewed 48 patients with incomplete paraplegia who underwent anterior decompression.[55] Fifty percent of patients who could not walk preoperatively regained the ability. Twelve of 32 patients with an impaired bladder function also improved. Conversely Esses et al comparing anterior decompression and instrumentation with posterior instrumentation in patients with thoracolumbar burst fractures in a prospective randomized study found no statistical difference in neurological recovery,[56] maintenance of reduction, or rate of hardware failure between the two methods.

Timing of Surgery

Vaccaro et al in a randomized prospective study revealed no substantial difference in outcome between early and late surgical decompression and stabilization of patients with spinal cord injury.[58]

Concerns for early surgical stabilization of the spine in the multiply injured patient include: (1) the possibility of aggravating pulmonary decompensation through the prone position; (2) blood loss incurred through spinal surgery; and (3) concerns that occult injuries especially to the intraabdominal viscera may be masked by early surgical intervention.

However, early surgical intervention may have its advantages. It may decrease morbidity and hospital costs.[59] Marshall et al found that in 134 patients treated surgically 4 patients deteriorated after treatment.[60] These patients were treated within 48 hours of surgery whereas no patients treated after 5 days experienced this complication. They, therefore, recommended refraining from surgery within the first 5 days. McLain et al prospectively studied 75 patients with spinal trauma and other injuries treated with surgical stabilization within 72 hours of injury.[61] The mean injury severity score for these patients was greater than or approached LD 50 (i.e. expected mortality 50%). Only two patients died postoperatively and no major complications were noted. Krengel et al found significant neurological improvement in their series of patients treated surgically within the first 24 hours.[62] The basis of all surgical interventions is the experimental studies by Delamarter showing the efficacy of early decompression in reversing cord injuries in dogs. In patients with complete motor and sensory paraplegia, however, surgical treatment was not found to alter the prognosis.

Burst Fractures

The literature abounds with controversies regarding the management of these fractures. Researchers have advocated both operative and nonoperative treatment. Internal fixation offers the possibilities of immediate stability, early ambulation, and theoretical prevention of late deformity. Nonoperative care offers the avoidance of a surgical intervention and its attendant morbidity. Controversy mainly surrounds the management of burst fractures with no neurological deficit.

Controversies in the management of these fractures (surgical and nonsurgical) revolve around the following points:

1. **Can neurological deterioration occur after injury?** Boerger and colleagues carried out experimental studies on the lumbar spines from calf cadavers.[40] Burst fractures were produced experimentally in the lumbar spine in these cadaveric models. Pressures within the spinal canal were recorded before injury, at the time of injury, and after injury. These studies revealed that the pressure within the spinal canal was highest at the time of the injury. They hypothesized that the energy that produces the fracture is also responsible for the injury to the spinal cord. However, neurological deterioration after injury has been reported. Davies et al reported neurological deterioration in 2 of their 32 patients with thoracolumbar fractures.[41] Denis et al in their series of 29 patients with burst fractures managed nonoperatively had six patients who developed neurological complications and four who exhibited neurological deficit.[42] Likewise Frankel et al in their series of 205 injuries at the thoracolumbar region identified two patients with neurological deterioration.[33] Thus, it is likely that neurological deterioration may evolve over the course of management of these fractures.
2. **Is there a relation between deficit and displacement of the spinal column?** Gertzbein et al reported on 1019 spinal fractures followed prospectively for 2 years in a multi-center study.[43,44] They concluded that there was a greater incidence of complete neurological deficit caused by fractures at the spinal cord level and a diminished incidence at the cauda equina level. For burst fractures there was a weakly positive relationship between canal compromise and neurological deficit including bladder function.
3. **Does canal remodeling occur without surgery?** Several authors have reported on remodeling of the spinal canal following burst fractures. Mumford et al reviewing 41 patients without neurological deficit found that canal compromise averaged 37% at initial injury.[45] At a 2-year follow-up the average improvement in canal compromise and midsagittal diameter was 22% and 11%, respectively. Krompinger et al reporting on 29 patients with thoracic and lumbar fractures treated nonoperatively found bony remodeling to have occurred in 11 of the 14 patients who were found to have a canal compromise of greater than 25% on initial evaluation.[46] Thus, regardless of treatment significant remodeling of the compromised spinal canal occurs (Figs. 12.**12**, 12.**13**).
4. **Does late deformity cause pain?** Gertzbein in his multi-center study found that a kyphotic deformity of greater than 32° at a 2-year follow up was associated with an increased incidence of significant back pain.[43] Other authors have not found this relationship. Weinstein et al in their long-term follow-up of 42 patients treated conservatively for thoracolumbar burst fractures found that at follow-up the average back pain score was 3.5 in a score from zero to 10.[35] There was an average kyphosis angle of 26.4° in flexion and 16.8° in extension. The degree of kyphosis did not correlate with pain or function at follow up. Similarly, Rechtine in his review found that there was more pain in the group of patients treated with fusions as compared to those that were treated nonsurgically.[34] Other studies have similarly failed to demonstrate any association between reported pain and radiographic parameters such as degree of kyphosis. The incidence of significant pain following kyphosis is reported to be around 10%.[40]
5. **Length of hospital stay:** In most studies the length of hospital stay is longer in the nonsurgical group as would be expected. However, there is a recent trend in early mobilization of patients with stable burst fractures. Boerger et al recommend that stable burst fractures may be treated with 2 or 3 days of bed rest for pain relief, followed by subsequent mobilization in a suitable orthosis.[40]
6. **Return to work:** The ability of patients with spinal fractures to return to work has been reported following both operative and nonoperative treatment. Mumford et al reported that 26 of 32 patients with a thoracolumbar fracture treated with a brace were able to return to work.[45] Sixty percent of the patients in their series returned to jobs at the same level of activity. Knight et al reported that nonoperatively treated patients with lumbar burst fractures returned to work in half the time needed by patients treated operatively.[47] Similarly good functional results have been obtained after surgery.

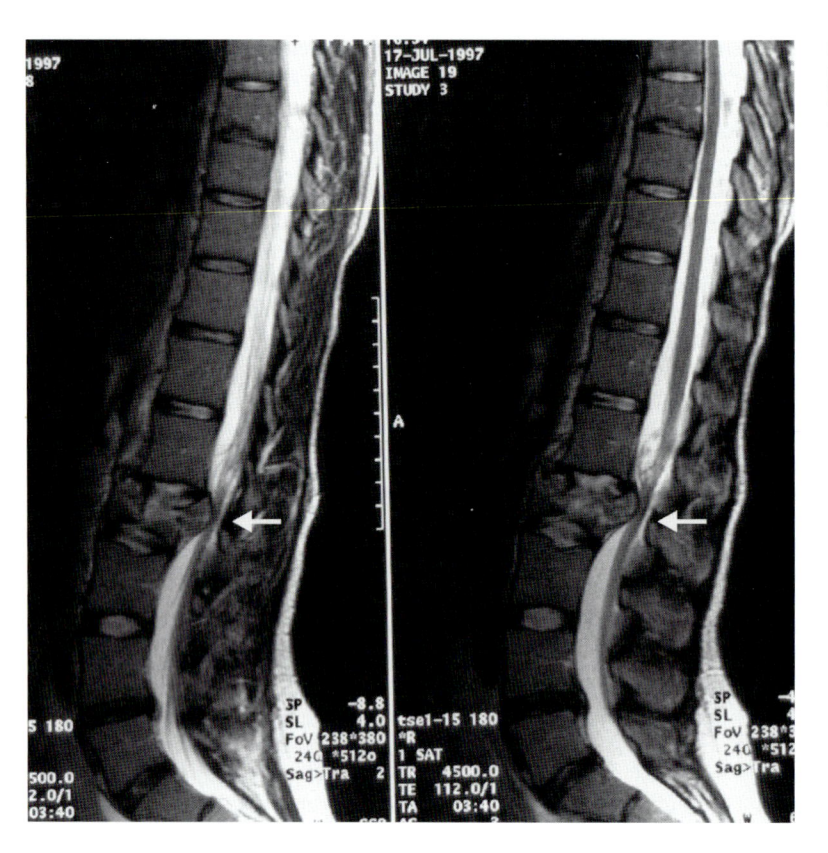

Fig. 12.**12** Sagittal MRI scan of a patient with a burst fracture of the lumbar spine showing canal encroachment (*arrows*) at L2.

McLain reported that 70% of patients treated surgically returned to full time work.[48] Fifty-four percent returned to previous employment without restriction. Work status correlated directly with neurological injury and not with the extent of surgical dissection, hardware failure, or surgical construct. Other studies have reported similar findings.

7. **Cost:** Wood et al in a randomized prospective study comparing operative and nonoperative treatment of burst fractures found that for a similar hospital stay, the average charge per injury for the group treated surgically was approximately $ 49 063 and that for the nonoperative group was $ 11 264.[49] The difference was statistically significant.

Early Ambulant Treatment of Thoracolumbar Burst Fractures

Early ambulant treatment of patients with burst fractures offers all the advantages of nonoperative treatment with the added benefit of a reduced hospital stay and hence a reduction in the hospital costs. The author is increasingly utilizing this method for the treatment of thoracolumbar burst fractures. The treatment is suitable for patients who have an isolated burst fracture without neurological deficit. The treatment consists of the application of a custom-fitted hyperextension thoracolumbar orthosis as soon as the patient is sufficiently pain free and able to sit up in bed. This is usually within a few days to a week after the injury. Following the application of the orthosis the patient is mobilized under the supervision of physiotherapists and allowed home as soon as he or she is independently mobile. The patient is then followed-up in the outpatients department at 4-weekly intervals with standing lateral radiographs of the spine to assess fracture healing. At the 3-month stage, depending on fracture healing, the orthosis is discontinued and a physical therapy program for back muscle strengthening is instituted. Wood et al in a randomized prospective study compared operative treatment with early ambulant nonoperative treatment of patients with thoracolumbar burst fractures.[49] In their study 27 patients were randomized to nonoperative treatment and 26 to surgical treatment, for thoracolumbar burst fractures without neurological deficit, with a mean follow-up of 44 months. The authors found no statistical significance in the amount of kyphosis, degree of pain, and the extent of canal compromise at the final follow-up between the two groups. The average cost of treatment in the surgical group was $ 49 063 and $ 11 264 in the nonoperative group ($p < 0.01$). The rates of return to work were no different in the two groups. There was a difference in the prevalence of complications between the two groups. Nineteen complications occurred in 16 of the 24 patients in the operative group compared with two complications in 3 of the 23 individuals treated nonoperatively.

Osteoporotic Vertebral Fractures

Osteoporosis is a systemic disease that results in progressive bone mineral loss and a vulnerability to fractures after minimal or no trauma.[63] The spinal column is often affected and it is estimated that about 700 000

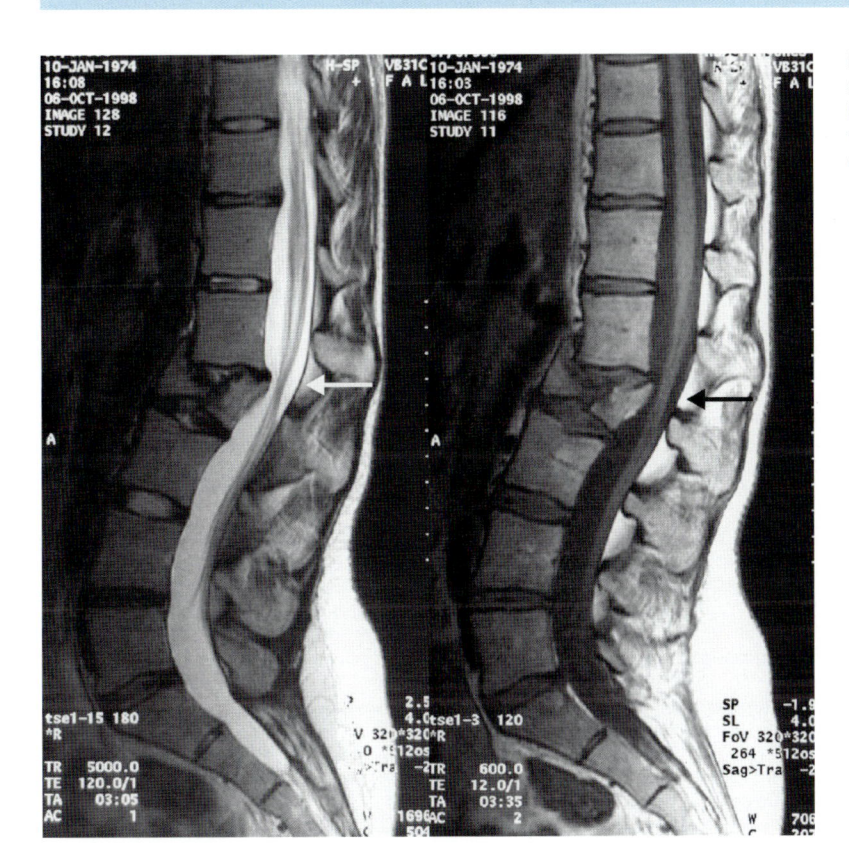

Fig. 12.13 Sagittal MRI scan of the same patient performed 1 year after injury showing remodeling of the fracture and restoration of the spinal canal dimensions (*arrows*).

osteoporotic vertebral fractures occur each year in the United States alone.[64] These fractures may be painful and could lead to progressive spinal deformity in the sagittal plane. Traditionally, osteoporotic vertebral fractures are treated nonoperatively with analgesics, bracing, and sometimes bed rest. However, nonoperative treatment does not prevent or restore sagittal plane deformity. To preserve sagittal spinal balance, and also relieve pain in these patients, two new treatments are increasingly being used. These include percutaneous vertebroplasty and kyphoplasty. Developed by Deramond et al in France,[65] percutaneous vertebroplasty entails injection of polymethylmethacylate cement into the collapsed vertebra. Although this does not reexpand the collapsed vertebra, reinforcing and stabilizing the fracture with cement seems to alleviate the pain.

The principal limitation of vertebroplasty is the tendency to cement extravasation, the rates of which are as high as 60% in metastases and 30% in osteoporotic fractures.[66] Kyphoplasty is a newer technique that involves the introduction of a canula into the vertebral body. This is then followed by the insertion of an inflatable bony tamp designed to reduce the vertebral body back towards its original height, creating a cavity within the body that is filled with bone cement.

Both these techniques are now increasingly prevalent in the United States and Europe although randomized trials comparing these treatments with the natural history of osteoporosis are required before their widespread use in the treatment of osteoporotic vertebral fractures.

Conclusion

The primary objectives of treating patients with spinal injury consist of the preservation of neurological function and the restoration of spinal stability while incurring minimal additional morbidity and cost. Spinal stability continues to be a poorly understood and controversial concept but is of paramount importance in terms of determining optimum treatment.

In the neurologically intact patient good results are obtained with both conservative and nonsurgical treatment. In patients with neural injury the potential for recovery may depend upon the initial insult at injury. **The higher the energy responsible for the injury** the more severe the degree of neurological deficit and spinal instability. Some improvement in neurological deficit in incomplete injuries may be expected whatever the modality of treatment.

Acknowledgement

Figure 12.**1** reprinted from *Eur J Radiol*, 2002, Vol. 42. J.M. Trivedi, Spinal trauma: therapy—options and outcomes, pp. 127–34, with permission from Elsevier.

References

1. Thurman DJ, Burnett CC, Jeppson L, Beaudoin DE, Sniezek JE. Surveillance of spinal cord injuries in Utah, USA. *Paraplegia.* 1994;32(10):665–669.
2. Benson DR, Keenen TL, Antony J. Unsuspected associated findings in spinal fractures. *J Orthop Trauma.* 1989;3:160.
3. Riggins RS, Kraus JF. The risk of neurologic damage with fractures of the vertebrae. *J Trauma.* 1977;7:126–133.
4. Stover SL, Fine PR. The epidemiology and economics of spinal cord injury. *Paraplegia.* 1987;25(3):225–228.
5. Browner BD, Levine AM, Jupiter JB, Trafton PG. Lower cervical spine injuries. In: *Skeletal Trauma.* 2nd ed. Philadelphia, PA: W.B. Saunders Company; 895–945.
6. Guttman L. History of the National Spinal Injuries Centre, Stoke Mandeville Hospital, Aylesbury. *Paraplegia.* 1967;5: 115–126.
7. Rivlin A, Tator CH. Effect of duration of acute spinal cord compression in a new acute spinal cord injury model in the rat. *Surg Neurol.* 1978;10:39–43.
8. Delamarter RB, Sherman JE, Carr JB. Volvo Award in experimental studies. Cauda equina syndrome: neurologic recovery following immediate, early or late decompression. *Spine.* 1991;16(9):1022–1029.
9. Bodner DR, Delamarter RB, Bohlman HH, Witcher M, Biro C, Resnick MI. Urologic changes after cauda equina compression in dogs. *J Urol.* 1990;143(1):186–190.
10. Dolan EJ, Tator CH, Endrenyi L. The value of decompression for acute experimental spinal cord compression injury. *J Neurosurg.* 1980;53:749–755.
11. Ducker TB, Solomon M, Daniel HB. Experimental spinal cord trauma III. Therapeutic effects of immobilization and pharmacologic agents. *Surg Neurol.* 1978;10(1):71–76.
12. Holdsworth FW. Fractures, dislocations and fracture-dislocations of the spine. *J Bone Joint Surg. Am.* 1970;52:1534–1551.
13. Denis F. The three-column spine and its significance in the classification of acute thoracolumbar spinal injuries. *Spine.* 1983;8:817–831.
14. Chance GQ. Note on a type of flexion fracture of the spine. *Br J Radiol.* 1948;21:452–453.
15. Anderson PA, Rivera FP, Maier RV, Drake C. The epidemiology of seatbelt-associated injuries. *J Trauma.* 1991;31:60–67.
16. Piepmeier JM, Lehmann KB, Lane JG. Cardiovascular instability following acute cervical spinal cord trauma. *Cent Nerv Sys Trauma.* 1985;2:153–160.
17. Eismont FG, Arena MJ, Green BA. Extrusion of intervertebral disc associated with traumatic subluxation or dislocation of cervical facets. *J Bone Joint Surg Am.* 1991;73:1555–1559.
18. Mahale YJ, Silver JR, Henderson NJ. Neurological complications of the reduction of cervical spine dislocations. *J Bone Joint Surg Br.* 1993;75:403–409.
19. Robertson PA, Ryan MD. Neurological deterioration after reduction of cervical spine subluxations. Mechanical compression by disc tissue. *J Bone Joint Surg Br.* 1992;74:224–227.
20. Lee AS, MacLean JCB, Newton DA. Rapid traction for reduction of cervical spine dislocations. *J Bone Joint Surg Br.* 1994;76: 352–356.
21. Star AM, Jones AA, Cotler JM, Balderston RA, Sinha R. Immediate closed reduction of cervical spine dislocation using traction. *Spine.* 1990;15:1068–1072.
22. Bracken MB, Shepard MJ, Collins WF, et al. A randomized controlled trial of methylprednisolone or naloxone in the treatment of acute spinal cord injury. Results of the Second National Acute Spinal Cord Injury Study. *N Engl J Med.* 1990; 322:1405–1411.
23. Bracken MB, Shepard MJ, Collins WF, et al. Methylprednisolone or naloxone treatment after spinal cord injury: 1 year follow-up data. Results of the Second National Acute Spinal Cord Injury Study. *J Neurosurg.* 1992;76:23–31.
24. Bracken MB, Shepard MJ, Holford TR, et al. Administration of metylprednisolone for 24 or 48 hours or tirilazad mesylate for 48 hours in the treatment of acute spinal cord injury. Results of the Third National Acute Spinal Cord Injury Randomized Controlled Trial. National Acute Spinal Cord Injury Study. *JAMA.* 1997;277:1597–1604.
25. Short DJ, El Masry WS, Jones PW. High dose methylprednisolone in the management of acute spinal cord injury. *J Spinal Disord.* 2000;38:273–286.
26. Coleman WP, Benzel D, Cahill DW, et al. A critical appraisal of the reporting of the National Acute Spinal Cord Injury Studies (II and III) of methylprednisolone in acute spinal cord injury. *J Spinal Disord.* 2000;13:185–199.
27. Hurlbert RJ. Methylprednisolone for acute spinal cord injury: an inappropriate standard of care. *J Neurosurg.* 2000; 93:1–7.
28. Geisler FH, Dorsey FC, Coleman WP. Recovery of motor function after spinal cord injury. A randomized placebo-controlled trial with GM-1 gangliozide. *N Engl J Med.* 1991;324: 1829–1838.
29. Anderson DK, Waters TR, Means ED. Pre-treatment with alpha tocopherol enhances recovery after experimental spinal cord injury. *J Neurotrauma.* 1988;5:61–67.
30. Shi RY, Lucas JH, Wolf A, Gross GW. Calcium antagonists fail to protect mammalian spinal neurons after physical injury. *J Neurotrauma.* 1989;6:261–278.
31. Nicoll EA. Fractures of the dorso-lumbar spine. *J Bone Joint Surg Br.* 1949;31:376–394.
32. Bedbrook GM. Treatment of thoraco-lumbar dislocations and fractures with paraplegia. *Clin Orthop.* 1975;43:112–127.
33. Frankel HL, Hancock DO, Hyslop G, Melzak J, Michaelis LS, Ungar GH, Vernon JD, Walsh JJ. The value of postural reduction in the initial management of closed injuries of the spine with paraplegia and tetraplegia. *Paraplegia.* 1969; 7(3):179–192.
34. Rechtine GR. Nonsurgical treatment of thoracic and lumbar fractures. American Academy of Orthopaedic Surgeons' Instructional Course lecture. 1999;48:413–416.
35. Weinstein JN, Collalto P, Lehmann TR. Thoraco-lumbar "burst" fractures treated conservatively: A long term follow-up. *Spine.* 1988;13(1);33–38.
36. Norton PL, Brown T. The immobilizing efficiency of back braces. *J Bone Joint Surg Am.* 1957;19:111–139.
37. Fidler MW, Plasmans CT. The effect of four types of support on segmental mobility of the lumbosacral spine. *J Bone Joint Surg Am.* 1983;65:943–947.
38. Nagel DA, Koogle TA, Piziali RL, Perkash I. Stability of the upper lumbar spine following progressive disruption and the application of individual internal and external fixation devices. *J Bone Joint Surg Am.* 1981;63:62–70.
39. White AA III, Panjabi MM. The problem of clinical instability in the human spine: A systematic approach. In: White AA, Panjabi MM, eds. *Clinical biomechanics of the spine.* 2nd ed. Philadelphia, PA: JB Lippincott; 1990:277–388.
40. Boerger TO, Limb D, Dickson RA. Does canal clearance affect neurological outcome after thoraco-lumbar burst fractures. *J Bone Joint Surg Br.* 2000;82:629–635.
41. Davies WE, Morris JH, Hill V. An analysis of conservative (nonsurgical) management of thoraco-lumbar fractures and fracture dislocations with neural damage. *J Bone Joint Surg Am.* 1980;62:1324–1328.
42. Denis F, Armsrong GWD, Searls K, Matta LL. Acute thoracolumbar burst fractures in the absence of neurologic deficit. A comparison between operative and nonoperative treatment. *Clin Orthop.* 1984;189:142–149.
43. Gertzbein SD. Scoliosis Research Society. Multicenter spine fracture study. *Spine.* 1992;17(5):528–540.
44. Gertzbein SD, Court-Brown CM, Marks P, Martin C, Fazl M, Schwartz M, Jacobs RR. The neurological outcome following surgery for spinal fractures. *Spine.* 1988;13(6):641–644.
45. Mumford J, Weinstein JN, Spratt KF, Goel VK. Thoracolumbar burst fractures: the clinical efficacy and outcome of nonoperative management. *Spine.* 1993;18(8):955–970.
46. Krompinger JW, Frederickson BE, Mino DE, Yuan HA. Conservative treatment of fractures of the thoracic and lumbar spine. *Orthop Clin North Am.* 1986;17(1):161–170.
47. Knight RQ, Stornelli DP, Chan DP, Devanny JR, Jackson KV. Comparison of operative versus nonoperative treatment of lumbar burst fractures. *Clin Orthop.* 1993;293:112–121.
48. McLain RF. Functional outcomes after surgery for spinal fractures: return to work and activity. *Spine.* 2004;15;29(4):470–477.
49. Wood K, Butterman G, Mehbod A, Garvey T, Jhanjee R, Sechriest V. Operative compared with nonoperative treatment

of a thoracolumbar burst fracture without neurological deficit: A prospective randomized study. *J Bone J Surg Am.* 2003; 85(5):773–781.
50. Dall BE, Stauffer ES. Neurologic injury and recovery patterns in burst fractures at the T12 or L1 motion segment. *Clin Orthop.* 1988;233:171–176.
51. Edwards CC, Levine AM. Early rod-sleeve stabilization of the injured thoracic and lumbar spine. *Orthop Clin North Am.* 1986;17:121–145.
52. Kaneda K, Abumi K, Fujiya M. Burst fractures with neurologic deficits of the thoraco-lumbar spine. Results of anterior decompression and stabilization with anterior instrumentation. *Spine.* 1984;9:788–795.
53. Bohlmann HH, Anderson PA. Anterior decompression and arthrodesis of the cervical spine. Long term motor improvement: I. Improvement in incomplete traumatic quadripareisis. *J Bone Joint Surg Am.* 1992;74:659–670.
54. Anderson PA, Bohlmann HH. Anterior decompression and arthrodesis of the cervical spine. Long term motor improvement: II. Improvement in incomplete traumatic quadriparesis. *J Bone Joint Surg Am.* 1992;74:671–682.
55. McAfee PC, Bohlmann HH, Yuan HA. Anterior decompression of traumatic thoraco-lumbar fractures with incomplete neurological deficit using a retroperitoneal approach. *J Bone Joint Surg Am.* 1985;67:89–104.
56. Esses SI, Botsford DJ, Kostuik JP. Evaluation of surgical treatment for burst fractures. *Spine.* 1990;15:667–673.
57. McLain RF, Sparling E, Benson DR. Early failure of short-segment pedicle instrumentation for thoraco-lumbar fractures. A preliminary report. *J Bone Joint Surg Am.* 1993;75: 162–167.
58. Vaccaro AR, Daugherty RJ, Sheehan TP, Dante SJ, Cotler JM, Balderston RA, Herbison GJ, Northup BE. Neurologic outcome of early versus late surgery for cervical spinal cord injury. *Spine.* 1997;22:2609–2613.
59. Schlegel J, Yuan H, Fredericksen B. Timing of operative management of acute spinal injuries. *Orthopaedic Transactions.* 1992;16:688.
60. Marshall LF, Knowlton S, Garfin SR, et al. Deterioration after spinal cord injury. A multicenter study. *J Neurosurg.* 1987;66: 400–404.
61. McLain RF, Benson DR. Urgent surgical stabilization of spinal fractures in polytrauma patients. *Spine.* 1999;24(16): 1646–1654.
62. Krengel WF, Anderson PA, Henley MB. Early stabilization and decompression for incomplete paraplegia due to a thoracic level spinal cord injury. *Spine.* 1993;18:2080–2087.
63. Riggs BL, Melton LJ III. Involutional osteoporosis. *N Engl J Med.* 1986;314:1676–1686.
64. Cooper C, Atkinson EJ, O'Fallon WM, Melton LJ III. The incidence of clinically diagnosed vertebral fractures: a population based study in Rochester, Minnesota, 1985–1989. *J Bone Miner Res.* 1992;7:221–227.
65. Deramond H, Darrason R, Galibert P. Percutaneous vertebroplasty with acrylic cement in the treatment of aggressive spinal angiomas. *Rachis.* 1989;1:143–153.
66. Well A, Chiras J, Simon JM, Rose M, Sola-Martinez T, Enkaoua E. Spinal metastases: indications for and results of percutaneous injection of acrylic cement. *Radiology.* 1996; 199:241–247.

13 Imaging in Chronic Spinal Cord Injury: Indications and Benefits

R. Bodley

Abbreviations

AXR	abdominal radiograph
US	ultrasound
IVP/U	intravenous pyelogram/urogram
MRI	magnetic resonance imaging
CTM	computed tomography myelogram
ERPF	effective renal plasma flow study (Tc-99m MAG3)
DREZ	dorsal root entry zone
PPMM	progressive posttraumatic myelomalacic myelopathy
PPCM	progressive posttraumatic cystic myelopathy
PCNL	percutaneous nephrolithotomy
EO	ectopic ossification
HO	heterotopic ossification
PAO	paraarticular ossification (osteopathy)
DVT	deep venous thrombosis
SCI	spinal cord injury

Introduction

With improvements in the management of patients with spinal cord injuries (SCI) over the past 60 years, the demographics have changed quite markedly.[1] With patients injured in their youth now surviving for many decades, there is an aging population of patients with SCI so the chronic changes in the body, particularly in the central nervous and renal systems, are becoming more important. In addition, there is a group of geriatric patients injured as a result of trauma exacerbating degenerative changes in the spine.

As the late complications of SCI are seen increasingly frequently, regular surveillance of both the renal tract and the central nervous system is important as the treatment of impending, potentially fatal complications can be implemented before damage has progressed too far.

Renal tract complications are particularly dangerous as they are often clinically silent but regular surveillance to detect early deterioration in renal function, particularly from reversible causes such as reflux or obstruction, can preempt problems. Follow-up protocols depend on the bladder management regimen but most centers advocate regular ultrasound with less frequent isotope function studies and urodynamics.

With the increasing ability to diagnose and treat the neurological complications, surveillance of the state of the spinal cord with MRI is also important and many centers now advocate checks every few years with sagittal mid-line T2W sections generally sufficient.

Imaging is critical in acute situations. In addition to suffering from the usual conditions, patients with spinal cord injury suffer others peculiar to, or particularly related to, the injury, which may be missed as their symptomatology is greatly altered by their paraplegic or quadriplegic status and they may often present as generally unwell but with no obvious cause or pathological focus.

This chapter discusses the role of radiology in routine surveillance of the CNS and the renal tract as well as in assessing specific conditions such as deteriorating neurology or renal function, pain, spinal instability, pressure sores, ectopic ossification, muscular spasm, spinal instability, airway problems, and elective operations on the renal tract (Table 13.1).

Table 13.1 Radiology is critical in:

Routine surveillance	Central nervous system
	Renal tract
Specific conditions	Deteriorating neurology
	Spinal instability
	The acutely unwell patient
	Deteriorating renal function
	Pressure sores
	Ectopic ossification
	Pain
	Muscular spasm
	Airway problems
	Elective management of the renal tract

Neurological System

Significant recovery of neurological function rarely commences more than 1 year after the accident, particularly in complete lesions. There is often, however, deterioration with time, the main heralding symptoms being loss of function, the loss of a reflex, or increasing pain or spasms. Any deterioration, however slight, in the limited function the patient possesses may make the difference between relative independence and the need for chronic care, so prompt and accurate diagnosis as well as regular surveillance to preempt problems is of paramount importance.

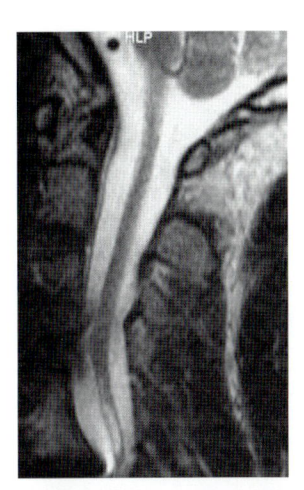

Fig. 13.**1** Sagittal T2W section showing atrophy.

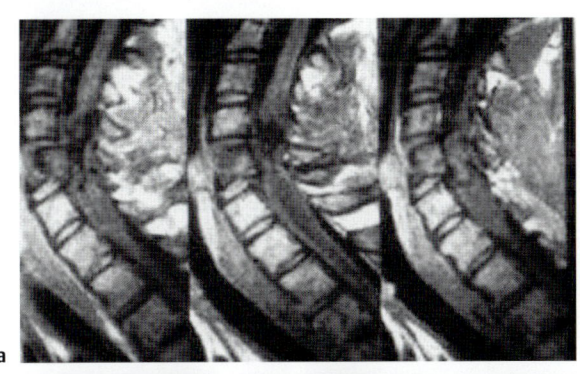

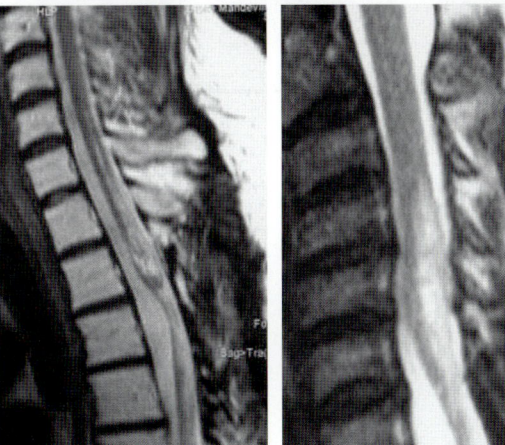

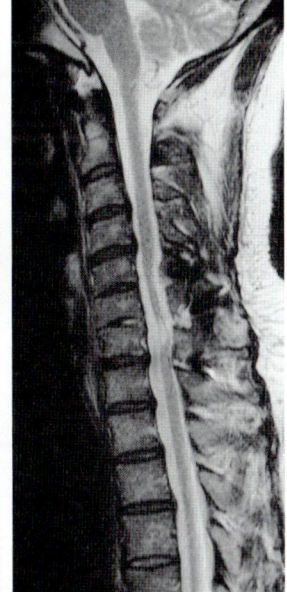

Fig. 13.**2** **Progressive post-traumatic myelomalacic myelopathy. a** Sagittal T1W sections showing changes at 3 months post-injury. **b** Sagittal T2W section showing a mixed signal change in the cord. **c** Sagittal T2W section showing posterior arachnoid tethering. **d** Sagittal T2W section showing myelomalacia.

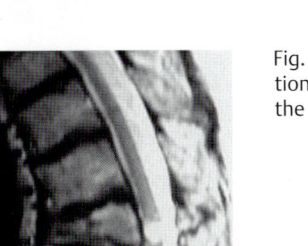

Fig. 13.**3** Sagittal T2W section showing a focal cyst at the injury site.

Cord Changes Post-SCI

Although in 1915 Holmes described six SCI patients whose neurological condition had deteriorated and who at surgery had intramedullary cysts extending several segments above or below the injury site, until MRI became available, there were few further reports of the changes.[2]

The three most important changes that have been noted in the cord are atrophy (Fig. 13.**1**), myelomalacia (Fig. 13.**2**; progressive posttraumatic myelomalacic or noncystic myelopathy [PTMM]), and cystic changes (progressive posttraumatic cystic myelopathy [PTCM], focal cyst [Fig. 13.**3**], and syringomyelia [Fig. 13.**4**]).

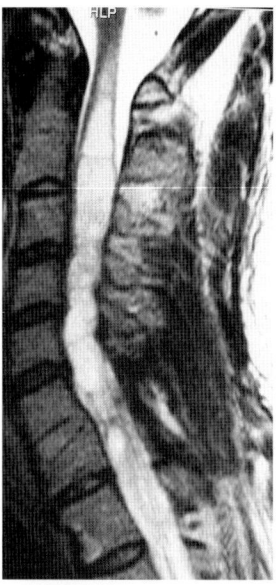

Fig. 13.**4** **Syringomyelia. a** Sagittal T2W section showing a flare at the rostral end indicating edema. **b** Axial T1W section. **c** Sagittal T1W sections showing "septa" that are probably decussating tracts. **d** Sagittal T2W section of a syrinx. **e** Posterior fixation clearly showing a syrinx. **f** Intraoperative US axial image showing the cyst.

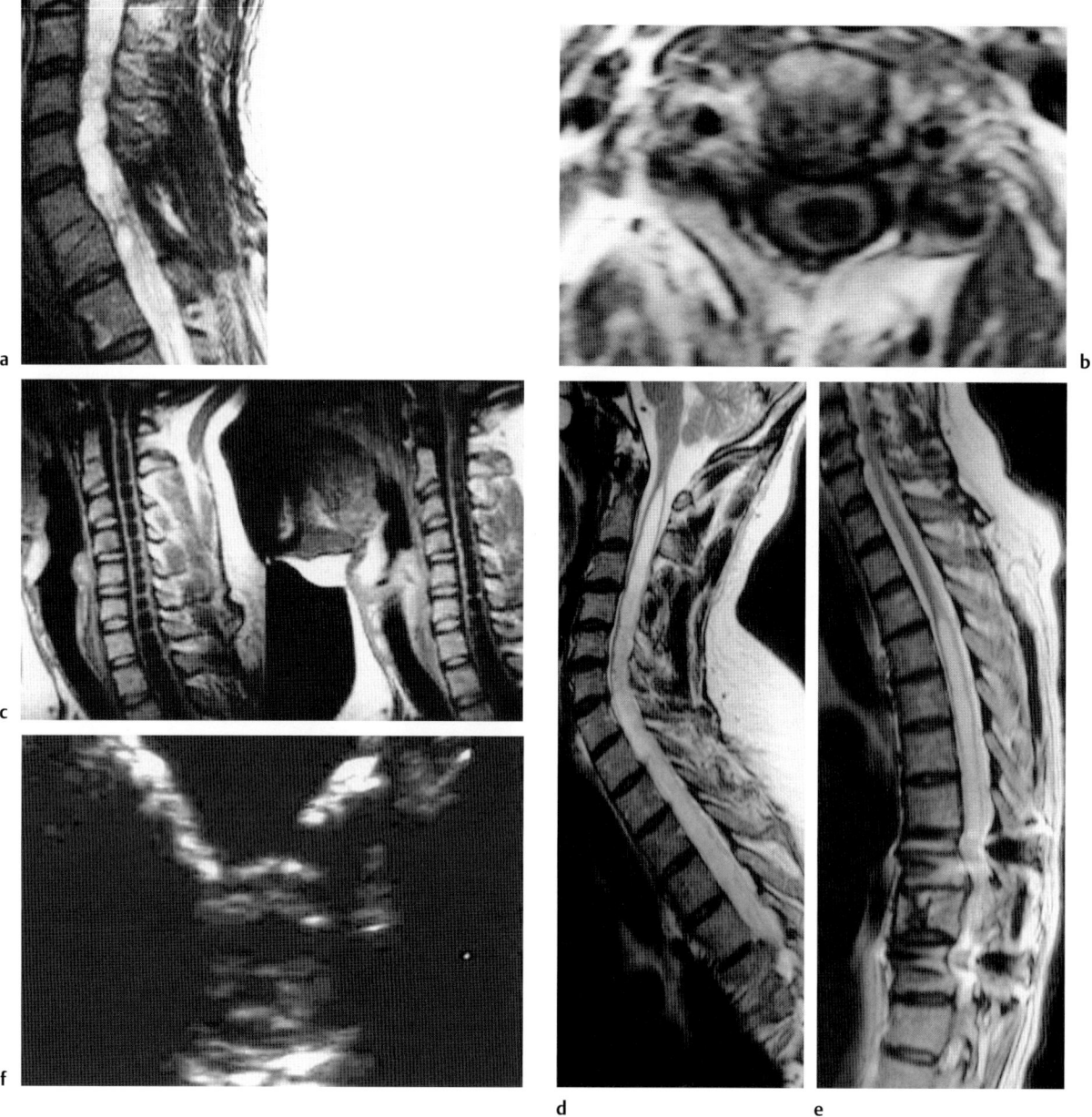

Understanding of all these conditions has been greatly impeded by a general lack of agreement on their definitions, both histologically and radiologically, in the various studies of their occurrence, and a true incidence is essentially unknown. Posttraumatic changes in the cord are difficult to study as there is no good animal model and there are few extensive patient series. The most comprehensive descriptions and insights into the pathophysiology are by Quencer and Squier.[3–5]

Wallerian degeneration with demyelination and subsequent gliosis is the main cause of irreversible proximal atrophy causing a loss of spinal cord substance and abnormal narrowing of the cord diameters. Other factors are still poorly understood and possibly relate to ischemia and focal inflammatory changes, a postulated mechanism that surgeons who decompress or physicians who administer high-dose corticosteroids within 6 hours of trauma are aiming to ameliorate.[6–8]

At the time of injury there may be an injection of crushed cord tissue from the site of maximum impact along shear planes in the cord. The cord then becomes edematous and the tissue undergoes necrosis and cyst formation, a process also probably involving liquefaction of parenchymal hematoma, ischemia, the release of intracellular enzymes, and mechanical damage from cord compression. Those cysts that develop macroscopically are eccentrically placed, are rarely contiguous with the central canal, and have been termed "contusion evolving to cavity."

The progression to syringomyelia, i. e., a cyst extending beyond the limits of bony damage, appears to involve arachnoid adhesions, presumably secondary to blood products and inflammatory changes at the time of injury. The inability of the cord to move freely and the consequent turbulent CSF flow dynamics, with high-pressure ballistic impulses particularly focused on the damaged parts of the cord, is thought to lead to the formation and propagation of the syrinx,[9–11] though in-vitro hydrodynamic studies are still incomplete and inconclusive. This leads to a "pre-syringomyelic" myelopathic state of reversible cord edema that develops into the two distinct conditions of PPMM and PPCM.[12–14] The radiological appearances may oscillate rapidly over a few weeks with no real contemporary correlation with the clinical picture (as shown by Milhorat in 1998 and from personal unpublished experience).[15] The histological changes are unknown.

CSF flow assessments in patients with Chiari malformations and post-traumatic cysts support these views and restoration of CSF dynamics with untethering of adhesions and an allograft expansile duraplasty is the basis of the most successful surgical approach for treatment,[16–23] shunting alone being less successful (Fig. 13.5).

The need for early operative restoration of normal alignment and the reduction of deformity, and restoration of canal capacity to normalize CSF function is still controversial with most studies being retrospective on symptomatic patients but there is a large body of conservative thinkers who feel that the risks of surgery for most patients do not often outweigh the risks of subsequent neurological change.[24–26]

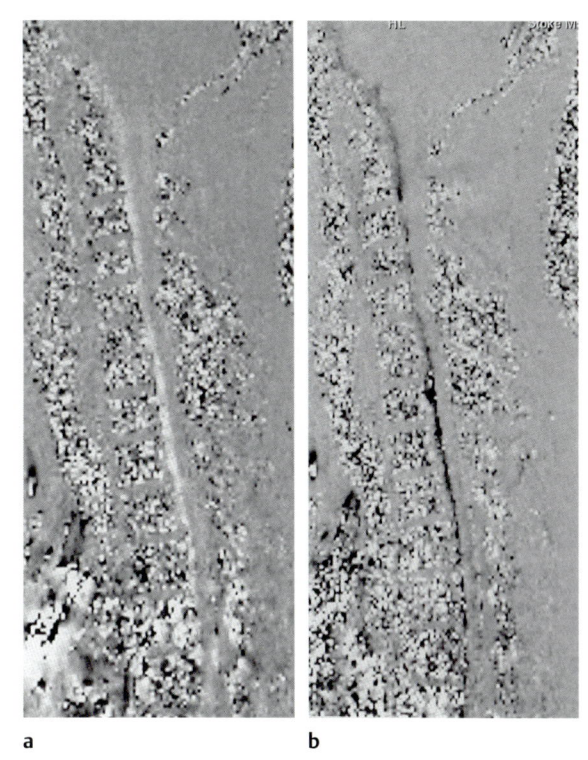

Fig. 13.**5** **CSF flow study**. The *white* (**a**) and *black line* (**b**) anterior to the cord is the pulsating CSF. There is no significant flow posteriorly indicating that the CSF is not moving, presumably as the result of posterior adhesions.

Reported Series

Atrophy

Cord measurements at different levels have been determined from pathological studies and CT myelography although the results are significantly different between the two methods depending on the window/level settings. Similar differences exist in measuring atrophy on T1 and T2 sequences (personal observations). From the pathological studies, a normal cervical cord A-P diameter is not less than 7.5 mm, and the thoracic cord 6.5 mm.[36] Some authors have assessed atrophy qualitatively so it is difficult to compare rates when the criteria are not given.

Using MRI, incidences of 7%,[37] 18%,[25] and 27% have been reported but the groups are heterogeneous and symptomatic and the techniques undefined so comparisons are virtually meaningless.[36]

Myelomalacic changes

In the literature there is often confusion between cysts, myelomalacia, and syringomyelia so comparisons of the different series is impossible. Some authors record all abnormal cystic-looking structures as posttraumatic spinal cord cysts (PTSCC),[38,39] however others distinguish between focal cysts, syrinxes, and myelomalacia.[25,36,37,40] Incidences for "syringomyelia" vary between 1%, 1.4%, and 3.2% using clinical criteria in the pre-MRI era and up to 59% using MRI.[39] The term "myelomalacia" has been used loosely to describe acute ischemic changes due to vascular stasis and perivascular edema or areas of degenerative change in the cord in which there are multiple small cysts and gliosis.

Examining a heterogeneous group of 87 patients, approximately one-third of whom had already undergone spinal surgery, Curati et al defined myelomalacia as areas of patchy low intensity on T1W images with corresponding high intensity on T2W images with signal intensities not quite the same as the surrounding CSF and syrinx as a low intensity linear or septate structure within the cord tissue on T1W sections together with areas of low signal in at least part of the cyst on the T2W sections—a change thought to be due to fluid motion—the overall signal characteristics being similar to those of the surrounding CSF.[25] No distinction between syringomyelia and a focal cyst was made. With these criteria, they found an incidence of myelomalacia in 37%, syringomyelia in 40%, atrophy in 18%, and persistent cord compression in 32%. This latter was found in approximately equal frequency in patients with total paraplegia, incomplete paralysis, and with minor signs only.

The confusion and heterogenicity in published series emphasizes the need for long-term, longitudinal, prospective studies to try to understand the pathogenesis of these entities.[41]

To date the most likely indicator of incidence is the study reported by Wang et al,[42] in which MR imaging was performed on a cohort of 153 consecutive patients, regardless of their symptomatology, who had had their SCI at least 20 years previously. Using the following definitions:

Atrophy: abnormal narrowing of the spinal cord in the sagittal plane two segments or more beyond the limits of the vertebral injury (< 7.5 mm in the cervical and < 6.5 mm in the thoracic cord—based on normals taken from measurements on a local population; Fig. 13.**1**).

Myelomalacia: an area of low T1W and high T2W signal intensity that is between that of normal spinal cord and the surrounding CSF with ill-defined contours and irregular shapes, occasionally appearing as a string of small cysts (Fig. 13.**2**).

Syrinx: an area with the same signal intensity as CSF which is usually tapered at one or both ends and which may appear loculated, with a well-defined contour and which extends beyond the length of maximal bony damage (Fig. 13.**4**).

Focal cyst: an area having the same signal intensity and contour definition as a syrinx, but with a round or oval shape and confined to the site of maximal bony protrusion into the spinal canal (Fig. 13.**3**).

Disruption: the complete absence of the spinal cord signal through the traumatized area.

They reported an incidence of
- atrophy in   62%,
- myelomalacia in   54%,
- syringomyelia in 22%,
- focal cysts in   9%,
- and disruption in 7%.

In a stable cyst or syrinx there is fluid equilibrium and in our experience, appearances may not change for many years though if there is no deteriorating neurology, few surgeons would recommend an operation. Life-style modification may be suggested, e. g., the avoidance of contact sports, which might aggravate the condition by increasing the ballistic impulses of the CSF.

In a hydrodynamically unstable cyst, however, there may be MRI abnormalities in the cord tissue surrounding the cyst. An increased T2W signal cephalad to the top of a syrinx (Fig. 13.**4a**) has been correlated with clinically progressive disease and its disappearance with resolution of the clinical problems post-operatively. This presumably represents edema from raised intra-cystic pressure and is analogous to the flare in the periventricular edema of hydrocephalus.[43,44]

Treatment

The treatment of syringomyelia is still controversial and generally reserved for symptomatic patients.[27,28] CT-guided cyst puncture as a temporary and predictive treatment has been described but most surgery to date has been myelotomy or shunt placement, sometimes with the aid of intraoperative US for restoration of CSF flow dynamics, which is now the favored approach.

Omental transposition and grafting has largely been discredited in controlled trials but a Chinese experience of 3000 patients claims return of some useful autonomic function.[29-31]

In refractory cases, cordotomy is offered but there is a general reluctance to accept this final step in the light of impending cord treatments aimed at reconnecting the pathways and promoting regeneration of the cord (see Chapter 17).

Post-operative assessments to confirm syrinx collapse or a return to normal of the cord signal can be rapidly performed in a brief examination as only two or three T1W or T2W sagittal mid-line sections are required. Occasionally shunt blockage is suspected and i. v. contrast enhancement may show chronic inflammatory reaction and perhaps infection around the tip (Fig. 13.**6**).

Imaging

The purpose of imaging in the chronic state is to assess the presence of remediable pathology. PPMM, PTCM, and syringomyelia are the only directly treatable complications but other pathologies may coexist, such as disk disease, tumors etc., and they would require as full a work-up as in any other patient.

Frequency of Investigation

Sequential studies have shown that changes in the cord can progress at various times and with surprising speed. A developing syrinx may become evident within 2–3 months (Fig. 13.**2a**), at which stage it has the features of PPMM.

Syrinx incidence is reported to be twice as common after 10 years as before and the author of this chapter has noted incidences of approximately 6% at 2 years, 9% at 5 years, 20% at 20 years, and 30% at 30 years (unpublished data) so it would seem prudent to scan at least before discharge from hospital so that a baseline is established,[25] and then at regular intervals, perhaps every 2–5 years, during the follow-up or at any other time if the neurological condition deteriorates (Table 13.**2**).

MRI

A spin-echo sagittal T2W, STIR, or FLAIR sequence of the whole of the cord (with axial T1W or T2W sections if inconclusive) are generally sufficient for diagnosis and take little more than a few minutes of room time. Most patients are relatively mobile and the short scan times mean that special precautions against pressure sores are rarely needed. There is a recent pictorial review of the MRI findings.[32]

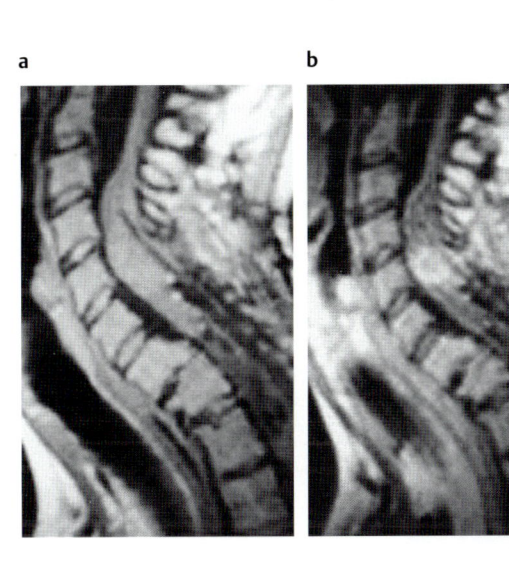

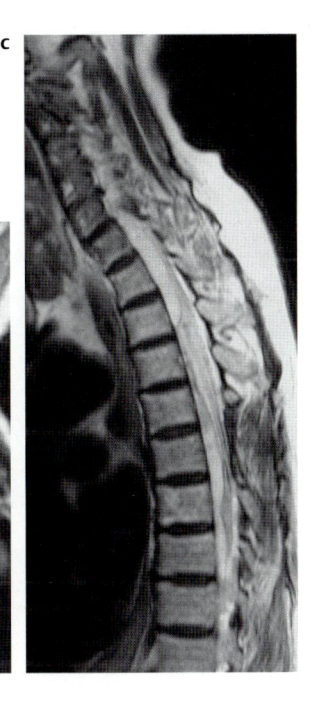

Fig. 13.6 Post-shunt complications. a Sagittal T1W section pre-gadolinium. **b** Section post-gadolinium showing inflammatory reaction at the end of the tube that settled with antibiotics. **c** Syrinx that is held open by adhesions despite shunting.

Table 13.2 Routine asymptomatic surveillance

System	Technique	Frequency	Benefit and Comment
CNS	MRI of the cord Sagittal T2 Axial T1	Prior to discharge then possibly every 5 years	Watch for early development of PPMM, PTCM and syringomyelia. Lifestyle modifications (e. g., decreased contact sport, etc.) may be advised. Only treat symptomatic patients.
Renal tract	US AXR (IVP not routinely indicated)	At the regular clinical review. Possibly less frequent if stable for 10 years	The frequency and use will depend on the bladder management technique. **Renal tract complications are the silent killer**. Monitor development of stones and hydronephrosis—useful as a baseline when symptoms suddenly change. Low threshold for nephrostomy if obstructed.
	ERPF/MAG 3 renography	Baseline, at 1 year then 5 yearly (depending on departmental capacity and bladder management technique)	Regular monitoring of renal function to pre-empt pressure-related effects from detrusor/sphincter dyssynergia. Deterioration should be investigated further.
	Urodynamics	Variable practice depending on the resources available	Not needed if the patient is catheterized or uses self-intermittent catheterization. Pressure-flow measurement generally sufficient. Cystourethrography is rarely performed as surveillance but when there is deteriorating function, to check for reflux

CSF flow studies are currently being assessed and may become useful predictors of surgical success if myelomalacic or syringomyelic states are present.

Contraindications to MRI Scanning

See Table 13.3.
In addition to the usual contraindications, phrenic pacemakers may be a problem, although there have been occasional cases of scans performed on patients with phrenic pacers with no demonstrable deleterious effects. With gunshot or shrapnel wounds it is wise to remove the fragments surgically prior to scanning unless they can be demonstrated as firmly fixed in the tis-

Table 13.3 Contraindications to MRI scanning

Absolute	General comments
SARS, phrenic pacing	Theoretically absolute. (Unsupported by manufacturers if patient or the equipment is damaged. No damage yet reported in practice, especially at low field strengths)
Intrathecal pumps	Mechanical: no problem Electronic: discuss, as control settings may be altered
Spinal fixation devices	No safety problem after 2 weeks postoperatively
	Variable artifact

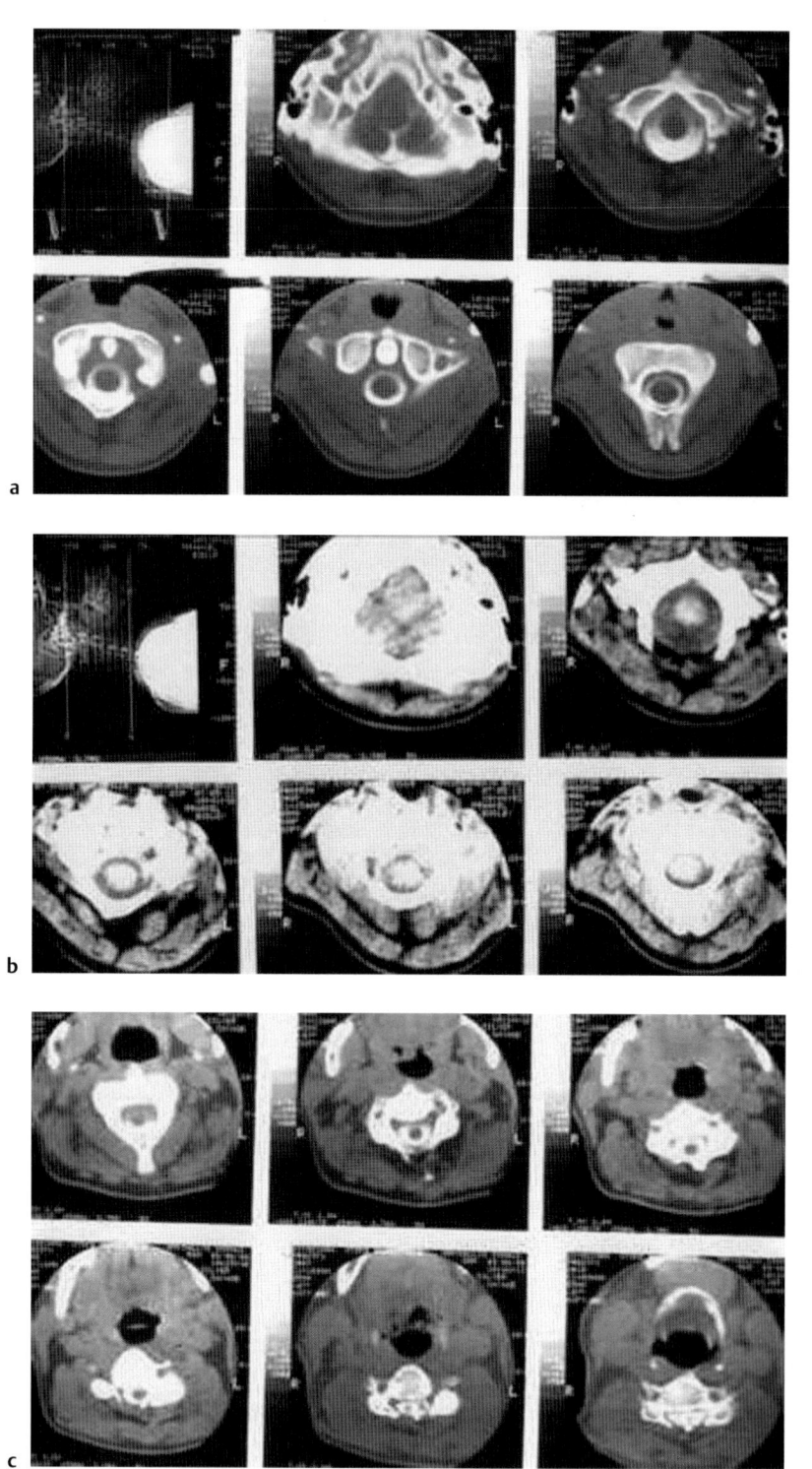

Fig. 13.7 **CT myelography. a** Axial sections immediately post-injection—note the dilated cord with surrounding contrast. **b** Sections 18 hours post-injection with contrast "reversal." **c** Atrophy.

sues. This is probably safe in the chronic state but caution is always appropriate. The problems are theoretically decreased in magnets with low field and low power gradient strengths and if the patient is introduced slowly into the magnet, any abnormal reaction should be reversible. It must be remembered, however, that sensation is very abnormal in these patients.

Sacral Anterior Root Stimulators are used to aid control of micturition and bowel function. A receiver is implanted subcutaneously and wires are tunneled through a laminectomy in the upper sacrum and clipped to the anterior roots of the sacral nerves S1–S4. This can act like a pacemaker and there are theoretical reasons for avoiding MRI, such as inadvertent activation of the bodily functions and heat damage to the roots themselves.[33]

At least one manufacturer, (Siemens, personal communication) refuses to support the scanning of patients with SARS on the grounds of potential damage to both patient and scanner, despite the inventor's own

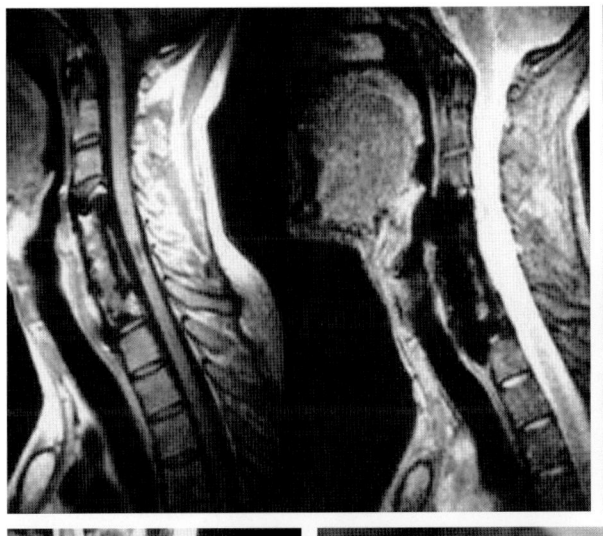

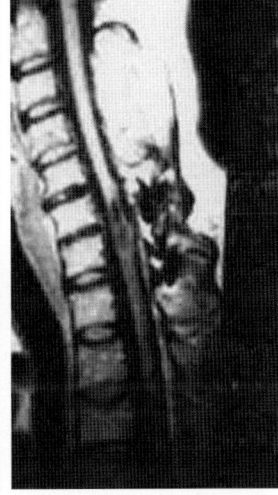

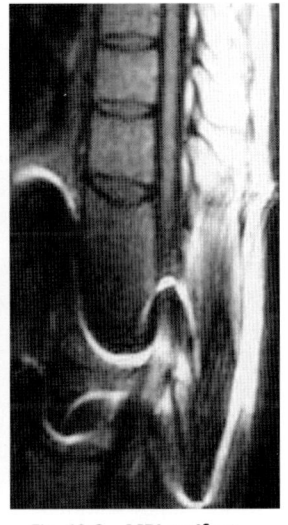

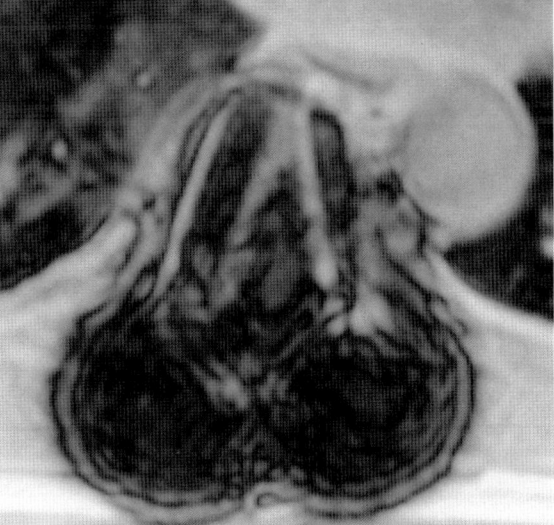

Fig. 13.8 MRI artifact post-stabilization.
a Titanium anterior fixation (minimal artifact).
b Stainless steel wire posterior fixation. **c** Steel Harrington rods—note the cord can still be usefully seen. **d** Titanium posterior fixation clearly showing a syrinx. **e** Gradient-echo T2 section with artifact (titanium screws).

experience in scanners with his implanted devices. We have scanned many patients on low (0.2T) and high (1.5T) systems with no untoward effects apart from occasional muscular contractions that were related to the orientation of the receiver to the magnetic field and which in all but one patient were stopped by changing the position of the patient on the table. It is, however, prudent not to examine these patients in high-field systems with rapid sequences using high gradients.

The use of titanium in stabilization procedures decreases metal artifact and in many cases excellent visualization of the cord and soft tissues is obtained (Fig. 13.**8**). Older and cheaper materials are associated with quite marked artifact, especially on gradient-echo T2W images, which may obscure some details but in most cases useful information can be seen and major complications delineated.

Persistent spasms may be treated with implanted intrathecal drug administration systems that have a subcutaneous combined pump and reservoir that are either gas or electronically driven. The reservoir should be emptied of active drug before scanning to prevent possible overdosage. Artifacts may arise from the reservoir but as this is situated on the anterior abdominal wall it rarely interferes with images of the spine. Programming should be checked after the scan.

CT Myelography

If MRI is contraindicated (Table 13.**3**), computed tomographic myelography (CTM) can give an accurate assessment of the spinal cord.[34,35] The contrast is preferably run up from below but if there is a spinal block, cisternal puncture (most comfortably approached via the posterior mid-line with the patient in left lateral decubitus) may be needed. Sections at 15–20 mm intervals, the length of the cord, are then performed.

In a myelopathy the contrast agent diffuses into areas of myelomalacia or cystic change over several hours. The rate at which this occurs is variable so that scanning of the whole cord at 6, 18, and 24 hours post myelography may be needed to show the characteristic contrast reversal (Fig. 13.**7**). There are false-positive and false-negative results and it can be difficult to differentiate myelomalacia from true cystic change.

Urological Investigations

Surveillance

The urological system is by far the most important in terms of long-term survival. It is largely because of the detailed attention to the urinary tract that the life expectancy of the patients with SCI has been increased and their quality of life enhanced. In the past 20–30 years this change has been so successful that deaths related to urological complications have fallen to fourth place behind cardiovascular and respiratory causes and suicide.[1]

Bladder contraction is under parasympathetic (S2–4) and the bladder neck and sphincter under sympathetic (T10–L2) and voluntary (S2–4) control so function after damage can be complex. Spinal cord lesions above T10 will "disconnect" the reflex areas from higher control giving an upper motor neuron reflexic bladder unless there is secondary ischemic damage to the lower cord and reflex arcs. Trauma below this will damage the conus or lower motor neurons; hence the reflexes are lost giving an atonic bladder. In most cases, the sphincter control is also damaged and detrusor–sphincter dyssynergia occurs when the bladder contracts against a closed sphincter causing a rise in pressure, poor upper tract emptying, the possibility of reflux and a trabeculated, neuropathic bladder.

Infection and reflux with consequent renal damage and stone formation are common sequelae (typically 3% renal and 11% bladder stones, some as early as 6 weeks) so long-term surveillance of the renal tract is needed in all patients, whether or not they are symptomatic although it may not be so critical after 10 years of normal radiological follow-up. The bladder management technique is controversial and depends on the level of injury, the aim being a "balanced," low pressure, regularly drained, and infection free bladder using either intermittent self-catheterization, indwelling catheters, or condom drainage after sphincter destruction (for a full review see reference 45).

Balloon dilatation and metal stenting of the external sphincter and prostate has been used with initial success although a long-term follow-up assessment is required. Complications with fixed Wallstents are unacceptably high but temporary nitinol and biodegradable stents give better results (Derry, personal communication). Women may prefer suprapubic to urethral catheterization although they do not have the same degree of problems as men with urethral catheters.

Annual or biennial assessment of the upper tracts with either IVU, US and plain films, or isotope studies have their advocates,[46,47] although the IVU is now rarely used routinely in most centers, especially when there is renal function impairment. If the upper tracts are dilated, a post-micturition view must be obtained,

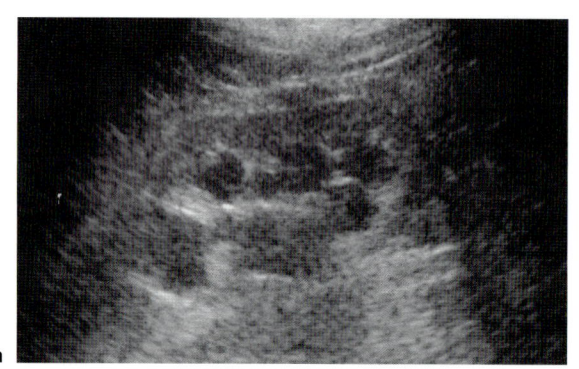

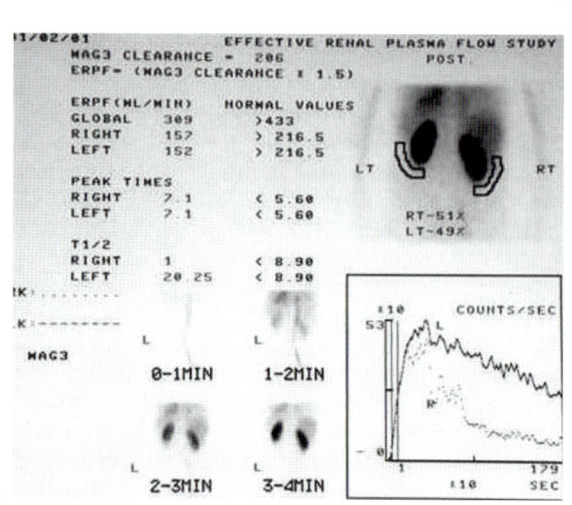

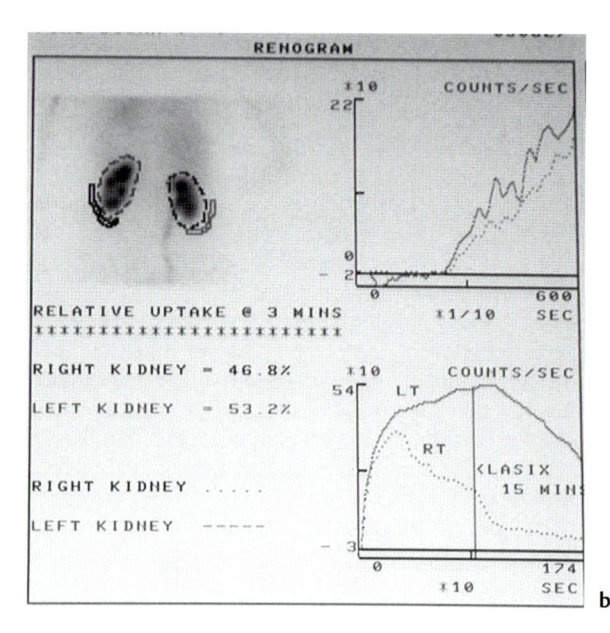

Fig. 13.9 The contribution of renography. a US showing moderate hydronephrosis. b Corresponding MAG3 study showing good equal function and delayed emptying. c ERPF study: poor left renal function (but the patient had a misleading, normal US)

if necessary after a trial with an indwelling catheter, to assess whether or not this is reversible.

A reasonable practice would be US at 1–2 year intervals with a renography or ERPF study as a baseline before discharge, at 1 year and every 5 years if stable (Table 13.**2**). Protocols vary with departmental capacity but the ERPF study is a critical method for assessing the function that US alone cannot provide. Urodynamics (Fig. 13.**9**) is occasionally advocated as a routine screening technique but is critical in assessing complications and planning the bladder management strategy.[48]

Patients with stones require access to the normal range of treatments such as extra-corporeal shock wave lithotripsy, percutaneous nephrolithotomy, or open surgical techniques.

Imaging in Specific Conditions

See Table 13.**4**.

Deteriorating Neurology

MRI or CTM is needed to differentiate between evolving PPMM, syrinx and atrophy, and other non-SCI-related causes.

Spinal Instability

Pain or instability, particularly if associated with changing neurology, is an indication for stabilization. MRI and CT studies allow for planning of the surgical approach and to assess bone stock and pedicle sizes. Liaison with the surgeon is crucial, as the studies often have to be tailored to the particular case. In some cases, instability is not evident on rapidly performed flexion and extension radiographs and careful positioning over pillows for at least 25–20 minutes before taking the film can reveal instability causing pain.

Local misalignment will lead to abnormal stresses in the compensating areas and scoliosis assessment is critical. Long cassettes are needed to compare the spine in the normal sitting or standing position with that in the recumbent position under traction to assess the correction possible.

A rare complication found in the thoracolumbar region is Charcot arthropathy with a pseudoarthrosis of the disk in which definitive exclusion of infection, e. g., tuberculosis may require vertebral biopsy. This complication is dealt with in Chapter 16.

The Acutely Unwell Patient

Such patients present a diagnostic challenge as there is often severe infection present but because of the abnormal sensation and autonomic function compromise, localizing the problem is very difficult. Often a nonspecific trawl is necessary, though the most common causes are the renal tract (see below), pressure sores, and orthopedic sepsis.

Deteriorating Renal Function and Renal Tract Complications

Any change in dilatation of the upper tracts should be investigated fully with US and ERPF/MAG3 studies (Fig. 13.**9**), particularly if acute and accompanied by symptoms ranging from a vague feeling of being unwell to overt infection. A SCI patient feeling "unwell" but not objectively very ill, in whom a dilated upper tract is noted as a new finding, must be assumed to have an obstructed kidney with urinary tract infection, possibly a frank pyonephrosis, until excluded, which is a reflection of the length of time from onset to presentation and the potentially fatal masking of symptoms. Stones are generally the cause and access to a full range of stone treatment techniques will be needed.

Cystography to assess for reflux may be required but autonomic dysreflexia is a hazardous complication of over-distending the bladder, particularly in quadriplegics. It is advisable not to instill more than 250–350 ml, with the investigation being terminated as soon as reflux is noted. In unstable patients where dysreflexia is likely, investigations should be terminated and the bladder drained as soon as headaches and/or sweating is experienced. In patients where this is a possibility, an automatic blood pressure recorder should be used and sublingual nifedipine or a GTN patch may be required to reverse the massive hypertension occasionally suffered.

Urodynamics has a pivotal role in problem bladder management.[49] Multi-channel analyzers that measure intravesical and intraabdominal pressures to give detrusor muscle activity, combined with pelvic floor electromyography and video cysto-fluoroscopy are now used to assess detrusor function. In most centers, the decision to perform a sphincterotomy is based on urodynamic assessment together with the presence of other factors such as vesicoureteric reflux, upper urinary tract abnormalities, symptomatic urinary infection, or autonomic symptoms.

With self-intermittent catheterization commonly practiced, traumatic urethral complications are associated with sometimes less than dextrous manipulation of anesthetic tissues. Urethrography, sometimes with catheter placement under screening control is required in this situation.

Pressure Sores

Anesthetic skin in a paralyzed patient is particularly prone to pressure sores so thin cushions and prolonged waits must be avoided (2 hours' immobility on a stretcher may take 2 days to recover). Once established, the depth of the injury is often much greater than expected from the surface. Secondary infection is

Table 13.4 Indications for specific investigations

Condition	Investigation	Benefits and comment
Deteriorating neurology	MRI	Differentiation of PPMM and syrinx (treatable) from atrophy and other nontreatable causes.
	Sagittal T1, T2, axial T1, CSF flow	Exclude non-neurological but treatable causes, e. g., disk, spinal stenosis.
	CTM with delayed scanning US (intraoperative)	Confirmation of syrinx cavity size and location.
Spinal instability	Plain films (flexion and extension, 30 min positioning) MRI	Assessment of mechanical instability. Long cassettes for scoliosis monitoring. Planning for choice of surgical options, e. g., pedicle screw size.
	CT Biopsy	May need guided biopsy to rule out infection, e. g., tuberculosis.
Acutely unwell	Routine CXR and AXR. US abdomen—especially renal tract evaluation CT chest, abdomen, and pelvis Nephrostomy PCNL	It must be remembered that advanced sepsis often presents as a nonspecific malaise, increased spasms, autonomic dysreflexia, etc. A newly demonstrated hydronephrosis, especially if associated with stones, needs a nephrostomy to exclude infection.
Deteriorating renal function	AXR, US, (rarely IVP)	Rule out obstruction, stones, etc.
	ERPF/MAG3 Urodynamics	Split function and handling assessment. Urodynamics for abnormal split function or high residual volumes in reflux voiders.
	Cystourethrography	Assessment of ureteric reflux.
Pressure sores, hip and joint problems	Plain films	Extent of involvement.
	MRI T1 ± gadolinium	Assessment of subcutaneous tissue damage (often conical and deep), osteomyelitis or septic arthritis.
	STIR Sinography ± CT	Delineation of sinus or fissure tract.
Ectopic ossification (HO, PAO)	US	Ultrasound is the earliest indicator of muscle and soft tissue pertubation, which is a precursor to EO. DVT can also be excluded in the same examination.
	Bone scintigraphy (isotope bone scan)	Bone scintigraphy is indicated where ultrasound skills are not available. It is probably most useful in monitoring activity prior to excision.
	CT	CT is more sensitive than plain radiography, which is not positive until 10+ days after the start of the process. Aim is to start treatment as soon as possible—bisphosphonates or radiotherapy (ideally within 5 days of onset).
Pain: nociceptive, spine, visceral	Plain film Plain film (flexion/extension) CT, MRI	To assess stability of spine or visceral problems; to assess the state of the spine, e. g., possible bone infection; to assist in the planning of surgery.
Pain: neuropathic, CNS	MRI	Size morphology and extent of PPMM or syrinx and its relation to the fracture. To look for arachnoid tethering, CSF flow abnormalities, etc. To confirm the level of the lesion prior to laminectomy for DREZ lesion or rhizotomy surgery.
Muscle spasms	US, AXR MRI	General health assessment. Cord assessment (rule out central cause or identify the site for laminectomy for posterior rhizotomy).
	Scintigraphy: cysternography, pump function	Assessment for intrathecal therapy (CSF pathway integrity). Level of blockage if pump fails.
Airway patency	AP and lateral tomography CT (very low dose spiral) with multi-planar reconstruction	Assessment of degree and level of tracheal stenosis.
Elective surgery of the renal tract.	US, AXR, plain films, IVP	To exclude ureteric reflux, stones, etc. Exclude spinal anomalies.
SARS, augmentation cystoplasty, artificial sphincter	Urodynamics, cystourethrogram	Aid surgical planning.

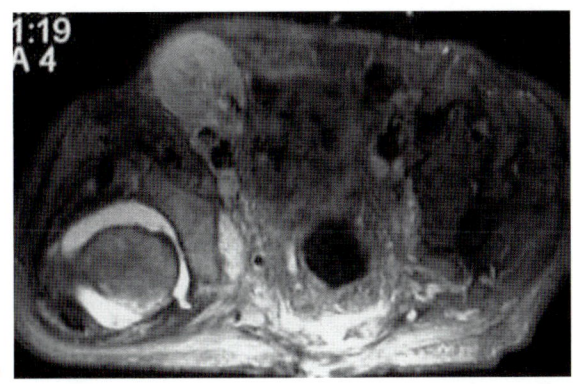

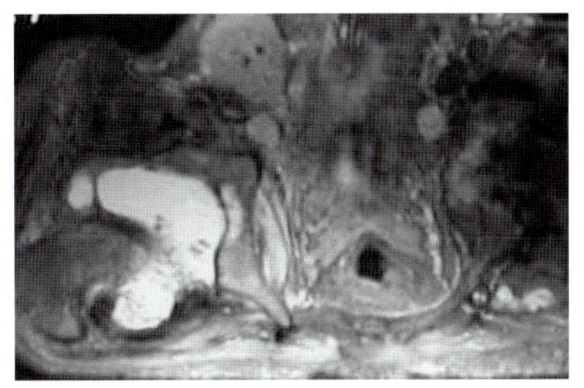

Fig. 13.**10** **a** Patient with a deep pressure sore, (?) osteomyelitis. **b** Large joint effusion, no evidence of osteomyelitis.

common and septic arthritis and osteomyelitis must often be excluded. STIR sequences are invaluable (Fig. 13.**10**) but sinography followed by CT will frequently be necessary.

Ectopic Ossification

Ectopic, heterotopic, or paraarticular ossification is an area of abnormal bone formation occurring in the denervated limb muscles, probably secondary to micro-trauma, commonly around the hips and knees, which generally presents in the second to fourth months post-injury as a thick, swollen leg. Differentiation from deep venous thrombosis is critical and this can be readily performed using Doppler ultrasound when assessment of the muscles can also be made.[50,51]

Ectopic ossification has a characteristic chaotic echo texture that replaces the normal lamellar structure of striated muscle (Fig. 13.**11**) and this finding is sufficient diagnostically to initiate treatment—radiotherapy, bisphosphonates, nonsteroidals, etc. Where the skill is available, this technique has been found to be more convenient, practical, and cheaper for early diagnosis than the three-phase isotope bone scan.[52]

Pain

This can be considered as nociceptive when a spinal or visceral cause should be sought, or neuropathic, when a central cause is likely. A full work-up of the whole patient including the spine and cord MRI may be necessary, with a special search for infection.

Many patients suffer from posturally related mechanical orthopedic problems (e. g., facet arthrosis), as a result of spinal malalignment, that will need standard assessments. Facet injections and denervation may be appropriate and kyphoplasty and vertebroplasty to correct deformity is being discussed in some centers.

Surgery to the dorsal roots and pain pathways in the cord (DREZ lesions) may be offered and MRI is needed for level identification.

Muscular Spasms

These can be a response to pain, the development of syringomyelia or other pathology and a full pain assessment may be needed. If no underlying cause can be found then intrathecal antispastic drugs can be given via an implanted pump and catheter. The most useful technique for assessing delivery system failure is scintigraphy (Fig. 13.**12**).[53]

Airway Problems

As well as problems that affect the lungs of normal people, patients with SCI have increased risks of tracheal stenosis after tracheostomy and of infections if their neurological level compromises normal respiratory activity. Low-dose CT of the trachea with multiplanar reconstruction is more informative than tracheal tomography.

Elective Management of the Renal Tract

Sacral Anterior Root Stimulators, artificial sphincters, sphincter stents, augmentation cystoplasties, etc., all require a careful urological workup to exclude anatomical abnormalities, reflux, renal disease, and stones.

Conclusion

With appropriate rehabilitation, a patient with a spinal cord injury can live an extremely fulfilled and useful life with the minimum of dependency on others. Regular surveillance and high-quality imaging of the neurological and urological systems is critical to this goal, but unwell patients are a diagnostic challenge that requires complex imaging and thought to resolve.

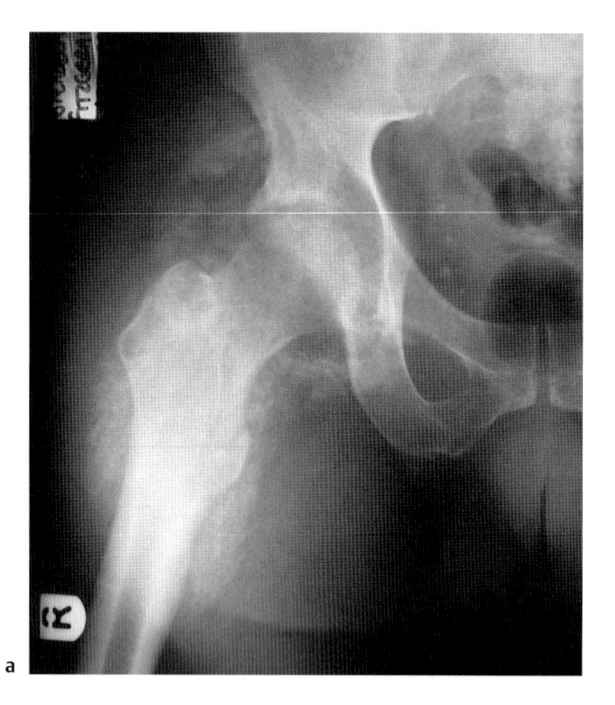

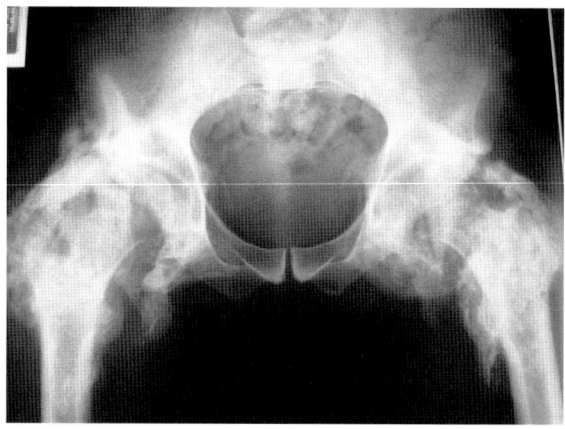

Fig. 13.**11 Ectopic ossification**. **a** Early EO. **b** Established EO. **c** US normal muscle. **d** US abnormal "chaotic" muscle structure 1 day after clinical suspicion. **e** Tc HMDP bone scintigram showing extent of abnormality 7 days after clinical suspicion. **f** CT of the hips showing calcification in the quads.

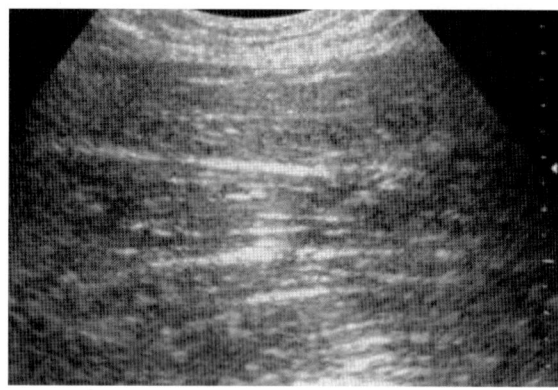

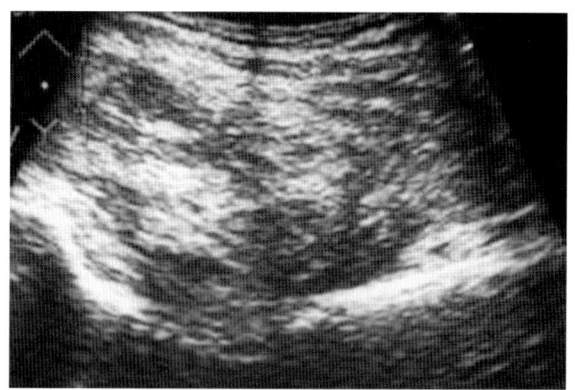

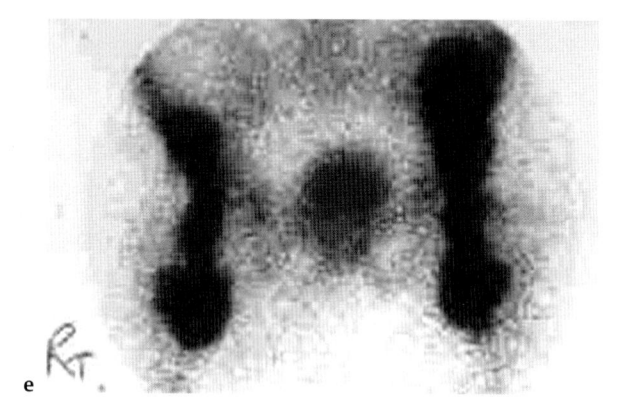

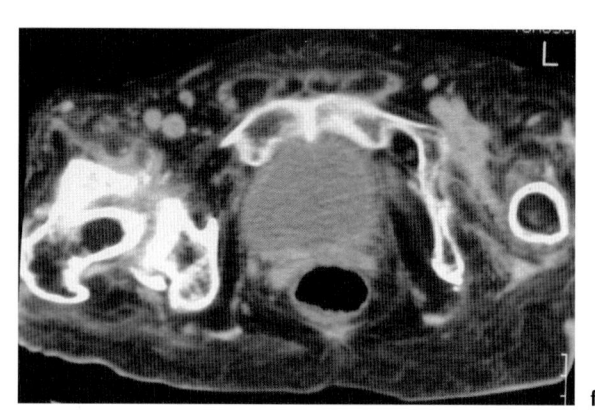

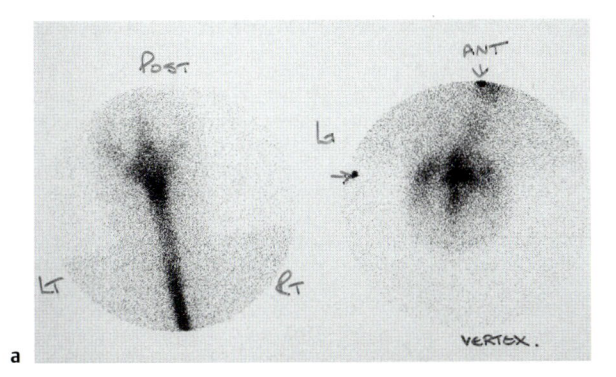

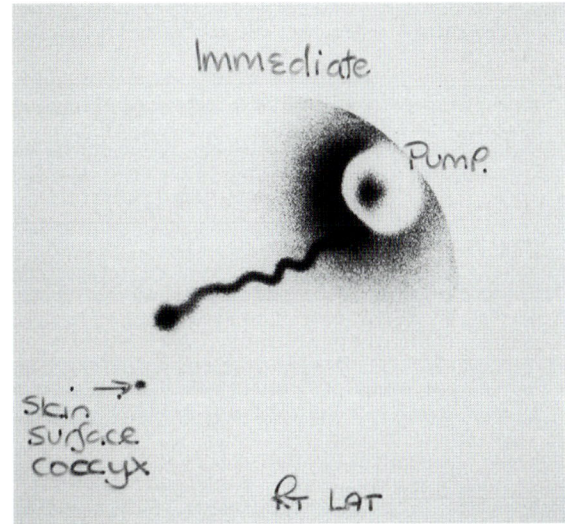

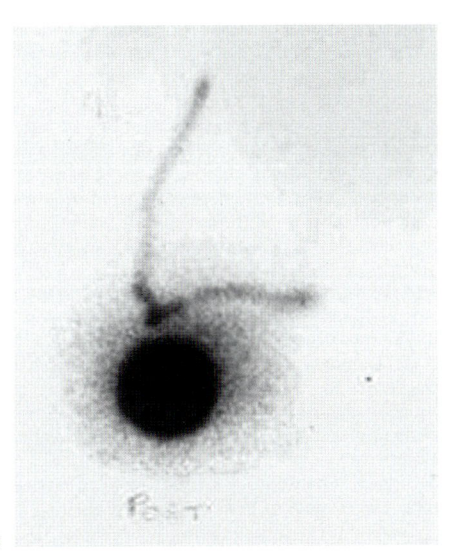

Fig. 13.**12** **Isotope pump studies (Tc-99m DTPA). a** Showing a normal study with activity around the brain. **b** Showing a block at the entry to the spinal canal. **c** Showing a block at the injury site in the mid-thoracic region.

Acknowledgement

Figures 13.**1**, 13.**2a–c**, 13.**3a, c, d**, 13.**5a, b** 13.**6a–c** and 13.**7a–c** reprinted from *Eur J Radiol*, 2002, Vol. 42. R. Bodley, Imaging in chronic spinal injury, pp. 135–53, with permission from Elsevier.

References

1. Weitzenkamp DA, Jones RH, Whiteneck GG, Young DA. Ageing with spinal cord injury: cross-sectional and longitudinal effects. *Spinal Cord*. 2001;39(6):301–309.
2. Holmes G. Goulstoman lecture on spinal injury of warfare. *BMJ*. 1915;2:769.
3. Quencer RM, Bunge RP. The injured spinal cord: imaging, histopathologic clinical correlates and basic science approaches to enhancing neural function after spinal cord injury. *Spine*. 1996;21(18):2064–2066.
4. Schwartz ED, Falcone SF, Quencer RM, Green BA. Post traumatic syringomyelia: pathogenesis, imaging and treatment. *AJR Am J Roentgenol*. 1999;173(2):487–492.
5. Squier M, Lehr R. Post traumatic syringomyelia. *J Neurosurg Psychiatry*. 1994;57:1095–1098.
6. O'Beirne J, Cassidy N, Raza K, Walsh M, Stack J, Murray P. Role of magnetic resonance imaging in the assessment of spinal injuries. *Injury*. 1993;24(3):149–154.
7. Silberstein M, Brown D, Tress B, Hennessey O. Suggested MRI criteria for surgical decompression in acute spinal cord injury. Preliminary observations. *Paraplegia*. 1992;30:704–710.
8. Bracken M, Shepard M et al. (1990) A randomised, controlled trial of Methylprednisolone or Naloxone in the treatment of acute spinal cord injury. *N Engl J Med*. 322:1405–1411.
9. Cho KH, Iwasaki Y, Imamura H, Hida K, Abe H. Experimental model of post traumatic syringomyelia: the role of adhesive arachnoiditis in syrinx formation. *J Neurosurg*. 1994; 80(1): 133–139.
10. Williams B. Post traumatic syringomyelia, an update. *Paraplegia*. 1990;28:296–313.
11. Brodbelt AR, Stoodley MA, Watling AM, Tu J, Jones NR. Fluid flow in an animal model of post-traumatic syringomyelia. *Eur Spine J*. 2003;12(3):300–306.
12. Falcone S, Quencer R, Green B, Patchen S, Post MJD. Progressive post traumatic myelomalacic myelopathy; imaging and clinical features. *AJNR Am J Neuroradiol*. 1994;15:747–784.
13. Fischbein MJ, Dillon WP, Cobbs C, Weinstein PR. The "presyrinx" state; a reversible myelopathic condition that precedes syringomyelia. *AJNR Am J Neuroradiol*. 1999;20(1):7–20.
14. Quencer R. The pre syringomyelic myelopathic state; a plausible hypothesis. *AJNR Am J Neuroradiol*. 1999;20(1):1–2.
15. Milhorat TH. Is reversible enlargement of the spinal cord a pre syrinx state? *AJNR Am J Neuroradiol*. 1999;20(1):21–22.
16. Tobimatsu Y, Mihei R, Kimura T, Suyama T, Tobimatsu H. A quantitative analysis of CSF flow in post-traumatic syringomyelia. *Seikeigeka Gakkai and Zasshi*. 1991;65(8);505–516.
17. Brugieres P, Iffenecker C, Hurth M, Parker F, Fuerxer F, Idy-Peretti I, Bittoun J. Dynamic MRI in the evaluation of syringomyelic cysts. *Neurochirurgie*. 1991;45(1):115–129.
18. Greitz D, Wirestam R, Franck A, Nordell B, Thomsen C, Stahlberg F. Pulsatile brain movement and associated hydrodynamic studies with magnetic resonance imaging. The Monro-Kellie doctrine revisited. *Neuroradiology*. 1992; 34(5):370–380.

19. Levy LM. Towards an understanding of syringomyelia; MR imaging of CSF flow and neuraxis motion. *AJNR Am J Neuroradiol.* 2000; 21(1):45–46.
20. Castillo M. Further explanations for the formation of syringomyelia; back to the drawing table. *AJNR Am J Neuroradiol.* 2000;21:1788–1789.
21. Falci SP, Lammertse DP, Best L, Starnes CA, Prenger EC, Stavros AT, Mellick D. Surgical treatment of post-traumatic cystic and tethered spinal cords. *Spinal Cord Med.* 1999;22(3):173–181.
22. David P, Tadie M. Treatment of syringomyelia. *Neurochiruigie.* 1999;45(1):130–137.
23. Ohata K, Gotoh T, Matsusaka Y, Morino M, Tsuyuguchi N, Sheikh N, Inoue Y, Hakuba A. Surgical management of syringomyelia associated with spinal adhesive arachnoiditis. *J Clin Neurosci.* 2001;8(1):40–42.
24. Perrouin-Verbe B, Lenne-Aurier K, Robert R et al. Post-traumatic syringomyelia and post-traumatic spinal stenois: A direct relationship: Review of 75 patients with a spinal cord injury. *Spinal Cord.* 1998;36:137–143.
25. Curati W, Kingsley E, Kendall B, Moseley I. MRI in chronic spinal cord trauma. *Neuroradiology.* 1992;35:30–35.
26. Vannemreddy SS, Rowed DW, Bharatwal N. Posttraumatic syringomyelia: predisposing factors. *Br J Neurosurg.* 2002; 16(3):276–283.
27. Nielsen OA, Biering-Sorensen F, Botel U et al. Post-traumatic syringomyelia. Clinical case of the month. *Spinal Cord.* 1999; 37:680–684.
28. Ronen J, Catz A, Spasser R, Gepstein R. The treatment dilemma in post-traumatic syringomyelia. *Disabil Rehabil.* 1999;21(9): 455–457.
29. Sgouros S, Williams B. A critical appraisal of pediculated omental graft transposition in progressive spinal cord failure. *Br J Neurosurg.* 1996;10(6):547–553.
30. Clifton FL, Donovan WH, Dimitrijevic MM et al. Omental transposition in chronic spinal cord injury. *Spinal Cord.* 1996;34: 193–203.
31. Xiongwei Zou. *Omentum transposition in the treatment of chronic SCI.* 42nd ISCoS Annual Scientific Meeting, Beijing, 2003.
32. PotterK, Saifuddin A. MRI of spinal cord injury. A pictorial review. *Br J Radiol.* 2003;76:347–352.
33. Dempsey M.F, Condon B. Thermal injuries associated with MRI. *Clin Radiol.* 2001;56:457–465.
34. Seibert CE, Barnes J, Dreisback JN, Swanson WB, Heck RJ. Accurate CT measurement of the spinal cord using metrizamide. *AJR.* 1980;136:777–780.
35. Quencer RM, Green BA, Eismont FJ. Post-traumatic spinal cord cysts: clinical features and characterisation with metrizamide computed tomography. *Radiology.* 1983;146: 415–423.
36. Nidecker A, Kocher M, Maeder M, Gratzi O, Zach G et al. MR imaging of chronic spinal cord injury. Association with neurologic function. *Neurosurg Rev.* 1991;14:169–179.
37. Yamashita Y, Takahashi M, Matsuno Y, Sakamoto Y, Oguni T et al. Chronic injuries of the spinal cord: Assessment with MR imaging. *Radiology.* 1990;175:849–854.
38. Backe H, Betz R, Mesgarzadeh M, Beck T, Clancy M. Post-traumatic spinal cord cysts evaluated by magnetic resonance imaging. *Paraplegia.* 1991;29:607–612.
39. Quencer R, Sheldon J, Post M, Diaz R, Montalvo B et al. Magnetic resonance imaging of the chronically injured cervical spinal cord. *AJNR.* 1986;7:457–464.
40. Sett P, Crockard A. The value of magnetic resonance imaging (MRI) in the follow-up management of spinal injury. *Paraplegia.* 1991;29:396–410.
41. Schurch B, Wichmann W, Rossier AB. Post-traumatic syringomyelia (cystic myelopathy): a prospective study of 449 patients with spinal cord injury. *J Neurol Neurosurg Psychiatry.* 1996;60(1):61–67.
42. Wang D, Bodley R, Gardner B, Frankel H. A clinical MRI study of the traumatised spinal cord more than 20 years following injury. *Paraplegia.* 1996;34(2):65–81.
43. Jinkins JR, Reddy S, Leite CC, Bazan C, Xiong L. MRI of parenchymal spinal cord signal change as a sign of active advancement in clinically progressive post traumatic syringomyelia. *AJNR Am J Neuroradiol.* 1998;19:177–182.
44. Quencer RM. Can MR help predict enlargement of post traumatic spinal cord cysts? *AJNR Am J Neuroradiol.* 1998;19(1): 192.
45. Labat JJ, Perrouin-Verbe B. Evolution and follow-up of lower urinary tract dysfunction in spinal cord injury patients. In: Corcos J, Schick E, eds. *Textbook of the Neurogenic Bladder.* London: Martin Dunitz; 2004.
46. Rao K, Hackler R, Woodlief R, Ozer M, Fields W. Real-time renal sonography in spinal cord injury patients: Prospective comparison with excretory urography. *J Urol.* 1986;135:72–77.
47. Klingensmith WC, Lammertse DP, Briggs DE, Smith WI, Roberts JF, Froelich JW, Sutherland JD. Tc 99 m MAG3 renal studies in spinal cord injured patients: normal range, reproducibility and change as a function of duration and level of injury. *Spinal Cord.* 1996;34:338–345.
48. Watanabe T, Rivas DA, Chancellor MB. Urodynamics of spinal cord injury. *Urol Clin North Am.* 1996;23(3):459–473.
49. Wyndaele JJ. Correlation between clinical neurological data and urodynamic function in spinal cord injured patients. *Spinal Cord.* 1997;35:213–216.
50. Bodley R, Jamous A, Short D. Ultrasound in the early diagnosis of heterotopic ossification in patients with spinal cord injury. *Paraplegia.* 1993;31:500–506.
51. Cassar-Pullicino VN, McClelland M, Badwan DA, McCall IW, Pringle RG, el Masry W. Sonographic diagnosis of heterotopic bone formation in spinal injury patients. *Paraplegia.* 1993; 31(1):40–50.
52. Subbarao JV, Garrison SJ. Heterotopic ossification: diagnosis and management, current concepts and controversies. *J Spinal Cord Med.* 1999;22(4):273–283.
53. Le Breton F, Davies JC, Monteil J, Vidal J, Munoz M, Dudognon P, Salle JY. Radioisotopic control for baclofen pump catheter failure. *Spinal Cord.* 2001;39:283–285.

14 Vertebral Fractures and Osteoporosis

P. Peloschek and S. Grampp

Introduction

Osteoporosis has been defined as "a chronic progressive disease characterized by low bone mass and microarchitectural deterioration of bone tissue, which leads to bone fragility and a consequent increase in fracture risk."[1,2]

Osteoporosis usually causes no symptoms unless a person has a fracture. Osteoporotic fractures tend to occur most commonly in sites of the skeleton that are rich in trabecular bone: the wrist, spine, and hip. Osteoporosis is a major risk factor for fractures of the hip, vertebrae, and distal forearm. Osteoporosis has lately been recognized as a disease of growing importance because demographic changes have led to an increased burden of morbidity and mortality due to osteoporotic fracturing. By the age of 80, 40% of women and 20% of men can be expected to have suffered an osteoporotic spine fracture. Osteoporosis can be prevented by lifestyle changes, and several effective drug treatments have recently become available to treat the disease by increasing bone density and reducing fracture incidence.

Vertebral fractures are the hallmark of osteoporosis, and occur with a higher incidence earlier in life than any other type of osteoporotic fracture (hip, forearm). About 60% of vertebral fractures occur without symptoms. Symptomatic and asymptomatic vertebral fractures are associated with increased morbidity and mortality. Morbidity, such as decreased physical function and social isolation, is associated with these fractures and has a significant impact on the patient's overall quality of life. After a lumbar vertebral fracture patients must remain in bed for approximately 1 month and suffer, on average, half a year of limited activity.[3]

Important factors in therapy management for prevention of both osteoporosis and osteoporotic fractures are preventive measures that can help estimate the risk of fracture. Measurement of bone density is, besides age, the best predictor of fracture risk and facilitates prevention and therapy that is not dependent on an actual fracture for a diagnosis.

Recently, considerable improvements have been made in therapeutic interventions to both increase bone density and reduce future fracture risk.[58,59] Such therapy regimens include the use of bisphosphonates (etidronate, alendronate, and risedronate) and the selective estrogen receptor modulator. These therapies have been added to hormone replacement therapy, which is known to be effective in preventing bone loss in post-menopausal women.

Definition

Osteoporosis

Decades ago, osteoporosis was only diagnosed if a low-trauma fracture occurred. A precise definition of osteoporosis in terms of bone densitometry was published by a working group of the WHO in 1994 (Table 14.**1**).[60] This definition is based on DXA measurements made in the lumbar spine, proximal femur, and forearm in menopausal white women. The WHO definition is as follows:

- Normal: bone mineral density (BMD) or bone mineral content (BMC) within 1 SD (score of 1T) of the young-adult reference mean;
- Low bone mass (osteopenia): a value for BMD or BMC lower than 1 SD (< 1T) below the young-adult mean, but not as low as 2.5 SDs (2.5T) below this value;
- Osteoporosis: a value for BMD or BMC 2.5 SDs (2.5T) or more below the young-adult mean;
- Severe (established) osteoporosis: a value for BMD or BMC 2.5 SDs (2.5T) or more below the young-adult mean and one or more "fragility fractures."

The SD of 2.5 was defined as the level of BMD in postmenopausal women that identifies 30% of these women as having osteoporosis and who were thought to suffer a vertebral fracture in their lifetime. The BMC is given in grams, and the area of the measured site in square centimeters. By dividing the BMC by the projected area, BMD is given in g/cm^2. It is very important to realize that the WHO definitions do not apply to all patients or to all sites measurable or to all techniques (e.g., QCT).[4–6]

T-Score and Z-Score

The T- and Z-scores were developed because of the variation in BMD measurement technology among differ-

Table 14.**1** WHO Definitions

WHO definition of osteoporosis	T-score
Normal	Score higher than 1T
Osteopenia	Lower than < 1T, but not as low as 2.5T
Osteoporosis	2.5T or less
Established osteoporosis	2.5T or less and one or more *fragility fractures*

ent manufacturers. Therefore, the BMD results are expressed as standard deviations from the referent mean.

The referent mean for a T-score is the bone mineral density of *young normal* individuals. The T-score is the number of standard deviations by which an individual's BMD differs from that of healthy young adults of the same sex. The lower the T-score, the more fragile the individual's bones are. The T-score is, therefore, a rough indication of the need for treatment in patients 20 years of age and older. In children and adolescents, the Z-score serves an analogous function.

The referent mean for a Z-score is the bone mineral density of *age-matched normal* individuals. The Z-score is the number of standard deviations by which an individual's BMD differs from that of healthy age-matched individuals of the same sex. Until peak bone mass has been reached (i.e., in children and young adults up to approximately 25 years), interpretation can be made only with comparison to an age-matched mean (Z-score).[7]

In calculating a change over time, the absolute BMD values (g/cm^2) must be used. Due to the slow bone mineral metabolism in individual patients, there must be an intervening period of at least 18–24 months between measures in longitudinal studies to ensure significant change has taken place.[8] Alternative methods of interpretation include determining a percentage or percentile of expected—age- or sex-matched—peak bone mass.

At all ages, the relative risk of fracture doubles for each unit decrease in the T-score, regardless of the skeletal location used to calculate that score. It should be remembered that bone mass is a continuous variable. Therefore, the purpose of a bone density measurement cannot be a qualitative diagnosis of osteoporosis as an all-or-nothing finding. The purpose is to achieve a quantitative assessment of fracture risk, which is itself a continuous variable. For radiologists who interpret and report bone density studies an understanding of the clinical background is important for the diagnosis and follow-up of osteoporosis in the patient, as is communication of the results to clinicians.

Vertebral Fragility Fracture

Although whether a patient suffers a fracture depends on a number of factors (tendency to fall, the nature of the fall), about 60–70% of bone strength is related to BMD and determines whether a fracture will occur.

The relative risk of a spinal fracture for every 1 SD reduction in age-adjusted mean BMD has been reported to be 2.3 g/m^2.[9] A vertebral fracture in a patient with osteoporosis is pathognomonic for severe or established osteoporosis. These kinds of pathological fractures, occurring without adequate trauma, are also called vertebral fragility fractures. Vertebral compression fractures in the thoracic or lumbar spine are a common clinical problem, particularly in elderly patients, despite the fact that about 60% of vertebral fractures occur without symptoms. Osteoporosis is the most common cause of compression fractures in this age group, but up to 39% of all bone metastases occur in the spine and such metastases may also result in a pathological fracture.

Differentiation from benign compression fractures due to osteoporosis often complicates the appropriate clinical staging and treatment planning in patients with known nonosseous malignancies in this age group.

In these patients, contrast-enhanced magnetic resonance imaging (MRI) can help to distinguish benign from malignant vertebral fractures. Basically, chronic benign compression fractures can be diagnosed by the absence of abnormal signal intensity in a compressed vertebral body. Problems could arise if an acute osteoporotic compression fracture has to be differentiated from a malignant compression fracture.

MR imaging findings, such as abnormal signal intensity of the pedicle or posterior element, an epidural or paraspinal mass, and a convex posterior border of the vertebral body, are useful for differentiation of metastatic from acute osteoporotic compression fractures of the spine.

Multiple compression fractures, retropulsion of a posterior bone fragment, a low-signal-intensity band on T1W and T2W images, and spared normal bone marrow signal intensity of the vertebral body are suggestive of acute osteoporotic compression fractures (see Chapter 15).[10–18]

Epidemiology and Outcome of Osteoporotic Spinal Fractures

Osteoporosis strikes mostly older women and is therefore an increasing problem for the Western world's aging population. In Europe, one in four women will be over 60 by 2010, and 1% of women aged 65 will suffer a spinal fracture each year. For men aged 65, at least one in 200 will suffer a spinal fracture within a year. By the age of 80, 40% of women and 20% of men can be expected to have suffered an osteoporotic spine fracture that causes chronic pain.[19]

After lumbar vertebral fractures, the mean number of bed days has been reported to be 25.8 and limited activity days, 158.5. Also, fractures of the thoracic vertebrae result in a substantial amount of illness and disability.[3]

The Radiologist's Role in Diagnosis

Screening during Routine Chest Radiography

Radiographic findings suggestive of osteopenia and osteoporosis are frequently encountered in daily radiological practice. It has been reported that, in most cases, spinal osteopenia becomes detectable on conventional radiographs only after a loss of at least 20–40% of the skeletal calcium.[21,22] The visual estimation of bone quality may, therefore, be inadequate for the quantification of osteopenia, but remains useful for detecting clinically important asymptomatic vertebral fractures that indicate a high risk for successive fractures.

At any rate, osteoporosis is still underdiagnosed and therefore undertreated; however, routine chest radiography still holds potential as a screening tool for revealing previously undiagnosed vertebral fractures.[23] Osteoporosis patients with one osteoporotic fracture anywhere in the body are predisposed to a 20% higher risk of developing an additional fracture, a risk that is on a par with the WHO criteria for the definition of fracture risk in osteopenia. To make the most of the screening potential of routine chest radiography, relevant vertebral fractures, defined as at least moderate to severe (loss of height of approximately 25% or greater) should be cited in chest reports. Especially in patients over 60 years old, in whom the prevalence of such fractures approaches 25%, routine chest radiographs could be used to screen patients for osteoporosis-related vertebral fractures. Unfortunately, compression fractures are very often not mentioned in radiology reports. It was reported recently that only 55% of vertebral fractures are mentioned in official radiology reports. Perhaps fully automated digital morphometry of the thoracic spine will increase the sensitivity of this screening method in routine clinical practice in the near future.

Diagnosis of Osteoporosis on Lateral Radiographs of the Spine

Since the majority of vertebral fractures do not come to clinical attention, radiographic diagnosis is considered to be the best way to identify and confirm the presence of osteoporotic vertebral fractures in clinical practice. Conventional lateral radiographs of the spine are visually evaluated by radiologists to identify vertebral fractures. The severity of such fractures should be assessed semiquantitatively, based on visual evaluation, or quantitatively, using different morphometric criteria. Surprisingly, there is still debate about what defines a vertebral fracture or what might be considered an anatomical variation on lateral spine radiographs since there are no good prospective studies of variations in vertebral morphology. Nevertheless, the identification of vertebral fractures is very important because the risk of suffering a subsequent fracture is 20% higher than with no history of fractures. The radiologist is thus in a strong position to guide the clinician in evaluating fracture risk.[24,25] Osteopenia and osteoporosis of the spine lead to increased radiolucency of the vertebrae, which may assume the radiographic density of the intervertebral disk space, or a vertical striation, and a "framed" appearance of the vertebrae, as well as increased (bi-) concavity of the vertebral endplates. These characteristics are summarized in the Saville index (Table 14.**2**).[26] Despite its significant relation to measured bone density, this index never gained widespread acceptance because it was prone to subjectivity and reader experience.[22,27]

Even though osteopenia may not be diagnosed reliably from spinal radiographs, osteoporosis-induced changes of the shape of vertebral bodies, as endplate impressions or crush fractures, are clearly visible in lateral views. These fractures should be described semiquantitatively as published by Genant et al:[28] the

Table 14.**2** Osteopenia score for vertebrae by Saville

Grade	Radiographic appearance of vertebral bodies
0	Normal bone density.
1	Minimal loss of density: endplates begin to stand out, giving a stencilled effect.
2	Vertical striation is more obvious: endplates are thinner.
3	More severe loss of density than grade 2: endplates becoming less visible.
4	Ghost-like vertebral bodies, density is no greater than soft tissue, no trabecular pattern is visible.

Table 14.**3** Genantsemi quantitative assessment of vertebral fractures

Grade	Radiographic deformation of vertebral shape
0	No deformation.
1	Mild deformation: approximately 20–25% reduction in anterior, middle, and/or posterior height.
2	Moderate deformation: approximately 25–40% reduction in anterior, middle, and/or posterior height.
3	Severe deformation: 40% and greater reduction in anterior, middle, and/or posterior height.

severity of a spinal fracture from T4 to L4 is solely assessed by visual determination of the extent of vertebral height reduction and morphological change, and vertebral fractures are differentiated from other nonfracture deformities. Vertebral heights are graded without direct measurements as normal, mildly deformed, moderately deformed, and severely deformed (Table 14.**3**).

In the near future, digital morphometry could increase the percentage of quantitatively reported thoracic and lumbar spine fractures. There is still a major role for radiologists in the careful assessment and diagnosis of vertebral fractures using standardized grading schemes such as the one described earlier.[28]

Bone Densitometry

Densitometric measurements are performed to predict the individual fracture risk. To increase the predictive value of densitometric measurements and to avoid unnecessary radiation exposure, only patients with suggestive anamnesis should undergo this examination. If the result would not alter therapeutic management, then the scan is not indicated. There are two major groups of individuals in whom bone densitometry is indicated.

The first group includes the screening population of healthy and asymptomatic individuals with a proven family history of osteoporotic fracture, slender build (BMI < 19 kg/m²), early menopause (< 45 years), or prolonged amenorrhea (> 1 year).

Table 14.4 Risk factors indicating bone densitometry (from Royal College of Physicians of London, 1999)

Strong risk factors	Estrogen or testosterone deficiency	Premature menopause—age < 45 years
		Prolonged secondary amenorrhea (> 1 year)
		Primary hypogonadism
	Corticosteroid therapy (prednisolone > 7.5 mg/day for > 6 months)	
	Family anamnesis of risk factors	
	Low body mass index (< 19 kg/m²)	
Disease with secondary osteoporosis (e. g., hyperparathyroidism, Cushing's, etc.)		
Radiographic evidence of osteopenia or vertebral deformity		
Low trauma fracture, particularly hip, wrist, and spine		
Monitoring response to therapy		

The other group includes patients who suffer from diseases or who undergo treatments that lead to bone mineral decrease. Endocrine disorders that result in estrogen deficiency, Cushing's disease, hyperparathyroidism, thyrotoxicosis, and hyperprolactinemia all indicate the need for osteodensitometric screening. In addition, patients who have been immobile for long periods of time, or with anorexia nervosa, bulimia, malabsorption diseases, and chronic liver/kidney disease should be scanned. Patients undergoing long-term treatment with corticosteroids (> 7.5 mg/d or more of prednisolone or equivalent dose for > 6 months), chronic heparin administration, or patients who take LHRH antagonists or anticonvulsants should undergo screening densitometry. The Royal College of Physicians published a case finding strategy that is summarized in Table 14.4.

If follow-up densitometries are planned, these should to be performed on the same scanner model for comparability and the same software version should be used for analysis. The referring clinician must know the site at which the bone was analyzed and should be advised that any follow-up required is best performed with the same machine at the same region and in the same season. Physiological, pathological, and therapeutic changes in mineralization are not more than 1–2% per year, but there are winter losses and summer gains in BMD, especially in more northerly latitudes.[20]

Serial measurements of bone density are most reliable when the highest possible test reproducibility is ensured by:[8]
- Using the identical densitometer for each serial exam.
- Daily calibrating routines that exceed minimum recommendations.
- Using a minimum number of expert and highly concentrated staff.
- Having an experienced osteoporosis researcher review every scan.

The routine follow-up interval to monitor therapy is recommended to be 2 years. To monitor borderline BMD results in perimenopausal women, when bone loss is greatest, a follow-up scan should be planned 1–2 years after menopause as bone density decrements may be in the range of 1–2% per annum. Within the 10 years following menopause, intervals of 2–3 years can be considered. Otherwise, a 4- to 5-year interval is thought to be sufficient.

In calculating the change over time, the absolute BMD values (g/cm²) must be used. When a BMD measurement has been made, a written report must be formulated that contains all the pertinent information for the referring clinician.[1] For this purpose, age-, sex-, and ethnicity-matched reference data should be provided. Available databases are predominantly drawn from a white, Caucasian, American-based population. Appropriate reference ranges for children and certain ethnic minorities are not readily available. As described earlier, results can be interpreted in terms of the standard deviations from the mean of either sex-matched peak bone mass (T-score) or age-matched BMD (Z-score).

Dual X-ray Absorptiometry

DXA is currently the most widely used method applied to bone densitometry.[31–35] The dual energy X-ray beams are required to correct bone density measurements for overlying soft tissue. Two principles are used to obtain dual X-ray energies: energy switching and k-edge filtration[20]. Scanners manufactured by Hologic (Bedford, Massachusetts, USA) use an energy switching system in which the X-ray tube potential is switched rapidly from 70–140 kVp. Scanners manufactured by General Electric/Lunar (Madison, Wisconsin, USA), Norland Medical Systems (Fort Atkinson, Wisconsin, USA), and Sopha (Buc Cedex, France) use a constant potential X-ray source, combined with a rare earth filter with energy-specific absorption characteristics (k-edge filtration). The X-ray beam is separated by the k-edge filter into two separate components of 'high' and 'low' energy photons (70 keV and 40 keV using cerium; 45 keV and 80 keV using a samarium filter).[29]

DXA also allows the combined evaluation of vertebral fracture status and bone mass density if lateral projections are obtained. The disadvantage of DXA is that upper thoracic vertebrae cannot be evaluated in a substantial number of patients due to poor imaging quality.[29,36–38]

The measurements provided by DXA are bone mineral content in grams, and projected area of the measured site in square centimeters. By dividing the BMC by the area, bone mineral density (BMD) is given in g/cm². As the DXA image is a two-dimensional image of a three-dimensional object, this is an "areal," rather than a true volumetric, density. The depth of the bones cannot be covered with a single PA projection.[39] To overcome this limitation, to some extent, bone mineral apparent density of the spine can be calculated.[40]

Standard DXA spinal measurements are performed in the posteroanterior projection, and both the spine and the proximal femur are most often measured. To assess early changes in trabecular bone density (i.e., due to cortisone therapy), densitometers were constructed to allow imaging of the spine in the lateral projection. Thus, measurements of vertebral morphometry may be made in lateral projections of the segments from T4 to L4 inclusively as fractures above T4 are unlikely to be of osteoporotic origin and the shape of L5 is subject to great morphologic variation.

Potential contributions from the mineral in ribs or iliac crests limit this application. In addition, the greater soft tissue thickness encountered when measuring BMC or BMD in the coronal plane decreases precision compared with measurements in the sagittal plane.

Lateral densitometry can be used to assess BMD in the body of the vertebra and thus eliminate the contribution from mineral in the predominantly cortical bone in the posterior vertebral complex. Trabecular bone is affected before cortical bone in estrogen or androgen deficiency and glucocorticoid excess, and this bone loss is first apparent in the vertebral bodies (lateral DXA), and later in the whole vertebrae (PA DXA).

Hyperparathyroidism and hyperthyroidism, in contrast, affect cortical bone before trabecular bone, so the bone loss they cause is apparent first in the PA DXA and later in the lateral DXA.

As all the calcium in the path of the X-ray beam will contribute to the BMD measured, the BMD will be falsely elevated if there is osteoarthritis with hyperostosis of the facet joints, degenerative disk disease with osteophytes, or a vertebral fracture.[41-45] Affected vertebra must be excluded from analysis. Therefore, it is recommended to perform additional conventional radiographs of the region where the DXA is performed to avoid possible artifacts, which may lead to falsely elevated results (see Case Study).

Because of these artifacts of the lumbar spine in the more elderly population (over 65 years), it has been suggested that only the proximal femur should be scanned.[46] However, the monitoring of change is best done with scans of the lumbar spine, if there are no artifacts.

The quantitative absorptiometric techniques used today apply very low radiation doses, which are similar to those of natural background radiation (2400 μSv per annum; about 7 μSv per day).[47,48] The applied doses are mostly less than 10% of chest radiography (50 μSv), and far lower than doses used in radiographic imaging methods to confirm the diagnosis of osteoporosis in patients at risk.

Posteroanterior or lateral lumbar densitometry can be combined with lateral spinal morphometry.

Quantitative Computed Tomography

With quantitative computed tomography (QCT) the bone mineral density of the spine can be determined and is given as the true volumetric density (mg/cm³) of trabecular or cortical bone. QCT has been used for assessment of vertebral fracture risk, measurement of age-related bone loss, and follow-up of osteoporosis and other metabolic bone diseases.

A software package available for computed tomography workstations allows the conversion of Hounsfield units to an absolute measurement of bone density of calcium in milligrams per cubic centimeter by including standards containing known amounts of test material in the field of view. With these standards, a calibration curve is constructed and the absolute volumetric density of the vertebra being examined is calculated. Further accuracy can be achieved by measuring at two X-ray energies and adjusting for the amount of soft tissue in the tissue volume examined.[29] Care is necessary in setting the cursor to avoid partial-volume averaging artifacts if the endplate or disk is included in the measured volume.

Because of the expense and radiation dose, very small-aperture alternatives for peripheral quantitative CT have been built and are available commercially. These machines may be used to measure skeletal sites in the extremities (e.g., distal radius, calcaneus) in the same way.

Quantitative Ultrasonography of Bone

The speed of ultrasound through calcaneal bone and the attenuation of the signal have been found to correlate well with BMD measurements and, at least in some populations, to predict fracture risk.[49] Anatomical, clinical, and other variables are potential causes of error.[4,50-54]

Radiographic Absorptiometry

Radiographic absorptiometry involves digitization and computed analysis of hand radiographs acquired with the inclusion of a standardized wedge used to calibrate bone density. Accuracy and precision are reported to be excellent. More recently, a system has been marketed that automates this analysis. The advent of computed radiography may facilitate the use of this method in centers without access to other technologies. However, the evidence base for its adoption is modest and outcome studies are lacking.[55,56]

Single-Photon Absorptiometry

In the early days of quantitative radiology, single-photon absorptiometry was used for bone mineral measurement, with measurement of bone size on radiographs of the hand or crude determinations of optical density from similar images. Single-photon absorptiometry is an effective technique for measurements of bone in the distal radius and ulna.[30] The challenge of measuring bone in the proximal femur and spine prompted new technological developments.

The Radiologist's Role in Therapy—Percutaneous Vertebroplasty

Percutaneous vertebroplasty has been developed as an effective technique for the treatment of painful vertebral compression fractures caused by osteoporosis, malignancy, and some benign bone tumors.

Because the pain of a compression fracture is alleviated by vertebroplasty, patients feel significant relief almost immediately. One of the risks, however, is that a small amount of orthopedic cement can leak out of the vertebral body. This does not usually cause a serious problem, unless the leakage moves into a potentially dangerous location, such as the spinal canal. Other possible complications include infection, bleeding, increased back pain, and neurological symptoms. Paralysis is extremely rare. Sometimes, the procedure causes another fracture in the spine or ribs. Vertebroplasty does not correct an osteoporosis-induced curvature of the spine, as kyphoplasty does. Patients with a healed vertebral fracture are not candidates for vertebroplasty.

During a vertebroplasty, a metal needle is passed into the vertebral body and a cement mixture, containing polymethylmethacrylate (PMMA), barium powder, tobramycin, and a solvent, are injected under imaging guidance by the physician. The procedure was originally developed in France in 1984.

It usually takes approximately 30–60 minutes to perform one level. More than one level can be performed if necessary during a single session.

In selecting appropriate patients for vertebroplasty, it is important to distinguish the pain caused by VCF from other numerous causes of back pain. Careful adherence to clinical and imaging selection criteria is crucial to procedural success.

Painful osteoporotic compression fractures of the spine in patients whose pain is refractory to conservative therapy are excellent indications for vertebroplasty. Ideally, the onset of symptoms was not earlier than 4 months before presentation. Symptoms include mid-line, *nonradiating* back pain that increases when weight-bearing and can be exacerbated by manual palpation of the spinous process of the involved vertebra. If patients have multiple fractures, MR imaging is helpful to document the age of some or all of the fractures, as edema within the marrow space of the vertebral body can be visualized on sagittal T2W images. Absolute contraindications for vertebroplasty include hemorrhagic diathesis and infection. Lesions with epidural extension require careful injection to prevent epidural overflow and spinal cord compression by the cement or displaced epidural tissue.

Conclusion

Every radiologist should be aware of osteoporosis as a "silent killer" in the elderly population, leading to a substantial amount of illness and disability. The radiologist should be aware that screening for osteoporosis is not restricted to bone densitometry and report suspected osteopenia or "asymptomatic" spinal fractures in spinal as well as in chest radiographs.

Radiologists must be familiar with the basic principles of a bone density examination and must ensure rigorous quality assurance with regard to the education of the staff involved. In addition, the radiologist should understand the clinical relevance of diagnosis and follow-up, as well as reporting to and communicating with clinicians.

Ten Things to Remember

1. Bone mineral density (BMD; g/cm^2) and risk fracture are continuous variables.
2. Bone mineral density depends on age, sex, lifestyle, metabolic disease, and medication and correlates indirectly with the risk of low trauma fractures of the spine, femur, forearm, and wrist.
3. After lumbar vertebral fractures, the mean number of bed days is reportedly 25.8 and limited activity days are 158.5.
4. The WHO has established criteria for normal BMD, low bone mass (osteopenia), osteoporosis, and severe (established) osteoporosis.
5. Bone densitometry results can be reported in terms of the standard deviations from the mean of either sex-matched peak bone mass (T-score) or age-matched BMD (Z-score), but for reporting change over time, the absolute BMD values (g/cm^2) must be used.
6. At all ages, the relative risk of fracture doubles for each unit decrease in T-score, regardless of the skeletal location used to calculate that score.
7. Osteoporosis can be diagnosed on chest and spinal radiographs and quantified with DXA, quantitative CT, and quantitative ultrasonography.
8. On lumbar spine radiographs, osteopenia should be reported semiquantitatively using the Saville index, and Genant's score should be applied in grading osteoporotic spinal fractures.
9. Patients with one osteoporotic fracture anywhere in the body have a 20% higher risk of developing a further fracture.
10. Vertebroplasty may be indicated in patients with acute vertebral instability fractures who present with mid-line, *nonradiating* back pain that increases when weight-bearing and can be exacerbated by manual palpation of the spinous process of the involved vertebrae.

Case Study

Patient: 81-year-old female patient with back pain and suspected osteoporosis.

Exam: Lumbar spine: sagittal (Fig. 14.**1**) and lateral (Fig. 14.**2**) view radiographs; p.a. DXA lumbar spine (L1-L4) report (Figs. 14.**3**, 14.**4**).

Findings: In the conventional radiograph of the lumbar spine the vertebral body of L1 shows a marked sclerotic internal structure with marked reduction of the vertebral height in the medial aspect. There is also a considerable reduction of the intervertebral space with spondylotic reactions in the segments TH 12/L1 and L1/2. The processus spinosus of the lumbar spine show significantly increased subchondral sclerosis (M. Baastrup).

The DXA of the vertebral body L1 shows a T-score of +1.2 and a Z-score of +3.61 equivalent to a pathological bone mineral density due to the underlying Paget's disease. The other vertebral bodies have a BMD between 0.843 g/cm² and 0.950 g/cm² equivalent to a T-score between –1.15 and –2.48 and a Z-score between 0.42 and 1.6.

Diagnosis: Paget's disease of the vertebral body L1. The other vertebral bodies have a T-score between –1.15 and –2.48, which is in the osteopenic range and above normal according to age-adjusted normal values. L1 must be excluded!

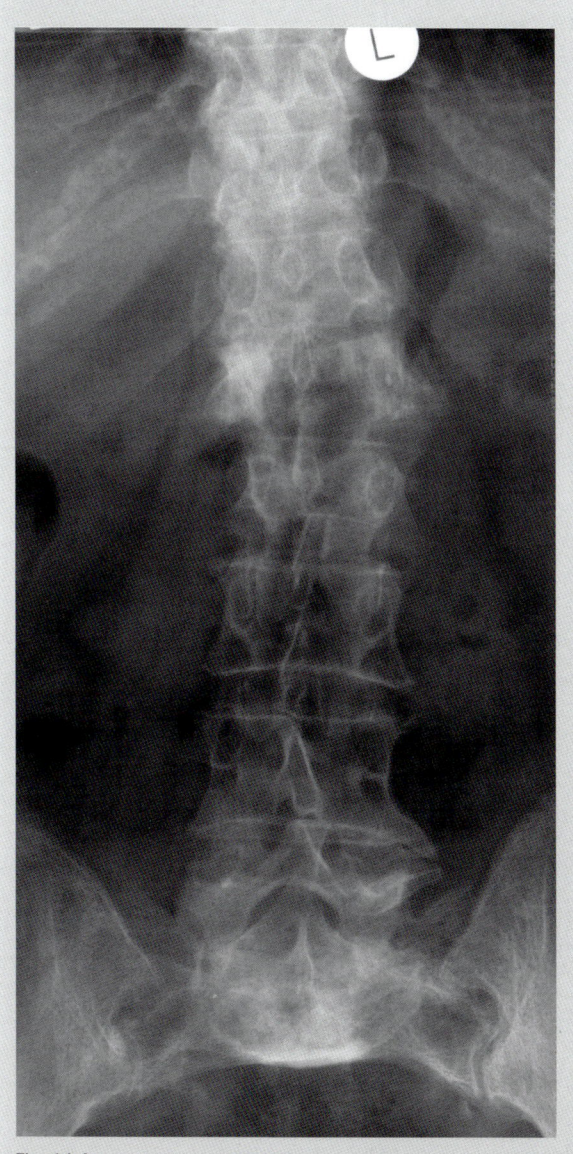

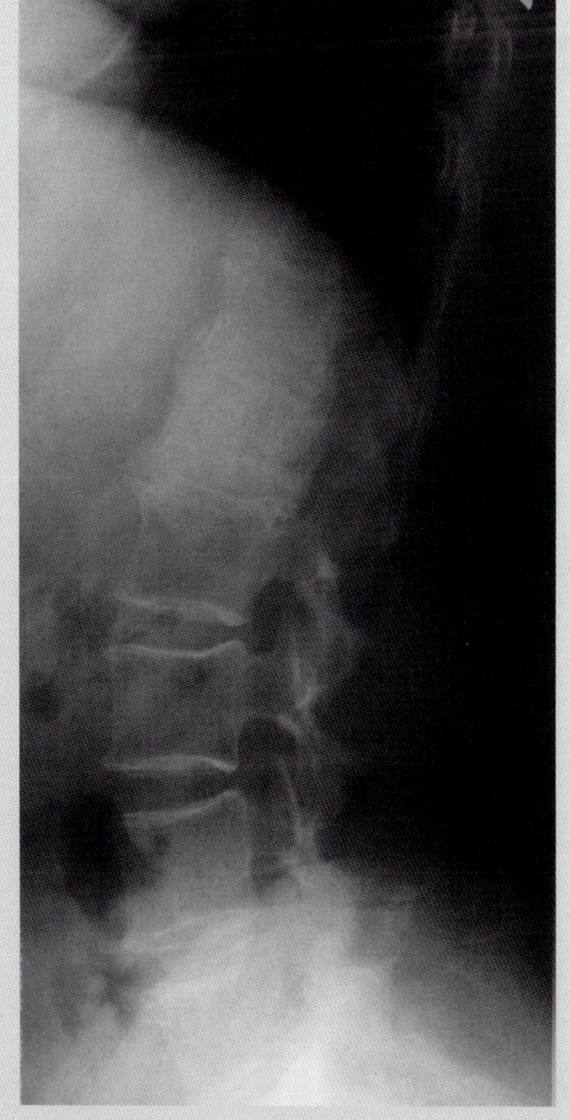

Fig. 14.**1**

Fig. 14.**2**

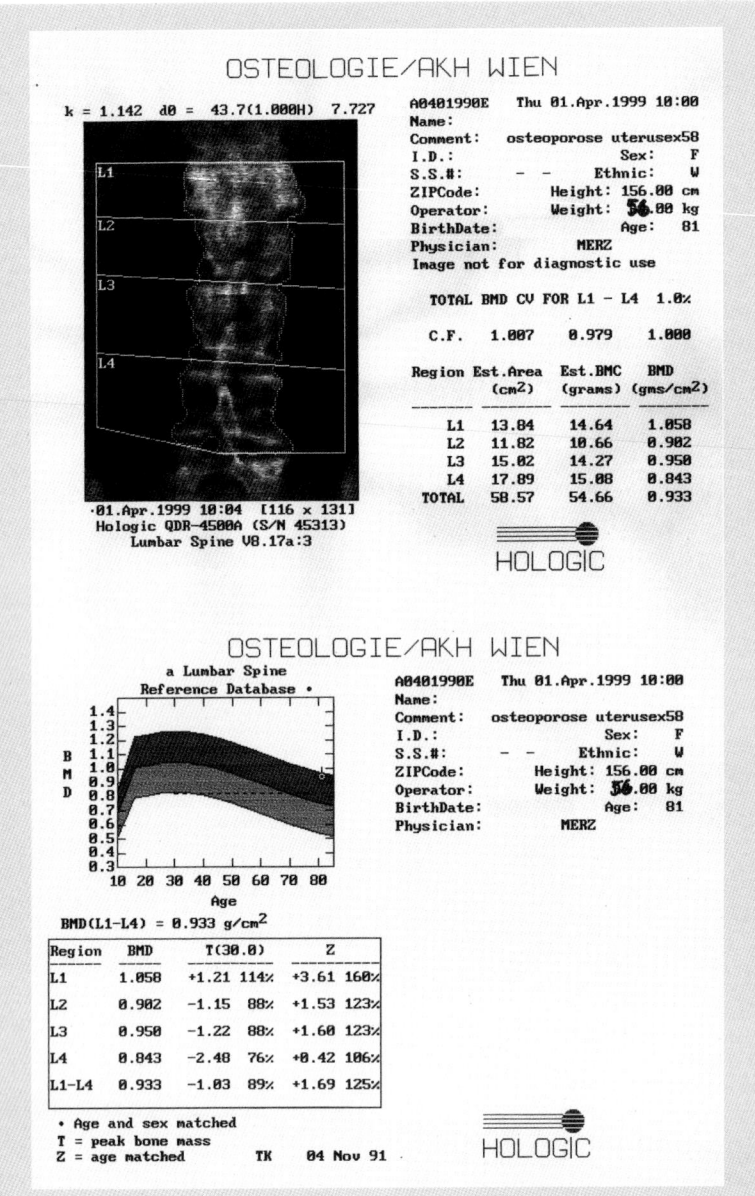

Fig. 14.3

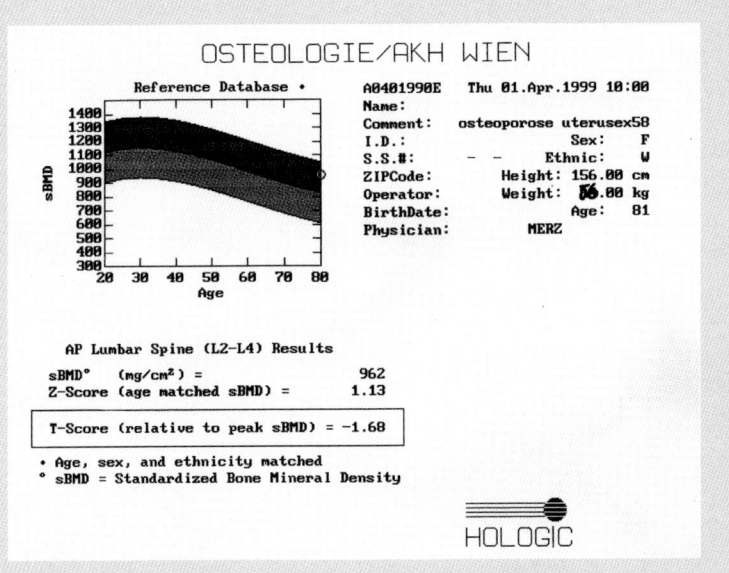

Fig. 14.4

References

1. Miller PD, Bonnick SL, Rosen CJ. Consensus of an international panel on the clinical utility of bone mass measurements in the detection of low bone mass in the adult population. *Calcif Tissue Int*. 1996;58(4):207–214.
2. Miller PD, et al. Clinical utility of bone mass measurements in adults: consensus of an international panel. The Society for Clinical Densitometry. *Semin Arthritis Rheum*. 1996;25(6):361–372.
3. Fink HA, et al. Disability after clinical fracture in postmenopausal women with low bone density: the fracture intervention trial (FIT). *Osteoporos Int*. 2003;14(1):69–76.
4. Grampp S, et al. Comparisons of noninvasive bone mineral measurements in assessing age-related loss, fracture discrimination, and diagnostic classification. *J Bone Miner Res*. 1997;12(5):697–711.
5. Faulkner KG, von Stetten E, Miller P. Discordance in patient classification using T-scores. *J Clin Densitom*. 1999;2(3):343–350.
6. Miller PD. Controversies in bone mineral density diagnostic classifications. *Calcif Tissue Int*. 2000;66(5):317–319.
7. Faulkner KG, et al. Simple measurement of femoral geometry predicts hip fracture: the study of osteoporotic fractures. *J Bone Miner Res*. 1993;8(10):1211–1217.
8. Gluer CC. Monitoring skeletal changes by radiological techniques. *J Bone Miner Res*. 1999;14(11):1952–1962.
9. Marshall D, Johnell O, Wedel H. Meta-analysis of how well measures of bone mineral density predict occurrence of osteoporotic fractures. *BMJ*. 1996;312(7041):1254–1259.
10. Jung HS et al. Discrimination of metastatic from acute osteoporotic compression spinal fractures with MR imaging. *Radiographics*. 2003;23(1):179–187.
11. Yuh WT, et al. Vertebral compression fractures: distinction between benign and malignant causes with MR imaging. *Radiology*. 1989;172(1):215–218.
12. Baker LL et al. Benign versus pathologic compression fractures of vertebral bodies: assessment with conventional spin-echo, chemical-shift, and STIR MR imaging. *Radiology*. 1990;174(2):495–502.
13. An HS et al. Can we distinguish between benign versus malignant compression fractures of the spine by magnetic resonance imaging? *Spine*. 1995;20(16):1776–1782.
14. Frager D et al. Subacute osteoporotic compression fracture: misleading magnetic resonance appearance. *Skeletal Radiol*. 1988;17(2):123–126.
15. Shih TT, Huang KM, Li YW. Solitary vertebral collapse: distinction between benign and malignant causes using MR patterns. *J Magn Reson Imaging*. 1999;9(5):635–642.
16. Tan SB, Kozak JA, Mawad ME. The limitations of magnetic resonance imaging in the diagnosis of pathologic vertebral fractures. *Spine*. 1991;16(8):919–923.
17. Cuenod CA et al. Acute vertebral collapse due to osteoporosis or malignancy: appearance on unenhanced and gadolinium-enhanced MR images. *Radiology*. 1996;199(2):541–549.
18. Herneth AM et al. Vertebral metastases: assessment with apparent diffusion coefficient. *Radiology*. 2002;225(3):889–894.
19. Reeve J, Silman A. Epidemiology of osteoporotic fractures in europe: towards biologic mechanisms. The European Prospective Osteoporosis Study Group. *Osteoporos Int*. 1997;7(Suppl 3):78–83.
20. Blake GM, Rea JA, Fogelman I. Vertebral morphometry studies using dual-energy X-ray absorptiometry. *Semin Nucl Med*. 1997;27(3):276–290.
21. Virtama P et al. Density of human carpal, metacarpal and digital bones. *Ann Med Exp Biol Fenn*. 1960;38:467–471.
22. Jergas M et al. Interobserver variation in the detection of osteopenia by radiography and comparison with dual X-ray absorptiometry of the lumbar spine. *Skeletal Radiol*. 1994;23(3):195–199.
23. Kim N et al. Underreporting of vertebral fractures on routine chest radiography. *AJR Am J Roentgenol*. 2004;182(2):297–300.
24. Ross PD et al. Pre-existing fractures and bone mass predict vertebral fracture incidence in women. *Ann Intern Med*. 1991;114(11):919–923.
25. Ross PD et al. A critical review of bone mass and the risk of fractures in osteoporosis. *Calcif Tissue Int*. 1990;46(3):149–161.
26. Saville PD. A quantitative approach to simple radiographic diagnosis of osteoporosis: its application to the osteoporosis of rheumatoid arthritis. *Arthritis Rheum*. 1967;10(5):416–422.
27. Garton MJ et al. Can radiologists detect osteopenia on plain radiographs? *Clin Radiol*. 1994;49(2):118–122.
28. Genant HK et al. Vertebral fracture assessment using a semiquantitative technique. *J Bone Miner Res*. 1993;8(9):1137–1148.
29. Blake GM, Fogelman I. Technical principles of dual energy X-ray absorptiometry. *Semin Nucl Med*. 1997;27(3):210–228.
30. Duppe H et al. A single bone density measurement can predict fractures over 25 years. *Calcif Tissue Int*. 1997;60(2):171–174.
31. Faulkner KG, Cann CE, Hasegawa BH. Effect of bone distribution on vertebral strength: assessment with patient-specific nonlinear finite element analysis. *Radiology*. 1991;179(3):669–674.
32. Faulkner KG et al. Noninvasive measurements of bone mass, structure, and strength: current methods and experimental techniques. *AJR Am J Roentgenol*. 1991;157(6):1229–1237.
33. Grampp S et al. Radiologic diagnosis of osteoporosis. Current methods and perspectives. *Radiol Clin North Am*. 1993;31(5):1133–1145.
34. Grampp S, Steiner E, Imhof H. Radiological diagnosis of osteoporosis. *Eur Radiol*. 1997;7(10):11–19.
35. Peel N, Eastell R. Measurement of bone mass and turnover. *Baillieres Clin Rheumatol*. 1993;7(3):479–498.
36. Baran DT et al. Diagnosis and management of osteoporosis: guidelines for the utilization of bone densitometry. *Calcif Tissue Int*. 1997;61(6):433–440.
37. Blake GM, Gluer CC, Fogelman I. Bone densitometry: current status and future prospects. *Br J Radiol*. 1997;70:177–186.
38. Compston JE, Cooper C, Kanis JA. Bone densitometry in clinical practice. *BMJ*. 1995;310(6993):1507–1510.
39. Genant HK et al. Noninvasive assessment of bone mineral and structure: state of the art. *J Bone Miner Res*. 1996;11(6):707–730.
40. Katzman DK et al. Clinical and anthropometric correlates of bone mineral acquisition in healthy adolescent girls. *J Clin Endocrinol Metab*. 1991;73(6):1332–1339.
41. Orwoll ES, Oviatt SK, Mann T. The impact of osteophytic and vascular calcifications on vertebral mineral density measurements in men. *J Clin Endocrinol Metab*. 1990;70(4):1202–1207.
42. Laskey MA et al. Short communication: heterogeneity of spine bone density. *Br J Radiol*. 1993;66(785):480–483.
43. Franck H, Munz M, Scherrer M. Evaluation of dual-energy X-ray absorptiometry bone mineral measurement—comparison of a single-beam and fan-beam design: the effect of osteophytic calcification on spine bone mineral density. *Calcif Tissue Int*. 1995;56(3):192–195.
44. Frohn J et al. Effect of aortic sclerosis on bone mineral measurements by dual-photon absorptiometry. *J Nucl Med*. 1991;32(2):259–262.
45. Jaovisidha S et al. Influence of spondylopathy on bone densitometry using dual energy X-ray absorptiometry. *Calcif Tissue Int*. 1997;60(5):424–429.
46. Kanis JA, Gluer CC. An update on the diagnosis and assessment of osteoporosis with densitometry. Committee of Scientific Advisors, International Osteoporosis Foundation. *Osteoporos Int*. 2000;11(3):192–202.
47. Kalender WA. Effective dose values in bone mineral measurements by photon absorptiometry and computed tomography. *Osteoporos Int*. 1992;2(2):82–87.
48. Huda W, Morin RL. Patient doses in bone mineral densitometry. *Br J Radiol*. 1996;69(821):422–425.
49. Kang C, Speller R. Comparison of ultrasound and dual energy X-ray absorptiometry measurements in the calcaneus. *Br J Radiol*. 1998;71(848):861–867.
50. Hans D et al. Ultrasonographic heel measurements to predict hip fracture in elderly women: the EPIDOS prospective study. *Lancet*. 1996;348(9026):511–514.
51. Hans D et al. Influence of anthropometric parameters on ultrasound measurements of Os calcis. *Osteoporos Int*. 1995;5(5):371–376.

52. Johansen A, Stone MD. The effect of ankle oedema on bone ultrasound assessment at the heel. *Osteoporos Int.* 1997;7(1):44–47.
53. Grampp S et al. Quantitative US of the calcaneus: cutoff levels for the distinction of healthy and osteoporotic individuals. *Radiology.* 2001;220(2):400–405.
54. Grampp S et al. Diagnostic agreement of quantitative sonography of the calcaneus with dual X-ray absorptiometry of the spine and femur. *AJR Am J Roentgenol.* 1999;173(2):329–334.
55. Yang SO et al. Radiographic absorptiometry for bone mineral measurement of the phalanges: precision and accuracy study. *Radiology.* 1994;192(3):857–859.
56. Kleerekoper M et al. Comparison of radiographic absorptiometry with dual-energy X-ray absorptiometry and quantitative computed tomography in normal older white and black women. *J Bone Miner Res.* 1994;9(11):1745–1749.
57. European Communities/European Foundation for Osteoporosis. *Building strong bones and preventing fractures.* Summary report on osteoporosis in the European Community-Action for prevention. Germany: European Communities/European Foundation for Osteoporosis; 1998: 3–12.
58. Royal College of Physicians. *Osteoporosis: guidelines for prevention and treatment.* London, UK: Royal College of Physicians; 1999: 63–70.
59. Royal College of Physicians. *Osteoporosis: Clinical guidelines for prevention and treatment. Update on pharmacological interventions and an algorithm for management.* London, UK: Royal College of Physicians; 2000: 1–16.
60. World Health Organization (WHO) Study Group. *Assessment of fracture risk and its application to screening for postmenopausal osteoporosis.* WHO Technical Report Series 843. Geneva, Switzerland: World Health Organization; 1994.

15 Vertebral Collapse—Benign or Malignant

A. M. Herneth

Introduction

Vertebral collapse is a serious condition, which is closely related to age.[1,2] According to the demographic changes of our society the incidence and prevalence of vertebral compression fractures are increasing. Vertebral compression fractures are associated with increased morbidity and mortality and thus, vertebral collapse has a significant impact on the patient's overall quality of life and on the patient's life expectancy.[3,4]

The causes of vertebral collapse are manifold, including benign and malignant conditions.[5–7] Most vertebral compression fractures are of benign origin caused by inadequate trauma in patients with osteoporosis or osteomalacia.[8] The International Osteoporosis Foundation estimated that at the age of 65 years 1% of women and 0.5% of men will sustain an acute vertebral compression fracture and the presence of an osteoporotic vertebral compression fracture increases the odds of subsequent fractures five fold.[9] Early diagnosis followed by appropriate therapy reduces the occurrences of subsequent fractures and other sequelae.[10]

Less frequently seen are vertebral compression fractures following metastatic, hematologic or neoplastic disease.[1,4] The spine represents the most frequent site of skeletal metastasis predominating in the thoracic and lumbar spine.[11] It is essential to differentiate benign from malignant vertebral collapse because their medical management and their outcome are substantially different.[1,4,12]

In general, the differentiation of pathological from benign vertebral compression fractures is based on distinct imaging findings such as replacement of fatty bone marrow, contrast enhancement, soft tissue compartments, and the shape and site of fracture.[1,11] However, separating benign from malignant vertebral compression fractures can be problematic in the acute setting, because within the first 8 to 12 weeks after the vertebral collapse the clinical presentation and radiological appearance are similar in both conditions. The problem in the differentiation arises from edema, hemorrhage, and the presence of repair tissue that accompanies acute benign fractures, which results in bone marrow changes which resemble metastatic disease.[13,14] Thus, the differentiation between benign or pathological vertebral compression fractures remains a challenge for the clinician and the radiologist involved.[14–16]

Although clinical evaluation, laboratory data, and imaging findings may be suggestive of either benign or pathological vertebral collapse, there are currently no absolute criteria available for definite diagnosis of one or the other type of fracture.[17,19] There is general agreement that definite diagnosis can only be established by obtaining a tissue specimen. This, however, requires a biopsy or another invasive procedure, which is inappropriate or even counterproductive in patients with multiple or subsequent vertebral compression fractures.[14,20–22] Thus, in these patients differentiation between benign or pathological vertebral compression fractures has to be based on imaging features, clinical presentation, and laboratory data.

In the following paragraphs the most important clinical findings and radiologic features for the differentiation of benign versus pathological vertebral collapse will be discussed.

Clinical Evaluation

Age

The patient's age is ambiguous for such differentiation, as most of the vertebral collapses occur in elderly people because the prevalence of both osteoporosis and metastatic disease increases with age.[23] In patients with known metastatic disease, up to 25% of vertebral compression fractures are of osteoporotic origin. On the other hand, in patients with moderate to severe osteoporosis up to 10% of vertebral collapses are of pathological origin.[11] It is also well known that a pathological vertebral compression fracture is frequently the first presentation of an otherwise occult primary tumor, thus the lack of a known neoplasm does not necessarily exclude a pathological vertebral compression fracture. Furthermore, patients with known metastatic disease in other locations than the spine may also suffer from benign vertebral collapse, following adjuvant therapy for the primary tumor.[7,10,24] Most of these adjuvant therapy concepts use chemotherapeutic agents and/or radiation, with either localized or generalized effects on bone metabolism.[3–5]

History of Trauma

In most patients with benign vertebral collapse a trauma history can be obtained. However, if such patients report inadequate trauma strength or if the fracture location does not match with the trauma mechanism the suspicion of a pathological compression fracture has to be raised.

Imaging Findings

In general, recognition of vertebral collapse presents no difficulties to the radiologist (Table 15.1). Most vertebral collapses are diagnosed on conventional radiographs, which are considered an adequate screening technique. The detection and diagnosis of vertebral collapse has improved significantly with the use of cross-sectional imaging, such as magnetic resonance imaging (MRI) or computed tomography (CT), mainly because of their multi-planar reconstruction (MPR) capabilities.[25,26] However, the differentiation between benign and pathological vertebral compression fractures remains a challenge to the radiologist because of their ambiguous appearance.[16,27–30] Thus, the radiologist and the clinician involved have to keep in mind that the accuracy of almost all imaging findings listed below is low because they can be found in both pathological and benign fractures or they occur infrequently (see Tab. 15.2).[23,31]

Fatty Bone Marrow

The best imaging clue for distinguishing benign from pathological fractures is the presence of fatty (yellow) bone marrow.[11] After adolescence, yellow bone marrow replaces the preexisting hematopoietic (red) bone marrow (Fig. 15.1). Yellow bone marrow has a distinctive (i. e., fatty) appearance on MRI presenting with hyperintense signals on T1W and T2W sequences and loss of signal on STIR and fat-saturated sequences.[32–34] On the other hand in metastatic disease tumor tissue, which in general lacks any fatty compartments, supersedes fatty bone marrow. Hence, the MRI appearance of osseous metastases presents with low-signal intensities on T1W images and high-signal intensities on STIR and T2W images.

Thus, yellow bone marrow and tumor tissue produce a distinctive natural contrast on T1W images, which can be easily depicted on MRI. It is safe to say that if fatty bone marrow is present in a vertebral collapse, vertebral metastasis can be excluded.[19,35]

Edema

Unfortunately, the reverse does not apply, because acute vertebral collapse presents with pronounced edema regardless of the underlying cause. Features favoring benign vertebral collapse include preservation of fatty bone marrow within the collapsed vertebral body and a typical, horizontal band-like pattern of the edema.[30] Signs suggesting pathological vertebral compression fractures include diffuse replacement of fatty bone marrow by edema typically throughout the entire vertebral body including the posterior elements.[36,37]

These two distinctive patterns are useful guidelines for differentiating benign from pathological vertebral compression fractures, however, they are infrequently present and they lack specificity.[23]

Table 15.1 Sensitivity and specificity of imaging techniques in the evaluation of acute vertebral compression fractures

		Sensitivity	Specificity
X-ray	AP	3	1
	lateral	4	1
CT	ax	3	2
	MPR sag.	5	2
MRI	T1	5	2
	#T1 + contrast	4	3
	##T2	4	3
	STIR	5	3
	in-/opposed phase	5	3
	proton density	4	3
	DWI (SI)	5	4
	DWI (ADC)	5	5
Scintigraphy		4	2
FTG-PET		4	4

\# Caution: contrast enhancement may mask replacement of fatty bone marrow.
\#\# Specificity may increase if *fluid sign* is present.

Table 15.2 Acute vertebral compression fractures: likelihood of imaging to indicate either benign or pathologic vertebral compression fractures

	Benign	Malignancy
Involvement of dorsal elements	1	4
Bulging/destruction of dorsal wall	1	4
Involvement of posterior half of vert. body	2	3
Soft tissue mass	2	3
Edema (diffuse)	2	3
Contrast enhancement	2	3
Single segment	3	3
Dislocation of intact dorsal wall	3	2
Edema (focal)	3	2
Multi-segmental	3	2
Involvement of anterior half of vert. body	3	2
Fatty bone marrow (remnants)	4	1
Fluid sign (if present)	5	0

Likelihood to be found in either benign or malignant vertebral compression fractures: 0 (not likely at all) to 5 (almost pathognomonic)

Other clinical features, such as pain, restricted mobility of the spine, neurological deficits or fatigue are common in patients with both benign and pathological vertebral compression fractures, and may therefore not be used for differentiation. Thus, clinical presentation may provide clues but not criteria for the differentiation of benign versus pathological vertebral collapse.

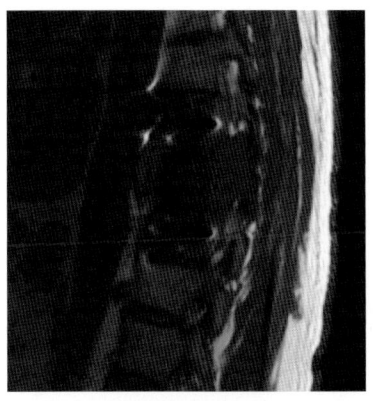

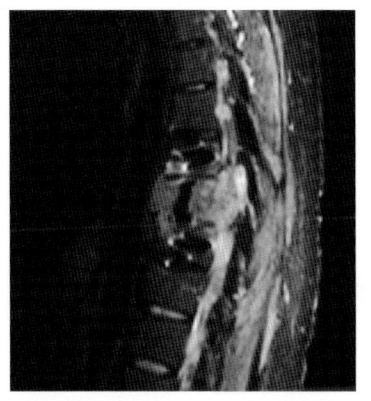

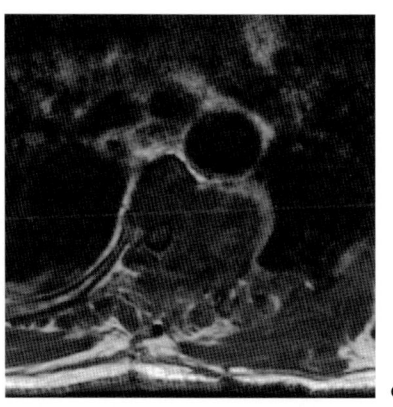

Fig. 15.1 Pathological vertebral compression fracture. A T1W image (**a**) before and (**b**) after (fat suppression) i. v. application of contrast material. **c** A T1W image in the axial plane. Convex deformation (bulging) of the posterior vertebral wall and involvement of the posterior vertebral elements as well as the marked enhancement after i. v. administration of gadolinium are almost pathognomonic for metastatic disease. The involvement of the dorsal vertebral structures is best delineated on the axial images.

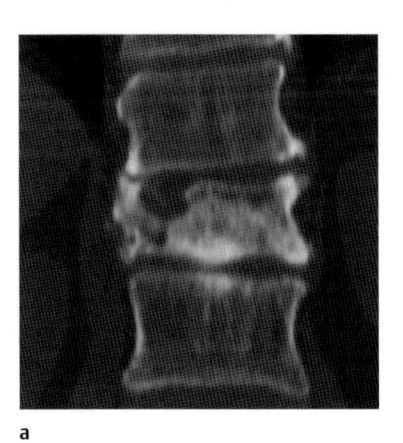

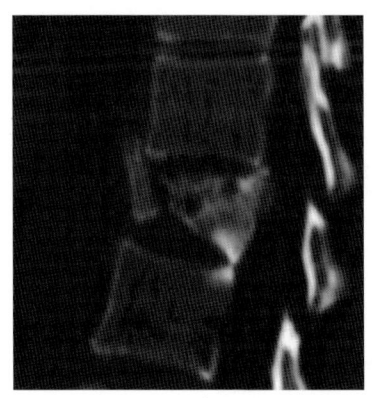

Fig. 15.2 Benign vertebral compression fracture of L1. The images show a multi-planar reconstruction in the coronal (**c**) and sagittal (**b**) planes. The patient was reported to have fallen from a ladder (adequate trauma). A wedge-shaped vertebral compression fracture is shown with a dislocated anterior vertebral wall and an intact posterior vertebral wall, which is a typical finding in post-traumatic vertebral compression fractures. Note the sclerotic appearance of the fractured vertebra following impaction. There is no soft tissue mass, edema, or hemorrhage present indicating an old vertebral compression fracture.

Shape—Extent of Fracture

Vertebral collapse can be of minimal extent (circumscribed vertebral endplate fracture), of moderate extent (loss of height less than 25%), or severe (up to 75% of height) or subtotal. However, the extent of fracture does not correlate with its cause.

Several different shapes of vertebral compression fractures are known, such as: (1) "wedge-shaped vertebrae" related to collapse of the anterior aspect of the vertebral body (Fig. 15.2); (2) "fish-bone vertebrae," which are characterized by intact anterior and posterior walls, and bi-concave deformities of the upper and lower vertebral endplate (Fig. 15.3); (3) "pancake vertebrae," which are flat-shaped remnants of vertebral bodies after subtotal vertebral compression fractures; and (4) "burst fractures," which are complex-shaped vertebral collapses with irregular margins and multiple fragments.[11] The first three types of fractures are frequently associated with benign collapses, and the latter two with pathological fractures.

Convex deformation of the posterior wall is frequently seen in metastatic disease and may serve as an indicator for pathological vertebral compression fractures (Fig. 15.4). However, in patients with extensive vertebral collapse displacement of the posterior wall may resemble such pathological deformation.

Although shape is a good indicator for distinguishing between benign and pathological collapse, this feature lacks specificity and is infrequently suitable for differentiation.

Contrast Material—Enhancement

Enhancement after intravenous administration of contrast material (i. e., gadolinium DTPA) can be used to identify vertebral metastases (Figs. 15.1, 15.4).[38] However, in an acute vertebral fracture such an enhancement is ambiguous, because acute benign vertebral compression fractures can also present with substantial enhancement.[30,39,40] This enhancement is probably due to the extravasation of gadolinium, which is presumed to be up to 30% at first pass.

In edema this extravasation derives benefit from stases of blood flow, neo-angiogenesis, and increased vascular permeability. Accordingly, enhancement after intravenous administration of contrast material is not

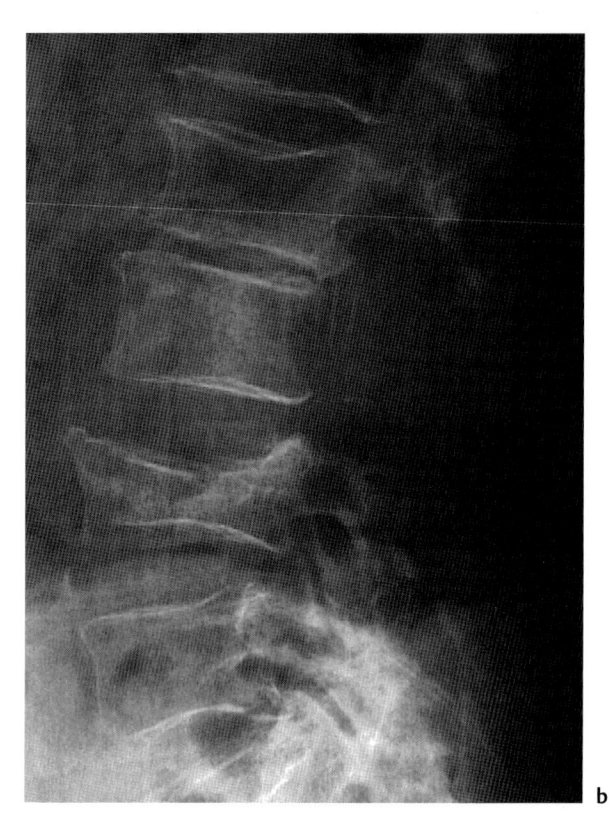

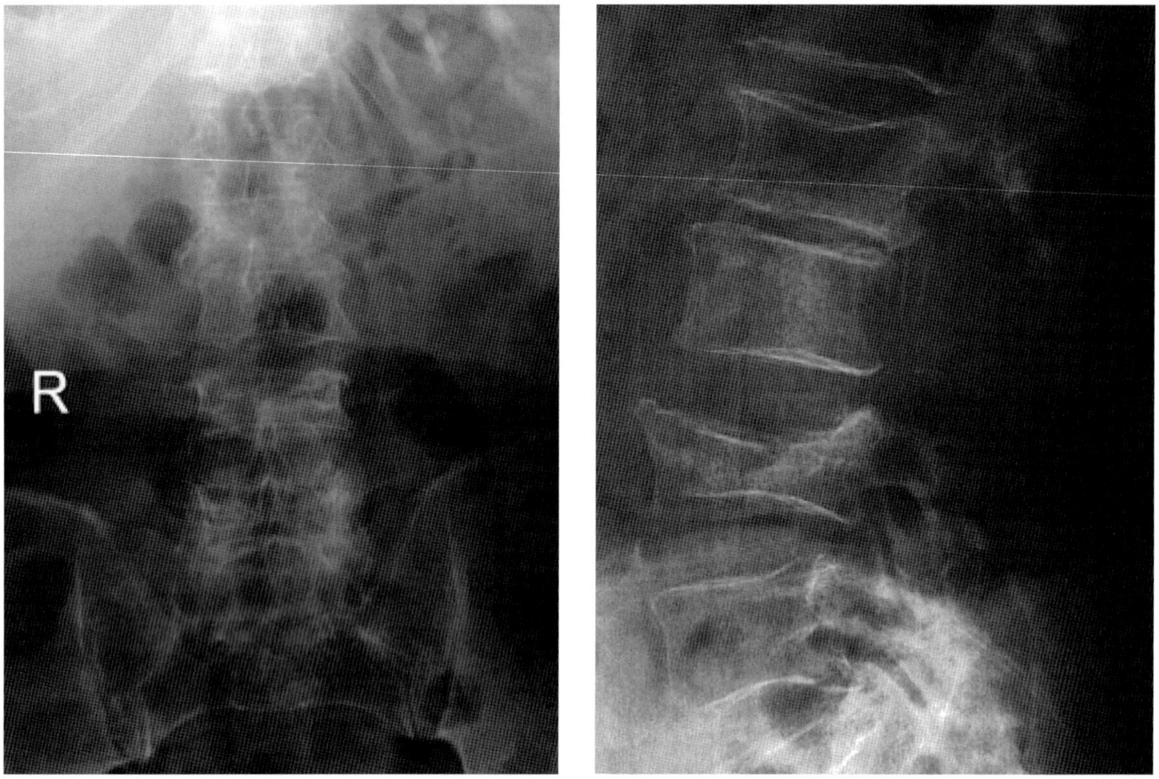

Fig. 15.3 Fish-bone shaped (old) benign vertebral compression fracture (L4) in a patient with vertebral metastases from renal cell carcinoma. An AP and lateral radiograph of the lumbar spine. The benign vertebral compression fracture is of post-actinic origin and occurred 7 years ago following radiation after surgical resection of the renal cell carcinoma. Note the large osteolytic metastases destroying the posterior elements of L2 and L3 following renal cell carcinoma.

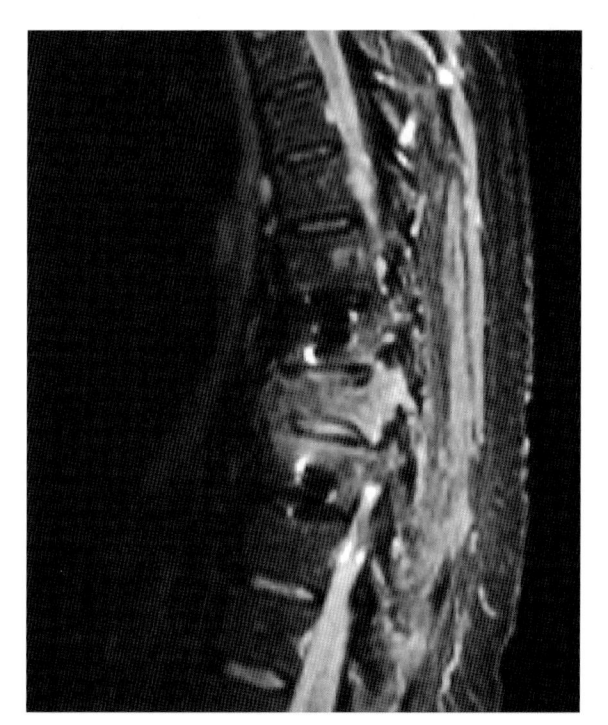

Fig. 15.4 Pathological vertebral compression fracture. T1W contrast-enhanced image with fat suppression. Fish-bone shaped pathological compression fracture in the lower thoracic spine presenting with pronounced contrast enhancement. Note the band-like reactive edema in the vertebral endplate of the adjacent vertebra, the preserved disks, and the susceptibility artifacts of the dorsal instrumentation.

a criterion to distinguish benign from malignant vertebral collapse, however, it may well serve as a distinctive parameter after edema has been absorbed. Unfortunately, bone marrow edema in benign acute vertebral compression fractures persists for up to 6 months, which may be due to neo-angiogenesis and new bone formation. Thus, the presence of edema and/or contrast enhancement in a short-term follow-up is an unequivocal finding.

Contrast Material—Dynamics

There are several articles in the literature reporting differences in the dynamics of contrast material according to the underlying cause of vertebral collapse.[41] Time-density curves in metastatic disease are considered to show rapid in- and out-flow of gadolinium, whereas benign vertebral collapse presents with a moderate incline and a plateau during the wash-out phase.[13,39] Although such patterns are strongly suggestive of one or the other cause of vertebral fractures, time-density curves often present with unequivocal shapes.

Site of Fracture

The site of fracture may also be used as an indicator for either benign or pathological collapse.[11] Metastatic disease frequently occurs in the posterior aspect of the vertebral body usually expanding into the posterior

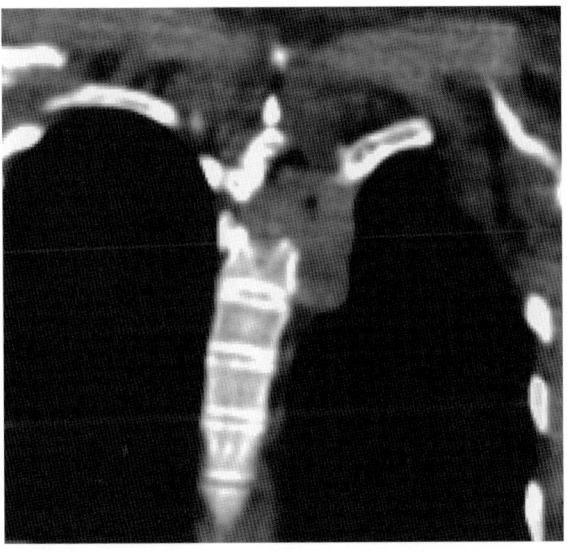

Fig. 15.5 **Pathological vertebral compression fracture.** Multi-detector CT images. **a** Multi-planar reconstruction in the coronal plane using the bone-window setting and an axial scan **b** using the lung window setting. Note the large soft tissue mass infiltrating the pleura (Pancoast tumor) destroying the dorsal vertebral elements and the corresponding rib.

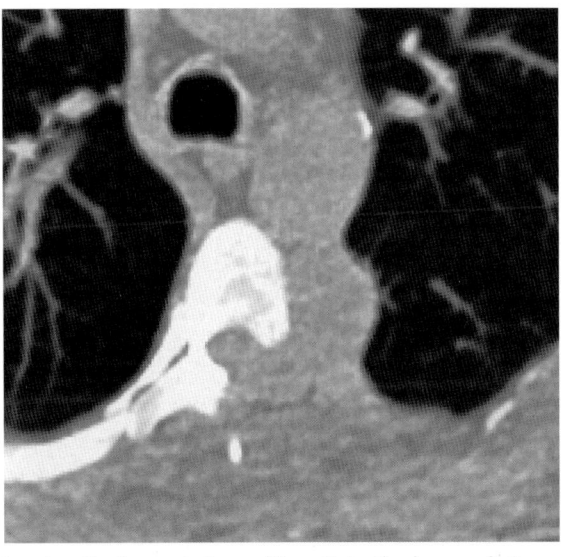

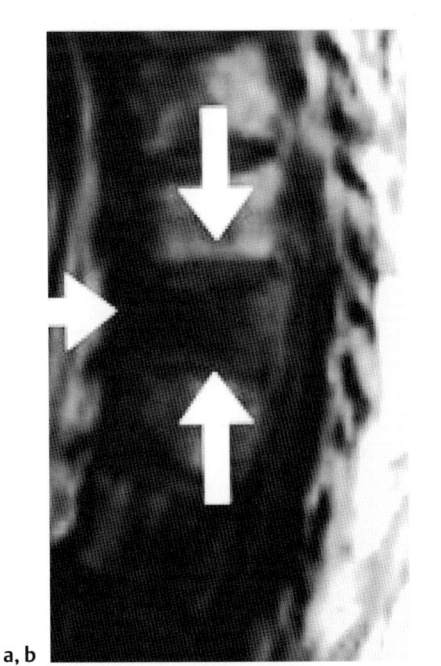

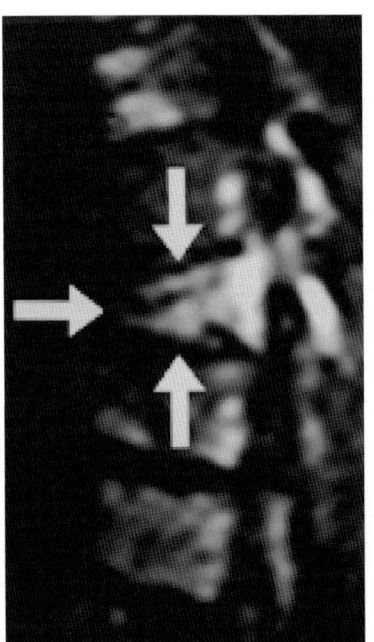

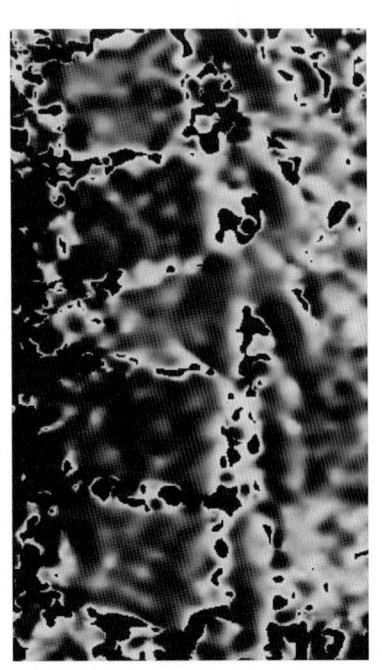

Fig. 15.6 **Pathological vertebral compression fracture of Th7. a** T1W image; **b** DWI (diffusion weighted image, b = 880 sec/mm); and **c** ADC (apparent diffusion coefficient) map in the sagittal plane. The wedge-shaped pathologic vertebral compression fracture is hypointense on the T1W images indicating replacement of regular fatty bone marrow. On the DWI this fracture is hyperintense demonstrating restricted diffusion, which is indicative for malignancy. Restricted diffusion corresponds with low signals on ADC maps. Note that fatty bone marrow also presents with low ADC values, which may resemble malignancy. [56]

vertebral structures (Fig. 15.4).[42,43] This typical pattern of involvement can be explained with the particular blood support of the vertebral bodies.[2] Destruction of the pedicles is almost pathognomonic for metastatic disease and can be easily depicted on MRI (Fig. 15.1) and CT (Fig. 15.5) and it is a well known but infrequent finding on plain radiographs (i. e., vanished eyes of the vertebra).

On the other hand collapse of the anterior aspects of the vertebral bodies is closely associated with osteoporosis, because mechanical strain is highest in this portion of the vertebral body (see Fig. 15.2). A good indicator for benign collapse is an intact posterior wall, even if it is displaced as is frequently observed in traumatic burst fractures. However, metastatic disease may occur in the anterior portion of the spine without destruction of the posterior wall and without involvement of the pedicles (Fig. 15.6).

Fluid-Sign (Osteonecrosis)

Baur and colleagues reported that in fractured vertebral bodies signal intensities isointense to that of cerebrospinal fluid adjacent to the vertebral endplate may be present.[44] Histological correlation demonstrated osteonecrosis, edema, and fibrosis in this area and this finding was significantly associated with osteoporosis. Although this feature seems to be highly suggestive for osteoporotic vertebral compression fractures, it was observed in less than 40% of cases and has also been present in pathological fractures.

Soft Tissue Mass

Many metastases present as soft tissue masses destroying the original structures.[43,45] Thus, the presence of soft tissue within and/or adjacent to the vertebral body is a good indicator for malignancy and is not a common finding with acute osteoporotic vertebral collapse (see Figs. 15.**1**, 15.**4**, 15.**5**).[1,14,46] Sometimes, trauma can be associated with paravertebral hematoma, which can resemble a soft tissue mass. However, hematoma has a distinct appearance on MRI and CT, which is dependent on the stage of resorption, and is rarely a problem for the radiologist.

Spondylodiskitis may also produce soft tissue masses adjacent to the vertebral column and within the intervertebral disk space. Furthermore, it frequently leads to destruction of the vertebral endplates, mimicking a vertebral compression fracture.[47] In addition these soft tissue masses show a marked enhancement after intravenous administration of contrast material. In such cases the clinical presentation, the patient's history, and the laboratory data can be reliably used for diagnosis.

New Imaging Methods

Diffusion Weighted Imaging

Within the last few years new imaging methods have been introduced for the differentiation of benign from pathological vertebral compression fractures. Although the data presented are promising large scale and multi-center trials have to be performed for a thorough evaluation.[48]

Diffusion weighted imaging (DWI) is a powerful imaging tool for appraisal of the tissue-specific diffusion capacity of biological tissue.[15,49,50] First attempts with semiquantitative evaluation of the diffusion capacity of benign and pathological vertebral compression fractures produced promising results for their differentiation.[33,51] The rationale of this technique is that in hypercellular metastatic tissue the diffusion capacity is substantially restricted, leading to increased signal intensities on DWI (Fig. 15.**6**).[52,53] On the other hand, in benign vertebral compression fractures the diffusion capacity remains unchanged resulting in a signal loss (Fig. 15.**7**).

Visual evaluation of DWI, however, may be misleading, because "T2 shine-through effects" and increased perfusion may resemble restricted diffusion.[18,54] This shortcoming can be overcome by calculating the 'Apparent Diffusion Coefficient' (ADC) and using appropriate sequence parameters.[15] The ADC correlates well with the diffusion capacity and may therefore, be considered a reliable and objective parameter in the evaluation of vertebral compression fractures.[22,55,54]

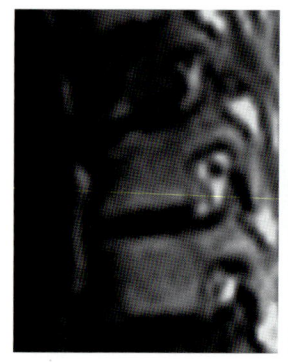

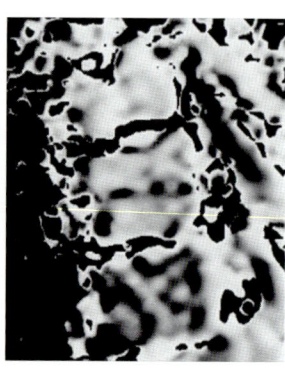

Fig. 15.**7** Benign vertebral compression fracture following an adequate trauma. **a** T2W image and **b** an ADC map. The regular fatty bone marrow has been replaced by post-traumatic edema. This signal change is indistinguishable from metastatic disease. However, the fracture presents with high signals on the ADC map indicating regular diffusion without evidence of malignancy.

FDG-PET

Radionuclides have also been used to differentiate benign from pathological vertebral compression fractures. Since a high fluorine-18 deoxy-glucose (FDG) uptake is characteristic for areas with high energy turn over (standard uptake value <2.5) (Fig. 15.**9**),[57] the use of FDG-Positron Emission Tomography (FDG-PET) may have potential value for differentiation between osteoporotic and pathological vertebral fractures.[58,59] One of the downsides of this method is its limited accuracy because acute osteoporotic fracture is often indistinguishable from metastatic disease (Fig. 15.**8**). Additionally, the limited spatial resolution of this diagnostic tool may lead to problems in the diagnosis of vertebral compression fractures, however, this limitation can be overcome by fusion imaging (CT/SPECT, PET-CT, MRI).

Such tandem tools provide images with a spatial resolution in the sub millimeter range and tissue-specific information which can be reliably used to differentiate osteoporotic vertebral compression fractures from metastatic disease.[60] Although this technique has a high potential in the evaluation of acute vertebral collapse, it is not commonly used because of its limited availability and relatively high costs. In addition, differentiation between inflammatory, post-traumatic, and malignant processes is sometimes difficult and may lead to problems in the differential diagnosis.[61]

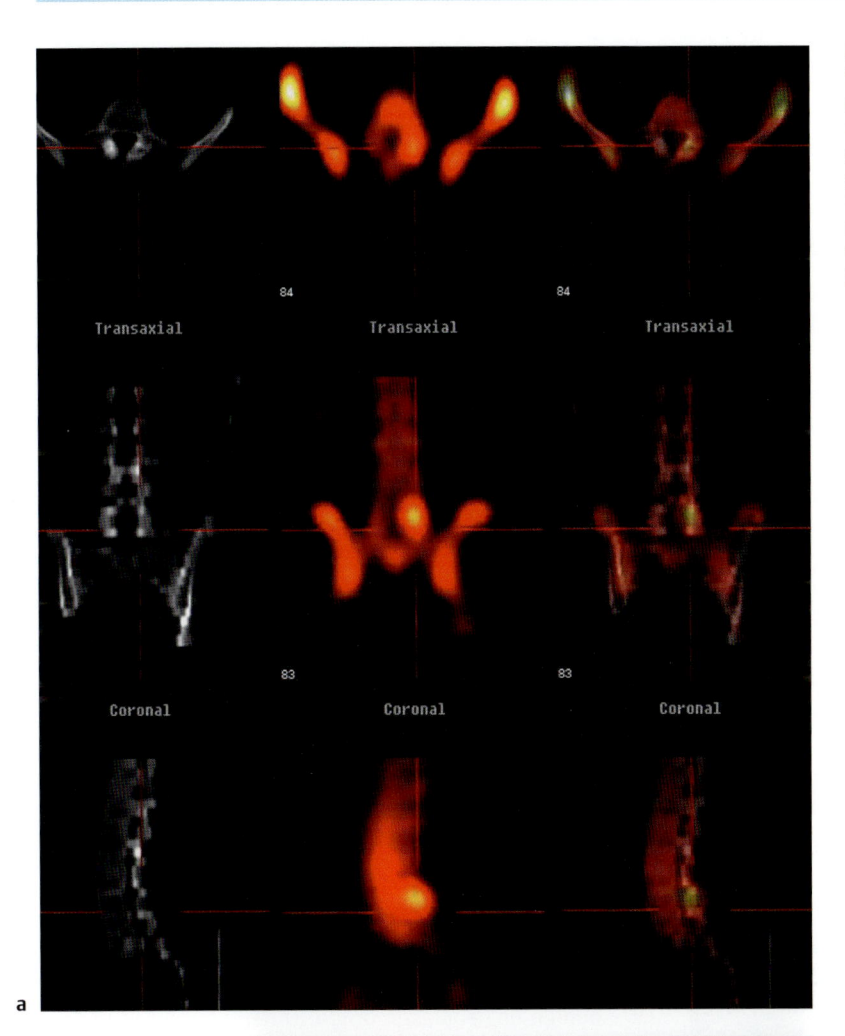

Fig. 15.**8** CT/SPECT (GEMS, Millenium VG with Hawkeye) shows high nuclide uptake within the left pedicle of L5, which is indistinguishable from osseous metastases. An additional CT shows a fracture of the left pedicle without any evidence of malignancy. (Courtesy of Drs. O Kienas and A. Kurtaran, Dept. of Nuclear Medicine, Medical University Vienna, Austria.)

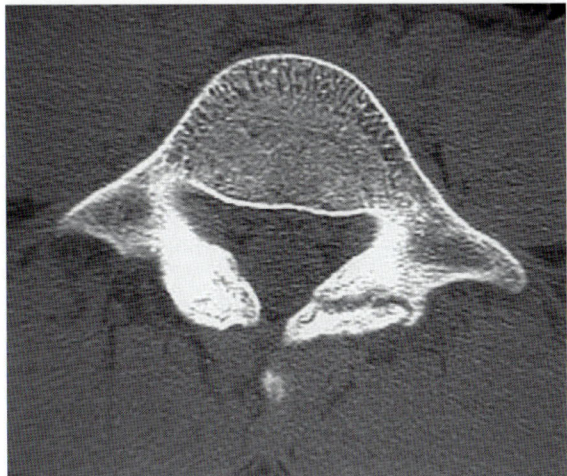

Scintigraphy

Bone scintigraphy with Tc-99mHDP is a well-established screening method for skeletal metastases (Fig. 15.**10**).[28,62,63] In general, skeletal metastases present with a rapid and pronounced uptake of radionuclides.[28,64] Unfortunately, acute vertebral compression fractures, many degenerative disorders, and inflammation show similar radionuclide dynamics.[65] Thus, scintigraphy lacks specificity in respect of differentiating benign from malignant vertebral compression fractures.

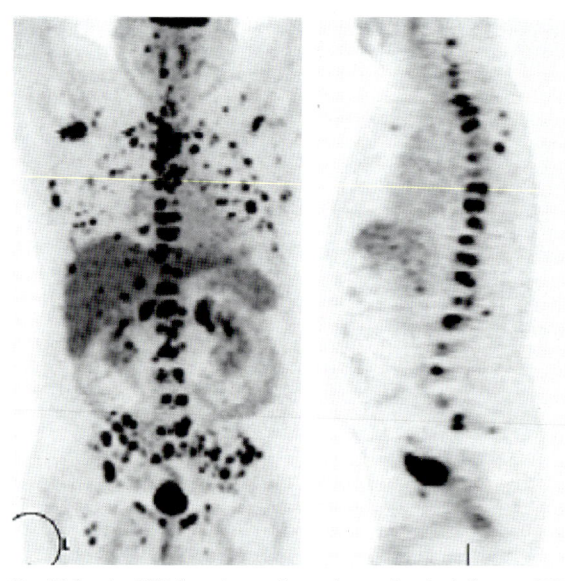

Fig. 15.**9** An MIP (maximum intensity projection) from a PET (positron emission tomography) in a patient with metastatic disease from a melanoma. The *dark areas* indicate high uptake in the osseous and hepatic metastases. (Courtesy of Dr. O Kienast, Dept. of Nuclear Medicine, Medical University Vienna, Austria.)

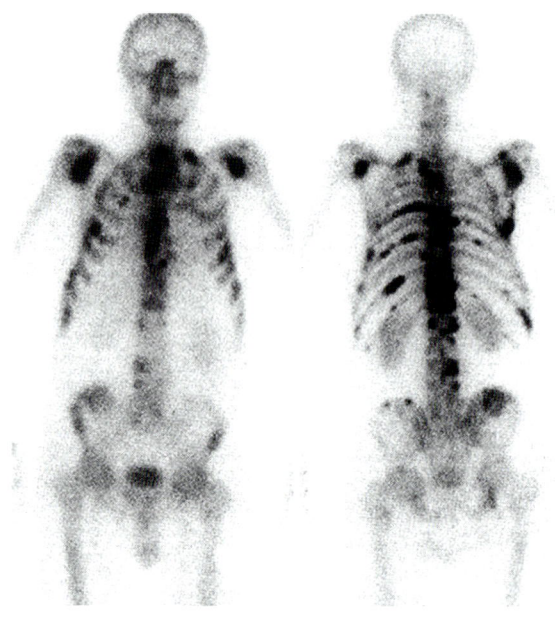

Fig. 15.**10** This bone scintigraphy shows a strong radionuclide uptake of the multiple osseous metastases in a patient with lung cancer. (Courtesy of Dr. O. Kienast, Dept. of Nuclear Medicine, Medical University Vienna, Austria.)

Biopsy

Tissue characterization is mandatory in patients with acute vertebral collapse of unknown origin.[20,21] Although some noninvasive techniques have been reported to have the potential for tissue characterization, histological evaluation is currently the only method for establishing a definite diagnosis. Thus, a representative specimen of the tissue of interest has to be obtained for such an evaluation.[66]

Minimally invasive procedures such as image-guided fine needle biopsy are easy to perform and yield sufficient material for an accurate diagnosis.[67] MRI has become the preferred imaging tool for such an intervention, because of its excellent soft tissue contrast, which can be used to guide the biopsy device directly into the tissue of interest.

This is of special interest in patients with acute pathological vertebral collapse. If in these patients the biopsy device is incorrectly positioned only debris instead of tumor tissue may be obtained, leading to false-negative results. With the introduction of MRI for guiding the biopsy device, the false-negative result rate as well as complications such as bleeding, infection, instability, and neurological sequelae have diminished.[68]

The transpedicular approach is best for the biopsy of intraosseous lesions. Dedicated skeletal biopsy tools are needed to get through this compact structure. Paravertebral tumor masses, however, can be reached directly without drilling through the pedicle. For both approaches a sound knowledge of the complex anatomy of the vascular, nerve, and bony structures is required.

Conclusion

Acute vertebral collapse is a severe condition of either benign or neoplastic origin. Differentiation of benign from pathological collapse is mandatory for establishing a diagnosis and initiating appropriate treatment. Such differentiation, however, remains a dilemma for the radiologist and the clinician involved, because the clinical presentation, the laboratory results, and the imaging findings are often ambiguous in these patients.

MRI has evolved as the imaging modality of choice for the evaluation of metastatic disease of the spine, because of its MPR capabilities and its excellent soft tissue contrast, which occurs after the fatty bone marrow of the vertebral body is displaced by neoplastic tissue. However, in acute vertebral collapse edema may also displace fatty bone marrow and thus, such edema may resemble a pathological condition.

In most cases accurate diagnosis can only be established after histological evaluation of an invasively obtained specimen. Although advanced biopsy techniques under sophisticated imaging guidance are used, the diagnostic accuracy has not yet reached 100%. Furthermore, there is a low but remaining risk of sometimes inevitable complications, which do occur after such invasive procedures.

References

1. Enderle A, Schmitt E, Zichner L. Diagnosis of focal spinal diseases – a critical review [in German]. *Z Orthop Ihre Grenzgeb.* 1981;119(2):193–205.
2. Batson OV. The function of the vertebral veins and their role in the spread of metastases. *Ann Surg.* 1940;112:56–72.
3. Aaron AD, Berg CD. Local Treatment of Bone Metastases. In: JR Harris et al, eds. *Diseases of the Breast.* Philadelphia, Pa: Lippincott Williams & Wilkins; 1996: 931–944.
4. Nielsen OS, Munro AJ, Tannock IF. Bone metastases: pathophysiology and mangement policy. *J Clin Oncol.* 1991; 9(3): 509–524.
5. Scheid V et al. Clinical course of breast cancer patients with osseous matastasis treated with combination chemotherapy. *Cancer.* 1986;58(12):2589–2593.
6. Porter RW, Miller CG. Back pain and trunk list. *Spine.* 1986;11(6):596–600.
7. Stierer M. Mammakarzinom. In: *Manual der chirurgischen Krebstherapie.* 1995:175–206.
8. Flemming DJ et al. Primary tumors of the spine. *Semin Musculoskelet Radiol.* 2000;4(3):299–320.
9. Grampp S et al. Radiologic diagnosis of osteoporosis. Current methods and perspectives. *Radiol Clin North Am.* 1993; 31(5):1133–1145.
10. Link TM et al. Spinal metastases. Value of diagnostic procedures in the initial diagnosis and follow-up [in German]. *Radiologe.* 1995;35(1):21–27.
11. Resnick D. Skeletal Metastases. In. Resnick D, Ed. *Bone and Joint Imaging.* Philadelphia, Pa: WB Saunders Co; 1996: 1076–1092.
12. Krempien B. Pathogenesis of bone metastasis and tumor osteopathies [in German]. *Radiologe.* 1995;35(1):1–7.
13. Kroon HM et al. MR imaging of edema accompanying benign and malignant bone tumors. *Skeletal Radiol.* 1994; 23(4):261–269.
14. Moulopoulos LA et al. MR prediction of benign and malignant vertebral compression fractures. *J Magn Reson Imaging.* 1996;6(4):667–674.
15. Herneth AM et al. The value of diffusion-weighted MRT in assessing the bone marrow changes in vertebral metastases [in German]. *Radiologe.* 2000;40(8):731–736.
16. Le Bihan DJ. Differentiation of benign versus pathologic compression fractures with diffusion-weighted MR imaging: a closer step toward the "holy grail" of tissue characterization? *Radiology.* 1998;207(2):305–307.
17. Conturo TE et al. Diffusion MRI: precision, accuracy and flow effects. *NMR Biomed.* 1995;8(7–8):307–332.
18. Finelli DA. Diffusion-weighted imaging of acute vertebral compressions: specific diagnosis of benign versus malignant pathologic fractures. *AJNR Am J Neuroradiol.* 2001;22(2):241–242.
19. Frager D et al. Subacute osteoporotic compression fracture: misleading magnetic resonance appearance. *Skeletal Radiol.* 1988;17(2):123–126.
20. Berning W, Freyschmidt J, Ostertag H. Percutaneous bone biopsy, techniques and indications. *Eur Radiol.* 1996;6(6): 875–881.
21. Fyfe IS, Henry AP, Mulholland RC. Closed vertebral biopsy. *J Bone Joint Surg Br.* 1983;65(2):140–143.
22. Leeds NE et al. Magnetic resonance imaging of benign spinal lesions simulating metastasis: role of diffusion-weighted imaging. *Top Magn Reson Imaging.* 2000;11(4):224–234.
23. Vogler JB, Murphy WA. Diffuse Marrow Diseases. In: Berquist TH, ed. *MRI of the Musculoskeletal System.* Philadelphia, Pa: Lippincott Williams & Wilkins; 2001:979–1028.
24. Lecouvet F et al. Long-term effects of localized spinal radiation therapy on vertebral fractures and focal lesions appearance in patients with multiple myeloma. *Br J Haematol.* 1997;96(4): 743–745.
25. Rupp RE, Ebraheim NA, Coombs RJ. Magnetic resonance imaging differentiation of compression spine fractures or vertebral lesions caused by osteoporosis or tumor. *Spine.* 1995;20(23):2499–2503; discussion 2504.
26. Hergan K et al. Onkologie. In: Czembirek H, Frühwald F, Kainberger F, eds. *Orientierungshilfe Radiologie.* Austria: Verlag der Österreichischen Ärztekammer; 2002:75–85.
27. Lauenstein TC et al. Whole-body MRI using a rolling table platform for the detection of bone metastases. *Eur Radiol.* 2002;12(8):2091–2099.
28. Savelli G et al. Bone scintigraphy and the added value of SPECT (single photon emission tomography) in detecting skeletal lesions. *Q J Nucl Med.* 2001;45(1):27–37.
29. Taoka T et al. Factors influencing visualization of vertebral metastases on MR imaging versus bone scintigraphy. *AJR Am J Roentgenol.* 2001;176(6):1525–1530.
30. Vanel D, Bittoun J, Tardivon A. MRI of bone metastases. *Eur. Radiol.* 1998;8(8):1345–1351.
31. Tan SB, Kozak JA, Mawad ME. The limitations of magnetic resonance imaging in the diagnosis of pathologic vertebral fractures. *Spine.* 1991;16(8):919–923.
32. Ballon D et al. Magnetic Resonance Bone Marrow Scanning Using Diffusion-Weighted Echo Planar Imaging. *Proceedings of the 8th ISMRM.* Denver, Co: 2000;209;2128.
33. Baur A et al. Diffusion-weighted MR imaging of bone marrow: differentiation of benign versus pathologic compression fractures [see comments]. *Radiology.* 1998;207(2):349–356.
34. Vanel D, Dromain C, Tardivon A. MRI of bone marrow disorders. *Eur Radiol.* 2000;10(2):224–229.
35. Daffner RH et al. MRI in the detection of malignant infiltration of bone marrow. *AJR Am J Roentgenol.* 1986;146(2):353–358.
36. Allgayer B et al. NMR tomography compared to skeletal scintigraphy after traumatic vertebral body fractures [in German]. *Rofo.* 1990;152(6):677–681.
37. Bonel H et al. Comparison of sequences for depicting bone marrow alterations in osteomyelitis applied in a low field strength magnetic resonance imaging system. *Magma.* 1998;7(1):1–8.
38. Cuenod CA et al. Acute vertebral collapse due to osteoporosis or malignancy: appearance on unenhanced and gadolinium-enhanced MR images. *Radiology.* 1996;199(2): 541–549.
39. Erlemann R et al. Musculoskeletal neoplasms: static and dynamic Gd-DTPA – enhanced MR imaging. *Radiology.* 1989; 171(3):767–773.
40. Lang P et al. Advances in MR imaging of pediatric musculoskeletal neoplasms. *Magn Reson Imaging Clin North Am.* 1998;6(3):579–604.
41. Verstraete KL et al. Static, dynamic and first-pass MR imaging of musculoskeletal lesions using gadodiamide injection. *Acta Radiol.* 1995;36(1):27–36.
42. Lecouvet FE et al. Vertebral compression fractures in multiple myeloma. Part I. Distribution and appearance at MR imaging. *Radiology.* 1997;204(1):195–199.
43. Ehara S, Shimamura T, Wada T. Single vertebral compression and involvement of the posterior elements in tuberculous spondylitis: observation on MR imaging. *Radiat Med.* 1997;15(3):143–147.
44. Baur A et al. Acute osteoporotic and neoplastic vertebral compression fractures: fluid sign at MR imaging. *Radiology.* 2002;225(3):730–735.
45. Moulopoulos LA et al. Bone lesions with soft-tissue mass: magnetic resonance imaging diagnosis of lymphomatous involvement of the bone marrow versus multiple myeloma and bone metastases. *Leuk Lymphoma.* 1999;34(1–2):179–184.
46. Yuh WT et al. Vertebral compression fractures: distinction between benign and malignant causes with MR imaging. *Radiology.* 1989;172[1]:215–218.
47. Shih TT, Huang KM, Li YW. Solitary vertebral collapse: distinction between benign and malignant causes using MR patterns. *J Magn Reson Imaging.* 1999;9(5):635–642.
48. Falcone S. Diffusion-weighted imaging in the distinction of benign from metastatic vertebral compression fractures: is this a numbers game? *AJNR Am J Neuroradiol.* 2002;23(1): 5–6.
49. Le Bihan D. Molecular diffusion, tissue microdynamics and microstructure. *NMR Biomed.* 1995;8(7–8):375–386.
50. Le Bihan DJ. Differentiation of benign versus pathologic compression fractures with diffusion-weighted MR imaging: a closer step toward the "holy grail" of tissue characterization? [editorial; comment]. *Radiology.* 1998; 207(2):305–307.

51. Spuentrup E et al. Diffusion-weighted MR imaging for differentiation of benign fracture edema and tumor infiltration of the vertebral body. *AJR Am J Roentgenol.* 2001; 176(2):351–358.
52. Herneth AM. Diffusion weighted imaging: have we found the "Holy Grail" of diagnostic imaging or is it still a game of numbers? *Eur J Radiol.* 2003;45(3):167–168.
53. Herneth AM, Guccione S, Bednarski M. Apparent diffusion coefficient: a quantitative parameter for in vivo tumor characterization. *Eur J Radiol.* 2003;45(3):208–213.
54. Castillo M et al. Diffusion-weighted MR imaging offers no advantage over routine noncontrast MR imaging in the detection of vertebral metastases. *AJNR Am J Neuroradiol.* 2000;21(5):948–953.
55. Zhou XJ et al. Characterization of benign and metastatic vertebral compression fractures with quantitative diffusion MR imaging. *AJNR Am J Neuroradiol.* 2002;23(1):165–170.
56. Herneth AM et al. Vertebral metastases: assessment with apparent diffusion coefficient. *Radiology.* 2002;225(3):889–894.
57. Schmitz A et al. FDG-PET findings of vertebral compression fractures in osteoporosis: preliminary results. *Osteoporos Int.* 2002;13(9):755–761.
58. Yang SN et al. Comparing whole body (18)F-2-deoxyglucose positron emission tomography and technetium-99 m methylene diphosphonate bone scan to detect bone metastases in patients with breast cancer. *J Cancer Res Clin Oncol.* 2002;128(6):325–328.
59. Stafford SE et al. Use of serial FDG PET to measure the response of bone-dominant breast cancer to therapy. *Acad Radiol.* 2002;9(8):913–921.
60. Beyer T et al. A combined PET/CT scanner for clinical oncology. *J Nucl Med.* 2000;41(8):1369–1379.
61. Fayad LM et al. Sacral fractures: a potential pitfall of FDG positron emission tomography. *AJR Am J Roentgenol.* 2003; 181(5):1239–1243.
62. Kao CH et al. Comparison and discrepancy of 18F-2-deoxyglucose positron emission tomography and Tc-99 m MDP bone scan to detect bone metastases. *Anticancer Res.* 2000; 20(3B):2189–2192.
63. McNeil BJ. Value of bone scanning in neoplastic disease. *Semin Nucl Med.* 1984;14(4):277–286.
64. Staudenherz A et al. Is there a diagnostic role for bone scanning of patients with high pretest probability for metastatic renal cell carcinoma? *Cancer.* 1999;85(1):153–155.
65. Stabler A et al. The nuclear magnetic resonance tomographic differentiation of osteoporotic and tumor-related vertebral fractures. The value of subtractive TR gradient-echo squences, STIR sequences and Gd-DTPA [in German]. *Rofo Fortschr Geb Roentgenstr Neuen Bildgeb Verfahr.* 1992; 157(3):215–221.
66. Gupta RK et al. Diagnostic value of image-guided needle aspiration cytology in the assessment of vertebral and intervertebral lesions. *Diagn Cytopathol.* 2002;27(4):191–196.
67. Phadke DM, Lucas DR, Madan S. Fine needle aspiration biopsy of vertebral and intervertebral disc lesions: specimen adequacy, diagnostic utility, and pitfalls. *Arch Pathol Lab Med.* 2001;125(11):1463–1468.
68. Jorda M et al. Fine needle aspiration cytology of bone: accuracy and pitfalls of cytodiagnosis. *Cancer.* 2000;90(1):47–54.

16 Neuropathic Osteo-Arthropathy of the Spine

A. Chevrot, A. Feydy, C. Vallée, J. L. Drapé

Introduction

Neuropathic osteoarthropathy (Charcot's) of the spine is a destructive condition of the spine secondary to a loss of the protective proprioceptive reflexes. Classically, it is due to nontraumatic causes including tabes dorsalis, syringomyelia, diabetes, mellitus, or spinal arteriovenous malformation.[2,3] It can be due to central nervous (CNS) system trauma. In the majority of CNS cases, it occurs in patients who have suffered from traumatic medullary lesions and is responsible for destruction of the vertebral bodies with considerable spinal deformity. Charcot's spine may also be found in patients with complete neurological lesions of the spinal cord. Traumatic spinal neuropathy is a condition that results as a loss of the feedback response from the desensitized components of the spine. Although spinal neuroarthropathy is a little-known complication of traumatic paraplegia,[1,2] it is easy to over-look in the follow-up of such patients.

Neuropathic (Charcot's) arthropathy of the spine is a relatively rare problem that, nonetheless, must always be considered in the differential diagnosis of any patient with degenerative lesions of one or more levels of the spine associated with diminished or absent protective sensation and significant bone destruction.

As care of spinally injured patients continues to improve, they live longer and lead a more active lifestyle. It is, therefore, expected that the incidence and prevalence of Charcot's joints will increase. In cases of established neuro-osteoarthropathy secondary infection may also rarely complicate the clinical and radiological scenario.

Mechanism

The factors predisposing patients to the development of a neuropathic joint are diminished pain and proprioceptive sensations with maintained mobility. These factors apply to the spine whether the patient is ambulant or nonambulant. The lack of proprioception and altered muscle tone lead to compromised stability of the spine and its natural curvatures. Progressive deformity of the spine (scoliosis, kyphosis, or both) appears below the traumatic level (Fig. 16.**1**).

Repeated microtrauma and macrotrauma increases joint mobility beyond the normal limits, and this leads to further damage, with the process culminating in severe instability and bone destruction (Fig. 16.**2**). This cascade leads to failure of supporting intervertebral disks, facet joints, and ligaments resulting in subluxation, dislocation, juxta-articular bone destruction with bony fragmentation, necrosis, sclerosis, and collapse.

The disorder is characterized in both the ambulant and nonambulant patient by biological inflammation and repair reaction to recurrent injury. Neuropathic osteoarthropathy of the spine may occur in isolation or in combination with neuropathic osteoarthropathy of other joints. The thoracolumbar junction and lumbar spine are most frequently affected (Fig. 16.**1**), and one or more vertebral segments may be involved (Fig. 16.**3**). In cases of previous posterior spinal fusion with Harrington instrumentation, Charcot's joint may occur just below the caudal end of the fusion and remote from the level of spinal cord injury.

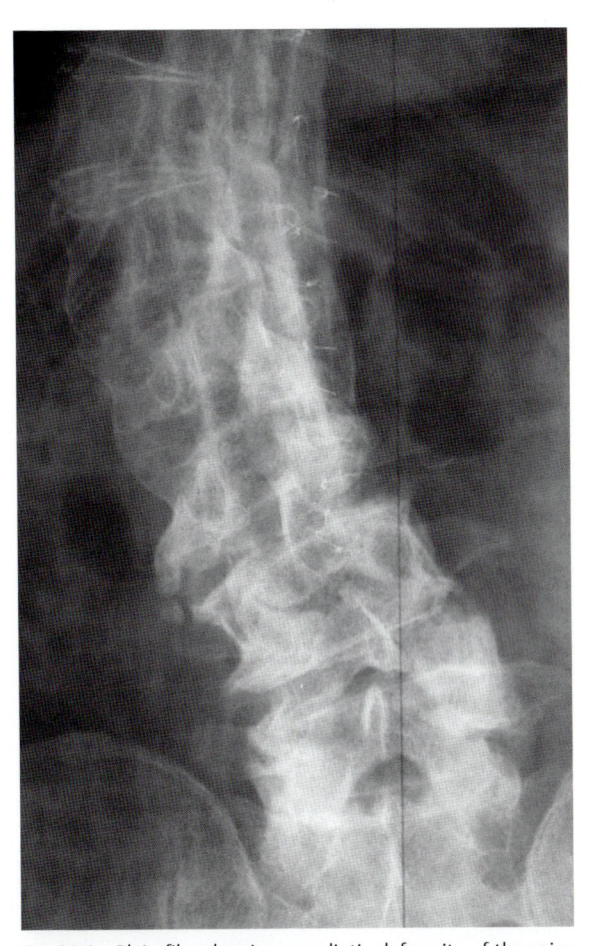

Fig. 16.**1** Plain film showing a scoliotic deformity of the spine (curvature) below a dorsal osteosynthesis for traumatic fractures.

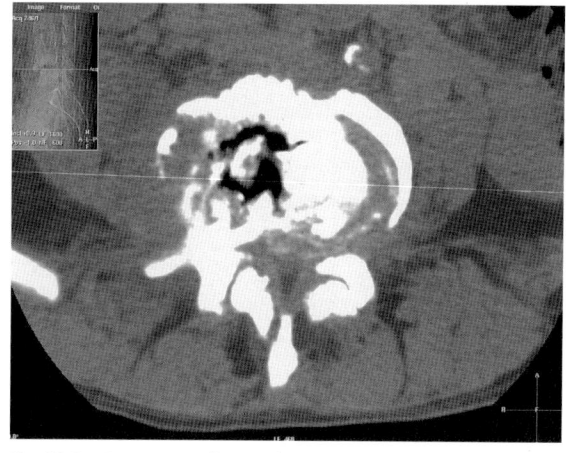

Fig. 16.**2** Destructive bone changes of the lumbar spine in a 47-year-old man with traumatic paraplegia. **a** Axial CT image at level L4 shows bone destruction with fragmentation and a vacuum phenomenon. **b** Axial gadolinium-enhanced T1W MRI image at level L4 shows vertebral and perivertebral inflammatory changes related to the repair reaction.

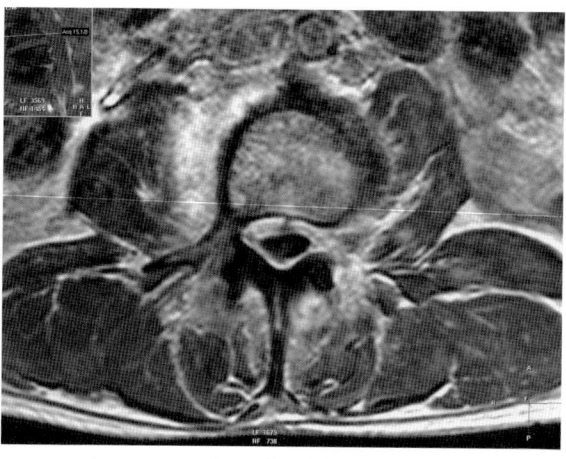

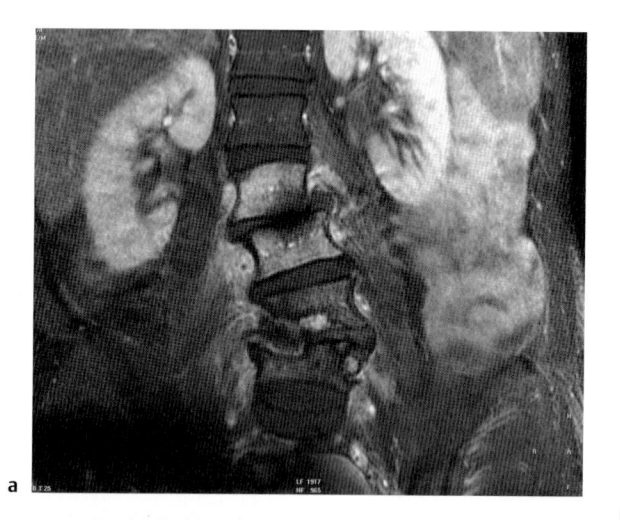

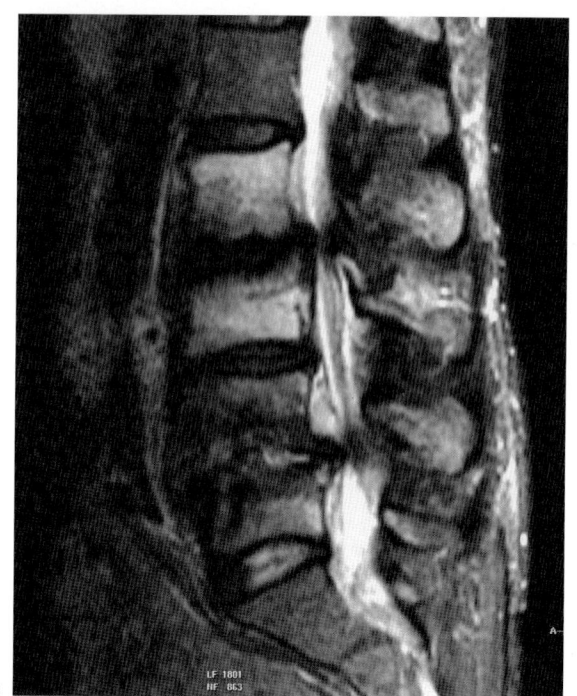

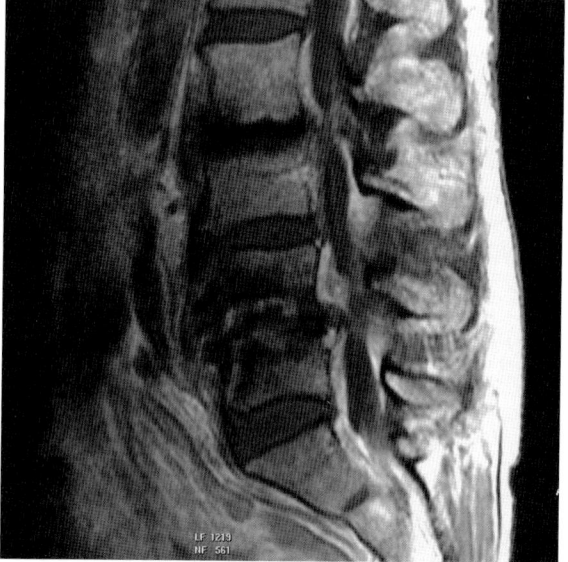

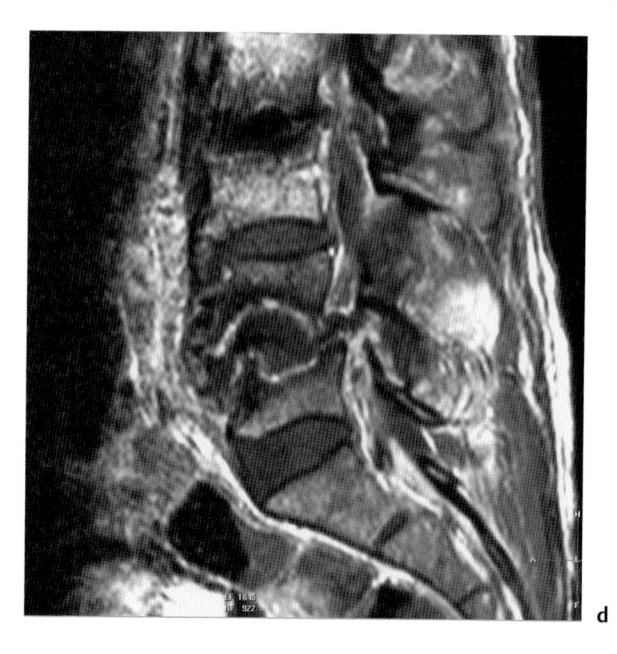

Clinical Findings

Neuropathic changes in the spine are often silent, delaying diagnosis and treatment, or may be mistaken for infection or degenerative disease. The diagnosis was made from 6 to 31 years after original spinal cord injury in a series of post-traumatic Charcot spines.[1]

Clinically progressive kyphosis leading to a severe kyphotic deformity, flexion instability leading to gross instability, and loss of height are suggestive. Traumatic spinal cord injury can also produce pain and further disability. In patients having complete paraplegia with levels of neurological injury ranging from T7 to T12, the common presenting symptoms of a neuropathic spine include back pain, loss of spasticity, a change in bladder function, and audible noises with motion of the unstable segments.

Imaging Findings

The radiological hallmarks of chronic neuropathic-osteoarthropathy are destruction, dislocation, disorganization, and debris. Spinal neuroarthropathy is a destructive process involving the disk space, the adjoining vertebral bodies, and the facet joints.[2,3,5]

Repeated follow-up imaging of the spine with plain films shows sagittal and/or coronal deformation with further progression of the deformity (Figs. 16.1 and 16.4). This type of complication may represent the first step of a Charcot's spine.

Radiologically, findings of either sclerosis or osteolysis may predominate (Figs. 16.4, 16.5). Indeed, the spinal changes are often initially thought to be due to vertebral osteomyelitis or metastatic destruction of a vertebra. Radiographs of the spine may show disk

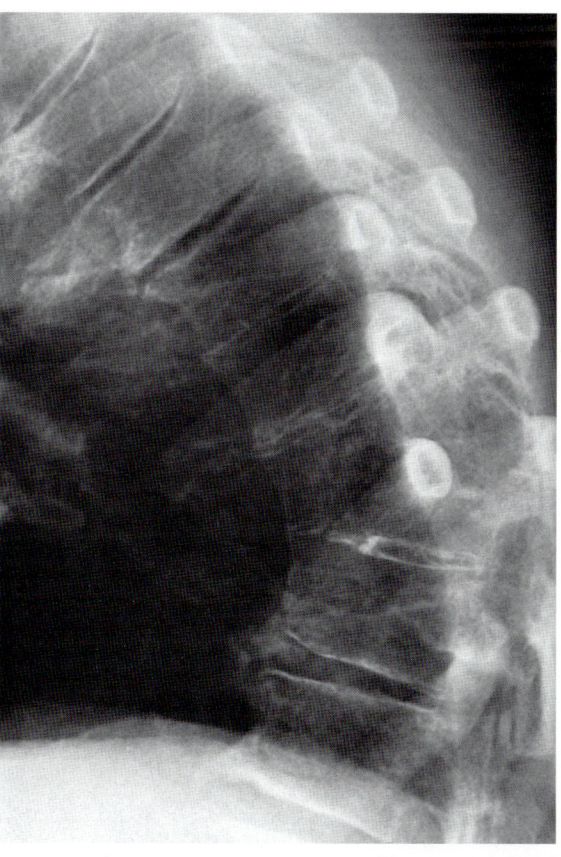

Fig. 16.4 Charcot's spine in a 58-year-old man. History of lower dorsal spine fracture at 18 years of age, followed by progressive spinal fusion. Absence of pain. Vertebral bone destruction at the L1–L2 level. **a** Radiograph. Dorsal spine lateral view shows an ankylosis of T8–T9–T10 vertebral bodies. **b** Thoracolumbar AP radiograph. Note the destruction associated with extensive perivertebral tumoral like bone formation.

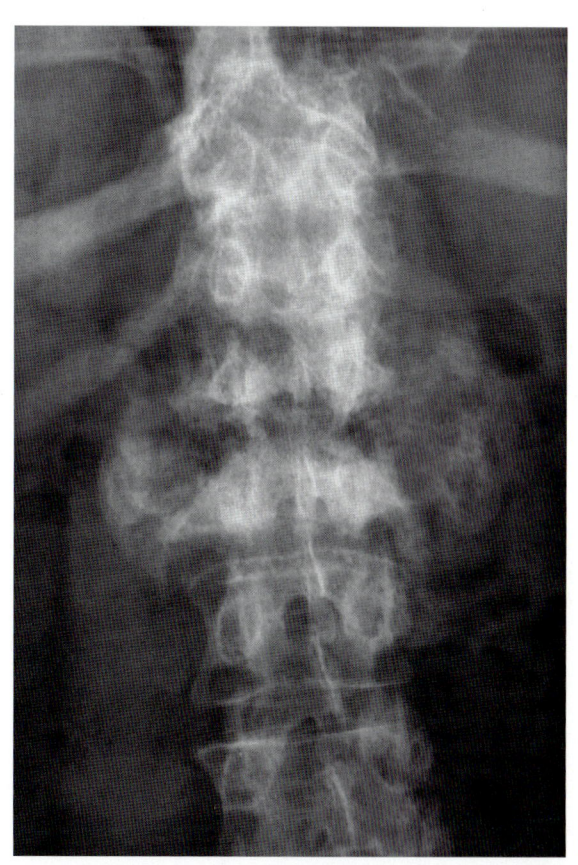

◁ Fig. 16.3 Destructive bone changes of the lumbar spine in a 52-year-old man with traumatic paraplegia. Spinal deformity with a dislocation at the L4–L5 level. Destructive vertebral lesions at the L4–L5 level. There is marked bone marrow edema of the L2–L5 vertebral bodies and inflammatory signal changes of the perivertebral soft tissues. **a** Coronal fat-saturated gadolinium-enhanced T1W MRI image. L4–L5 destruction involving predominantly the right side of the disk space and vertebral endplates but also early changes are present at L2/L3 levels. **b** Sagittal T1W MRI image showing destruction of L4–L5. **c** Sagittal fat-saturated T2W MRI image showing destruction of L4–L5. Marked bone marrow edema of the L2 and L3 vertebral bodies. **d** Sagittal fat-saturated gadolinium-enhanced T1W MRI image. Note the rim enhancement surrounding a liquid or necrotic area in the L4/5 disk space.

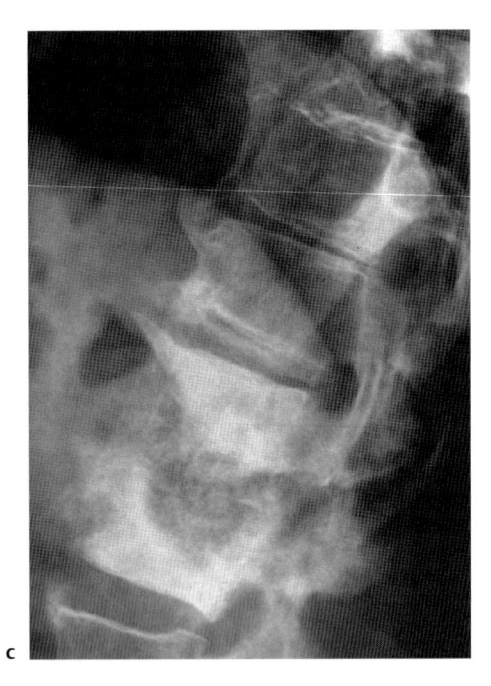

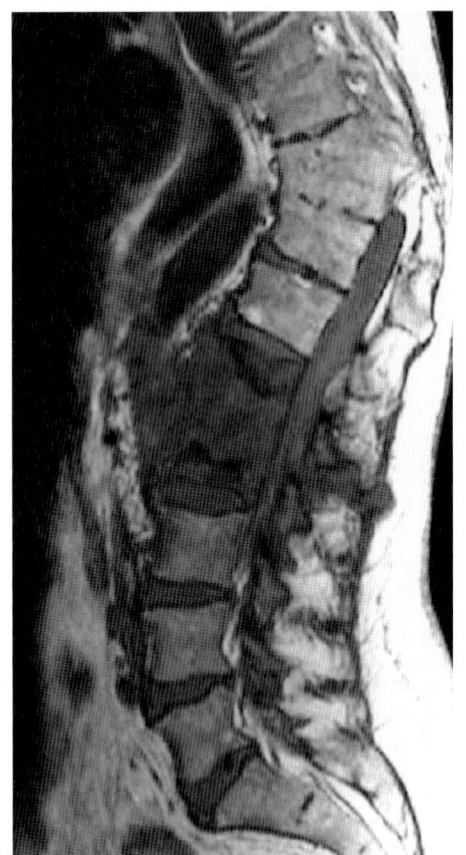

Fig. 16.4 c Thoracolumbar lateral radiograph. Pseudoarthrosis of L1–L2 with a typical "ball and socket" appearance. Compare with the CT scan performed 6 months later (see g and h). d Sagittal T2W MRI of the cervicodorsal spine. Note the normal pattern of the spinal cord above the chronic fracture in the lower thoracic spine. e Sagittal T1W MRI of the lumbar spine. Ankylosis of T8–T9–T10 related to the previous healed fracture. Very low signal intensity of the L1 and L2 vertebral bodies. f Sagittal gadolinium-enhanced T1W MRI of the lumbar spine. There is no enhancement of the space between the L1 and L2 destroyed vertebral bodies.

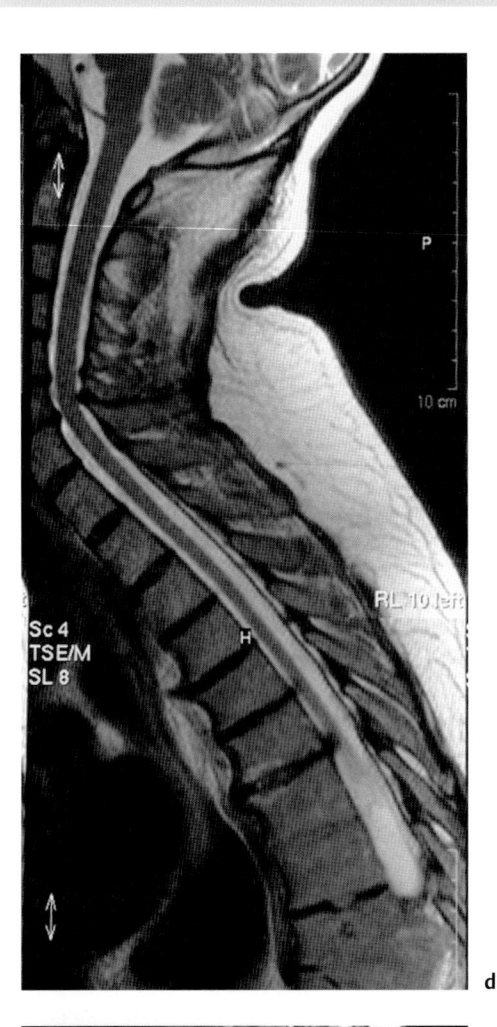

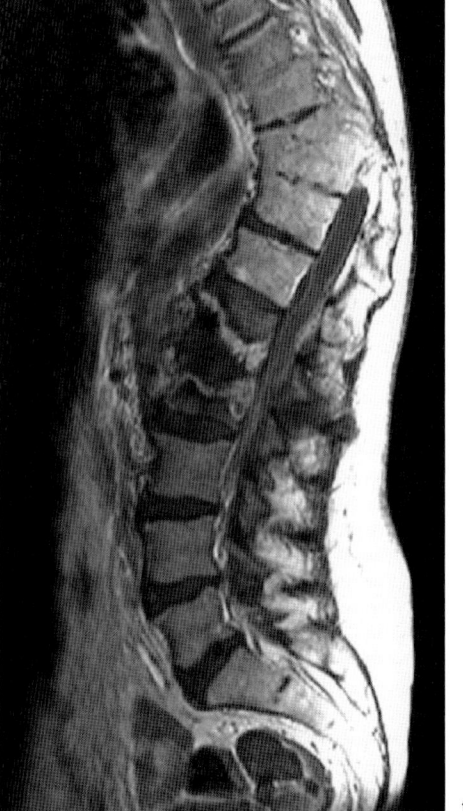

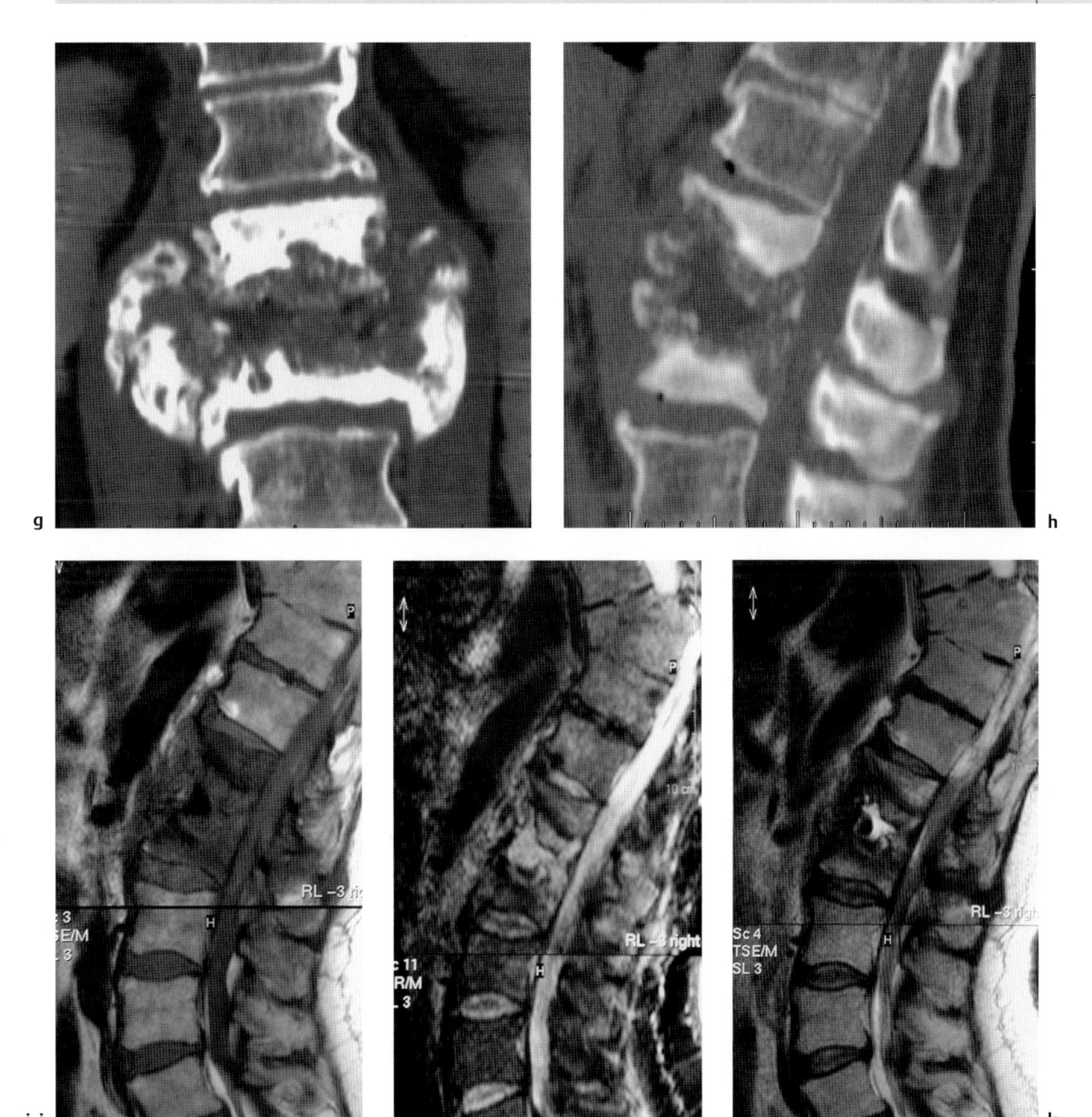

Fig. 16.4 **g** Lumbar CT performed 6 months after previous examinations (plain films and initial MRI). Coronal image shows a pseudotumor-like pattern with destructive changes and bone formation. Note the spots of radiolucency indicating vacuum phenomenon. **h** Lumbar CT, sagittal image. **i–m**: Follow-up lumbar MRI performed 1 year after the initial MRI showing chronic destructive changes at the L1–L2 level. Fluid signal of the L1–L2 disk space. **i** Sagittal T1W image. **j** Sagittal fat-saturated T2W image. **k** Sagittal T2W image.

space narrowing (Fig. 16.6), vertebral lysis or sclerosis, subluxations, abrupt curvature, and often paraspinal soft-tissue calcifications. Large hypertrophic marginal osteophytes may form (Fig. 16.4). Computed tomographic (CT) changes of neuropathic osteoarthropathy of the spine are those of sclerosis and destruction of all three vertebral columns including destruction of the facet joints (Fig. 16.2). Osseous fragments typically extend beyond the confines of the vertebral body margins into paraspinous and erector spinae musculature and into the spinal canal.[6] Bone debris and effusion may result in a paraspinous mass containing calcifications (Fig. 16.7), but a large enhancing solid paraspinous or epidural mass is typically lacking. The presence of vertebral body sclerosis and osseous fragmentation are further imaging findings that help differentiate a neuropathic spine from other processes.[7]

Neuropathic destructive changes in the vertebral bodies may lead to fracture, followed by additional changes, including bone sclerosis, large osteophytes, and a loss of disk space. A large paraspinal mass can develop because of improper fracture healing. At the

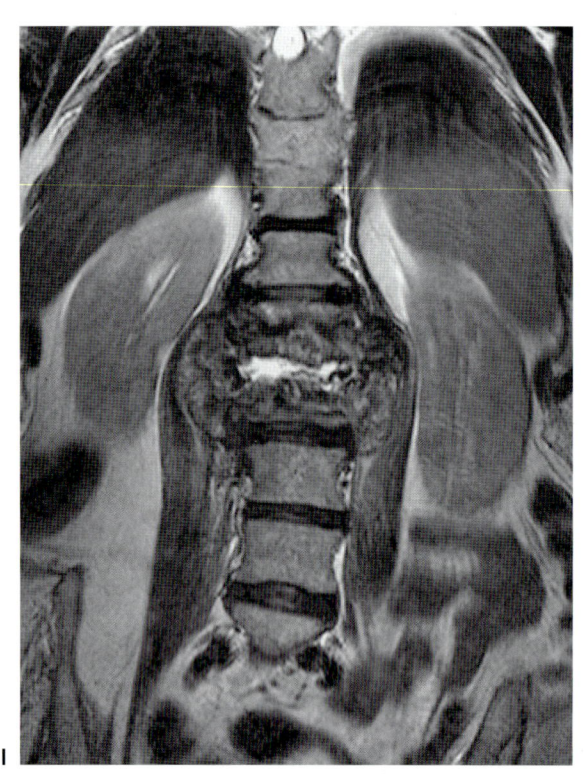

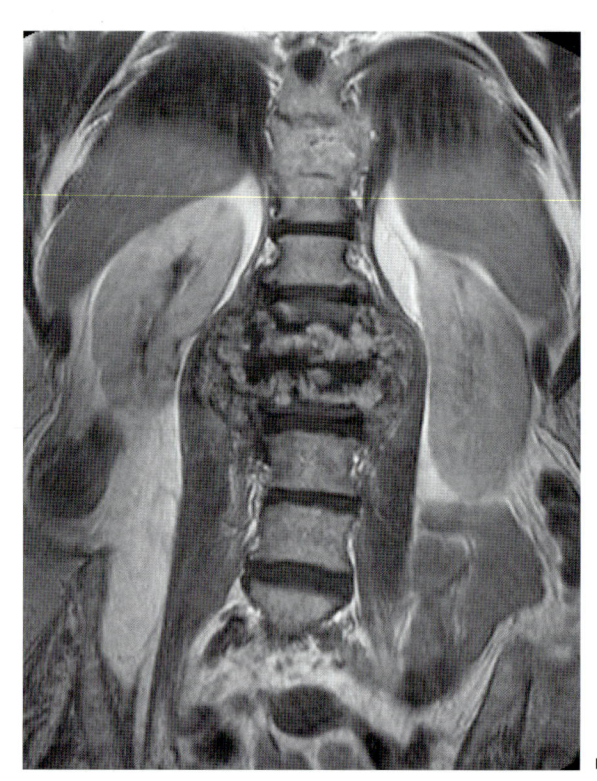

Fig. 16.4 **l** Coronal T2W image. **m** Coronal gadolinium-enhanced T1W image.

end stage of this process, a pseudoarthrosis may form. A severe joint destruction with a "ball and socket" pseudoarthrosis may be finally observed (Fig. 16.4).

On plain radiographs and CT scans, the finding of the neuropathic spine may be similar to those of disk space infection, severe degenerative disease, and skeletal metastasis.[8] Magnetic resonance imaging (Fig. 16.3, 16.4), shows characteristic hypointensity of signal on T1W and T2W images, which is not specific enough to differentiate the neuropathic spine from infection.[8]

Differential Diagnosis

Infection must be considered as a possible etiology in cases of Charcot's spine with destructive lesions. An infectious process must be excluded especially in patients with other known chronic infections. Scintigraphic techniques include technetium 99 and indium 111 bone scans. CT and MRI with gadolinium injection are used in the extensive work-up and are helpful, although not always diagnostic.

Sclerosis and osseous destruction in vertebral osteomyelitis are typically limited to the adjacent endplates. Extensive osseous fragmentation is not an expected imaging finding in typical bacterial vertebral osteomyelitis or metastatic disease of the spine. Granulomatous infection of the spine may result in calcifications in the paraspinous soft tissues and may simulate axial

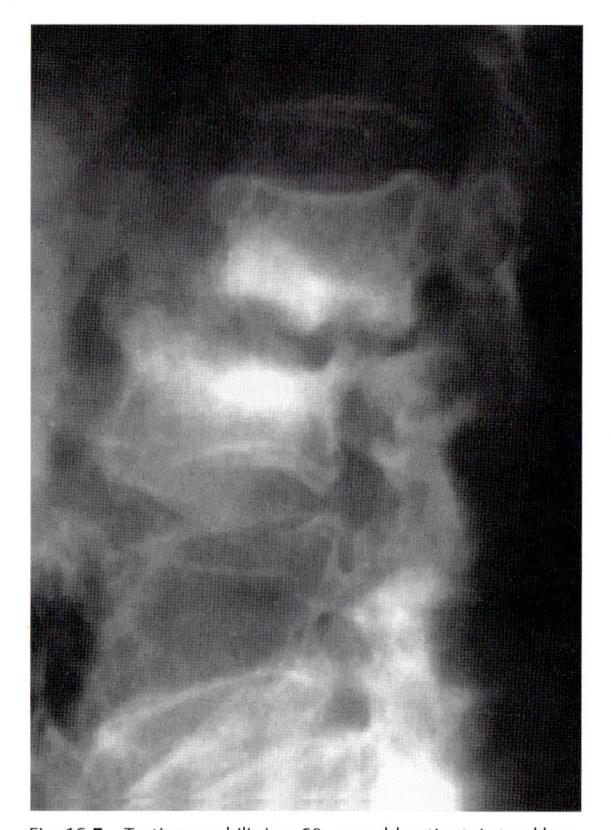

Fig. 16.5 Tertiary syphilis in a 69-year-old patient. Lateral lumbar plain film shows chronic changes at the L3-L4 level with a destruction of the disk space and a bone sclerosis of the vertebral endplates.

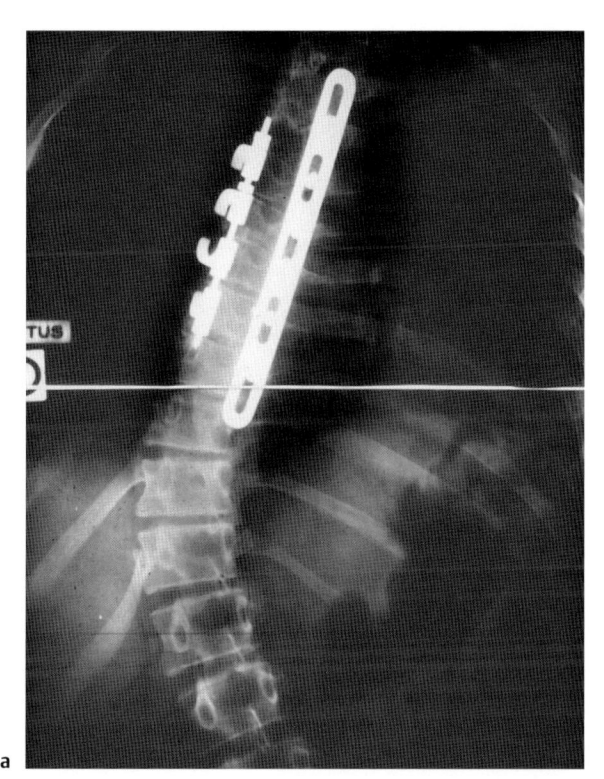

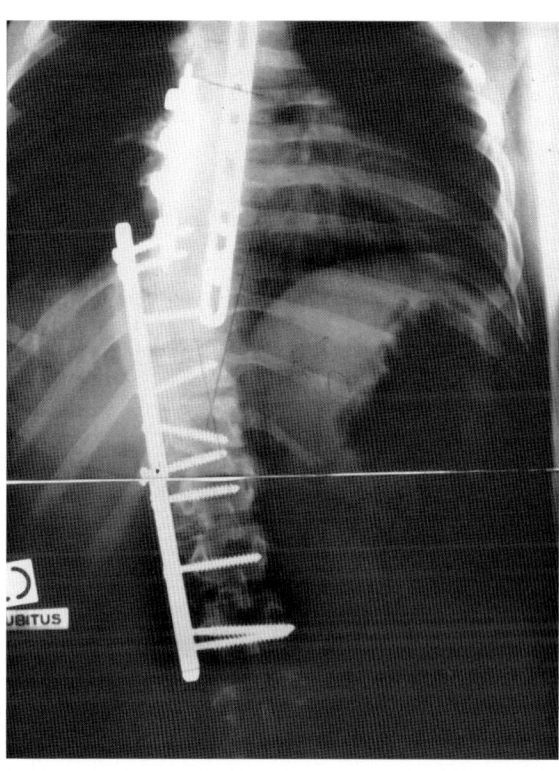

Fig. 16.**6** Previous posterior spinal fusion with instrumentation for dorsal fracture in an 35-year-old patient. **a** AP plain film of the thoracolumbar junction shows a spinal scoliotic deformity. **b** Follow-up shows a Charcot's joint pattern just below the fusion at the thoracolumbar junction. A preventive lumbar osteosynthesis with instrumentation was performed.

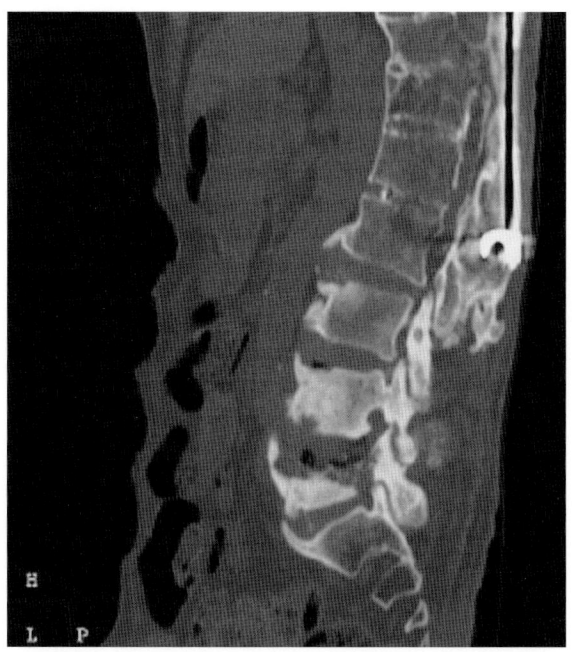

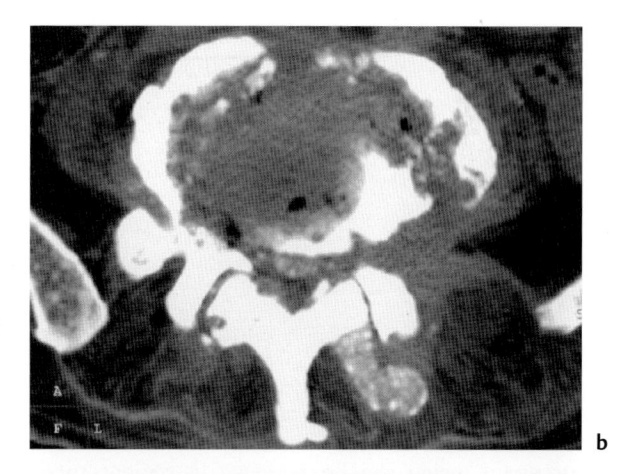

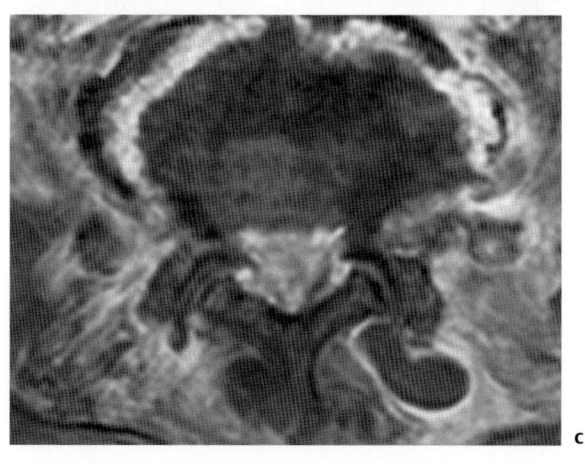

Fig. 16.**7** Paraplegia for 20 years in a 59-year-old patient complaining of back pain. **a** Sagittal CT image shows a spinal fusion with ankylosis of the thoracolumbar junction including also L1 and L2. Advanced bony destruction of L5 and sclerosis of L4 and L5 vertebral bodies with a vacuum phenomenon. **b** Axial CT image at the L4–L5 level. Destructive changes and partially calcified cyst posteriorly close to the left facet joint. **c** Axial fat-saturated gadolinium-enhanced T1W MR image at the same level. Extensive perivertebral soft tissue inflammatory changes. Peripheral enhancement of the articular cyst.

neuropathic osteoarthropathy; however, fragmentation of the facet joints would not be expected.[6]

On radiographs, CT, and MRI, the most helpful findings for diagnosis of spinal neuropathic arthropathy are vacuum disk, debris, disorganization, facet involvement, and spondylolisthesis. Diffuse signal intensity patterns in vertebral bodies and rim enhancement of disks on gadolinium-enhanced MR images are also suggestive of the diagnosis of spinal neuropathic arthropathy.[8] Findings that are not helpful to differentiate spinal neuropathic arthropathy from disk space infection include endplate sclerosis and erosions, osteophytes, paraspinal soft-tissue mass, and decreased disk height.[8] Closed needle and even open surgical biopsies are often necessary to finally confirm the diagnosis (see Fig. 16.**4**). Superimposed infection of Charcot's spine is very rare but may be considered as a possible etiology in some progressively destructive lesions. Extensive investigations and surgical treatment are warranted in these patients.[9,10]

The other causes of neuropathic changes in the spine such as tertiary syphilis, syringomyelia, and diabetes, must be ruled out on clinical grounds because of their specific treatment (see Fig. 16.**5**).

Ankylosing spondyloarthritis and diffuse idiopathic skeletal hyperostosis, ossifying diathesis that commonly affects the vertebral skeleton also lead to spinal ankylosis. These diseases predispose the spine to abnormal stresses and fracture. Fracture through an ankylosed segment with continued motion at the site of fracture can result in pseudoathrosis. Pseudoarthrosis can also develop at the junction of the fused and mobile spine secondary to chronic abnormal stresses.

Scheuermann's kyphosis is an uncommon autosomal dominant disease that manifests itself as a progressive thoracic skeletal deformity.[11]

Treatment

Immobilization of the affected joint is an essential element of treatment. With the use of combined anterior and posterior fusion with extensive debridement, autogenous grafting, and posterior instrumentation, successful fusion can be achieved in patients with Charcot's arthropathy of the spine. However, the surgical technique is demanding, the rehabilitation must be carefully supervised, and the post-operative complication rate remains high. The possibility of developing secondary levels of arthropathy below a previously successful fusion must be considered.[12]

Spinal arthrodesis is used successfully to correct the deformity, stabilize the spine, restore sitting balance, and prevent complications resulting from neuropathic arthropathy.[13,14] Surgery consists typically of reduction of the deformation, posterolateral spinal fusion with hooks and pedicular screws, and a posterior lumbar interbody fusion (e. g. Cotrel-Dubousset instrumentation) (Fig. 16.**6**).

References

1. Standaert C, Cardenas DD, Anderson P. Charcot spine as a late complication of traumatic spinal cord injury. *Arch Phys Med Rehabil.* 1997;78(2):221–225.
2. Crim JR, Bassett LW, Gold RH, Mirra JM, Mikulics M, Dawson EG, Eckhardt JJ. Spinal neuroarthropathy, after traumatic paraplegia. *AJNR Am J Neuroradiol.* 1988;9(2):359–362.
3. Park YH, Taylor JA, Szollar SM, Resnick D. Imaging findings in spinal neuroarthropathy. *Spine.* 1994;19(13):1499–1504.
4. Vialle R, Parker F, Lepeintre JF, Rodesch G, Tassin JL, Tadie M. Late spinal dislocation after treatment of spinal arteriovenous malformation. A case of Charcot spinal arthropathy. *Neurochirurgie.* 2004;50(6):647–651.
5. Harrison MJ, Sacher M, Rossenblum BR, Rothman AS. Spinal Charcot arthropathy. *Neurosurgery.* 1991;28(2):273–277.
6. Jones EA, Manaster BJ, May DA, Disler DG. Neuropathic osteoarthropathy: diagnostic dilemmas and differential diagnosis. *Radiographics.* 2000;20:279–293.
7. Kapila A, Lines M. Neuropathic spinal arthropathy: CT and MR findings. *J Comput Assist Tomogr.* 1987;11(4):736–739.
8. Wagner SC, Schweitzer ME, Morrison WB, Przybylski GJ, Parker L. Can imaging findings help differentiate spinal neuropathic arthropathy from disk space infection? Initial experience. *Radiology.* 2000;214(3):693–699.
9. Pritchard JC, Coscia MF. Infection of a Charcot spine. A Case report. *Spine.* 1993;18(6):764–767.
10. Suda Y, Saito M, Shioda M, Kato H, Shibasaki K. Infected Charcot spine. *Spinal Cord.* 2005;43(4):256–259.
11. Komar JC, James J, Little JW. Scheuermann's kyphosis following cervical spinal cord injury. *J Spinal Cord Med.* 2003;26(1):92–94.
12. Brown CW, Jones B, Donaldson DH, Akmakjian J, Brugman JL. Neuropathic (Charcot) arthropathy of the spine after traumatic spinal paraplegia. *Spine.* 1992;17(6 Suppl):1038.
13. Arnold PM, Baek PN, Stillerman CB, Rice SG, Mueller WM. Surgical management of lumbar neuropathic spinal arthropathy (Charcot joint) after traumatic thoracic paraplegia: report of two cases. *J Spinal Disord.* 1995;8(5):357–362.
14. Wirth CR, Jacobs RL, Rolander SD. Neuropathic spinal arthropathy. A review of the Charcot spine. *Spine.* 1980;5(6):558–567.

17 The Future: Trends and Developments in Spinal Cord Regeneration

A. E. Osman, D. J. Short, V. N. Cassar-Pullicino, H. Imhof, W. S. El Masry

Introduction

Many strategies are being explored to enhance recovery of spinal cord function.[1] Everyone in the field of spinal cord injury (SCI) hopes that one day there will be a cure for the paralysis that follows a spinal cord lesion. Basic science has enhanced our understanding of the pathophysiology of traumatic spinal cord damage (Fig. 17.1) and demonstrated the efficacy of various interventions to improve neurological function following experimental spinal cord injury.[2] The International Spinal Research Trust (ISRT) proposed a research strategy in 1996 to effectively direct resources by identifying areas in spinal cord research that would require particular attention.[1] These areas are to:
- Minimize immediate harmful responses to SCI;
- Enhance trophic influence and blocking of inhibitory influence;
- Correct reconnection of damaged axons and targets;
- Optimize the function of surviving fibers (in the case of incomplete damage).

At this stage it is likely that individuals, with existing SCI, will need a combination of available therapies to restore maximum function.[2,3] A single treatment to cure spinal paralysis has not emerged from research done to date. Whatever is involved in translating interventions from experimental models to humans,[3,4] there remains the fundamental clinical challenge, and ultimate responsibility to patients, to know how to ask (let alone answer) the question "Does it really work?" We are still coming to an understanding of long-observed changes following acute cord insult—"spinal shock" and have recognized the need for better clinical evaluation.[5–8] What follows is not a comprehensive coverage but an introduction to some of the aspects of this evolving area.

Spinal Cord Research

Research to find a cure and to optimize the outcome, has to involve all the phases of care that follow inevitably from trauma to a person and the consequent physiological dysfunction of spinal cord "interruption"—beginning with effective handling at the scene of the accident, during acute care, and through rehabilitation.

At the cord level research focuses on four main areas:
1. Neuroprotection
2. Regeneration
3. Transplantation
4. Rehabilitation

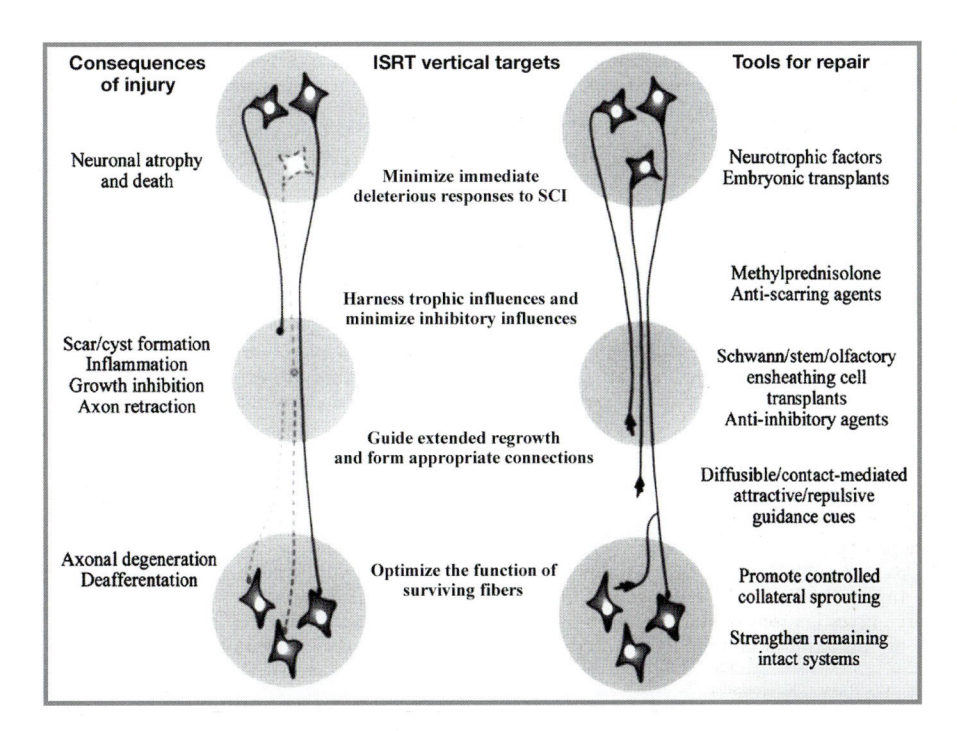

Fig. 17.1 ISRT research strategy—summary of the events subsequent to spinal cord injury.

Neuroprotection

Mechanical trauma inflicts direct neuronal damage but a large amount of axonal disruption and cellular death appears to result from secondary pathophysiological events. There is an evolving understanding of an "injury-triggered-cascade" of mechanisms, their complexity, and interactions.[9-11] What actually happens in vivo in humans remains largely conjectured by extrapolation from this. Mention of a few of pathophysiological processes currently in focus may be appropriate[9]:

- Vascular mechanisms; loss of microcirculation, small vessel disruption, and hemorrhage, failure of autoregulation, and glutamate-mediated excitotoxicity;[10]
- Oxygen free radical formation and cell membrane lipid peroxidation;
- Apoptosis, the term for programmed cell death. This contrasts with necrotic death of cells at the site of trauma, which releases cell contents that cause a secondary inflammatory reaction.

Apoptotic demise of neurons and oligodendrocytes has been demonstrated postmortem in human SCI.[12] Other work suggests a time course for this process of a few hours to 3 weeks, maximal around day 8 post-injury.[13,14]

On the basis of the evolving data of these pathophysiological mechanisms, it is possible to introduce experimentally efficacious interventions—glutamate receptor antagonists, agents affecting free radical formation and lipid peroxidation, inflammatory response modulators, targeting the molecular apoptotic pathway. (Specific agents are detailed in the referenced articles.)

Clinical trials in acute spinal cord injury are possible but difficult—the methylprednisolone and GM-1 ganglioside (Sygen) experience has been instructive.[15-19] Randomized controlled trial design, execution, and reporting standards have moved on from those of the National Acute Spinal Cord Injury Studies (NASCIS) with the intention of improving the value of trial results as evidence of clinical effectiveness.[20] The patterns of neurological loss (spinal cord level and completeness), the natural history of recovery and relevant outcome measures, which were considered in detail for the Sygen research remain a crucial "trial design challenge."[18]

Regeneration

Is it possible to get CNS neurons to grow and regenerate? Two concepts had emerged from basic research: injured neurons lacked the intrinsic ability to regenerate; the CNS environment was not permissive to regeneration.[21,3]

Experiments have demonstrated that neurons can become "regeneration-capable" and regeneration-associated genes in the cell body up-regulated by the application of trophic factors to the cell body and also to the injured axon.[21,3]

Various strategies have been effective in facilitating "permissiveness to regeneration" at the injury site: providing a "cellular bridge" using Schwann cells, olfactory ensheathing glial cells, fetal tissue, stem cells; opposing axonal growth inhibitory molecules within the glial scar, e.g., effect of chondroitinase ABC on chondroitin sulfate proteoglycans; direct application of trophic factors such as NT3 or antibody to inhibitors—IN-1 antiNogo-A antibody.[3]

The question above then has to be refined to "Is it possible to get CNS neurons to regenerate, grow, and make functionally effective, useful connections? Is it vital that these axons reconnect to their proper target sites?" Significant functional restoration has been possible in some rodent model experiments—some of those reported using olfactory ensheathing cell transplants have done so.[22-25]

Some thought has been directed towards the possible application of signaling molecules or guidance cues and trophic factors to direct neuronal growth/axonal sprouting.[2,3]

Transplantation

Transplantation or cellular therapies have a number of possible applications:[26]

- Replacing cell populations lost following injury, such as motor neurons or inhibitory interneurons;
- Bridging across the damaged area, e.g., Schwann cells, olfactory ensheathing glia;
- Providing therapeutic molecules (neurotrophic factors, neurotransmitters) by a cellular "minipump" function, e.g., autologous fibroblasts transfected to produce NT3 inserted at the injury site; adrenal medullary transplants (encapsulated chromaffin cells) in the spinal cord in humans to treat pain.

Stem Cells

The question to implant exogenous cells or to mobilize a patient's endogenous cells is still being tested by different scientists.[27]

Figure 17.**2** summarizes application ideas for stem cells and transplant or progenitor cells to the site of injury in the spinal cord.[27]

Over the last 10 years olfactory ensheathing cell transplantation (OEC) has emerged as a leading candidate for therapeutic transplantation using a cell-based strategy.

Rehabilitation

The potential for rehabilitative strategies to influence neuronal plasticity or to utilize spinal control networks is still largely unquantified and uncharacterized, although the possible functional improvements that

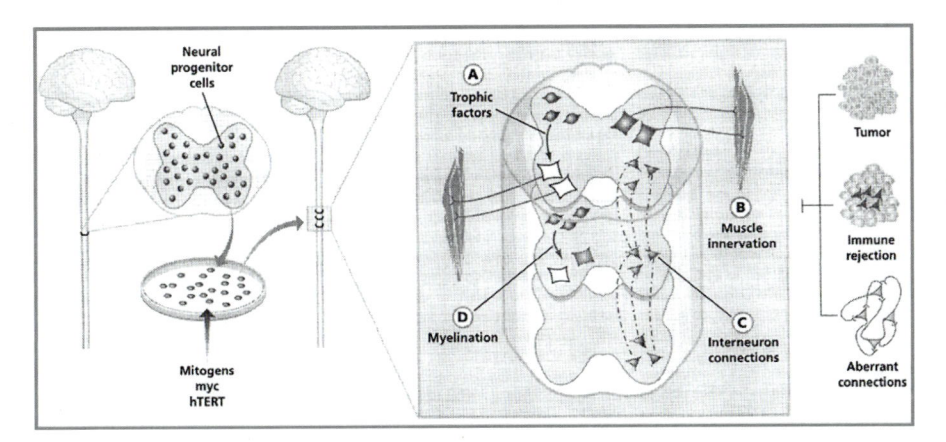

Fig. 17.2 Rothstein and Snyder:[27] Potential applications of stem cells. (Reprinted from *Nature Biotechnology*, 2004, Vol. 22, pp. 283 by Rothstein, et al., with permission from Nature Publishing Group.)

have been demonstrated are quite "large."[4] Synergistic approaches involving this aspect and actual cord interventions need to be explored. Conversely any trial of a "cure" for spinal cord injury must control for these influences. Much more practical clinical research is necessary to complement "laboratory-based" initiatives.

It is unlikely that any cure treatment will result in immediate or complete recovery of all functions. Rehabilitation is expected to be a crucial part of any cure treatment strategy.

Future Trends—Role of Imaging

From what has been outlined above the future has to be multidisciplinary within and between scientists and clinicians. To benefit humans with spinal cord injury, initiatives have to encompass the wider context of spinal injury management and rehabilitation—to integrate constructively rather than produce confusing contradictions.

There seem to be numerous experimental possibilities, making hope not unrealistic. Already, some interventions have been, or are being, tried in humans—embryo transplants, OECs, activated macrophages. (A suggested starting place on the internet for current information would be the International Campaign for the Cure of Paralysis: www.campaignforcure.org)

However, bringing effective and relatively safe treatments into mainstream medical practice involves consideration of producing translational experimental data, and certainly going through the established and appropriate procedures required by regulatory authorities.[3,4,26]

The question "Does this really work, will it harm me doctor?" remains.

The ability to better "quantitate" the clinical neurological deficit is one essential component to evaluating the effect of treatment;[6-8] functional MRI could link with this.[28]

Imaging would appear to have the potential to make some fundamentally important, if not essential contributions to progress.[29] A brief search of publications leads to some questions about turning possibilities into clinical practicality. Can post-injury structure and function cord changes be "seen" and the pathophysiology of human in vivo secondary processes be clarified?[30] Can interventions be monitored for effectiveness?[31,32] Could the modality that defines the lesion be used to direct the treatment—MRI-guided introduction of cell transplants sounds ridiculous…? Is the technology there to "reference" subsequent scans over time so that the same "slice" of tissue is being viewed and changes are not due to positional/technical factors? What is required is a focused and dedicated MRI approach to work in tandem with the evolving clinical research.

The clinical value of MRI continues to improve providing prognostic information and increasingly sensitive changes seen in cervical spondylotic myelopathy,[33,34] and newer MRI sequences can be applied to traumatic spinal cord injury. Without doubt diffusion and perfusion imaging as well as ultra-fast MRI sequences will have a role to play. Furthermore, the role of contrast MRI studies and MRI spectroscopy will possibly provide valuable prognostic information before and during the treatment as well as during rehabilitation periods.

Conclusion

Spinal cord researchers are now taking a more multidisciplinary approach. Imaging has an important role in taking forward experimental work but could be vital in the final analysis of what does and does not work in cord regeneration.

References

1. Ramer LM, Ramer MS, Steeves JD. Setting the stage for functional repair of spinal vord injuries: a cast of thousands. *Spinal Cord.* 2005;43:134–161.
2. Ramer MS, Harper GP, Bradley EJ. Progress in spinal cord research. *Spinal Cord.* 2000;38,449–474.
3. Fawcett J. Repair of spinal cord injuries: where are we, where are we going? *Spinal Cord.* 2002;40:615–623.
4. Dietrich WD. Confirming an experimental therapy prior to transfer to humans: what is the ideal? *J Rehabil Res Dev.* 2003;40(4):63–69.

5. Ditunno JF, Little JW, Tesslar A, Burns AS. Spinal shock revisited: a four-phase model. *Spinal Cord.* 2004;42:383–395.
6. Ellaway PH, Anand P, Bergstrom EMK et al. Towards improved clinical and physiological assessments of recovery in spinal cord injury: a clinical initiative. *Spinal Cord.* 2004;42: 325–337.
7. Martinez-Arizala A. Methods to measure sensory function in humans versus animals. *J Rehabil Res Dev.* 2003;40(4):35–39.
8. Thomas CK. Physiological methods to measure motor function in humans and animals with spinal cord injury. *J Rehabil Res Dev.* 2003;40(4):25–33.
9. Sekhon LHS, Fehlings MG. Epidemiology, demographics, and pathophysiology of acute spinal cord injury. *Spine.* 2001;26: 2–12.
10. Park E, Velumian AA, Fehlings MG. The role of excitotoxicity in secondary mechanisms of spinal cord injury: A review with emphasis on the implications of white matter degeneration. *J Neurotrauma.* 2004;21(6):754–774.
11. Profyris C, Cheema SS, Zang D, Azari MF, Boyle K, Petratos S. Degenerative and regenerative mechanisms governing spinal cord injury. *Neurobiol Dis.* 2004;25(3):415–436.
12. Newcombe REA, Blumbergs PC, Manavis J, Jones NR. A human study of apoptosis in acute and chronic compressive myelopathy. *J Bone Joint Surg Br.* 2003;85:283.
13. Crowe MJ, Bresnahan JC, Shuman SL, Masters JN, Beattie MS. Apoptosis and delayed degeneration after spinal cord injury in rats and monkeys. *Nat Med.* 1997;3(1):73–76.
14. Shuman SL, Bresnahan JC, Beattie MS. Apoptosis of microglia and oligodendrocytes after spinal cord contusion in rats. *J Neurosci Res.* 1997;50(5):798–808.
15. Bracken MB et al. A randomised controlled trial of Methylprednisolone or Naloxone in the treatment of acute spinal cord injury. Results of the second National Acute Spinal cord Injury Study. *N Engl J Med.* 1990;322:1405–1411.
16. Short DJ, El Masry WS, Jones PW. High dose Methylprednisolone in the management of acute signal cord injury – Systemic review from clinical perspective. *Spinal Cord.* 2000; 38:273–286.
17. Geisler FH, Coleman WP, Grieco G, Poonian D, and the Sygen[R] Study Group. Recruitment and early treatment in a multicenter study of acute spinal cord injury. *Spine.* 2001;26: 58–67.
18. Geisler FH, Coleman WP, Grieco G, Poonian D, and the Sygen[R] Study Group. Measurement and recovery patterns in a multicenter study of acute spinal cord injury. *Spine.* 2001, 26:68–86.
19. Geisler FH, Coleman WP, Grieco G, Poonian D, and the Sygen[R] Study Group. The Sygen[R] Multicenter Acute Spinal Cord Injury Study. *Spine.* 2001;26:87–98.
20. Altman DG, Schulz KF, Moher D et al. The revised CONSORT statement for reporting randomised trials: explanation and elaboration. *Ann Intern Med.* 2001;134:663–694.
21. Kwon BK, Tetzlaff W. spinal cord regeneration. From gene to transplants. *Spine.* 2001;26:13–22.
22. Keyvan-Fouladi N, Raisman G, Li Y. functional repair of the corticospinal tract by delayed transplantation of olfactory ensheathing cells in adult rats. *J Neurosci.* 2003; 23(28):9428–9434.
23. Li Y, Decherchi P, Raisman G. Transplantation of olfactory ensheathing cells into spinal cord lesions restores breathing and climbing. *J Neurosci.* 2003;23(28):727–731.
24. Resnick DK, Cechvala CF, Yan Y, Witwer BP, Sun D, Zhang S. Adult olfactory ensheathing cell transplantation for acute spinal cord injury. *J Neurotrauma.* 2003;20(3):279–285.
25. Garcia-Alias G, Lopez-Vales R, Fores J, Navarro X, Verdu E. Acute transplantation of olfactory ensheathing cells or Schwann cells promotes recovery after spinal cord injury in the rat. *J Neurosci Res.* 2004;75(5):632–641.
26. Sagen J. Cellular therapies for spinal cord injury: What will the FDA need to aprove moving from the laboratory to the human? *J Rehabil Res Dev.* 2003; 40(4):71–79.
27. Rothstein JD, Synder EY. Reality and immortality-neural stem cells for therapies. *Nat Biotechnol.* March 2004;22(3):283–285.
28. Stroman PW, Kornelsen J, Bergman A, Krause V, Ethans K, Malisza KL, Tomanek B. Noninvasive assessment of the injured human spinal cord by means of functional magnetic resonance imaging. *Spinal Cord.* 2004;42(2):59–66.
29. Quencer RM. Advances in imaging of spinal cord injury, implications for treatment and patient evaluation. *Prog Brain Res.* 2002;137:3–8.
30. Schwartz ED, Hackney DB. Diffusion-weighted MRI and the evaluation of spinal cord axon integrity following injury and treatment. *Exp Neurol.* 2003;184(2):570–589.
31. Schwartz ED, Shumsky JS, Werhli S, Tessler A, Murray M, Hackney DB. Ex vivo MR determined apparent diffusion coefficients correlate with motor recovery mediated by intraspinal transplants of fibroblasts genetically modified to express BDNF. *Exp Neurol.* 2003;182(1):49–63.
32. Lee IH, Bulte JW, Schweinhardt P, Douglas T, Trifunovski A, Hofsted C, Olson L, Spenger C. In vivo magnetic resonance tracking of olfactory ensheathing glia grafted into the rat spinal cord. *Exp. Neurol.* 2004;187(2):509–516.
33. Suri A, Chabbra Ravinder PS, Mehta Veer S, Gaikwad S, Pandey Ram M. Effect of intramedullary signal changes on the surgical outcome of patients with cervical spondylotic myelopathy. *Spine J.* 2003:33–45.
34. Demir A, Ries M, Moonen Crit et al. Diffusion-weighted MR imaging with apparent diffusion coefficient and apparent diffusion tensor maps in cervical spondylotic myelopathy. *Radiology.* October 2003:37–43.

Index

Page numbers in *italics* refer to illustrations only

A

ABCS approach 93–97
Abdominal assessment 6
Abscess, retropharyngeal 159
Absorptiometry
  dual X-ray (DXA) 206–207
  radiographic 207
  single-photon 207–208
Acutely unwell patient, imaging 197, 198
Airway patency assessment 198, 199
Alar ligaments 16
Alignment, normal 93–94
  cervicocranium 67–68
  lower cervical spine (C3–C7) 68–69
  see also Malalignment
Andersson lesion 173
Ankylosing spondylitis *44–45*, 48, 88–89, 155, 230
  cervical spine injuries 158–159
  elderly patients 170, 173
  pseudoarthrosis 163–164
  thoracolumbar spine injuries 160–164
  see also Rigid spine
Ankylosis 229
  in neuropathic osteoarthropathy *225, 226*
  see also Ankylosing spondylitis
Annulus fibrosus 31, 149
  nondegenerative disk pathology 24–26
  tears 152–153
  vertebral compression fracture and 28
  see also Intervertebral disks
Anterior longitudinal ligaments *see* Longitudinal ligaments
Anterolisthesis 88
AO (comprehensive) fracture classification system 58–60
  reproducibility 62
  type A injuries 58–59
  type B injuries 60
  type C injuries 60
Apical ligament 16–17
Articular cyst 229
Artificial sphincter 198, 199
ASIA/IMSOP classification 8
Atlanto-axial joint 15–18
  dislocation, childhood 119–120
  instability 134
  rotary displacement 71
  rotatory fixation (AARF), childhood 121–122
Atlanto-occipital joint 15–18

condylar fracture 15–16, *20*
dissociation (AOD) *15*
  childhood 118
Atlanto-occipital membrane
  anterior 16
    rupture *23*
  posterior 17–18
Atlas fracture 18–22, *42*
  ankylosing spondylitis and 158
  anterior arch 18–19, *22*
  burst fracture *22*
  childhood 118
  Jefferson fracture 19–20, 118
  lateral mass 20–21
  posterior arch 21–22
    extension trauma 21–22
    flexion trauma 21
Atrophy, spinal cord *189, 190, 191, 192*
Atypical Scheuermann's disease 145, 150
Augmentation cystoplasty 198, *199*
Avulsion fracture
  anterior arch of C1 *19*
  vertebral margin 29–30
    compression 29
    traction 30
Axis fracture 22–24
  childhood 119, *128*
  hangman's fracture 23–24, 88, *91, 97*
  odontoid fracture 22–23, 119, *120*
    ankylosing spondylitis and 158
  signs of 95–96
    fat axis body 71, 95, *96*
    Harris' ring disruption 94, *95*
  see also C2

B

Beaver's sign 6
Biomechanical instability (BI) 9
Biopsy
  neuropathic osteoarthropathy diagnosis 230
  vertebral collapse investigation 220
Birth injury 117
Bladder
  assessment 6
  function 196
  management 196–197
Bone marrow edema *42, 43*
Bone mineral density (BMD)
  dens fracture and *22*
  densitometry 205–206
    indications 206

dual X-ray absorptiometry (DXA) 206–207
quantitative CT 207
quantitative ultrasonography of bone 207
radiographic absorptiometry 207
single-photon absorptiometry 207–208
T-score and Z-score 203–204
see also Osteoporosis
Bony integrity abnormalities 95–96
  see also Vertebral injury
Brachial plexus injury 43
Bradycardia 5
Brown–Sequard syndrome 6, *51*
Bulbocavernous reflex 178
Burst fracture 56, *57*, 59, 81, *82, 83–85*, 176, 215
  atlas ring *22*
  C5 78, *81–82*
  C7 *37*
  childhood 125
  early ambulant treatment 184–185
  L1 *11*, 84
  length of hospital stay 184
  neurological deficit related to displacement 183
  neurological deterioration 183
  pain related to late deformity 183–184
  return to work 184
  spinal canal remodeling 183
  surgical treatment 92, 182–185

C

C1
  development 115
  fracture *see* Atlas fracture
  pseudospreading 114–115
C1/2 instability 134
C2
  childhood injuries 118–119
    Salter–Harris type 1 injury *120*
  fracture *see* Axis fracture
  malalignment 69–71
  pseudosubluxation on C3 70
    childhood 115, *116*
  spondylolysis 119, *156*
  subluxation 119
C2/3
  fracture dislocation *49*
  hyperextension injury *25*
C3, osteophyte avulsion *41*
C3/4 injury *129, 168*
C4 fracture *102*

C

C4/5
  disk disruption *158*
  jumped and locked facet *90*
  posterior ligamentous complex injury *129*
C5
  fracture *130*
    burst fracture 78, *81–82*
    malalignment 79
C5/6
  disk disruption *159*
  facet dislocation *128*
  hyperflexion sprain *86*
C6
  congenital spondylolysis 116, *117*
  facet fracture *105, 108*
  malalignment 73, 76–77
  transverse process fracture *43, 105, 108*
C6/7 fracture dislocation *44–45*, 80, *106*
C7
  burst fracture *37*
  compression fracture 79
  dislocation *39*
  transverse fracture *163*
Calcifications
  heterotrophic *1*
  prostatic *7*
Canadian C-spine rule 36, 47–48, 51
Canal encroachment 10
Cardiovascular system assessment 5
Carotid artery dissection *109*
Cartilage abnormalities 96
Cellular therapies 232
Central cord syndrome *41, 157*
  cervical 75–76
Centrum 113
Cerebrospinal fluid (CSF)
  flow dynamics 191
  leakage *43*
Cervical spine
  central cord syndrome 75–76
  malalignment 66
    case studies 69–80
    radiographic signs 66–67
    normal alignment 67–69
    C3–C7 68–69
    cervicocranium 67–68
  trauma 15–33
    atlanto-axial joint 15–18
    atlanto-occipital joint 15–18, 118
    atlas fracture 18–22
    axis fracture 22–24
    childhood injuries 118–122
    elderly patients 166–170
    intervertebral disks 24–27
    rigid spine and 157–160
    vertebral injury 27–33
Cervicocranium
  malalignment *69*
  normal alignment 67–68
Chance-type fractures 86–87, *88–89*
  childhood 123, *124*
Charcot's joints *see* Neuropathic osteoarthropathy
Chest radiography, osteoporosis screening 204–205
Childhood injuries *see* Pediatric spine
Chronic overuse injury *see* Overuse of spine

Clefts, congenital 145
Clivus avulsion *17*
Cognitive function assessment 7
Comprehensive classification system *see* AO (comprehensive) fracture classification system
Compression fracture *20*, 27–29, 56, *57*, 176
  benign 214, *215*, 218
  C7 79
  childhood 125, 133
  elderly patients 170, *171*
  imaging modalities 214
  L1 *83*, 215
  L4 *216*
  osteoporotic *171*, 172–173, 204
  pathological 214, *215–217*
  percutaneous vertebroplasty 185, 208
  T7 *217*
  vertebral endplate *28*, 29
  wedge 79, 133, 170
  see also Vertebral collapse
Computed tomographic angiography (CTA) 100
  vertebral artery injuries 106–107, 111
Computed tomography (CT) 4, 40, 47–51, 98
  elderly patients 167, 171
  multi-detector (MD-CT) 51, 81, 156, 162, 167
  myelography *194*
  quantitative (QCT), bone mineral density measurement 207
  rigid spine 156, 162
  spondylolysis 137–138
  see also Computed tomographic angiography (CTA)
Condylar fracture 15–16, *20*
  classification 15
Congenital clefts 145
Congenital spondylolisthesis 73
Congenital spondylolysis 116–117
Consciousness, assessment of 7
Cord compression 10, *157*, 175
  ankylosing spondylitis and 158
Cruciform ligament 17
CT imaging *see* Computed tomography
Cystic changes, spinal cord 189, 190–192

D

Denis classification 56–57, 176
  reproducibility 62
Dens fracture *19*, 71
  bone density analysis *22*
  elderly patients 167, *168*
Densitometry, bone 205–206
  indications 206
Detrusor-sphincter dyssynergia 7
Development, vertebral column 113–114, 149–150
Diabetes 230
Diffusion weighted imaging (DWI) 218
Disks *see* Intervertebral disks
Dislocation
  cervical 178–179

  atlanto-axial, childhood 119–120
  C7 *39*
  extension-dislocation injuries 88–89
  flexion-dislocation injuries 87
  hyperextension 75, 76
  unilateral interfacetal (UID) 77, 80
  see also Fracture dislocations
Dissection
  carotid artery *109*
  vertebral artery *107*
Disseminated idiopathic skeletal hyperostosis (DISH) *92*, 155, 230
  cervical spine injuries 159–160
  elderly patients 169–170, 173
  pseudoarthrosis 163–164
  thoracolumbar spine injuries 160–164
  see also Rigid spine
Distraction
  extension injuries 87–88
  flexion injuries 85–87, 176, 177
    Chance-type fractures 86–87, *88–89*, 123, *124*
    hyperflexion sprain 85–86
    surgical stabilization 177
Dual X-ray absorptiometry (DXA) 206–207

E

Ectopic ossification, imaging 198, 199, *200*
Edema
  bone 151
  bone marrow *42, 43*
  Schmorl's nodes and 150
  soft tissue *41, 42, 49*
  spinal cord *37*, 101, 103–104
    neurological outcome and 104
  vertebral body *130*
  vertebral collapse and 214, 215–216
Effendi type II traumatic spondylolisthesis 72
Elderly patients 166
  cervical spine injuries 166–170
    biomechanical characteristics 166
    clinical features 166–167
    dens fracture 167, *168*
    hyperextension injury 167, *168*
    imaging techniques 167
    radiological features 167–170
    rigid spine and 167–170
    SCIWORA 167
  thoracolumar spine injuries 170–174
    biomechanical characteristics 170
    clinical features 170–171
    fractures related to rigid segments 173
    imaging features 172–174
    imaging techniques 171
    Kummell-type vertebral collapse *172*, 173
    osteoporotic compression fracture *171*, 172–173
    pathological fracture secondary to neoplasm 173–174

Electrophysiological assessment 7
Endplate 149
   compression fracture *28, 29, 78*
   lesions, Scheuermann's disease 150–152
Epidemiology of spinal trauma 175
   osteoporotic fractures 204
Epidural bleeding 17–18, *45*
   ankylosing spondylitis and 158
Extension injuries 87–89
   dislocation 88–89
   distraction injury 87–88
   "fingerprints" of 88
   intervertebral articulation *28*
   simple injuries 87

F

Facet joint injuries 30–32
   articular process fractures *32, 33*
   C5/6 dislocation *128*
   C6 fracture *105, 108*
   locked facet 77, 80
      unilateral *90, 94*
Fat axis body 71, 95, *96*
Fatty bone marrow 214
"Fingerprints" of vertebral injury 88, 136
"Fish vertebra" 173, 215, *216*
Flexion injuries 83–87, 176
   anterior atlanto-occipital membrane rupture 23
   burst fractures 83–85
   distraction injuries 85–87, 176, *177*
      Chance-type fractures 86–87, *88–89, 123, 124*
      hyperflexion sprain 85–86
      surgical stabilization *177*
   "fingerprints" of 88
   flexion-dislocation injuries 87
   posterior atlanto-axial membrane rupture *18*
   rotation and 178
   simple injuries 83
   surgical stabilization *177*
Fluid-sign 218
Fluorine-18 deoxy-glucose PET (FDG-PET) 218–219
Focal cyst 189, 192
"Footprints" of vertebral injury 93–97
Foreign bodies 48, *50*
Fracture classification 55–64, 175–176
   imaging modality influence 60–61
   need for 63–64
   reproducibility problems 61–62
   thoracolumbar spine fractures 55–60
      AO (comprehensive) classification 58–60
      load-sharing classification 57–58
      three-column concept 56–57
      type A injuries 58–59
      type B injuries 60
      type C injuries 60
Fracture dislocations 55, *57*
   C2/3 *49*
   C6/7 44–45, 80, *106*
   rigid spine and *169*

Fracture-separation, pedicolaminar 77
Fractures 95–96
   see also specific fractures; Vertebral injury
Frankel's classification 8

G

Grisel's syndrome 122

H

Hangman's fracture 23–24, 88, *91*, 97
Harris' ring of C2 94
   disruption 94, 95
Hemarthrosis 32
Hematoma 102, *103*, 107–108, *110*, 218
   ankylosing spondylitis and 158
   elderly patient *168*
Hematomyelia 100
Hemorrhage
   alar ligaments 16
   apical ligament *17*
   disk rupture and *26*
   epidural 17–18, *45*
      ankylosing spondylitis and 158
   into intervertebral foramina 31–32
   longitudinal ligaments *25, 26, 30*
   spinal cord *25*, 101, 103–104
      MRI features 101–102
   subdural 31
   within facet joint meniscus 32
Herniation, nucleus propulsus *29*, 150, 152, 156, 178–179
Heterotrophic calcifications 1
Hyperextension injury 75–76, *92*
   C2/3 *25*
   dislocation 75, 76
   elderly patients 166, *167, 168*
   hyperextension sprain 88, *91*
   lower cervical spine 75–76
   rigid spine and *159, 160*
   traction injury 30
Hyperflexion injury
   elderly patients 167
   hyperflexion sprain 74, 85–86
Hyperkyphotic angulation *74, 78*
Hypotension 178

I

Imaging 4–5, 36, 81, 98
   acutely unwell patient 197, 198
   airway patency assessment 198, 199
   approaches 47–48, 51–52
   chronic spinal cord injury 192–195
   ectopic ossification 198, 199, *200*
   elderly patients
      cervical spine 167–170
      thoracolumbar spine 171
   future trends 233
   indicators of high risk for injury 82–83
   modalities 38–40
      compression fractures 214
      influence on fracture classification 60–61

      pros and cons 40
      type of injury and 52
   muscle spasm investigation 198, 199
   neurological deterioration 197, 198
   neuropathic osteoarthropathy 225–228
   pain investigation 198, 199
   pressure sores 197–199
   renal tract complications 197, 198
      elective management 198, 199
   rigid spine 156–157
   spinal instability 197, 198
   spondylolysis and 137–138
   technical considerations 48–50
   vertebral collapse 214–220
   see also Computed tomography (CT); Magnetic resonance imaging (MRI); Radiography
Impaction fractures 58–59
Instability 55–56, 62
   biomechanical (BI) 9
   degrees of 56
   following childhood injury 134
   imaging 197, 198
   physiological (PI) 10
   signs of 98
   see also Stability
International Spinal Research Trust (ISRT) 231
Intervertebral disks 24–27, 149–150
   degeneration 27, 152–153
      pathology 27
   herniation *125*, 150, 152, 156, 178–179
   nondegenerative pathology 24–27
      axial loading 24
      extension trauma 25–26
      flexion trauma 26–27
      nonaxial loading 24–27
      staging 25
   post-traumatic changes 60–61
   vertebral compression fracture and 28–29
   widening of *75, 76, 87, 88*
Intervertebral foramina 30–32
   bone fragment *38*
Ischemia, post-traumatic 100–101
Isotope pump studies *201*

J

Jefferson fracture 19–20
   childhood 118
   pseudo Jefferson fracture 114–115
   without Jefferson effect *21*
Joint space abnormalities 96
Jumped and locked facet *90*

K

Klippel-Feil syndrome 157, *158*
Kummell-type vertebral collapse *172, 173*
Kyphoplasty 185
Kyphosis 60, *85*, 225, 230

L

L1
  burst fracture *11*, 84
  compression fracture 83, *215*
  Paget's disease 209–210
L1/2
  bone destruction *225*
  flexion distraction injury 87
  pseudoarthrosis *226*
L2, Chance fracture *124*
L3, post-operative spondylolysis *143*
L4
  compression fracture *216*
  fragmentation *224*
L4/5
  bone destruction *224*
  dislocation *224*
L5, spondylolysis *140–141*, 142
Lap-belt injuries 86–87
  pediatric 123
Late complications 188
Level of injury 2
Load-sharing fracture classification system 57–58
Locked facet 77, 80
  unilateral *90*, 94
Longitudinal ligaments 24
  anterior 16
    degenerative pathology 27, *28*
    hemorrhage *25*, *30*
    trauma 16, 25
  posterior 26
    disruption *130*
    hemorrhage *25*, *26*
    ossification of (OPLL) *160*, 169–170

M

Magnetic resonance angiography (MRA) 100
  vertebral artery injuries 106–110, *111*
Magnetic resonance imaging (MRI) 40, 47–48, 51, 52, 81
  acute spinal cord injuries 4, 100–101
    hemorrhage 101–102
  artifact, post-stabilization *195*
  categorization scheme *61*
  chronic spinal cord injury 192–195
    contraindications 193–195
  elderly patients 167, 171
  future trends 233
  influence on fracture classification 60–61
  neurovascular injuries 100
  osteoporosis 204
  prognostic role in neurological outcome 103–104
  rigid spine 156–157, 162
  spondylolysis 137, *138*
  vertebral artery injuries 106–110, *111*
Major injury, signs of 98
Malalignment 94
  cervical spine 66
    case studies 69–80
    radiographic signs 66–67

Management
  bladder 196–197
  neuropathic osteoarthropathy 230
  renal tract complications 198, *199*
  spinal cord injury 9–12
    role of surgery 11–12
  syringomyelia 192
    postoperative complications 192, *193*
  trauma 178–185
    burst fractures 92, 182–185
    initial management 178–179
    nonsurgical management 180–181
    pharmacological intervention 180
    surgical treatment 181–185
Metastasis 173–174, 215–218, *220*
Methylprednisolone 180
Missed spinal injuries 2
Motor evoked potentials (MEPs) 7
MRI *see* Magnetic resonance imaging (MRI)
Multiple myeloma 173–174
Muscle spasm investigation 198, *199*
Myelomalacia 189, 191–192

N

Naked facets *76*, 86, *87*, 96
Naloxone 180
Neoplasms 147
  pathological fracture and 173–174
Nerve conduction studies 7
Neurological deterioration 183, 188–195
  cord changes following spinal cord injury 10, 189–191
    atrophy 189, *190*, 191, 192
    cystic changes 189, 190–192
    myelomalacia 189, 191–192
    syringomyelia 189–190, 191–192
  imaging 197, *198*
Neuronal regeneration 232
Neuropathic osteoarthropathy 223, *224*
  clinical findings 225
  differential diagnosis 228–230
  imaging findings 225–228
  mechanism 223
  treatment 230
Neuroprotection 232
Neurovascular injuries 100
  vertebral artery injury 100, 104–111
  see also Hemorrhage
Nonaccidental injury (NAI), children 118
Nuclear medicine studies
  fluorine-18 deoxy-glucose PET (FDG-PET) 218–219
  isotope pump studies *201*
  spondylolysis *138*
Nucleus propulsus 149
  herniation *29*, 150, 152, 156, 178–179
  nondegenerative disk pathology 24–27

  vertebral compression fracture and 28–29
  see also Intervertebral disks

O

Odontoid fracture 22–23
  ankylosing spondylitis and 158
  childhood 119, *120*
Olfactory ensheathing cell (OEC) transplantation 232
Orthotic management 180–181
Os odontoideum 119, *121*
  instability and 134
Ossification
  ectopic, imaging indications 198, 199, *200*
  posterior longitudinal ligament (OPLL) *160*
    elderly patients 169–170
  spine *44–45*, 48
    during development 114, 149–150
Osteoarthropathy *see* Neuropathic osteoarthropathy
Osteoid osteoma 147
Osteonecrosis 218
Osteopenia 204, *205*
Osteophyte avulsion *41*
Osteoporosis 203
  case study 209–210
  compression fracture *171*, 172–173, 204
    semiquantitative assessment 205
    treatment 185, 208
  definition 203
  epidemiology of spinal fractures 204
  radiography 204–205
    diagnosis 205
    screening 204–205
  vertebral fragility fracture 204
  see also Bone mineral density (BMD)
Overuse of spine 145
  chronic 149
  disk degeneration and 152–153
  Scheuermann's disease and 150–152

P

Paget's disease 209–210
Pain investigation 198, *199*
"Pancake" vertebra 215
Pancoast tumor *217*
Paraplegia *42*, *162*, 229
  traumatic *224*
Paravertebral ligamentous ossification 169–170
  see also Disseminated idiopathic skeletal hyperostosis (DISH); Ossification
Pars interarticularis defect *141*, 142
Pediatric spine 113
  birth injury 117
  cervical spine injuries 118–122
    atlanto-axial dislocation 119–121
    atlanto-axial rotatory fixation (AARF) 121–122

atlanto-occipital dissociation (AOD) 118
  C1 fractures 118
  C2 injury 118–119
  os odontoideum 119, 121
nonaccidental injury (NAI) 118
normal variants 114–117
  congenital spondylolysis 116–117
  pseudo Jefferson fracture 114–115
  pseudosubluxation of C2 on C3 115, 116
  vertebral pseudowedging 115–116
physeal injury 126–127, 128–130
prognosis following injury 133–134
SCIWORA 131, 132
slipped vertebral apophysis 132
spondylolysis 132
thoracolumbar spine injuries 123–125
vertebral column development 113–114, 149–150
Pedicle defect 116
Pedicolaminar fracture-separation 77
Penetrating injuries 48, 51
Percutaneous vertebroplasty 185, 208
  contraindications 208
Pharmacological intervention 180
Physeal injury 126–127, 128–130
Physiological instability (PI) 10
Pillar fracture 76
Positron emission tomography (PET) 218–219, 220
Posterior longitudinal ligaments see Longitudinal ligaments
Predental space, widening of 96, 97
Pressure sores 197–199
Progressive post-traumatic cystic myelopathy (PTCM) 189, 191
Progressive post-traumatic myelomalacic myelopathy (PTMM) 189, 191
Prostatic calcifications 7
Pseudo Jefferson fracture 114–115
Pseudoarthrosis 163–164
  in neuropathic osteoarthropathy 226, 228
Pseudospondylolysis 142
Pseudospreading of C1 114–115
Pseudosubluxation of C2 on C3 70
  childhood 115, 116
Pseudowedging 115–116

Q

Quantitative CT (QCT), bone mineral density measurement 207
Quantitative ultrasonography of bone 207

R

Radiographic absorptiometry 207
Radiography 4–5, 38–40, 47–48, 81
  elderly patients 167, 171
  osteoporosis 204–205
    diagnosis 205
    screening 204–205

rigid spine 156
spondylolysis 138
Radiological assessment see Imaging
Recumbency, treatment by 180
Regeneration 232
Rehabilitation 232–233
Renal cell carcinoma metastases 216
Renal tract complications 188
  elective management 198, 199
  imaging 197, 198
  routine surveillance 193
  urological investigations 196–197
Renography 196, 197
Research see Spinal cord research
Respiratory system assessment 5–6
  airway patency 198, 199
Retropharyngeal abscess 159
Rheumatoid arthritis 97
Rigid spine 155
  cervical spine injuries 157–160
  elderly patients 167–170, 173
  imaging 156–157
  mechanisms 155–156
  pseudoarthrosis 163–164
  thoracolumbar spine injuries 160–164
  see also Ankylosing spondylitis; Disseminated idiopathic skeletal hyperostosis (DISH)
Ring apophysis 149–150
Rotary injuries 89–92
  atlanto-axial displacement 71
  atlanto-axial rotatory fixation (AARF) 121–122
  "fingerprints" of 88
  flexion and 178
  grinding injury 92
  treatment 92

S

Sacral anterior root stimulators (SARS)
  imaging applications 198, 199
  MRI scanning and 194–195
Sacral fracture 46–47
Salter–Harris type I injury 119, 120, 127, 128
Salter–Harris type III injury 127, 129
Salter–Harris type IV injury 130
Saville index 205
Scheuermann's disease 150–152, 230
  atypical 145, 150
Schmorl's nodes 150, 151, 171
Scintigraphy 219, 220
SCIWORA (spinal cord injury without radiologic abnormality) 4, 48
  childhood 127, 131, 132
  elderly patients 167
Sclerotic pars defect 141
Scoliosis 133, 223, 229
"Scotty dog" collar 143, 144
Seat-belt injuries 56, 57
Semiconscious patient assessment 3
Sensation, assessment of 2–3
Shearing injuries 92–93
  "fingerprints" of 88
Shock, spinal 5, 128
Single-photon absorptiometry 207–208

Slipped vertebral apophysis 132
Soft tissue abnormalities 96–97
  edema 41, 42, 49
  masses 218
Somatosensory evoked potentials (SSEPs) 7
Spina bifida occulta
  spondylolysis and 136, 144
  type I 144
  type II 144
  type III 144
Spinal canal remodeling 183
Spinal cord injury (SCI)
  acute stage assessment 2–5, 100–101
    associated injuries 3–4
    conscious patient 2–3
    MRI prognostic role 103–104
    radiological assessment 4–5
    semiconscious/unconscious patient 3
  biomechanical instability (BI) 9
  blunt trauma 48
  canal encroachment 10
  chronic state assessment 192–195
    CT myelography 195
    frequency of investigation 192, 193
    MRI 192–195
  classification of 103
    ASIA/IMSOP classification 8
    Frankel's classification 8
  cord compression 10, 157, 175
    ankylosing spondylitis and 158
  effects of 1–2
  late complications 188
  level of injury 2
  management 9–12
    role of surgery 11–12
  missed spinal injuries 2
  natural history of 11
  neurological damage 10, 189–191
    examination and documentation standards 7–8
    see also Neurological deterioration
  pathophysiology 175
  penetrating injuries 48, 51
  physiological instability (PI) 10
  secondary injury 9
  spinal cord changes
    atrophy 189, 190, 191, 192
    cystic changes 189, 190–192
    myelomalacia 189, 191–192
    syringomyelia 189–190, 191–192
  subacute stage/long term assessment 5–7
    abdomen 6
    cardiovascular system 5
    cognitive functions 7
    consciousness 7
    electrophysiological assessment 7
    respiratory system 5–6
    urinary system 6–7
  transection 103
  without radiologic abnormality (SCIWORA) 4, 48
    childhood 127, 131
    elderly patients 167

Spinal cord research 231–233
  neuroprotection 232
  regeneration 232
  rehabilitation 232–233
  research strategy 231
  transplantation 232
Spinal overuse see Overuse of spine
Spinal shock 5, 178
Spinal trauma epidemiology 175
Spinous processes
  fractures 33
  rotation 80
Split fractures 59
Spondylodiskitis 173, 218
Spondylolisthesis 136–137, *142*, 146
  classification 146
  congenital 73
  traumatic 72, *103*
Spondylolysis 132, 136, *139–141*
  C2 119, *156*
  C6, congenital 116–117
  differential diagnosis 145–147
    congenital clefts 145
    neoplasms 147
    overuse of spine 145
    spondylolisthesis 146
  image interpretation 142–145
    imaging anatomy 142
    signs 143–145
  indications for imaging 137–138
  investigation techniques 138
  post-operative *143*
  spina bifida occulta and 136, *144*
Spondyloptosis 136, *146*
Spondylosis deformans 167–169
Sports injuries
  chronic overuse injuries 149
  disk degeneration and 152–153
  Scheuermann's disease 150–152
  spondylolysis 136
Stab wound *51*
Stability 98
  concept of 62
  see also Instability
Stem cells 232, *233*
Steroid therapy 180
Stress reaction *145*
Subluxation
  anterior 74
  T12 *103*
Surgical treatment 181–185
  burst fractures 92, 182–185
  choice of approach 181–182
  indications for 181
  osteoporotic vertebral fractures 185, 208
  spinal cord injury 11–12
  timing of 182
Surveillance, renal tract complications 193
Syphilis, tertiary *228*, 230
Syringomyelia 189–190, 191–192, 230
  treatment 192
    post-operative complications 192, *193*

T

T7 fracture *173*, 217
T8 fracture *43*
T11/12, hyperextension injury *92*
T12
  subluxation *106*
  vertebral collapse *172*
T12/L1 rotary "grinding" injury *92*
T-score 203–204
Teardrop fracture 29, 30, 85
Tectorial membrane 17–18
Tertiary syphilis *228*, 230
Thoracolumbar spine
  childhood injuries 123–125
  fracture classification 55–60
  injuries with rigid spine 160–164
  trauma in elderly patients 170–174
Three-column fracture classification system 56–57, 176
Torticollis 71, 121–122
Tracheal stenosis assessment 198, *199*
Traction 178–179
Transplantation 232
Transverse ligament, tear 17, *18*
Treatment see Management; Surgical treatment

U

Ultrasonography, quantitative 207
Unconscious patient assessment 3
Unilateral interfacetal dislocation (UID) 77, 80
Urinary system assessment 6–7
Urodynamics 197
Urological investigations 196–197

V

Vacuum phenomenon *224*, *227*, *229*
Vascular injury 100, 104
  vertebral artery 100, 104–111
  see also Hemorrhage
Vertebral artery 104
  injury 100, 104–111
    dissection *107*
    imaging 106–111
    occlusion *105*, *110*
    symptoms 106
    thickening *108*
Vertebral collapse 213
  biopsy 220
  clinical evaluation 213–220
    age 213
    trauma history 213–214
  imaging findings 214–219
    alternative imaging methods 218–219
    contrast material–dynamics 216
    contrast material–enhancement 215–216
    edema 214
    fatty bone marrow 214
    fluid-sign (osteonecrosis) 218
    shape–extent of fracture 215
    site of fracture 216–217
    soft tissue mass 218
  Kummell-type *172*, *173*
  see also Compression fracture
Vertebral column development 113–114, 149–150
Vertebral endplate 149
  compression fracture 28, 29, 78
  lesions, Scheuermann's disease 150–152
Vertebral injury 27–33
  facet joints 30–32, *33*
  "fingerprints" of 88, 136
  "footprints" of 93–97
  growth plate injuries *126*
  imaging 81
  indicators of high risk for injury 82–83
  intervertebral foramina 30–32
  mechanisms of injury 83–93, 176–178
    extension injuries 87–89
    flexion injuries 83–87, 176–178
    rotary injuries 89–92, 178
    shearing injuries 92–93
  nonsurgical management 180–181
  osteoporotic fractures *171*, 172–173, 203
    epidemiology 204
    fragility fracture 204
  slipped vertebral apophysis 132
  surgical treatment 181–185
    choice of approach 181–182
    indications for 181
    timing of 182
  see also specific fractures
Vertebroplasty 185, 208
  contraindications 208

W

Wedge compression fracture 215, *217*
  C7 79
  childhood 133
  elderly patients 170
  see also Compression fracture
"Windswept" appearance 93

X

X-rays 4–5
  see also Radiography

Y

Yellow bone marrow 214

Z

Z-score 203–204